Clinical Manual of Child and Adolescent Psychopharmacology

Fourth Edition

Clinical Manual of Child and Adolescent Psychopharmacology

Fourth Edition

Edited by

Molly McVoy, M.D.

Ekaterina Stepanova, M.D., Ph.D.

Robert L. Findling, M.D., M.B.A.

AMERICAN PSYCHIATRIC ASSOCIATION PUBLISHING

Note: The authors have worked to ensure that all information in this book is accurate at the time of publication and consistent with general psychiatric and medical standards, and that information concerning drug dosages, schedules, and routes of administration is accurate at the time of publication and consistent with standards set by the U.S. Food and Drug Administration and the general medical community. As medical research and practice continue to advance, however, therapeutic standards may change. Moreover, specific situations may require a specific therapeutic response not included in this book. For these reasons and because human and mechanical errors sometimes occur, we recommend that readers follow the advice of physicians directly involved in their care or the care of a member of their family.

Books published by American Psychiatric Association Publishing represent the findings, conclusions, and views of the individual authors and do not necessarily represent the policies and opinions of American Psychiatric Association Publishing or the American Psychiatric Association.

If you wish to buy 50 or more copies of the same title, please go to www.appi.org/specialdiscounts for more information.

Fourth Edition

Manufactured in the United States of America on acid-free paper
27 26 25 24 23 5 4 3 2 1

American Psychiatric Association Publishing
800 Maine Avenue SW, Suite 900
Washington, DC 20024-2812
www.appi.org

Library of Congress Cataloging-in-Publication Data

Names: McVoy, Molly, editor. | Stepanova, Ekaterina (Psychiatrist), editor. | Findling, Robert L, editor. | American Psychiatric Association Publishing, issuing body.

Title: Clinical manual of child and adolescent psychopharmacology / edited by Molly McVoy, Ekaterina Stepanova, Robert L. Findling.

Description: Fourth edition. | Washington, DC : American Psychiatric Association Publishing, [2024] | Includes bibliographical references and index.

Identifiers: LCCN 2023022897 (print) | LCCN 2023022898 (ebook) | ISBN 9781615374892 (paperback ; alk. paper) | ISBN 9781615374908 (ebook)

Subjects: MESH: Mental Disorders—drug therapy | Child | Psychopharmacology—methods | Psychotropic Drugs—therapeutic use | Adolescent

Classification: LCC RJ504.7 (print) | LCC RJ504.7 (ebook) | NLM WS 350.33 | DDC 615.7/80835—dc23/eng/20230630

LC record available at https://lccn.loc.gov/2023022897

LC ebook record available at https://lccn.loc.gov/2023022898

British Library Cataloguing in Publication Data

A CIP record is available from the British Library.

Contents

List of Tables

List of Figures

Contributors

Boris Birmaher, M.D.
Distinguished Professor of Psychiatry, University of Pittsburgh Medical Center, Pittsburgh, Pennsylvania

Chiara Davico, M.D.
Division of Child and Adolescent Neuropsychiatry, Department of Public Health and Pediatrics, University of Turin, Turin, Italy

Roxanne Demarest, P.A.-C.
Physician Assistant, Nationwide Children's Hospital, Columbus, Ohio

David I. Driver, M.D.
Child Psychiatry Branch, National Institute of Mental Health, National Institutes of Health, Bethesda, Maryland

Mina K. Dulcan, M.D.
Pritzker Department of Psychiatry and Behavioral Health, Ann and Robert H. Lurie Children's Hospital of Chicago; Professor of Psychiatry and Behavioral Sciences and Pediatrics, Northwestern University Feinberg School of Medicine, Chicago, Illinois

Robert L. Findling, M.D., M.B.A.
Department of Psychiatry, Virginia Commonwealth University, Richmond, Virginia

Nitin Gogtay, M.D.
Chief, Division of Research, and Deputy Medical Director, American Psychiatric Association, Washington. D.C.

Pablo H. Goldberg, M.D.
Associate Clinical Professor of Psychiatry, Columbia University Irving Medical Center/NewYork-Presbyterian Morgan Stanley Children's Hospital, CUIMC/ Herbert Pardes Building of the New York State Psychiatric Institute, New York, New York

Laurence Greenhill, M.D.
Professor of Psychiatry, Voluntary Faculty, University of California at San Francisco, San Francisco, California

Peter S. Jensen, M.D.
Adjunct Professor, University of Arkansas for Medical Sciences, Little Rock, Arkansas; Board Chair and Founder, The REACH Institute, New York, New York

Christopher J. Keary, M.D.
Assistant Professor, Harvard Medical School, Boston, Massachusetts

Sarah Lytle, M.D.
Assistant Professor of Psychiatry, University Hospitals, Cleveland Medical Center, Case Western Reserve University, Cleveland, Ohio

Daniele Marcotulli, M.D., Ph.D.
Division of Child and Adolescent Neuropsychiatry, Department of Public Health and Pediatrics, University of Turin, Turin, Italy

Christopher J. McDougle, M.D.
Professor, Harvard Medical School, Boston, Massachusetts

Molly McVoy, M.D.
Associate Professor in Psychiatry, Division of Child and Adolescent Psychiatry Fellowship, University Hospitals/Case Western Reserve University, Cleveland, Ohio

Basim Mikhail, M.D.
Consultant Psychiatrist, Al Minya, Egypt

Baris Olten, M.D.
Child and Adolescent Psychiatry Fellow, Akron Children's Hospital, Akron, Ohio

Michelle L. Palumbo, M.D.
Instructor, Harvard Medical School, Boston, Massachusetts

Stephanie Pope, M.D.
Assistant Professor, Case Western Reserve University School of Medicine, Cleveland, Ohio

Judith L. Rapoport, M.D.
Child Psychiatry Branch, National Institute of Mental Health, National Institutes of Health, Bethesda, Maryland

Manivel Rengasamy, Ph.D.
Assistant Professor, University of Pittsburgh, Pittsburgh, Pennsylvania

Moira A. Rynn, M.D.
Consulting Professor and Chair of the Department of Psychiatry and Behavioral Sciences, Duke University School of Medicine, Durham, North Carolina

Lawrence Scahill, M.S.N., Ph.D.
Professor, Marcus Autism Center and Emory University, Atlanta, Georgia

Lauren Schumacher, M.D.
Assistant Clinical Professor, Division of Child and Adolescent Psychiatry, Department of Psychiatry, University of California San Francisco, San Francisco, California

Ekaterina Stepanova, M.D., Ph.D.
Chair, Child and Adolescent Psychiatry, Virginia Commonwealth University, Richmond, Virginia

Griffin Stout, M.D.
Child and Adolescent Psychiatry Attending, Nationwide Children's Hospital, Columbus, Ohio

Tiffany Thomas-Lakia, M.D.
Child and Adolescent Psychiatrist, Akron Children's Hospital, Akron, and Senior Instructor, Case Western Reserve University School of Medicine, Cleveland, Ohio

Benedetto Vitiello, M.D.
Division of Child and Adolescent Neuropsychiatry, Department of Public Health and Pediatrics, University of Turin, Turin, Italy; Department of Mental Health, Johns Hopkins Bloomberg School of Public Health, Baltimore, Maryland

Paula K. Yanes-Lukin, Ph.D.
Assistant Professor of Clinical Psychology in the Division of Child and Adolescent Psychiatry at Columbia University Medical Center/New York State Psychiatric Institute, New York, New York

Solomon G. Zaraa, D.O.
Director, Inpatient Psychiatric Services, University Hospitals Rainbow Babies and Children's Hospital; Assistant Professor, Psychiatry, Case Western Reserve University School of Medicine, Cleveland, Ohio

Disclosures

The following contributors have indicated a financial interest in or other affiliation with a commercial supporter, manufacturer of a commercial product, and/or provider of a commercial service as listed below:

Boris Birmaher, M.D.
Salary: University of Pittsburgh, University of Pittsburgh Medical Center/ Western Psychiatric Institute and Clinic. Research funding: National Institute of Mental Health. *Royalties:* Random House, Lippincott Williams & Wilkins, Wolters Kluwer.

Chiara Davico, M.D.
Consultant: Roche, Lundbeck Pharmaceuticals.

Robert L. Findling, M.D.
Research support, consultant, and/or honoraria: Acadia, Adamas, Aevi, Afecta, Akili, Alkermes, Allergan, American Academy of Child and Adolescent Psychiatry, American Psychiatric Association Publishing, Arbor, Axsome, Daiichi-Sankyo, Emelex, Gedeon Richter, Genentech, Idorsia, Intra-Cellular Therapies, Kempharm, Luminopia, Lundbeck, MedAvante-ProPhase, Merck, MJH Life Sciences, National Institutes of Health, Neurim, Otsuka, PaxMedica, PCORI, Pfizer, Physicians Postgraduate Press, Q BioMed, Receptor Life Sciences, Roche, Sage, Signant Health, Sunovion, Supernus Pharmaceuticals, Syneos, Syneurx, Takeda, Teva, Tris, and Validus.

Laurence Greenhill, M.D.
Salary: Kaiser Permanente Medical Group. *Honoraria and Travel Support:* The Klingenstein Third Generation Foundation Scientific Advisory Board.

Christopher J. Keary, M.D.
Advisory Board: Ovid Therapeutics, Biogen. Research funding: Ovid Therapeutics.

Daniele Marcotulli, M.D., Ph.D.
Consultant: Ethos, Ltd.

Christopher J. McDougle, M.D.
Consultant: Precidiag, Receptor Life Sciences, Sage Therapeutics, Acadia Pharmaceuticals. *Royalties:* Oxford University Press, Springer Publishing.

Molly McVoy, M.D.
Research funding: The Hartwell Foundation, Allergan Pharmaceuticals, National Institute of Mental Health, Case Western Reserve University. *Salary:* Case Western Reserve University.

Michelle L. Palumbo, M.D.
Research funding: Otsuka Pharmaceutical Inc.

Moira A. Rynn, M.D.
Consultant: Allergan (DSMB), Abbvie (DSMB), Otsuka America Pharmaceutical, IngenioRx. *Advisory Board:* Allergan (DSMB), Abbvie (DSMB)

Ekaterina Stepanova, M.D., Ph.D.
Research support: Psychnostics, LLC and Supernus.

Benedetto Vitiello, M.D.
Consultant: Medice, Angelini, Menari Pharmaceuticals.

The following contributors stated that they had no competing interests during the year preceding manuscript submission:

Roxanne Demarest, P.A.-C.; David I. Driver, M.D.; Nitin Gogtay, M.D.; Pablo H. Goldberg, M.D.; Peter S. Jensen, M.D.; Sarah Lytle, M.D.; Baris Olten, M.D.; Stephanie Pope, M.D.; Manivel Rengasamy, Ph.D.; Judith L. Rapoport, M.D.; Lawrence Scahill, M.S.N., Ph.D.; Lauren Schumacher, M.D.; Griffin Stout, M.D.; Tiffany Thomas-Lakia, M.D.; Paula K. Yanes-Lukin, Ph.D.; Solomon G. Zaraa, D.O.

Foreword

The most essential resource for anyone prescribing psychotropic medications for children and adolescents is an up-to-date, efficient, accessible, and trustworthy reference book. We have that here in the fourth edition of the *Clinical Manual of Child and Adolescent Psychopharmacology*. In the 5 years since the publication of the third edition, there has been impressive growth in our knowledge of using medications for emotions, cognition, and behavior in youth, and it is all right here. Bob Findling, the senior editor, is both a pediatrician and a child and adolescent psychiatrist, with broad and deep experience and expertise in pediatric psychopharmacology research and clinical practice. He is joined in this editorial effort by Drs. McVoy and Stepanova, and all are experienced child and adolescent psychiatric clinicians and educators.

The chapters, organized by disorders and syndromes, retain the structure of the previous edition, each written by acknowledged experts and thoroughly updated in this new edition. Several new chapter coauthors have been added to bring fresh perspectives. The clinical wisdom and experience of the authors supplement the balanced presentation of the findings of research studies. Clinical Pearls and summary tables in each chapter greatly enhance the value of this book for busy clinicians who are seeking efficient guidance on evidence-based treatments. How to select a medication and the practical management of side effects are covered well, in addition to treatment recommendations that go beyond medications. I was delighted to discover that the references are in author-date format rather than being numbered; this is a great help for readers like me who want to know quickly who wrote what and when.

This book should be on the shelves (and in the hands) of trainees and clinicians not only in child and adolescent psychiatry but also in pediatrics, because pediatric practitioners are increasingly expected to address patient mental health issues, including psychopharmacology. Others who treat children, including advanced practice nurses, physician assistants, and general psychiatrists, will also benefit greatly. In addition, other mental health professionals and those who direct programs serving children would benefit from the wisdom in this concise reference.

Mina K. Dulcan, M.D.

Preface

The field of pediatric psychopharmacology is complex and constantly changing, with new studies being published regularly, leading to more and more treatment options becoming available for the management of mental health conditions. In light of the ever-increasing demand to deliver mental health care, it can be difficult for busy providers to spend the additional time necessary for navigating the vast variety of studies so they can stay current with evidence-based treatment. For that specific reason, it remains our priority to continue to provide clinicians with the most recent evidence-based information and disseminate data-driven best treatment practices.

This fourth edition of the *Clinical Manual of Child and Adolescent Psychopharmacology* is consistent with the structure of the previous edition, in which each chapter describes treatment options for a particular diagnosis. All of the chapters have been updated with the newest research in pediatric psychopharmacology and not only provide a background for the medications discussed but also focus on how to practically use these new data to inform treatment in a clinical setting. Our goal was to make it easy for providers to find a comprehensive summary of evidence-based treatments. As in the previous editions, leading clinician-scientists with extensive research and clinical experience contributed to writing this book. One of the major changes from the previous edition is the addition of another editor, Ekaterina Stepanova, M.D., Ph.D., who is an expert clinician and scientist in mood and disruptive behavior disorders. She is a leader in the field, currently serving as director of child and adolescent psychiatry at Virginia Commonwealth University School of Medicine.

Despite the constantly growing data in the field of child and adolescent psychiatry, many providers continue to prescribe medications "off label." Although we acknowledge that there may be circumstances when this is necessary, we encourage providers to look carefully at the most current evidence available and to develop an appropriate treatment plan based on that evidence. For that purpose, it is especially important to review the acute and longitudinal trials as well as head-to-head comparisons of the medications. It is also vital to understand the methodology and the quality of these trials in order to accurately interpret the results. In this edition, we have attempted not only to provide comprehensive reviews of the evidence for treating mental health disorders in children and adolescents but also to help readers understand the difference between methodological approaches among the various clinical trials.

We are living during exciting times when the knowledge of how to treat psychiatric disorders in children and adolescents is expanding rapidly. Although the growing research field helps bridge the gap in understanding the treatment options, it can be daunting for providers to keep up with the pace of change. It may be especially difficult to interpret trials that seem methodologically similar, yet yield different results. In this edition, we strive to help providers understand the best clinical practices and be able to interpret the results of the clinical trials, all leading to providing better patient care.

Molly McVoy, M.D.
Ekaterina Stepanova, M.D., Ph.D.
Robert L. Findling, M.D., M.B.A.

1

Developmental Aspects of Pediatric Psychopharmacology

Chiara Davico, M.D.

Daniele Marcotulli, M.D., Ph.D.

Benedetto Vitiello, M.D.

Pediatric psychopharmacology is the science behind the therapeutic use of psychotropic agents in youth. Clinicians prescribing psychotropics to children and adolescents must be familiar with developmental psychopathology and the interaction between medication and the developing organism, in addition to the general principles of psychopharmacology. It is well recognized that mere extrapolation to children of information acquired from adults is insufficient to guide rational pharmacotherapy. Differences in how the developing organism affects the drug (pharmacokinetics), how the developing brain reacts to the drug (pharmacodynamics), and how psychopathology manifests during development can have clinically important implications for both efficacy and safety. Over the years, progress in pediatric psychopharmacology research has provided a foundation on which evidence-based pharmacotherapy can be built. In addition, special ethical and legal considerations apply when treating children for purposes of either clinical care or research.

In this chapter, we aim to describe the specific aspects of pediatric psychopharmacology that make it a distinct discipline at the crossroads of child and adolescent psychiatry, neurology, pediatrics, and pharmacology.

Pharmacokinetics and Metabolism

Pharmacokinetics determines the availability of a drug at the site of action and thus directly influences the intensity and duration of the pharmacological activity (Smits et al. 2022). The basic pharmacokinetic processes of absorption, distribution, metabolism (biotransformation), and excretion are all influenced by development (see Table 1–1 for essential terms). Because knowledge of a drug's pharmacokinetics is critical for identifying its therapeutic dosage range and frequency of administration, pediatric pharmacokinetics studies should precede and inform clinical trials aimed at testing the drug's efficacy in children.

Children have smaller body sizes than adults but have a greater proportion of liver and kidney parenchyma when adjustment for body weight is made. Compared with adults, children also have relatively more body water, less fat, and less plasma albumin to which drugs can bind. These structural characteristics can result in a smaller volume of distribution for drugs, greater drug extraction during the first pass through the liver following oral administration, lower bioavailability, and faster metabolism and elimination. These differences mean that simply decreasing adult doses based on child weight may result in undertreatment. Adjusting by body surface area would control for both weight and height, but this approach is usually reserved for drugs with a narrow therapeutic index, such as antineoplastics, and is seldom used in pediatric psychopharmacology.

Adolescence is characterized by marked growth in body size and by redistribution of body compartments. Differences between sexes become more pronounced. In males, the percentage of total body water increases and that of body fat decreases, whereas in females, the opposite occurs. These changes can contribute to sex differences in pharmacokinetics. For example, higher serum

Table 1–1. Essential pharmacokinetics terminology

Term	Definition
Absorption	Process by which a drug is absorbed from the site of administration into the systemic circulation
Liver first-pass extraction	Drug metabolism that occurs when a drug goes through the liver soon after intestinal absorption, before reaching the systemic circulation
Bioavailability	Proportion of administered drug that reaches the systemic circulation
Area under the curve (AUC)	Concentration of drug plasma as a function of time
Metabolism (biotransformation)	Phase I: cytochrome P450 (CYP)–mediated oxidation; hydroxylation
	Phase II: conjugation reactions (glucuronidation, sulfation, acetylation)
Volume of distribution (V_d)	Apparent volume in which the drug is distributed after absorption (V_d = dose absorbed/C_p)
Concentration in plasma (C_p)	Drug quantity for unit of plasma (C_p = dose absorbed/V_d)
Peak plasma concentration (C_{max})	Highest plasma concentration
Time to C_{max} (T_{max})	Time it takes from drug administration to reach C_{max}
Clearance (plasma clearance [CL])	Volume of plasma completely cleared of the drug in a unit of time; the cumulative result of drug removal that occurs in the liver, kidney, and other parts of the body (e.g., lungs, skin, bile); CL = dose absorbed/AUC
Elimination half-life ($t_{1/2}$)	Time that it takes, after full drug absorption and distribution in the body, for C_p to be reduced by 50%; a function of CL and V_d ($t_{1/2} = 0.693 \cdot V_d/CL$)
Steady-state plasma concentration	Stable C_p between doses that is achieved when the rate of elimination equals the rate of absorption; usually achieved after about four half-lives during constant drug administration

concentrations of risperidone have been found in males than in females (Calarge and Miller 2011). Faster metabolism in females may also account for this difference.

Drug metabolism consists of biotransformations that turn the drug into derivative products (metabolites) that are more polar and therefore more easily eliminated. Not all drugs undergo metabolism; lithium, for instance, is excreted unchanged through the kidneys. Drug metabolism typically includes a Phase I, during which medications undergo enzymatic oxidative or hydrolytic transformations, and a Phase II, during which conjugates are formed between the drug or its metabolites and glucuronic acid, sulfate, glutathione, or acetate. The Phase I oxidative processes are mediated by cytochrome P450 (CYP) microsomal enzymes, which are concentrated in the liver but present in small quantities in other tissues as well.

The CYP system matures rapidly after birth (van Groen et al. 2021). For instance, liver microsomes demonstrate only 1% of the adult CYP2D6 activity in the fetus, but this rate increases to about 20% of the adult activity by 1 month after birth. The immaturity of the CYP2D6 system at birth is one of the possible explanations for the syndrome of irritability, tachypnea, tremors, and increased muscle tone that has been observed in newborns of mothers taking selective serotonin reuptake inhibitors (SSRIs) (Chambers et al. 1996). An alternative explanation is that the syndrome represents a withdrawal reaction from the SSRI. In any case, the CYP metabolizing capacity is well developed by age 3 years (van Groen et al. 2021). Because children have proportionally greater liver parenchyma than adults, the weight-adjusted metabolic capacity is greater in childhood. Nonetheless, the activity of some CYP systems appears to be age dependent. For example, drugs metabolized by CYP1A2 tend to show a higher concentration in children following administration of equal doses by weight (Fekete et al. 2020).

The two most important CYP enzymes in pediatric psychopharmacology are CYP3A4 and CYP2D6, which are involved in the metabolism of most psychotropics, as summarized in Table 1–2. Genetic polymorphism has been associated with CYP2D6. About 7%–10% of whites, 1%–8% of Blacks, and 1%–3% of East Asians are poor metabolizers. Poor metabolizers have higher drug concentrations in plasma and other body tissues. For example, the mean elimination half-life of atomoxetine is about 5 hours in children or adults who are extensive metabolizers, but it is 22 hours in poor metabolizers (Sauer et al.

Table 1–2. Selected compounds relevant to pediatric pharmacotherapy that are metabolized by cytochrome P450 (CYP) enzymes

CYP enzyme	Genetic polymorphism	Substrates		Inhibitors	Inducers
CYP3A4	None	Alprazolam	Lurasidone	Clarithromycin	Carbamazepine
		Aripiprazole	Mirtazapine	Erythromycin	Dexamethasone
		Brexpiprazole	Nefazodone	Fluoxetine	Oxcarbazepine
		Bupropion	Pimozide	Fluvoxamine	Phenobarbital
		Buspirone	Quetiapine	Grapefruit juice	Phenytoin
		Citalopram	Ritonavir	Indinavir	Primidone
		Erythromycin	Saquinavir	Ketoconazole	Rifampin
		Escitalopram	Sertraline	Nefazodone	St. John's wort (*Hypericum perforatum*)
		Esketamine	Ziprasidone	Ritonavir	
		Ethinyl estradiol	Zolpidem		Topiramate
		Indinavir			

Table 1–2. Selected compounds relevant to pediatric pharmacotherapy that are metabolized by cytochrome P450 (CYP) enzymes *(continued)*

CYP enzyme	Genetic polymorphism	Substrates		Inhibitors	Inducers
CYP2D6	Yes (poor metabolizers: 7%–10% of whites, 1%–8% of Blacks, and 1%–3% of East Asians; ultrafast metabolizers: 1%–3% of whites)	Amitriptyline Aripiprazole Atomoxetine Brexpiprazole Desipramine Dextromethorphan Fluoxetine Haloperidol	Imipramine Nortriptyline Olanzapine Paroxetine Perphenazine Risperidone Venlafaxine Viloxazine	Amitriptyline Bupropion Clomipramine Desipramine Fluoxetine Haloperidol Imipramine Lamotrigine Nortriptyline Paroxetine Viloxazine	
CYP1A2	None	Agomelatine Amitriptyline Caffeine Clozapine	Fluvoxamine Olanzapine Theophylline	Ciprofloxacin Erythromycin Fluvoxamine Viloxazine	Carbamazepine Modafinil Tobacco smoke

Table 1–2. Selected compounds relevant to pediatric pharmacotherapy that are metabolized by cytochrome P450 (CYP) enzymes *(continued)*

CYP enzyme	Genetic polymorphism	Substrates		Inhibitors	Inducers
CYP2C9	Yes (poor metabolizers: 6%–12% of whites, 4% of Blacks, and 3% of East Asians)	Fluoxetine Fluvoxamine	Ibuprofen Naproxen	Fluoxetine Fluvoxamine Modafinil Sertraline	Carbamazepine Rifampin
CYP2C19	Yes (Poor metabolizers: 1%–3% of whites, 1%–3% of Blacks, and 20% of East Asians)	Amitriptyline Citalopram Clomipramine	Diazepam Escitalopram Imipramine	Fluoxetine Fluvoxamine Modafinil	
CYP2B6	Yes (reported in white and Japanese populations)	Bupropion Esketamine			Clonazepam Diazepam

2005). The clearance of risperidone in children and adolescents is fourfold greater in extensive CYP2D6 metabolizers than in poor metabolizers (Sherwin et al. 2012). Being a poor metabolizer can have safety implications, as shown by a case of death in a child with CYP2D6 genetic deficiency and unusually high plasma levels of fluoxetine (Sallee et al. 2000). Assaying for genetic polymorphism is not a standard procedure in pediatric psychopharmacology, but it can be considered for individual patients receiving long-term treatment with drugs metabolized by CYP enzymes with genetic polymorphism (e.g., CYP2D6, CYP2C19) or drugs with a low therapeutic index (e.g., tricyclic antidepressants [TCAs]); patients with treatment resistance or poor tolerability; or in cases of polypharmacy.

Possible medication interactions and medication-food interactions must be taken into account because some medications or foods can inhibit, induce, or compete with specific CYP enzymes (see Table 1–2). For example, fluoxetine, bupropion, and lamotrigine inhibit CYP2D6 activity and, when used concomitantly with risperidone, can increase risperidone serum levels. Especially important are those genetic polymorphisms and medication interactions that involve drugs with potential toxicities at high plasma concentration. Poor metabolizer status or the concomitant administration of another medication that competes with or inhibits the metabolism of the first agent would result in increased plasma concentrations. For example, toxic levels of TCAs could develop in poor metabolizers of CYP2D6; concomitant administration of fluvoxamine (an inhibitor of CYP3A4) and pimozide (metabolized by CYP3A4) could lead to high levels of pimozide and QTc interval prolongation; and oral contraceptives can induce CYP enzymes and thus increase drug metabolism and elimination.

The main route of drug elimination is through the kidneys, whereas bile, lungs, and skin account for a much smaller portion of elimination. Absolute clearance is usually lower in children than in adults, but weight-adjusted clearance can be greater. Because of the faster elimination, a drug plasma half-life can be shorter in children than in adults. Pharmacokinetics can be influenced by the dose of medication and the duration of treatment, as shown with sertraline in adolescents (Axelson et al. 2002). After a single dose of sertraline 50 mg in adolescents, the mean half-life was about 27 hours, but at steady state, after repeated administrations, the mean half-life decreased to about 15 hours. In addition, the steady-state half-life was found to be longer (about

20 hours) after administration of higher doses (100–150 mg). The clinical implication is that lower dosages (50 mg/day) should be given in two divided doses daily to ensure consistent treatment and prevent withdrawal, whereas higher dosages can be given once daily.

The pharmacokinetics of a number of commonly prescribed medications, such as escitalopram, aripiprazole, quetiapine, risperidone, lurasidone, and lithium, was found to be similar in children as in adults (Findling et al. 2008, 2010, 2015; Rao 2007; Thyssen et al. 2010). However, considerable intersubject variability was observed, suggesting that significant individual differences in the time course of the pharmacological effects may occur clinically.

In the case of medications such as methylphenidate and amphetamines, whose short half-lives result in a short duration of action and the consequent need for multiple daily doses, a variety of extended-release formulations have been developed. The first generation of extended-release methylphenidate consisted of tablets with different coatings of immediate- and slower-release medication. However, because of the large intersubject variability in absorption, the onset of action may be delayed in the morning and/or the therapeutic effect may attenuate in the afternoon. The second generation of biphasic extended-release formulations provided an initial bolus of medication to be absorbed immediately, followed by a second with more gradual release. The plasma pharmacokinetics curve thus shows an acute initial peak at about 1.5 hours after dosing, followed by a second peak about 3 hours later. The rationale behind these biphasic release formulations lies in the observation that optimal clinical effect occurs when the plasma level of methylphenidate is on the rise (Swanson et al. 2003). These extended-release preparations can be administered once daily in the morning because they allow adequate control of ADHD symptoms for up to 12 hours. Similarly, prolonged-release formulations of lithium (e.g., extended-release lithium carbonate and lithium sulfate) have been approved for use in the pediatric population. Extended-release lithium formulations might have more consistent serum lithium concentrations and fewer adverse events and thus might improve adherence to therapy, but direct comparison studies between regular and extended-release formulations are lacking.

Plasma levels are used as an indication ("surrogate marker") of drug concentration at the site of action, which, in the case of psychotropics, is not easily accessible. In fact, plasma drug levels are a rather incomplete reflection of the drug concentration in the brain, as also suggested by the rather low correlation between plasma level and clinical effects that is observed for most, but not all, drugs. Proton magnetic resonance spectroscopy has allowed the brain level of several medications, such as lithium and fluoxetine, to be directly measured. A direct correlation between serum and brain lithium levels was reported in both children and adults; younger subjects, however, had a lower brain-to-serum ratio, suggesting that they may need higher maintenance serum lithium concentrations than adults to achieve therapeutic lithium concentrations in the brain (Moore et al. 2002).

Pharmacodynamics

Although the exact mechanism of action responsible for the therapeutic effects of many psychotropics remains unknown, the basic biochemical activity of these medications is generally considered to be similar across ages. For instance, SSRIs block the reuptake of serotonin in both children and adults, and the antidepressant effect of these agents was found to be associated with the degree of inhibition of the serotonin transporter in platelets (Axelson et al. 2005). However, the possible effects of development on the intensity and specificity of this pharmacological activity have not been systematically evaluated.

Most psychotropics act through neurotransmitters, such as dopamine, serotonin, and norepinephrine, whose receptors undergo major changes during development (Rho and Storey 2001). Receptor density tends to peak between the ages of 3 and 6 years and then gradually declines to reach adult levels in late adolescence (Chugani et al. 2001). Recent evidence suggests that typical and fast-acting antidepressants act by binding the brain-derived neurotrophic factor receptor TrkB, which not only is developmentally regulated but also has a fundamental effect on neuronal survival and plasticity (Casarotto et al. 2021). The impact of these developmental changes on drug activity and the possible clinical implications have not been fully elucidated, but the observed differences between children and adults in the efficacy and safety of a number of psychotropics support the notion that development has a significant influence on the effects of psychotropic medications. For example, amphetamine-like stimulants are more likely to induce euphoria in adults than in children, and antipsychotics are more likely to induce metabolic effects in children than in adults (Correll et al. 2009).

Although not yet applicable to clinical care, brain imaging technology has been used to assess medication effects on neural circuits. For example, in youth with bipolar disorder, treatment with quetiapine was associated with normalization of the functional connectivity between brain regions involved in cognitive processing (Li et al. 2022).

Pharmacodynamics is expected to be significantly determined by genetic factors, and pharmacogenetics holds much appeal and promise to explain intersubject variability in drug effects and thus help clinicians personalize treatment. Although the theoretical rationale for applying pharmacogenetics to pediatric psychopharmacology is strong, the clinical data are still rather limited (Maruf et al. 2021; Rossow et al. 2020). Nonetheless, a number of guidelines about the clinical implementation of pharmacogenomic testing for psychoactive drugs have been published (https://cpicpgx.org/publications), and databases collecting up-to-date pharmacogenomic knowledge, including information regarding psychoactive drugs used in the pediatric population, are available online (www.pharmgkb.org/labelAnnotations).

Few pharmacogenomics-guided therapy prescription trials have been conducted, and their results are mixed (Papastergiou et al. 2021; Vande Voort et al. 2022). Thus, at this time, there is not sufficient evidence to recommend the routine use of pharmacogenetics tests in pediatric psychopharmacology (American Academy of Child and Adolescent Psychiatry 2020).

The only exception to the use of carbamazepine is in patients of Asian ethnicity because of their greater risk of Stevens-Johnson rash in those with *HLA-B* polymorphism *HLA-B*1502*, which is more common among Asian populations. Otherwise, genetic testing should be reserved for clinical situations in which there is concern that the tolerability or efficacy of the medication will be influenced by genetically determined functioning of metabolizing enzymes, such as CYP2D6.

Of great interest is research on mechanism-targeted interventions. As neuroscience sheds light on the pathogenesis of a disorder, opportunities arise to engage and modify specific biological targets in order to correct the pathogenetic mechanisms. This approach is already possible for conditions such as fragile X syndrome, Rett syndrome, and Down syndrome, whose underlying genetic and biochemical pathogenesis has been elucidated. This work can provide the model for a new generation of targeted interventions (Vitiello 2021).

Efficacy

As in adults, efficacy in children is ascertained primarily through controlled clinical trials. The theoretical framework of this methodology is the same across ages, but there are important differences when it is applied to pediatric samples. A distinctive characteristic is that the evidence for treatment effect often comes from adult informants, such as parents and teachers, rather than directly from the child. This is especially the case with young children or those with neurodevelopmental disorders such as intellectual development disorder (intellectual disability), autism spectrum disorder, or disruptive behavior disorders. This particular feature of pediatric pharmacology makes drug evaluations more complex and time-consuming for children than for adults, in both research and practice settings. Clinicians must integrate information from a variety of sources and arrive at a determination about therapeutic benefit.

Various rating instruments have been developed and validated for assessing treatment effects. In the absence of biological markers of disease and treatment effects, clinicians must rely on changes in clinical symptoms to gauge response. Although symptom rating scales have been introduced primarily for research purposes, with the goal of quantifying psychopathology at different points in time, they can and should be applied to usual clinical practice because they help the clinician measure and document the patient's condition prospectively. Thus, rating scales that are sensitive to medication effects are available in common child psychiatric disorders such as ADHD (e.g., Conners 2008; DuPaul et al. 2016), depression (e.g., Poznanski and Mokros 1996), and anxiety (e.g., Research Units on Pediatric Psychopharmacology Anxiety Study Group 2002). In some cases, scales originally developed for adults have been applied to pediatric psychopharmacology, such as the clinical trials of antipsychotics in early-onset schizophrenia that used the Positive and Negative Syndrome Scale with success (Kay et al. 1987). Further research is needed to develop measures of the core symptoms of autism that are sensitive to possible treatment effects of medications.

Besides effects on symptoms, it is relevant to document the overall level of functioning before and during treatment. Some scales of global functioning are available, including the Children's Global Assessment Scale for children and adolescents ages 6–17 years—along with its adaptation to children with autism spectrum disorder (Shaffer et al. 1983; Wagner et al. 2007)—and the Health of the Nation Outcome Scales for Children and Adolescents, a clinician report scale regarding general health and social functioning (Pirkis et al. 2005).

For some medications, continuity of efficacy from childhood to adulthood has been consistently found, such as for serotonin reuptake inhibitors (e.g., SSRIs) in OCD, stimulants in ADHD, and clozapine in schizophrenia (Kasoff et al. 2016). Remarkable differences have been observed for other medications; most notably, none of the placebo-controlled trials of TCAs has shown superiority of the active medication in children, and among the SSRIs, only fluoxetine and escitalopram have been found to be better than placebo in more than one study (Zhou et al. 2020). It is unclear whether the inability to consistently demonstrate antidepressant efficacy in youth for all of the SSRIs found to be effective in adults can be ascribed to some intrinsic difference in pharmacological activity or, more likely, to methodological issues in the pediatric clinical trials.

The increasing body of research in child and adolescent psychopharmacology has allowed evidence-based clinical practice guidelines and treatment algorithms to be developed. Treatment algorithms consist of step-by-step instructions on how to treat individual patients based on their symptoms and history of previous treatment. Algorithms are therefore more detailed and specific than general treatment guidelines or practice parameters. Practice guidelines and algorithms have been developed for ADHD, depression, bipolar disorder, and other conditions (Cheung et al. 2018; National Institute for Health and Care Excellence 2020; Penfold et al. 2022; Wolraich et al. 2019).

The magnitude of the treatment effect relative to a control is often expressed in standard deviation units using the *effect size.* Among the most common ways of computing an effect size is with Cohen's *d* or Hedges' *g*, either of which shows the difference in outcome measure between the study groups divided by the pooled standard deviation at the end of treatment (Rosenthal et al. 2000). Compared with placebo, stimulant medications have a large effect size (≥0.8) in decreasing symptoms of ADHD (Cortese et al. 2018). In the trials that detected a statistically significant difference between an SSRI and placebo, the SSRI had a medium effect size (0.5–0.7) in major depression (March et al. 2004) and in OCD (Pediatric OCD Treatment Study Team 2004). Meta-analyses of all available pediatric clinical trials, however, have consistently reported a small effect size for SSRIs in depression and a medium to large effect size in OCD and anxiety disorders (Locher et al. 2017; Zhou et al. 2020).

The effect size is a purely mathematical computation to quantify a difference between means and, as such, is at times used to quantify the difference from pretreatment to posttreatment within the same treatment group. When this is done, a large effect size often emerges because it includes the time effect. In the absence of a control condition and because of the consequent inability to distinguish treatment effect from time effect, the pre- to posttreatment effect size has limited meaning and cannot be taken as an index of treatment effect.

In addition to the effect size, a useful index of magnitude of the therapeutic benefit is the *number needed to treat* (NNT), which is the number of patients who need to be given the treatment for one more improved patient to be added to the number of those on the control condition who are expected to improve. For example, in the Treatment for Adolescents With Depression Study (March et al. 2004), 61% of patients treated with fluoxetine had improved by the end of the 12-week treatment, compared with 35% of those who received placebo. The NNT was 4, which indicates that, on average, four patients had to be treated for one patient to improve more than the placebo condition. The smaller the NNT, the greater the relative efficacy of the treatment. Clinical trials have shown that the NNTs of psychotropic medications, although variable across studies, are often quite favorable and compare well with those of other nonpsychiatric drugs used in pediatrics or general medicine (Leucht et al. 2012).

Because most psychiatric conditions are chronic or recurrent, treatment is often prolonged in time. Progress has been made in assessing the long-term effectiveness of pharmacotherapy in ADHD and some mood disorders (DelBello et al. 2021; Maia et al. 2017), but more research is needed to evaluate the effectiveness of pharmacotherapy beyond 1 year of treatment. An especially important issue for pediatric psychopharmacology is whether early treatment with successful control of symptoms translates distally into better "real-life" functional outcomes, such as higher educational and occupational attainment. This type of research poses considerable challenges from a methodological and implementation perspective, given the practical difficulties of conducting long-term randomized controlled trials and the limitations of uncontrolled observational studies for inferring causality. In this regard, analyses of population-based databases have recently provided useful information—for example, by documenting that pharmacotherapy of ADHD in childhood was associated with greater likelihood of entering high school education (Jangmo et al. 2019).

Safety

Safety considerations are paramount in pediatric psychopharmacology. Pharmacological treatment during a period in which the body undergoes marked developmental changes may result in toxicities not seen in adults. For example, prolonged administration of phenobarbital to young children to prevent recurrence of febrile seizures impairs their cognitive development (Farwell et al. 1990), and the risk of valproic acid–induced hepatotoxicity is much higher for children younger than 2 years than later in life (Bryant and Dreifuss 1996).

A general concern is that administration of agents acting on the neurotransmitter systems during development may interfere with brain maturation and result in unwanted long-lasting changes. Although some studies in animals suggest lasting effects of early medication exposure (Ansorge et al. 2004), no correlates of detectable adverse outcomes have emerged in humans. A high level of suspicion is, however, warranted when treating children with medications, especially if treatment is prolonged in time. Different types of adverse effects can occur (Vitiello et al. 2003). Some, such as rash or dystonias, emerge acutely upon initial brief drug exposure, whereas others, such as tardive dyskinesia or metabolic syndrome, are the result of chronic treatment. Some toxicities, such as lithium-induced tremor, are related to drug dosage and/or plasma concentrations; others, such as withdrawal dyskinesias, emerge after drug discontinuation. Some adverse effects may be anticipated based on the medication's mechanism of action, but others, such as the increased suicidality seen with antidepressant treatment, may be unexpected and even paradoxical.

As in assessing efficacy, the assessment of safety in pediatric psychopharmacology depends in large part on monitoring and reporting by parents and other adults. From the clinician's perspective, the identification of treatment adverse effects depends on the level of detail and accuracy with which the relevant information is elicited and collected from the child and their caregivers (Greenhill et al. 2004). Over the years, more information has become available on the long-term safety of psychotropic medications in children. Although limited by the fact that most of the studies have been observational in nature, the available data provide some guidance to clinicians. The paragraphs that follow provide examples of safety issues that pertain to commonly used psychotropics.

Chronic administration of methylphenidate and amphetamines to children for the treatment of ADHD has been found to cause a dose-related delay in physical growth in both weight and height. After 14 months of treatment, children treated with stimulant medication for ADHD had grown on average 1.2 cm less in height than peers treated with behavior therapy (MTA Cooperative Group 2004). The deficit in height growth was found to persist in continuously medicated children despite caloric supplementation (Waxmonsky et al. 2020). The mechanism underlying the interference of stimulants with skeletal growth is unclear, but it does not seem merely to be the result of a caloric deficit.

Stimulants have adrenergic effects, and concern has been raised about adverse cardiovascular outcomes, including sudden death (Gould et al. 2009). However, a number of retrospective analyses have not found any association between stimulant treatment and adverse cardiac events (Cooper et al. 2011). Moreover, prospective analyses of children treated for up to 10 years did not find an increased risk for hypertension, although stimulants have a detectable effect on heart rate even with long-term use (Vitiello et al. 2012).

Because stimulant medications are drugs of potential abuse, concerns have been raised about the possibility that treatment in childhood may sensitize the brain and thus make substance abuse and dependence more likely in adolescence and adulthood. The feasibility of mounting randomized, well-controlled studies to address this issue is questionable, and researchers have relied on naturalistically treated samples. Most of these studies have not found an increased risk of substance abuse after treatment with stimulants (Biederman et al. 2008; McCabe et al. 2016).

Differences in tolerability have been observed across age and type of development. Preschoolers with ADHD have lower tolerability to methylphenidate than older children (Childress et al. 2022; Wigal et al. 2006). Moreover, long-lasting effects of methylphenidate on human striatal and thalamic blood flow have been observed in children but not in adults, suggesting age-dependent effects of the drug on brain circuitry (Schrantee et al. 2016). Children with autism spectrum disorder or other pervasive developmental disorders with ADHD symptoms are more sensitive to methylphenidate, as indicated by an 18% treatment discontinuation rate due to intolerable adverse events (most commonly irritability) (Masi et al. 2022; Research Units on Pediatric Psychopharmacology Autism Network 2005). Youth exposed to second-generation antipsychotics are more prone to weight gain than adults (Correll et al. 2009).

Antidepressant treatment of children and adolescents has been associated with a slight but statistically significant increased risk of suicidality (i.e., suicidal ideation and suicide attempt), although not of suicide (Hammad et al. 2006). Subsequent analyses found strong evidence for suicide-related behavior only for patients treated with venlafaxine (Zhou et al. 2020). However, close monitoring of adolescents taking antidepressants is still warranted. A significant association was found between age and emergence of suicidality during antidepressant treatment, with an increased risk compared with placebo for patients younger than 25 years, a neutral effect for those ages 25–64 years, and a protective effect for patients older than 64 (Stone et al. 2009). These data demonstrate the interaction between development and pharmacological effect, although the biological underpinnings of this interaction remain unknown.

Safety is a relative concept, and possible risks of pharmacotherapy must be weighed against possible risks of untreated psychopathology. Decisions about prescribing medications must also take into account the availability of effective nonpharmacological interventions. Although it is generally found to be somewhat less effective at decreasing symptoms of ADHD or depression in children and adolescents, psychotherapy can be considered in lieu of medication for patients with mild depression or in combination with medications for those with more severe illness. Psychotherapy, used either sequentially (i.e., starting first with psychotherapy, then adding medication if insufficient) or in combination (i.e., starting both psychotherapy and medication concurrently), may reduce the medication dosage needed to control symptoms. Consideration should be given to using psychosocial interventions as first-line treatment, especially in young children. In any case, carefully monitoring children receiving psychotropics and documenting both positive and negative outcomes have emerged as critically important components of rational pharmacotherapy.

Ethical Aspects

Children should be given as much explanation as they can reasonably understand about their condition and possible therapeutic options, but they cannot give legal consent for treatment, which is the responsibility of the parents. Parents are also instrumental in implementing pharmacotherapy by ensuring appropriate administration of prescribed medication and by reporting possible treatment-emergent adverse effects. Parental permission is required for child participation in research, and such participation is subject to special regulations over and above those required for adults (Office for Human Research Protections 2018).

Only scientifically sound research investigations that use valid methodology and are posited to add new knowledge about important health issues can be ethically acceptable (Vitiello 2003). Pediatric research can be divided into two broad categories based on whether it presents the prospect of direct benefit to the individual participant. *Prospect of direct benefit* refers to the fact that each participant has the potential to derive a health benefit from participation. General acquisition of knowledge relevant to the child's condition does not satisfy the requirement of direct benefit. To be ethically acceptable, research with the prospect of direct benefit must show a favorable balance between anticipated benefits and foreseeable harms. A study that tests the efficacy of a treatment intervention usually has potential for direct benefit to the research participants. In this case, the main criterion for determining whether the study is ethically acceptable is the risk-benefit ratio. The presence of a placebo arm in a randomized clinical trial is usually considered acceptable in child psychiatry conditions. Placebo does not equal absence of treatment and has been associated with substantial improvement, especially in the case of mood and anxiety disorders.

Pharmacological research that *does not offer a prospect of direct benefit* includes pharmacokinetics and pharmacodynamics studies. To examine the acceptability of a study in this category, one must determine whether such a study has the potential for generating essential knowledge relevant to the disorder or condition of the participants. If the information that the study will acquire is not relevant to the child's disorder or condition (e.g., a pharmacokinetics study in healthy children who are at no increased risk for the condition being targeted by the treatment), then the research can be conducted only if it entails no more than minimal risk. *Minimal risk* means that the "probability and magnitude of harm or discomfort anticipated in the research are not greater in and of themselves than those ordinarily encountered in daily life risk for harm not greater than ordinarily encountered in daily life or during the performance of routine physical or psychological examinations or tests" (Office for Human Research Protections 2018, 45 C.F.R, Subpart A, Section 46.102[j]). The prevailing interpretation is that the daily life, examinations, and tests of a normal child are to be used as reference, but a precise quantification of risk in ordinary daily life is not easy and remains a matter of discussion (Wendler et al. 2005).

If the study aims to acquire information relevant to the child's condition (e.g., pharmacokinetics of a medication for ADHD being studied in children with ADHD), then the research risk cannot be greater than a "minor increase over minimal risk." A *minor increase over minimal risk* can be considered acceptable only if 1) it presents "experiences to the subjects that are commensurate with those inherent in their actual or expected medical, dental, psychological, social, or educational situations" (Office for Human Research Protections 2018, 45 C.F.R., Subpart D, Section 46.406[b]) and 2) the study has the potential to generate new knowledge considered of "vital importance" for understanding or treating the child's disorder or condition.

Research that is not otherwise approvable based on these criteria but offers an opportunity to understand, prevent, or alleviate a serious problem affecting the health or welfare of children can be referred to the U.S. Secretary of Health and Human Services for further review under regulations at 45 C.F.R., Subpart D, Section 46.407 (Office for Human Research Protections 2018) and 21 C.F.R. 50.56 (U.S. Food and Drug Administration 2001). Studies in which psychotropic medications may be given to children who are physically and mentally healthy for the purpose of understanding the medication's mechanisms of action on the brain would fall into this category because a nontherapeutic administration of a pharmacological compound would generally be considered to pose more than minimal risk. For example, the protocol for a brain MRI study of healthy children age 9 years or older receiving a single oral dose of dextroamphetamine was referred in 2004 by the institutional review board of the National Institute of Mental Health under regulations at 45 C.F.R. 46.407 (Couzin 2004). This study was reviewed and approved by the Pediatric Ethics Subcommittee of the FDA Pediatric Advisory Committee in September 2004. The reviewers determined that a single administration of dextroamphetamine 10 mg to a child age 9 years or older entails more than minimal risk because the potential adverse effects are more than those expected in a routine visit to a doctor, but the risk is limited to a minor increase over minimal risk. That being the case, and because the study had the potential to generate important information on the effects of a medication commonly used in children, the research was eventually approved.

The process of informing parents and children about the aims, procedures, and potential risks and benefits of research participation; the presence of alternative treatments; and the rights of research participants is critical for obtaining their informed permission and assent. In general, children age 7 years or older are able to provide assent, and this is often documented in writing with an appropriate assent form. With proper communication and explanation by researchers, parents can achieve a good understanding of both research procedures and participant rights. By age 16, youth generally have a level of understanding similar to that of their parents (Vitiello et al. 2007).

Several public and private websites provide detailed information about child participation in research and the process of determining whether a particular project is ethically acceptable (Office for Human Research Protections 2016).

Regulatory Aspects

A number of psychotropic medications currently have pediatric indications approved by the FDA and other regulatory agencies, whereas others are used off-label for indication or age (Table 1–3). The off-label use of a drug is not in itself inappropriate, because it is often supported by considerable empirical evidence and is consistent with treatment guidelines. However, patients and their family need to be informed that a medication is being prescribed for an off-label use so that they can make fully informed decisions.

Research in pediatric psychopharmacology has greatly expanded in the past 20 years thanks to a number of publicly funded clinical research networks and several seminal legislative and regulatory initiatives (Vitiello and Davico 2018). In particular, financial incentives have been provided to pharmaceutical companies for conducting pediatric research (Best Pharmaceuticals for Children Act 2002). This legislation and its subsequent reauthorizations and expansions have substantially changed the industry's approach to pediatric pharmacology, including also pediatric psychopharmacology. In parallel, legislation was enacted giving the FDA the authority to request that the industry conduct pediatric studies of a drug, even prior to its approval for adult use, when there are reasons to expect that it may be used also in children (Pediatric Research Equity Act 2003).

Table 1–3. Pediatric indications approved by the FDA and off-label use of selected psychotropic medications

Medication	FDA-approved indication(s)	Relative child age, *years*	Off-label use and child age, *years*
Agomelatine	None		MDD: ≥7
Amphetamines	ADHD	≥3	
Aripiprazole	Schizophrenia	≥13	Aggression
	Bipolar disorder	≥10	Tourette's disorder
	"Irritability" in autism	5–16	
Asenapine	Bipolar disorder	≥10	Schizophrenia
Atomoxetine	ADHD	≥6	ADHD: <6
Brexpiprazole	Schizophrenia	≥13	
Bupropion	None		MDD: ≥6
			ADHD: ≥6
Carbamazepine	Epilepsy	From infancy	Mania, aggression
Citalopram	None		OCD, other anxiety disorders: ≥6
			MDD: ≥6
Clomipramine	OCD	≥10	
Clonidine	ADHD	≥6	Tourette's disorder
Dexmethylphenidate	ADHD	≥6	ADHD: <6

Table 1–3. Pediatric indications approved by the FDA and off-label use of selected psychotropic medications *(continued)*

Medication	**FDA-approved indication(s)**	**Relative child age, *years***	**Off-label use and child age, *years***
Duloxetine	GAD	≥7	MDD: ≥6
Escitalopram	MDD	≥12	MDD: 6–11
Fluoxetine	MDD	≥8	MDD: <8
	OCD	≥7	Other anxiety disorders: ≥6
Fluvoxamine	OCD	≥7	Other anxiety disorders: ≥6
Guanfacine	ADHD	≥6	Tourette's disorder
Haloperidol	Psychosis, Tourette's disorder, hyperactivity, severe behavioral problems, explosive hyperexcitability	≥3	
Lamotrigine	Epilepsy	≥2	Depression in bipolar disorder
Lisdexamfetamine	ADHD	≥6	ADHD: <6
Lithium	Bipolar disorder (acute and maintenance treatment)	≥7	Aggression, prevention of suicidal behavior
Lurasidone	Schizophrenia	≥13	
	Bipolar I depression	≥10	
Methylphenidate	ADHD	≥6	ADHD: <6
Olanzapine	Schizophrenia	≥13	Aggression, Tourette's disorder, anorexia nervosa
	Bipolar disorder	≥10	

Table 1–3. Pediatric indications approved by the FDA and off-label use of selected psychotropic medications *(continued)*

Medication	FDA-approved indication(s)	Relative child age, *years*	Off-label use and child age, *years*
Oxcarbazepine	Epilepsy	≥4	Mania, aggression
Paroxetine	None		OCD, other anxiety disorders: ≥6
			MDD: ≥6
Pimozide	Tourette's disorder	≥12	
Quetiapine	Schizophrenia	≥13	Aggression
	Bipolar disorder	≥10	Tourette's disorder
Risperidone	Schizophrenia	≥13	Aggression
	Bipolar disorder	≥10	Tourette's disorder
	"Irritability" in autism	5–16	
Sertraline	OCD	≥6	OCD, anxiety disorders: ≥6
			MDD: ≥6
Valproate	Epilepsy	From infancy	Mania, aggression
Venlafaxine	None		MDD: ≥6
Viloxazine	ADHD	≥6	

Note. GAD = generalized anxiety disorder; MDD = major depressive disorder.

Conclusion

Pediatric psychopharmacology is a relatively new field of clinical pharmacology that has recently undergone a rapid expansion due to intense research activity. It is also the object of frequent debate and, at times, controversy in the media and the general public. The therapeutic value of several psychotropic medications is now well documented for both the short and intermediate term. Knowledge gaps remain, especially in the understanding of the long-term impact of pharmacotherapy with respect to both efficacy and safety. Practicing rational pharmacotherapy requires integration of knowledge at different levels, including developmental psychopathology, pharmacology, and drug regulation and bioethics, and a considerable investment of time on the part of the treating clinician and the child's parents.

Clinical Pearls

- Simply decreasing adult medication dosages on the basis of child weight can result in undertreatment because of faster drug elimination in children.
- Assessing treatment effects and safety requires collection and integration of data from different sources (i.e., child, parent, teacher).
- Safety is paramount, and a high level of suspicion is warranted when prescribing medication for children, especially at the beginning of treatment and when multiple medications are prescribed and taken concurrently.
- Younger children and children with neurodevelopmental disorders, such as autism spectrum disorder and intellectual developmental disorder (intellectual disability), tend to be more sensitive to the adverse effects of medications.
- Children should have their condition explained to the extent that they can understand, and whenever possible, their assent to treatment should be obtained.

References

American Academy of Child and Adolescent Psychiatry: Clinical Use of Pharmacogenetic Tests in Prescribing Psychotropic Medications for Children and Adolescents. Washington, DC, American Academy of Child and Adolescent Psychiatry, 2020. Available at: https://www.aacap.org/AACAP/Policy_Statements/2020/Clinical-Use-Pharmacogenetic-Tests-Prescribing-Psychotropic-Medications-for-Children-Adolescents.aspx. Accessed February 5, 2022.

Ansorge MS, Zhou M, Lira A, et al: Early life blockade of the 5-HT transporter alters emotional behavior in adult mice. Science 306(5697):879–881, 2004 15514160

Axelson DA, Perel JM, Birmaher B, et al: Sertraline pharmacokinetics and dynamics in adolescents. J Am Acad Child Adolesc Psychiatry 41(9):1037–1044, 2002 12218424

Axelson DA, Perel JM, Birmaher B, et al: Platelet serotonin reuptake inhibition and response to SSRIs in depressed adolescents. Am J Psychiatry 162(4):802–804, 2005 15800159

Best Pharmaceuticals for Children Act of 2002, Pub. L. No. 107–109, 115 Stat. 1408

Biederman J, Monuteaux MC, Spencer T, et al: Stimulant therapy and risk for subsequent substance use disorders in male adults with ADHD: a naturalistic controlled 10-year follow-up study. Am J Psychiatry 165(5):597–603, 2008 18316421

Bryant AE III, Dreifuss FE: Valproic acid hepatic fatalities III: U.S. experience since 1986. Neurology 46(2):465–469, 1996 8614514

Calarge CA, Miller D: Predictors of risperidone and 9-hydroxyrisperidone serum concentration in children and adolescents. J Child Adolesc Psychopharmacol 21(2):163–169, 2011 21486167

Casarotto PC, Girych M, Fred SM, et al: Antidepressant drugs act by directly binding to TRKB neurotrophin receptors. Cell 184(5):1299–1313, 2021 33606976

Chambers CD, Johnson KA, Dick LM, et al: Birth outcomes in pregnant women taking fluoxetine. N Engl J Med 335(14):1010–1015, 1996 8793924

Cheung AH, Zuckerbrot RA, Jensen PS, et al: Guidelines for Adolescent Depression in Primary Care (GLAD-PC) part II: treatment and ongoing management. Pediatrics 141(3):e20174082, 2018 29483201

Childress AC, Foehl HC, Newcorn JH, et al: Long-term treatment with extended-release methylphenidate treatment in children aged 4 to <6 years. J Am Acad Child Adolesc Psychiatry 61(1):80–92, 2022 33892111

Chugani DC, Muzik O, Juhász C, et al: Postnatal maturation of human GABA-A receptors measured with positron emission tomography. Ann Neurol 49(5):618–626, 2001 11357952

Conners CK: Conners, 3rd Edition. Toronto, ON, Canada, Multi-Health Systems, 2008

Cooper WO, Habel LA, Sox CM, et al: ADHD drugs and serious cardiovascular events in children and young adults. N Engl J Med 365(20):1896–1904, 2011 22043968

Correll CU, Manu P, Olshanskiy V, et al: Cardiometabolic risk of second-generation antipsychotic medications during first-time use in children and adolescents. JAMA 302(16):1765–1773, 2009 19861668

Cortese S, Adamo N, Del Giovane C, et al: Comparative efficacy and tolerability of medications for attention-deficit hyperactivity disorder in children, adolescents, and adults: a systematic review and network meta-analysis. Lancet Psychiatry 5(9):727–738, 2018 30097390

Couzin J: Human subjects research: pediatric study of ADHD drug draws high-level public review. Science 305(5687):1088–1089, 2004 15326317

DelBello MP, Tocco M, Pikalov A, et al: Tolerability, safety, and effectiveness of two years of treatment with lurasidone in children and adolescents with bipolar depression. J Child Adolesc Psychopharmacol 31(7):494–503, 2021 34324397

DuPaul GJ, Power TJ, Anastopoulos AD, Reid R: ADHD Rating Scale–5 for Children and Adolescents: Checklists, Norms, and Clinical Interpretation. New York, Guilford, 2016

Farwell JR, Lee YJ, Hirtz DG, et al: Phenobarbital for febrile seizures: effects on intelligence and on seizure recurrence. N Engl J Med 322(6):364–369, 1990 2242106

Fekete S, Hiemke C, Gerlach M: Dose-related concentrations of neuroactive/psychoactive drugs expected in blood of children and adolescents. Ther Drug Monit 42(2):315–324, 2020 32195989

Findling RL, Kauffman RE, Sallee FR, et al: Tolerability and pharmacokinetics of aripiprazole in children and adolescents with psychiatric disorders: an open-label, dose-escalation study. J Clin Psychopharmacol 28(4):441–446, 2008 18626272

Findling RL, Landersdorfer CB, Kafantaris V, et al: First-dose pharmacokinetics of lithium carbonate in children and adolescents. J Clin Psychopharmacol 30(4):404–410, 2010 20531219

Findling RL, Goldman R, Chiu Y-Y, et al: Pharmacokinetics and tolerability of lurasidone in children and adolescents with psychiatric disorders. Clin Ther 37(12):2788–2797, 2015 26631428

Gould MS, Walsh BT, Munfakh JL, et al: Sudden death and use of stimulant medications in youths. Am J Psychiatry 166(9):992–1001, 2009 19528194

Greenhill LL, Vitiello B, Fisher P, et al: Comparison of increasingly detailed elicitation methods for the assessment of adverse events in pediatric psychopharmacology. J Am Acad Child Adolesc Psychiatry 43(12):1488–1496, 2004 15564818

Hammad TA, Laughren T, Racoosin J: Suicidality in pediatric patients treated with antidepressant drugs. Arch Gen Psychiatry 63(3):332–339, 2006 16520440

Jangmo A, Stålhandske A, Chang Z, et al: Attention-deficit/hyperactivity disorder, school performance, and effect of medication. J Am Acad Child Adolesc Psychiatry 58(4):423–432, 2019 30768391

Kasoff LI, Ahn K, Gochman P, et al: Strong treatment response and high maintenance rates of clozapine in childhood-onset schizophrenia. J Child Adolesc Psychopharmacol 26(5):428–435, 2016 26784704

Kay SR, Fiszbein A, Opler LA: The Positive and Negative Syndrome Scale (PANSS) for schizophrenia. Schizophr Bull 13(2):261–276, 1987 3616518

Leucht S, Hierl S, Kissling W, et al: Putting the efficacy of psychiatric and general medication into perspective: review of meta-analyses. Br J Psychiatry 200(2):97–106, 2012 22297588

Li W, Lei D, Tallman MJ, et al.: Pretreatment alterations and acute medication treatment effects on brain task-related functional connectivity in youth with bipolar disorder: a neuroimaging randomized clinical trial. J Am Acad Child Adolesc Psychiatry 61(8):1023–1033, 2022 35091050

Locher C, Koechlin H, Zion SR, et al: Efficacy and safety of selective serotonin reuptake inhibitors, serotonin-norepinephrine reuptake inhibitors, and placebo for common psychiatric disorders among children and adolescents: a systematic review and meta-analysis. JAMA Psychiatry 74(10):1011–1020, 2017 28854296

Maia CR, Cortese S, Caye A, et al: Long-term efficacy of methylphenidate immediate-release for the treatment of childhood ADHD. J Atten Disord 21(1):3–13, 2017 25501355

March J, Silva S, Petrycki S, et al: Fluoxetine, cognitive-behavioral therapy, and their combination for adolescents with depression: Treatment for Adolescents With Depression Study (TADS) randomized controlled trial. JAMA 292(7):807–820, 2004 15315995

Maruf AA, Stein K, Arnold PD, et al: CYP2D6 and antipsychotic treatment outcomes in children and youth: a systematic review. J Child Adolesc Psychopharmacol 31(1):33–45, 2021 33074724

Masi G, Pfanner C, Liboni F, et al: Acute tolerability of methylphenidate in treatment-naïve children with ADHD: an analysis of naturalistically collected data from clinical practice. Paediatr Drugs 24(2):147–154, 2022 35137333

McCabe SE, Dickinson K, West BT, Wilens TE: Age of onset, duration, and type of medication therapy for attention-deficit/hyperactivity disorder and substance use during adolescence: a multi-cohort national study. J Am Acad Child Adolesc Psychiatry 55(6):479–486, 2016 27238066

Moore CM, Demopulos CM, Henry ME, et al: Brain-to-serum lithium ratio and age: an in vivo magnetic resonance spectroscopy study. Am J Psychiatry 159(7):1240–1242, 2002 12091209

MTA Cooperative Group: National Institute of Mental Health Multimodal Treatment Study of ADHD follow-up: changes in effectiveness and growth after the end of treatment. Pediatrics 113(4):762–769, 2004 15060225

National Institute for Health and Care Excellence: The NICE Guideline on the Assessment and Management of Bipolar Disorder in Adults, Children and Young People in Primary and Secondary Care, No. 185. Leicester, UK, British Psychological Society and Royal College of Psychiatrists, 2020

Office for Human Research Protections: Information on Special Protections for Children as Research Subjects. Rockville, MD, Office for Human Research Protections, 2016. Available at: https://www.hhs.gov/ohrp/regulations-and-policy/guidance/special-protections-for-children/index.html. Accessed February 7, 2022.

Office for Human Research Protections: Protection of Human Subjects. 45 C.F.R. 46 (Subparts A–D). Rockville, MD, Office for Human Research Protections, 2018. Available at: https://www.hhs.gov/ohrp/regulations-and-policy/regulations/45-cfr-46/index.html. Accessed February 7, 2022.

Papastergiou J, Quilty LC, Li W, et al: Pharmacogenomics guided versus standard antidepressant treatment in a community pharmacy setting: a randomized controlled trial. Clin Transl Sci 14(4):1359–1368, 2021 33641259

Pediatric OCD Treatment Study Team: Cognitive-behavior therapy, sertraline, and their combination for children and adolescents with obsessive-compulsive disorder: the Pediatric OCD Treatment Study (POTS) randomized controlled trial. JAMA 292(16):1969–1976, 2004 15507582

Pediatric Research Equity Act of 2003, Pub. L. No. 108-155, 117 Stat 1936

Penfold RB, Thompson EE, Hilt RJ, et al: Development of a symptom-focused model to guide the prescribing of antipsychotics in children and adolescents: results of the first phase of the Safer Use of Antipsychotics in Youth (SUAY) clinical trial. J Am Acad Child Adolesc Psychiatry 61(1):93–102, 2022 34256967

Pirkis JE, Burgess PM, Kirk PK, et al: A review of the psychometric properties of the Health of the Nation Outcome Scales (HoNOS) family of measures. Health Qual Life Outcomes 3(76):76, 2005 16313678

Poznanski EO, Mokros HB: Manual for the Children's Depression Rating Scale—Revised. Los Angeles, CA, Western Psychological Services, 1996

Rao N: The clinical pharmacokinetics of escitalopram. Clin Pharmacokinet 46(4):281–290, 2007 17375980

Research Units on Pediatric Psychopharmacology Anxiety Study Group: The Pediatric Anxiety Rating Scale (PARS): development and psychometric properties. J Am Acad Child Adolesc Psychiatry 41(9):1061–1069, 2002 12218427

Research Units on Pediatric Psychopharmacology Autism Network: Randomized, controlled, crossover trial of methylphenidate in pervasive developmental disorders with hyperactivity. Arch Gen Psychiatry 62(11):1266–1274, 2005 16275814

Rho JM, Storey TW: Molecular ontogeny of major neurotransmitter receptor systems in the mammalian central nervous system: norepinephrine, dopamine, serotonin, acetylcholine, and glycine. J Child Neurol 16(4):271–280, discussion 281, 2001 11332462

Rosenthal R, Rosnow R, Rubin DB: Contrasts and Effect Sizes in Behavioral Research. Cambridge, UK, Cambridge University Press, 2000

Rossow KM, Aka IT, Maxwell-Horn AC, et al: Pharmacogenetics to predict adverse events associated with antidepressants. Pediatrics 146(6):e20200957, 2020 33234666

Sallee FR, DeVane CL, Ferrell RE: Fluoxetine-related death in a child with cytochrome P-450 2D6 genetic deficiency. J Child Adolesc Psychopharmacol 10(1):27–34, 2000 10755579

Sauer JM, Ring BJ, Witcher JW: Clinical pharmacokinetics of atomoxetine. Clin Pharmacokinet 44(6):571–590, 2005 15910008

Schrantee A, Tamminga HG, Bouziane C, et al: Age-dependent effects of methylphenidate on the human dopaminergic system in young vs adult patients with attention-deficit/hyperactivity disorder: a randomized clinical trial. JAMA Psychiatry 73(9):955–962, 2016 27487479

Shaffer D, Gould MS, Brasic J, et al: A Children's Global Assessment Scale (CGAS). Arch Gen Psychiatry 40(11):1228–1231, 1983 6639293

Sherwin CM, Saldaña SN, Bies RR, et al: Population pharmacokinetic modeling of risperidone and 9-hydroxyrisperidone to estimate CYP2D6 subpopulations in children and adolescents. Ther Drug Monit 34(5):535–544, 2012 22929407

Smits A, Annaert P, Cavallaro G, et al: Current knowledge, challenges and innovations in developmental pharmacology: a combined conect4children Expert Group and European Society for Developmental, Perinatal and Paediatric Pharmacology white paper. Br J Clin Pharmacol 88(12):4965–4984, 2022 34180088

Stone M, Laughren T, Jones ML, et al: Risk of suicidality in clinical trials of antidepressants in adults: analysis of proprietary data submitted to US Food and Drug Administration. BMJ 339:b2880, 2009 19671933

Swanson J, Gupta S, Lam A, et al: Development of a new once-a-day formulation of methylphenidate for the treatment of attention-deficit/hyperactivity disorder: proof-of-concept and proof-of-product studies. Arch Gen Psychiatry 60(2):204–211, 2003 12578439

Thyssen A, Vermeulen A, Fuseau E, et al: Population pharmacokinetics of oral risperidone in children, adolescents and adults with psychiatric disorders. Clin Pharmacokinet 49(7):465–478, 2010 20528007

U.S. Food and Drug Administration: Additional safeguards for children in clinical investigations of FDA-regulated products. Fed Regist 66:20598, 2001

Vande Voort JL, Orth SS, Shekunov J, et al: A randomized controlled trial of combinatorial pharmacogenetics testing in adolescent depression. J Am Acad Child Adolesc Psychiatry 61(1):46–55, 2022 34099307

van Groen BD, Nicolaï J, Kuik AC, et al: Ontogeny of hepatic transporters and drug-metabolizing enzymes in humans and in nonclinical species. Pharmacol Rev 73(2):597–678, 2021 33608409

Vitiello B: Ethical considerations in psychopharmacological research involving children and adolescents. Psychopharmacology (Berl) 171(1):86–91, 2003 12677353

Vitiello B: Targeting the core symptoms of autism spectrum disorder with mechanism-based medications. J Am Acad Child Adolesc Psychiatry 60(7):816–817, 2021 33212159

Vitiello B, Davico C: Twenty years of progress in paediatric psychopharmacology: accomplishments and unmet needs. Evid Based Ment Health 21(4):e10, 2018 30352885

Vitiello B, Riddle MA, Greenhill LL, et al: How can we improve the assessment of safety in child and adolescent psychopharmacology? J Am Acad Child Adolesc Psychiatry 42(6):634–641, 2003 12921470

Vitiello B, Kratochvil CJ, Silva S, et al: Research knowledge among the participants in the Treatment for Adolescents With Depression Study (TADS). J Am Acad Child Adolesc Psychiatry 46(12):1642–1650, 2007 18030086

Vitiello B, Elliott GR, Swanson JM, et al: Blood pressure and heart rate over 10 years in the multimodal treatment study of children with ADHD. Am J Psychiatry 169(2):167–177, 2012 21890793

Wagner A, Lecavalier L, Arnold LE, et al: Developmental disabilities modification of the Children's Global Assessment Scale. Biol Psychiatry 61(4):504–511, 2007 17276748

Waxmonsky JG, Pelham WE III, Campa A, et al: A randomized controlled trial of interventions for growth suppression in children with attention-deficit/hyperactivity disorder treated with central nervous system stimulants. J Am Acad Child Adolesc Psychiatry 59(12):1330–1341, 2020 31473291

Wendler D, Belsky L, Thompson KM, Emanuel EJ: Quantifying the federal minimal risk standard: implications for pediatric research without a prospect of direct benefit. JAMA 294(7):826–832, 2005 16106008

Wigal T, Greenhill L, Chuang S, et al: Safety and tolerability of methylphenidate in preschool children with ADHD. J Am Acad Child Adolesc Psychiatry 45(11):1294–1303, 2006 17028508

Wolraich ML, Hagan JF Jr, Allan C, et al: Clinical practice guideline for the diagnosis, evaluation, and treatment of attention-deficit/hyperactivity disorder in children and adolescents. Pediatrics 144(4):e20192528, 2019 31570648

Zhou X, Teng T, Zhang Y, et al: Comparative efficacy and acceptability of antidepressants, psychotherapies, and their combination for acute treatment of children and adolescents with depressive disorder: a systematic review and network meta-analysis. Lancet Psychiatry 7(7):581–601, 2020 32563306

2

Attention-Deficit/ Hyperactivity Disorder

Lauren Schumacher, M.D.
Laurence Greenhill, M.D.

ADHD is a frequently occurring childhood-onset neurodevelopmental disorder with prevalence estimates of 7.2%–9.4% (Danielson et al. 2018; Thomas et al. 2015; Wolraich et al. 2019). ADHD costs the United States between $143 billion and $266 billion per year due to lost productivity and income, health care, and education (Doshi et al. 2012). ADHD is a chronic disorder. Follow-up studies of children first diagnosed with ADHD in primary school suggest that 60%–80% will continue to meet the full DSM-IV-TR criteria (American Psychiatric Association 2000) for ADHD throughout their teenage years. The estimated point prevalence in adults is 4.4%, with continued significant symptoms and impairment (Kessler et al. 2006; Swanson et al. 2017).

Diagnosis

First described in the nineteenth century, ADHD is a heterogeneous disorder characterized by a persistent, developmentally inappropriate pattern of gross motor overactivity, inattention, and impulsivity that impairs academic, social, and family function. DSM-5 (American Psychiatric Association 2013, 2022) subdivides the disorder into three presentations: predominantly hyperactive/impulsive, predominantly inattentive, and combined. The term *presentation* describes the shifting symptom picture over development better than *subtype* (Lahey and Willcutt 2010). Two-thirds of young children with ADHD have symptoms that also meet criteria for other childhood psychiatric disorders, including anxiety disorders, depression, oppositional defiant disorder (ODD), conduct disorder (CD), mood disorders, learning disorders, sleep disorders, and tic disorders (Molina et al. 2009; Reale et al. 2017). These comorbid psychiatric conditions are thought to increase the impairment associated with ADHD.

The DSM-5 age-at-onset criterion requires that the child present with ADHD symptoms before 12 years of age. Symptom criteria require the persistence of six or more symptoms of inattentiveness or hyperactivity/impulsivity for at least 6 months to a degree that is inconsistent with developmental level and negatively impacts social and academic/occupational activities. Five symptoms are required for adults age 17 years or older. DSM-5 also requires that symptoms cause impairment in more than one setting and are not better explained by a different disorder.

Diagnostic Procedures

Consensus guidelines for making the ADHD diagnosis have been published by the American Academy of Pediatrics (AAP; Wolraich et al. 2019) and the American Academy of Child and Adolescent Psychiatry (AACAP; Pliszka and AACAP Work Group on Quality Issues 2007). Because ADHD is so prevalent, the AACAP recommends that screening for ADHD be part of any patient's mental health assessment. Such screening can be accomplished by having the practitioner ask questions about inattention, impulsivity, and hyperactivity and whether such symptoms cause impairment. If ADHD is suspected, parents and teachers can fill out ADHD rating scales. A positive screen on a rating scale, however, does not constitute a definitive ADHD diagnosis.

A medical history should be obtained by the clinician during the diagnostic evaluation. Positive findings on this screening interview should be followed by referral to a pediatrician for a physical examination. If the patient's medical examination and history are unremarkable, no additional laboratory or neurological testing is required. Because neuropsychological testing has limited sensitivity and/or specificity for ADHD, it is not a requirement for making the ADHD diagnosis. However, neuropsychological testing may be helpful when a comorbid learning disorder is suspected (Pliszka and AACAP Work Group on Quality Issues 2007).

The child or adolescent should be interviewed to further assess for ADHD symptoms and to help determine whether other psychiatric disorders are present that would better explain the symptoms causing impairment. Although it is helpful to interview a preschool- or school-age child with the parent present, older children and adolescents should be interviewed alone because they are more likely to discuss symptoms of substance use, suicidal ideation or behavior, or depression when the parents are absent.

Most children with ADHD have at least one other major psychiatric disorder (Reale et al. 2017). Inquiries should be made about symptoms of ODD, CD, depression, anxiety disorders, tic disorders, substance use disorders, learning disorders, and mania. Parent-scored symptom checklists, such as the Child Behavior Checklist (a component of the Achenbach System of Empirically Based Assessment; Achenbach and Ruffle 2000), and rating scales, such as the revised Swanson, Nolan, and Pelham rating scale (SNAP-IV; Swanson 1992) and the Vanderbilt ADHD Diagnostic Rating Scale (Wolraich et al. 2003), may pick up these symptoms. In addition, the clinician should obtain information about the patient's family history, prenatal history, developmental milestones, medical history, and detailed school history.

Diagnostic Controversy

ADHD diagnosis has been controversial because there are no confirmatory laboratory tests. Although the diagnosis of ADHD remains a clinical one, there are ongoing efforts to define the neurobiological correlates of the diagnosis through neuroimaging and peripheral biomarkers (Scassellati et al. 2012), among other modalities. However, this remains a relatively new area of scientific research in terms of clinical application, and this literature should be followed over time.

The diagnosis of ADHD has been revised five times since 1970, with the most recent criteria published in DSM-5 (Box 2–1). These revisions have been made as new data have emerged. ADHD subtypes have been shown to be unstable over time (Lahey and Willcutt 2010), and the DSM-IV criteria (American Psychiatric Association 1994) underrepresented impulsivity. ADHD criteria thresholds for adults requiring six symptom criteria also may exclude those who are highly impaired but have fewer endorsed symptoms, and children with onset between ages 7 and 12 years do not show different outcomes (Kieling et al. 2010), suggesting that the requirement for having ADHD by age 7 may be too low. The DSM-5 criteria revisions may have led to an increased prevalence estimate of the disorder (McKeown et al. 2015; Vande Voort et al. 2014).

Box 2–1. Attention-Deficit/Hyperactivity Disorder

A. A persistent pattern of inattention and/or hyperactivity-impulsivity that interferes with functioning or development, as characterized by (1) and/or (2):

   1. **Inattention:** Six (or more) of the following symptoms have persisted for at least 6 months to a degree that is inconsistent with developmental level and that negatively impacts directly on social and academic/occupational activities:

      Note: The symptoms are not solely a manifestation of oppositional behavior, defiance, hostility, or failure to understand tasks or instructions. For older adolescents and adults (age 17 and older), at least five symptoms are required.

      a. Often fails to give close attention to details or makes careless mistakes in schoolwork, at work, or during other activities (e.g., overlooks or misses details, work is inaccurate).
      b. Often has difficulty sustaining attention in tasks or play activities (e.g., has difficulty remaining focused during lectures, conversations, or lengthy reading).
      c. Often does not seem to listen when spoken to directly (e.g., mind seems elsewhere, even in the absence of any obvious distraction).
      d. Often does not follow through on instructions and fails to finish schoolwork, chores, or duties in the workplace (e.g., starts tasks but quickly loses focus and is easily sidetracked).

e. Often has difficulty organizing tasks and activities (e.g., difficulty managing sequential tasks; difficulty keeping materials and belongings in order; messy, disorganized work; has poor time management; fails to meet deadlines).
f. Often avoids, dislikes, or is reluctant to engage in tasks that require sustained mental effort (e.g., schoolwork or homework; for older adolescents and adults, preparing reports, completing forms, reviewing lengthy papers).
g. Often loses things necessary for tasks or activities (e.g., school materials, pencils, books, tools, wallets, keys, paperwork, eyeglasses, mobile telephones).
h. Is often easily distracted by extraneous stimuli (for older adolescents and adults, may include unrelated thoughts).
i. Is often forgetful in daily activities (e.g., doing chores, running errands; for older adolescents and adults, returning calls, paying bills, keeping appointments).

2. **Hyperactivity and impulsivity:** Six (or more) of the following symptoms have persisted for at least 6 months to a degree that is inconsistent with developmental level and that negatively impacts directly on social and academic/occupational activities:

   Note: The symptoms are not solely a manifestation of oppositional behavior, defiance, hostility, or a failure to understand tasks or instructions. For older adolescents and adults (age 17 and older), at least five symptoms are required.

   a. Often fidgets with or taps hands or feet or squirms in seat.
   b. Often leaves seat in situations when remaining seated is expected (e.g., leaves his or her place in the classroom, in the office or other workplace, or in other situations that require remaining in place).
   c. Often runs about or climbs in situations where it is inappropriate. (**Note:** In adolescents or adults, may be limited to feeling restless.)
   d. Often unable to play or engage in leisure activities quietly.
   e. Is often "on the go," acting as if "driven by a motor" (e.g., is unable to be or uncomfortable being still for extended time, as in restaurants, meetings; may be experienced by others as being restless or difficult to keep up with).
   f. Often talks excessively.
   g. Often blurts out an answer before a question has been completed (e.g., completes people's sentences; cannot wait for turn in conversation).

h. Often has difficulty waiting his or her turn (e.g., while waiting in line).
i. Often interrupts or intrudes on others (e.g., butts into conversations, games, or activities; may start using other people's things without asking or receiving permission; for adolescents and adults, may intrude into or take over what others are doing).

B. Several inattentive or hyperactive-impulsive symptoms were present prior to age 12 years.
C. Several inattentive or hyperactive-impulsive symptoms are present in two or more settings (e.g., at home, school, or work; with friends or relatives; in other activities).
D. There is clear evidence that the symptoms interfere with, or reduce the quality of, social, academic, or occupational functioning.
E. The symptoms do not occur exclusively during the course of schizophrenia or another psychotic disorder and are not better explained by another mental disorder (e.g., mood disorder, anxiety disorder, dissociative disorder, personality disorder, substance intoxication or withdrawal).

Specify whether:

(F90.2) **Combined presentation:** If both Criterion A1 (inattention) and Criterion A2 (hyperactivity-impulsivity) are met for the past 6 months.

(F90.0) **Predominantly inattentive presentation:** If Criterion A1 (inattention) is met but Criterion A2 (hyperactivity-impulsivity) is not met for the past 6 months.

(F90.1) **Predominantly hyperactive/impulsive presentation:** If Criterion A2 (hyperactivity-impulsivity) is met and Criterion A1 (inattention) is not met for the past 6 months.

Specify if:

In partial remission: When full criteria were previously met, fewer than the full criteria have been met for the past 6 months, and the symptoms still result in impairment in social, academic, or occupational functioning.

Specify current severity:

Mild: Few, if any, symptoms in excess of those required to make the diagnosis are present, and symptoms result in no more than minor impairments in social or occupational functioning.

Moderate: Symptoms or functional impairment between "mild" and "severe" are present.

Severe: Many symptoms in excess of those required to make the diagnosis, or several symptoms that are particularly severe, are present, or the symptoms result in marked impairment in social or occupational functioning.

Source. Reprinted from American Psychiatric Association: *Diagnostic and Statistical Manual of Mental Disorders*, 5th Edition, Text Revision, Washington, DC, American Psychiatric Association, 2022.

Treatment

The AAP clinical practice guidelines recommend that treatment of ADHD include use of FDA-approved medication, evidence-based behavioral interventions (e.g., parent training in behavior management), and educational interventions for those age 6 years or older. For children younger than 6 years, behavioral and educational interventions are the first-line treatment, with methylphenidate as a second-line treatment option (Wolraich et al. 2019). FDA-approved medications for ADHD include stimulant medications, selective norepinephrine reuptake inhibitors, and α_2-adrenergic agonists. Bupropion and modafinil are other medications used for ADHD, although they are not FDA approved for this indication.

These recommendations are largely influenced by the National Institute of Mental Health (NIMH)–sponsored Multimodal Treatment Study of Children With ADHD (MTA). This parallel-design, double-blind, randomized controlled trial (RCT) compared 579 children ages 7–10 years diagnosed with combined-type ADHD who were randomly assigned to one of the following four treatment strategies for 14 months: stimulant medication alone, behavioral treatment alone, their combination, or community care (MTA Cooperative Group 1999b, 1999a). Children treated with medication (alone or combined) had significant improvements in inattention and hyperactivity compared with behavioral treatment alone or community care. Although there were no significant differences in the primary outcomes of core ADHD symptoms between the combined and medication-alone groups, the combined group required lower dosages of medication and had significant improvement in some secondary outcomes (social skills, oppositionality, internalizing symptoms, parent-child relations, and reading achievement scores). Details of pharmacological treatment of ADHD are discussed in later sections.

Psychosocial Treatments

In addition to medication, parent training in behavioral management, behavioral classroom interventions, and school accommodations are recommended as part of ADHD treatment (Wolraich et al. 2019). Behavioral interventions use strategies to increase desired behaviors and decrease undesired behaviors. For instance, parent training in behavioral management teaches parents methods to strengthen parent-child relationships and skills to manage problem behaviors. Behavioral classroom interventions employ strategies such as using a daily report card to track and reward desired classroom behaviors. Other psychosocial treatments studied for ADHD include cognitive training, which involves repeated practice to develop a targeted skill such as working memory or attention, and neurofeedback, which teaches patients to increase attention through visualization of brain activity with electroencephalography. In a meta-analysis of pharmacological and nonpharmacological treatments for ADHD, behavioral therapy was superior to placebo but inferior to stimulants (Catalá-López et al. 2017). Behavioral therapy in combination with stimulants outperformed stimulants and nonstimulant medications alone. Neurofeedback and cognitive training did not separate from placebo.

Stimulant Medications

The FDA has approved numerous stimulant medications for the treatment of ADHD. Fourteen racemic (*d-*,*l-*)-methylphenidate medications, two dexmethylphenidate medications, four dextroamphetamine medications, eight mixed amphetamine salts, and one lisdexamfetamine medication, some of which are also available in generic formulations, have been approved for children and adolescents ages 6 years or older. The duration of action and dosing for these medications are described in Table 2–1. All dextroamphetamine and methylphenidate preparations are structurally related to the catecholamines (dopamine and norepinephrine). The term *psychostimulant* used for these compounds refers to their ability to increase CNS activity in some but not all brain regions. In neuroscience-based nomenclature, they are referred to as dopamine and norepinephrine reuptake inhibitors and releasers or norepinephrine-dopamine–releasing agents.

Table 2–1. Stimulant medications used in the treatment of ADHD

Medication	Duration of action, *hours*	Pediatric dosage, *mg*[a]		Adult dosage, *mg*	
		Starting	Typical	Starting	Typical
Dexmethylphenidate					
Focalin (Novartis)[b]; generic available	5–6[c]	2.5 bid	2.5–10 bid	5 bid	5–10 bid
Focalin XR (Novartis)[d]; generic available	12; dual pulse	5 qAM	5–30 qAM	10 qAM	10–40 qAM
***d,l*-Methylphenidate hydrochloride**					
Short-acting (immediate release)					
Methylin Chewable Tablets (Mallinckrodt); generic available	3–5	5 bid or tid	10–20 tid	10 bid or tid	10–20 tid
Methylin Oral Solution (Mallinckrodt)	3–5	5 bid or tid	10–20 tid	10 bid or tid	10–20 tid
Ritalin (Novartis); generic available	3–5	5 bid or tid	10–20 tid	10 bid or tid	10–20 tid
Intermediate-acting					
Metadate ER (Upstate); generic available	3–8; single pulse	20 qAM	20–60 qAM	20 qAM	20–80 qAM
Long-acting					
Adhansia XR (Adlon)[d]	8–16	25 qAM	25–70 qAM	25 qAM	25–85 qAM
Aptensio XR (Rhodes)[d]	12	10 qAM	10–60 qAM	No adult data	No adult data

Table 2–1. Stimulant medications used in the treatment of ADHD *(continued)*

Medication	Duration of action, *hours*	Pediatric dosage, *mg*[a]		Adult dosage, *mg*	
		Starting	Typical	Starting	Typical
Long-acting (continued)					
Concerta (Janssen)[e]; generic available	10–12; ascending single pulse	18 qAM	18–72 qAM	18 or 36 qAM	18–72 qAM
Cotempla XR-ODT (Neos)[f]	12	17.3 qAM	8.6–51.8 qAM	No adult data	No adult data
Daytrana (Noven)[f]	10–12; transdermal single pulse	10 (patch) qd×9 hours, off 15 hours	10–30 (patch) qd×9 hours, off 15 hours	10 (patch) qd×9 hours, off 15 hours	10–30 (patch) qd×9 hours, off 15 hours
Jornay PM (Ironshore)[d]	7–12	20 qAM	20–100 qPM	20 qAM	20–100 qAM
Metadate CD (UCB)[d]; generic available	8–10; dual pulse	20 qAM	20–60 qAM	20 qAM	20–80 qAM
QuilliChew ER (Pfizer)	12	20 qAM	20–60 qAM	No adult data	No adult data
Quillivant XR (Pfizer)	12	20 qAM	20–60 qAM	No adult data	No adult data
Ritalin LA (Novartis)[d]; generic available	8–10; dual pulse	10–20 qAM	10–60 qAM	10–20 qAM	10–80 qAM

Table 2–1. Stimulant medications used in the treatment of ADHD *(continued)*

Medication	Duration of action, *hours*	Pediatric dosage, *mg*[a]		Adult dosage, *mg*	
		Starting	Typical	Starting	Typical
d-Amphetamine					
Short-acting					
Dextroamphetamine generic[g]	4–6	5 qAM or bid	5–20 bid	5 bid	5–20 bid
ProCentra solution (Independence)	6	5 qAM or bid	5–20 bid	5 bid	5–20 bid
Zenzedi (Arbor)	4–6	5 qAM or bid	5–20 bid	5 bid	5–20 bid
Long-acting					
Dexedrine Spansule (Amedra); generic available	8–12	5 qAM	10–40 qAM	5 qAM	10–40 qAM
Amphetamine mixed salts (*d*-and *l*-isomers)					
Short-acting					
Adderall (Teva)[g]; generic available	4–6	5 qAM or bid	5–20 bid	5 qAM or bid	5–20 bid
Long-acting					
Adderall XR (Shire)[d,g]	10–12; dual pulse	5 qAM	5–30 qAM	5 qAM	5–60 qAM
Adzenys ER suspension (Neos)	10–12	6.3 qAM	6.3–18.8 qAM	12.5 qAM	12.5 qAM

Table 2–1. Stimulant medications used in the treatment of ADHD *(continued)*

Medication	Duration of action, *hours*	Pediatric dosage, *mg*[a]		Adult dosage, *mg*	
		Starting	Typical	Starting	Typical
Long-acting (continued)					
Adzenys XR-ODT (Neos)	10–12	6.3 qAM	6.3–18.8 qAM	12.5 qAM	12.5 qAM
Dyanavel XR suspension (Tris)	13	2.5–5 qAM	2.5–20 qAM	2.5–5 qAM	2.5–20 qAM
Evekeo (Arbor)	10	5 qAM or bid	5–40 qAM	No adult data	No adult data
Evekeo ODT (Arbor)	10	5 qAM or bid	5–40 qAM	No adult data	No adult data
Mydayis (Shire)[d]	16	12.5 qAM	12.5–25 qAM	12.5 qAM	12.5–50 qAM
Lisdexamfetamine					
Vyvanse (Shire)[g] capsule and chewable tab	13–14	30 qAM	30–70 qAM	30 qAM	30–70 qAM

[a]Dosage for children age 6 years or older.
[b]Focalin and Focalin XR should not be taken with antacids or other drugs that decrease gastric acidity.
[c]Limited data.
[d]Contents of capsule can be sprinkled on small amount of applesauce or ice cream to disguise bitter taste and given immediately. Pharmacokinetics is identical whether the beads are swallowed whole or sprinkled on food.
[e]Some generic formulations (manufactured by Mallinckrodt and Kudco) may not be therapeutically equivalent to the brand-name product. The generic formulation that is manufactured by Janssen and marketed by Actavis is bioequivalent (www.fda.gov/drugs/drugsafety/ucm422568.htm).
[f]FDA approved only for use in children ages 6–17 years.
[g]Dextroamphetamine, mixed amphetamine salts, lisdexamfetamine: Taking the drugs with ascorbic acid or fruit juice decreases their absorption, whereas alkalinizing agents such as sodium bicarbonate increase their absorption.

The RCTs considered by the FDA in their approval process revealed that stimulants are highly effective in reducing ADHD symptoms, with an effect size of about 1 (Wolraich et al. 2019). As shown in Table 2–2, about 70% of ADHD participants responded to stimulants, whereas less than 13% experienced a response to placebo. Higher response rates can be achieved if individuals whose symptoms do not respond to one medication then try a stimulant of a different class. For instance, in the MTA study, 73% of participants responded to methylphenidate and another 10% responded to dextroamphetamine (MTA Cooperative Group 1999b). Symptoms return when stimulant medications are stopped (Coghill et al. 2014). A meta-analysis of 62 methylphenidate treatment RCTs of 3 months (or less) revealed large effect sizes when ratings were made by teachers and moderate effect sizes when ratings were made by parents (Schachter et al. 2001). A meta-analysis of 133 double-blind RCTs of medication for ADHD in 10,068 children and adults found that at 12 weeks, all medications examined (amphetamine, methylphenidate, atomoxetine, clonidine, guanfacine, modafinil, and bupropion) were superior to placebo in youth with regard to clinician-rated ADHD symptoms (Cortese et al. 2018). Amphetamines had an effect size of 1.02 (95% CI, 1.19–0.85), and methylphenidate had an effect size of 0.78 (95% CI, 0.93–0.62). Amphetamine was more efficacious than methylphenidate, guanfacine, atomoxetine, and modafinil, whereas methylphenidate was more efficacious than atomoxetine. A meta-analysis of 190 randomized trials including 52 different treatments, both pharmacological and nonpharmacological, and 26,114 subjects with ADHD found that stimulants, nonstimulants, and behavioral therapy were significantly more efficacious than placebo (Catalá-López et al. 2017). Stimulants outperformed nonstimulants and behavioral therapy. Methylphenidate and amphetamine had similar efficacy. Combination treatment with stimulants and behavioral therapy was superior to stimulants alone.

Compared with placebo, psychostimulants have a significantly greater ability to reduce externalizing ADHD symptoms such as overactivity (e.g., fidgetiness, off-task behavior during direct observation), classroom-disruptive behavior (e.g., constant requests of the teacher during direct observation), and parent- and teacher-rated inattention. Both types of stimulants have been shown to improve child behavior during parent-child interactions and problem-solving activities with peers. The behavior of children with ADHD has a tendency to elicit negative, directive, and controlling behavior from their par-

Table 2–2. Representative controlled studies of stimulant medication for ADHD

Study	*N*	Age range, *years*	Design	Drug (dosage*)	Duration	Response	Comments
Castellanos et al. 1997	20	6–13	Crossover	MPH (45 mg bid), DEX (22.5 mg bid)	9 weeks	ADHD + TD	Dosage-related tics at high dosages
Childress et al. 2015	107	6–12	Crossover	R-AMPH (Evekeo; 10–40 mg/day); PBO	2 weeks	$P<0.0001$ for all time points 0.45–10 hours	R-AMPH effective with single daily dose 0.45–10 hours following administration; well tolerated
Coghill et al. 2014	157	6–17	Randomized withdrawal	LDX (30, 50, or 70 mg/day); PBO	6 weeks	Treatment failure: LDX 15.8%, PBO: 67.5%	LDX efficacy maintained over long-term periods
Douglas et al. 1995	17	6–11	Crossover	MPH (0.3, 0.6, 0.9); PBO	4 weeks	70% (behavior)	No cognitive toxicity at high dosages; linear dose-response curves
Elia et al. 1991	48	6–12	Crossover	MPH (0.5, 0.8, 1.5); PBO; DEX (0.25, 0.5, 0.75)	6 weeks	MPH, 79%, DEX: 86%	Response rate for two stimulants: 96%

Table 2–2. Representative controlled studies of stimulant medication for ADHD *(continued)*

Study	*N*	Age range, *years*	Design	Drug (dosage*)	Duration	Response	Comments
Fernández de la Cruz et al. 2015	579	7–9	Parallel	MPH (<0.8 tid)	14 weeks (4 months)	MPH 77%, DEX: 10%, none 13%	Treatments targeting ADHD symptoms helpful for improving irritability in children with ADHD; moreover, irritability did not appear to influence response to treatment
Findling et al. 2013	269	13–17	Parallel, followed by open-label	LDX (30, 50, 70 mg/day)	52 weeks	Change from baseline (SD) ADHD-RS-IV −26.2 ($P<0.001$)	TEAEs (≥5%) such as upper respiratory tract infection (21.9%), decreased appetite (21.1%), headache (20.8%), decreased weight (16.2%), irritability (12.5%), and insomnia (12.1%)

Table 2–2. Representative controlled studies of stimulant medication for ADHD *(continued)*

Study	*N*	Age range, *years*	Design	Drug (dosage*)	Duration	Response	Comments
Findling et al. 2014	461	6–17	Parallel	Stimulant + GXR (1–4 mg qAM or qPM) + PBO (qAM or qPM); stimulant + PBO	9 weeks	Least-squares change vs. PBO: GXR qAM + stimulant −2.4, *P*=0.001; GXR qPM + stimulant −2.2, *P*=0.003	GXR added to stimulant reduced oppositional symptoms in subjects whose symptoms had suboptimal response to stimulant alone
Gadow et al. 1995	34	6–12	Crossover (ADHD + tic)	MPH (0.1, 0.3, 0.5); PBO	8 weeks	MPH 100%	No nonresponders in terms of behavior; physician motor tic ratings showed two minimal increases while subjects were taking drug; only effects over 8 weeks of treatment studied
Gillberg et al. 1997	62	6–12	Parallel	MAS (17 mg); PBO	60 weeks	70%; 27%–40% improved	No dropouts, but only 25% of placebo group at 15-month assessment
Greenhill et al. 2001	277	6–12	Parallel	Long-acting MPH; PBO	3 weeks	70%	Mean total daily dosage 40 mg; FDA registration

Table 2–2. Representative controlled studies of stimulant medication for ADHD *(continued)*

Study	*N*	Age range, *years*	Design	Drug (dosage*)	Duration	Response	Comments
Greenhill et al. 2002	321	6–16	Parallel	MPH-MR (Metadate ER; 20, 60 mg qd); PBO (tid)	3 weeks	MPH-MR 64%, PBO 27%	Mean MPH-MR dosage 40.7 mg/day (1.28 mg/kg/day)
Greenhill et al. 2006a	97	6–17	Parallel	*d*-MPH-ER (Focalin LA; 5–30 mg qd); PBO	7 weeks	*d*-MPH-ER 67.3%, PBO 13.3%	Mean *d*-MPH-ER dosage 24 mg/day
Greenhill et al. 2006b	165	3–5.5	Crossover	IR MPH (1.25, 2.5, 5, 7.5 mg tid); PBO (tid)	70 weeks	88%; ES = 0.4–0.8	Optimal IR MPH dosage 14.22 ± 8.1 mg/day (0.7 ± 0.4 mg/kg/day); treatment effect sizes less than in school-age children
Klein et al. 1997	84	6–15	Parallel	MPH (1.0)	5 weeks	MPH, 59%–78%, PBO 9%–29%	MPH reduced CD symptoms

Table 2–2. Representative controlled studies of stimulant medication for ADHD *(continued)*

Study	*N*	Age range, *years*	Design	Drug (dosage*)	Duration	Response	Comments
Levin et al. 2015	126	18–60	Parallel	MAS (60 mg, 80 mg); PBO with CBT	13 weeks	Abstinence in past 3 weeks: 30.2% (80 mg) vs. 17.5% (60 mg) vs. 7% (PBO)	Robust doses of MAS + CBT effective for co-occurring ADHD and cocaine use disorder, both improving ADHD symptoms and reducing cocaine use
Manor et al. 2012	200	6–13	Parallel	PS-Omega3 vs. PBO	15 weeks + 15-week extension phase	ADHD-Index (P=0.020); Global: restless/impulsive (P=0.014); DSM-IV inattentive (P=0.027); and DSM-IV total score (P=0.044) markedly reduced in PS-Omega3 group vs. PBO group	PS-Omega3: reduced ADHD symptoms in children; preliminary analysis suggested that this treatment may be especially effective in a subgroup of hyperactive-impulsive, emotionally and behaviorally dysregulated ADHD children

Table 2–2. Representative controlled studies of stimulant medication for ADHD *(continued)*

Study	*N*	Age range, *years*	Design	Drug (dosage*)	Duration	Response	Comments
McElroy et al. 2015	260	18–55	Parallel	LDX (30, 50, 70 mg)	14 weeks	50 mg (P=0.008) vs. 70 mg ($P\leq$0.001) vs. 30 mg (NS)	Efficacy demonstrated for active drug groups compared with placebo group in decreased binge-eating days, binge-eating cessation, and global improvement
McGough et al. 2006	97	6–17	Crossover	MPH transdermal worn 9 hours/day (12.5, 18.75, 25, 37.5 cm^2); PBO	2 weeks	79.8%	MPH transdermal system well tolerated and significantly more efficacious than PBO; FDA registration trial
MTA Cooperative Group 1999b	579	7–9	Parallel	MPH (<0.8 tid)	14 weeks (4 months)	MPH 77%, DEX 0%, none: 13%	NIMH-sponsored multisite, multimodal study supports stimulant medication use in ADHD
Musten et al. 1997	31	4–6	Crossover	MPH (0.3, 0.5)	3 weeks	MPH>PBO	MPH: improvement in attention in preschoolers

Table 2–2. Representative controlled studies of stimulant medication for ADHD *(continued)*

Study	*N*	Age range, *years*	Design	Drug (dosage*)	Duration	Response	Comments
Newcorn et al. 2013	333	6–12	Parallel	GXR (1–4 mg qAM, PBO qPM); GXR (PBO qAM, 1–4 mg qPM); PBO	8 weeks	GXR qAM = GXR qPM; both >PBO	Once-daily GXR monotherapy effective whether administered in morning or evening
Philipsen et al. 2015	419	18–58	Parallel	MPH (average 48.8 mg)	12 months	ES 0.5 for MPH vs. PBO	Psychological interventions resulted in better outcomes during a 1-year period when combined with MPH vs. PBO
Rapport et al. 1994	76	6–12	Crossover	MPH (5, 10, 15, 20 mg); PBO	5 weeks	94% (behavioral), 53% (attention)	MPH normalized behavior more than academic performance; higher dosages better; linear dose-response curve

Table 2–2. Representative controlled studies of stimulant medication for ADHD *(continued)*

Study	*N*	Age range, *years*	Design	Drug (dosage*)	Duration	Response	Comments
Rommel et al. 2015	232 twin pairs	16–20	NA	Energy expenditure based on self-reports of PA frequency, intensity, and duration	4 years	ES small (0.02) for hyperactivity/ impulsivity (0.21); inattention reduced (0.19)	Regular exercise in adolescents significantly associated with reduced ADHD symptom levels in early adulthood
Scahill et al. 2015	62	Mean 8.5	Parallel	Guanfacine XR (1–4 mg/day) vs. PBO	8 weeks	Cohen's d=1.57	ER guanfacine shown to be safe and effective for reducing hyperactivity, impulsiveness, and distractibility in children with ASD
Schachar et al. 1997	91	6–12	Parallel	MPH (33.5 mg); PBO	52 weeks	ES 0.7 SD	15% side effects: affective symptoms, overfocusing led to dropouts
Spencer et al. 1995	23	18–60	Crossover	MPH (1 mg/kg/ day)	7 weeks	MPH 78%, PBO 4%	MPH at 1 mg/kg/day led to improvement in adults equivalent to that seen in children

Table 2–2. Representative controlled studies of stimulant medication for ADHD *(continued)*

Study	*N*	Age range, *years*	Design	Drug (dosage*)	Duration	Response	Comments
Swanson et al. 1998	29	7–14	Crossover	MAS (5, 10, 15, 20 mg); PBO, MPH	7 weeks	100%	Adderall peak at 3 hours; MPH at 1.5 hours
Tannock et al. 1995a	40	6–12	Crossover	MPH (0.3, 0.6); ADHD + anxiety	2 weeks	70%	Activity level better in both groups; working memory not improved in anxious children
Tannock et al. 1995b	28	6–12	Crossover	MPH (0.3, 0.6, 0.9); PBO	2 weeks	70%	Effects on behavior: dose-response curve linear but effects on response inhibition U-shaped; suggests dosage adjustment on objective measures

Table 2–2. Representative controlled studies of stimulant medication for ADHD *(continued)*

Study	*N*	Age range, *years*	Design	Drug (dosage*)	Duration	Response	Comments
Vitiello et al. 2012	579	7–9	Parallel and naturalistic	MPH equivalents 22.6–38.1 mg	14 months	Heart rate in medication alone (84.2 bpm) and combined medication/behavioral modification (84.6 bpm) groups was higher vs. behavioral modification–only group (79.1 bpm) at 14 months	Risk of prehypertension or hypertension over 10-year observation not increased with stimulant use; suggests cardiovascular safety requires monitoring, starting with baseline health status before stimulants
Wigal et al. 2004	132	6–17	Parallel	*d*-MPH (2, 5, 10); *d,l*-MPH (5, 10, 20); PBO	4 weeks	*d*-MPH 67%, *d,l*-MPH 49%	Average *d*-MPH dosage (18.25 mg) as safe and effective as half of the average *d,l*-MPH dose (32.14 mg)
Wilens et al. 2006	177	13–18	Parallel	OROS MPH (18, 36, 54, 72 mg qd); PBO	2 weeks	OROS MPH 52%, PBO 31%	OROS MPH well tolerated and effective in adolescents at total daily dosage of up to 72 mg; FDA trial evidence for adolescents 72 mg

Table 2–2. Representative controlled studies of stimulant medication for ADHD *(continued)*

Study	*N*	Age range, *years*	Design	Drug (dosage*)	Duration	Response	Comments
Wilens et al. 2015	314	13–17	Parallel	Guanfacine XR (1–7 mg) vs. PBO	13 weeks	ES=0.52	GXR associated with statistically significant improvements in ADHD symptoms in adolescents

Note. *Dosages are listed in milligrams/kilogram/dose and medication or PBO is given twice daily (bid) unless otherwise stated.
ADHD-RS-IV=ADHD Rating Scale–IV; ASD=autism spectrum disorder; bpm=beats per minute; CBT=cognitive-behavioral therapy; CD=conduct disorder; DEX=dextroamphetamine; ER=extended release; ES=effect size; GXR=guanfacine extended release; IR=immediate release; LA=long-acting; LDX=lisdexamfetamine; MAS=mixed amphetamine salts (Adderall); MPH=methylphenidate; MPH-MR=modified-release methylphenidate; NA=not applicable; NIMH=National Institute of Mental Health; NS=nonsignificant; OROS=osmotic-release oral system; PA=physical activity; PBO= placebo; PS=phosphatidylserine; R-AMPH=racemic-amphetamine; TD=Tourette's disorder; TEAE=treatment-emergent adverse event; XR= extended release.

ents and peers. When these children are started on a regimen of stimulants, their mother's rate of disapproval, commands, and control diminishes to the extent seen between mothers and their children who do not have ADHD. Hyperactive children with CD show reductions in aggressive behavior when treated with stimulants, as observed in structured and unstructured school settings. Stimulants also can reduce the display of covert antisocial behaviors such as stealing and property destruction (Hinshaw et al. 1992). Although there is some evidence that stimulants may improve neurocognitive impairments associated with ADHD, findings are inconsistent (Wang et al. 2015).

Mechanism of Psychostimulant Action

Psychostimulants are thought to release catecholamines and to block their reuptake. Methylphenidate blocks dopamine and norepinephrine reuptake, increasing concentrations in the synaptic cleft. The amphetamines both block dopamine and norepinephrine reuptake and induce release of dopamine (Hodgkins et al. 2012).

Neuroimaging

Early brain imaging studies reported psychostimulant effects on glucose metabolism. In PET and ^{18}F-labeled PET studies carried out in adults with ADHD, stimulant treatment was associated with increased brain glucose metabolism in the striatal and frontal regions (Ernst and Zametkin 1995), but other studies (Matochik et al. 1994) have been unable to find a change in glucose metabolism during acute and chronic stimulant treatment. A 2012 meta-analysis of 55 studies revealed growing evidence of ADHD-related dysfunction in multiple neuronal systems involved not only in higher-level cognitive functions but also in sensorimotor processes, including the visual system, and in the default network. This finding extended our neurobiological models of ADHD pathophysiology beyond those focused on prefrontal-striatal circuits (Cortese et al. 2012) and led to a theory that ADHD resulted from a "breakthrough" of resting-state default mode activity into active cognitive processes, disrupting them (Sonuga-Barke and Castellanos 2007).

During treatment with ^{11}C-labeled methylphenidate, the drug's concentration in the brain is maximal in the striatum, an area rich in dopamine terminals where the dopamine transporter resides. Significant differences in the pharmacokinetics of [^{11}C]methylphenidate and [^{11}C]cocaine (Volkow et al.

1995) have been found in adults with cocaine addiction. Although both drugs rapidly concentrate in the striatum, methylphenidate is cleared more slowly than cocaine. This may explain why oral methylphenidate does not reinforce as powerfully as does snorted or injected cocaine and does not lead to as much self-administration as does cocaine.

On the other hand, therapeutic doses of oral methylphenidate have been shown to significantly increase extracellular dopamine in the human brain. As Volkow et al. (2001) noted, "DA [dopamine] decreases the background firing rates and increases signal-to-noise in target neurons[;] we postulate that the amplification of weak DA signals in subjects with ADHD by methylphenidate would enhance task-specific signaling, improving attention and decreasing distractibility" (p. 1).

Functional MRI data have shown that psychostimulants can be effective in suppressing activation in the default mode or task-negative neural circuit (Peterson et al. 2009). This neural circuit becomes increasingly deactivated as attentional demands increase. Failure to suppress or deactivate this circuit is associated with attentional lapses (Weissman et al. 2006). Children with ADHD show impaired suppression of the task-negative circuit during attentionally demanding tasks; psychostimulants seem to normalize this suppression and improve task performance. Other functional MRI studies suggest that psychostimulants may have direct effects on affective circuits, offering a potential explanation for the palliative effect that psychostimulants can have on emotional impulsivity in hyperactive children (Posner et al. 2011a, 2011b). In an additional meta-analysis, Hart et al. (2014) found consistency across the potential site of action of stimulants, demonstrating increased activation in the bilateral inferior frontal cortex/insula during inhibition and time discrimination, key areas of cognitive control.

Psychostimulant Treatment Studies

A variety of RCTs of ADHD medications, including those based on stimulants (methylphenidate and amphetamine) and nonstimulants, have contributed to the rich evidence base for the efficacy and safety of these preparations in the treatment of ADHD in youth, as shown by the sample of 35 ADHD RCTs listed in Table 2–2. Details of the individual medications are given in the sections that follow.

Methylphenidate, Short-Acting Preparations

Pharmacokinetics. Methylphenidate constitutes the active ingredient of the majority of stimulant medications prescribed in the United States. With the exception of the two dexmethylphenidate products (Focalin and Focalin XR; methyl α-phenyl-2-piperidineacetate hydrochloride), methylphenidate is used in its racemic form, which is composed of the *d-* and *l-threo* enantiomers. The *d-threo* enantiomer is more pharmacologically active than the *l-threo* enantiomer.

Methylphenidate absorption into the systemic circulation is rapid after the immediate-release (IR) tablet is swallowed, such that effects on behavior can be seen within 30 minutes. The plasma concentration peaks by 90 minutes, with a mean half-life of about 3 hours and a 3- to 5-hour duration of action.

If children take one methylphenidate dose just after breakfast, most will require a second dose at lunch (which for young children must be given by the school nurse) and a third dose just after school in the afternoon to prevent loss of effectiveness as well as rebound crankiness and tearfulness. Long-duration preparations of methylphenidate overcome the need for multiple daily doses, and these preparations are now the mainstay of practice.

Metabolism and excretion. In humans, methylphenidate is metabolized extrahepatically via de-esterification to α-phenylpiperidine acetic acid (or ritalinic acid), an inactive metabolite. About 90% of radiolabeled methylphenidate is recovered from the urine.

Dosage and administration. IR tablets may be utilized to augment long-duration forms to provide a boost in the morning or to smooth withdrawal in the late afternoon. Treatment may be initiated with either IR or long-duration preparations. If one starts with a long-duration methylphenidate such as osmotic-release oral system (OROS) methylphenidate (Concerta), it should be initiated with the lowest option (18 mg) in the morning. The total daily dose may be increased by adding additional 18-mg caplets at the morning administration, up to 54 mg for children (three caplets) and 72 mg (four caplets) for adolescents and adults.

Efficacy: clinical trials. Multiple RCTs, in addition to more than a half-century of clinical use, support methylphenidate's safety and efficacy (Pliszka and AACAP Work Group on Quality Issues 2007). The MTA study used a double-blind, placebo-controlled titration protocol to determine each child's optimal methylphenidate dosage, which was delivered in a three-times-daily dosing schedule (Greenhill et al. 2001; MTA Cooperative Group 1999b). School-age children with ADHD demonstrated a greater than 75% response rate to methylphenidate. Both the medication alone and the combined medication + behavioral treatment groups showed significant improvements in inattention and hyperactivity compared with behavioral treatment alone and community care. The medication-alone group, on average, required higher dosages of methylphenidate (37.7 mg/day) compared with the combined group (31.2 mg/day) (MTA Cooperative Group 1999b).

The Preschool ADHD Treatment Study (PATS), carried out with a similar titration trial and subsequent RCT methylphenidate optimization scheme, was conducted with 165 preschoolers with ADHD by the same investigators as the MTA study (Greenhill et al. 2006a, 2006b, 2006c). The mean *best* IR methylphenidate total daily dose varied by age, with preschoolers doing best at 14.4 ± 0.75 mg/day (0.75 mg/kg/day) and school-age children in the MTA doing best at 31.2 ± 0.55 mg/day (0.95 mg/kg/day). IR effect sizes were greater in school-age children (1.2 according to teachers and 0.8 according to parents at 30 mg/day) than in preschoolers (0.8 according to teachers and 0.5 according to parents at 14 mg/day), but optimal total daily doses were higher in the former. The preschoolers also had higher rates of adverse effects. On the basis of these findings, the AAP clinical practice guidelines recommend parent training in behavioral management and behavioral classroom interventions as first-line approaches for preschoolers and methylphenidate treatment as a second line approach (Wolraich et al. 2019).

Follow-up studies with the preschool ADHD sample 3 and 6 years after study completion revealed that 70.9% of the sample continued taking an indicated ADHD medication for as long as 6 years after completing the PATS protocol (Vitiello et al. 2015).

Medication interactions. Methylphenidate interacts with monoamine oxidase inhibitors (e.g., isocarboxazid, phenelzine, selegiline, and tranylcypromine), as well as antibiotics with similar activity (linezolid), leading to blood pressure elevations and an increase in methylphenidate serum concentrations. In addition, phenytoin, phenobarbital, tricyclic antidepressants, and warfarin increase the serum concentrations of methylphenidate. The effects of centrally acting antihypertensives (i.e., guanadrel, methyldopa, and clonidine) can be reduced by methylphenidate.

Methylphenidate, Long-Duration Preparations

Long-duration preparations deliver methylphenidate over the school day from a single morning administration. This approach is a mainstay of clinical practice in the United States (Chou et al. 2012). Long-duration formulations differ in the number and shape of stimulant pulses that they release over time into the blood circulation. Long-duration methylphenidate medications include single-pulse formulations such as extended-release (ER) Metadate; the dual-pulse beaded methylphenidate products such as Metadate CD, long-acting (LA) Ritalin, Focalin XR, Aptensio XR, Quillivant XR, and QuilliChew ER; and complex-release formulations, such as Concerta (OROS methylphenidate), that simulate a triple-pulse delivery system.

Single-pulse methylphenidate sustained-release preparations. Single-pulse, sustained-release methylphenidate formulations (Methylin ER and Metadate ER) are formulated in a wax-matrix preparation to prolong release. They have a slower onset of action than IR methylphenidate, produce lower serum concentrations, and have a 6- to 8-hour duration of action. Clinicians regard these as less effective in practice than the newer long-duration products. Clinicians administer them twice daily or give them with an IR tablet in the morning to compensate for the slow onset of action.

Dual-pulse, beaded methylphenidate preparations. Beaded methylphenidate products (Ritalin LA) are an ER formulation with a dual-pulse release profile that use a proprietary SODAS (Spheroidal Oral Drug Absorption System) technology involving a mixture of IR and delayed-release (DR) beads. These preparations help young children who have difficulty swallowing pills, because the capsule can be opened and the tiny medication spheres can be sprinkled into applesauce or yogurt.

Each dual-pulse capsule contains various proportions of IR methylphenidate beads and half as enteric-coated DR beads. For example, Ritalin LA's 50% proportion of each mimics the use of IR methylphenidate given in two doses, 4 hours apart. Given once daily, Ritalin LA exhibits a lower second-peak concentration, higher interpeak minimum concentrations, and less peak-to-peak trough fluctuation in serum concentration of methylphenidate than two administrations of IR methylphenidate tablets given 4 hours apart. This effect may be due to the earlier onset and more prolonged absorption of the DR beads. The efficacy of Ritalin LA in ADHD treatment was established in one controlled trial involving 134 children ages 6–14 years (Biederman et al. 2003).

Single-isomer dexmethylphenidate (Focalin, Focalin XR). Dexmethylphenidate hydrochloride (Focalin and Focalin XR) is the *d-threo* enantiomer of racemic methylphenidate. The drug's plasma concentration increases rapidly after ingestion, reaching a maximum in the fasted state at about 1–1.5 hours postdose (Quinn et al. 2004). Plasma levels of dexmethylphenidate are comparable with those achieved by a milligram dose of IR methylphenidate twice that of the single enantiomer; that is, plasma levels of dexmethylphenidate 10 mg are equivalent to methylphenidate 20 mg. This is thought to be related to the lack of efficacy of the *l-threo* enantiomer, with racemic methylphenidate having half the dose of *d-threo* methylphenidate compared with dexmethylphenidate.

Focalin XR is an ER form of dexmethylphenidate that uses the same proprietary SODAS technology as Ritalin LA. Each Focalin XR capsule contains a 1:1 mixture of IR beads and DR beads. In a single dose, Focalin XR capsules in strengths of 5 mg, 10 mg, and 20 mg provide the same amount of dexmethylphenidate as Focalin at dosages of 2.5 mg, 5 mg, and 10 mg bid.

IR dexmethylphenidate (5 mg, 10 mg, or 20 mg total daily dose) was compared with placebo in a multicenter, 4-week, parallel-group study of 132 patients (Keating and Figgitt 2002). Patients treated with dexmethylphenidate showed a statistically significant improvement in SNAP-ADHD teacher-rated symptom scores from baseline compared with patients who received placebo.

The long-duration preparation (Focalin XR) was demonstrated to be effective in a randomized, double-blind, placebo-controlled, parallel-group study of 103 pediatric patients ages 6–17 years (Greenhill et al. 2006c). Using the mean change from baseline scores on teacher-rated Conners' ADHD/DSM-IV Scales, the study reported a significantly greater decrease in ADHD scores for youth taking active Focalin XR than for youth receiving placebo. The drug's effectiveness for adult ADHD was reported in a 5-week, randomized, double-blind, parallel-group, placebo-controlled study of 221 adults ages 18–60 years whose signs and symptoms met DSM-IV criteria for ADHD on the DSM-IV ADHD Rating Scale (ADHD-RS) (Spencer et al. 2007b).

Signs and symptoms of ADHD were far fewer for adults taking daily doses of 20 mg, 30 mg, and 40 mg than for those randomly assigned to placebo.

OROS methylphenidate (Concerta). The OROS methylphenidate caplet uses an osmotic delivery system to produce ADHD symptom reduction for up to 12 hours (Swanson et al. 2004). IR methylphenidate is applied to the outside of the OROS caplet to provide immediate drug benefits in the first 2 hours after it is swallowed. Its long-duration component is delivered by an osmotic pump (OROS) that gradually releases the drug from an internal reservoir over a 12-hour period, producing a slightly ascending methylphenidate serum concentration curve. Taken once daily, it mimics the serum concentrations produced by taking IR methylphenidate three times daily, but with less variation (Modi et al. 2000). Long-duration preparations containing the beaded dual-pulse technology show a greater release concentration in the morning than does OROS, but they do not last as long in the afternoon (Swanson et al. 2004).

Two double-blind, placebo-controlled RCTs have tested the efficacy and safety of OROS methylphenidate compared with IR methylphenidate for children with ADHD (Swanson et al. 2003). Another multisite trial showed efficacy for Concerta over placebo in adolescents when the upper limit of the dosage range of Concerta was extended to 72 mg/day (Wilens et al. 2006). In addition, OROS methylphenidate was demonstrated in a small study (N=6) to have a longer duration of effect in reducing ADHD-induced driving impairments in the evening than IR methylphenidate given three times daily (Cox et al. 2004). A 2012 study demonstrated increased efficacy (66.1%), superior satisfaction, and equivalent safety for OROS methylphenidate compared with IR methylphenidate in a tolerable forced-titration scheme from IR methylphenidate to OROS methylphenidate (Chou et al. 2012), reinforcing the value of the OROS preparation.

Multilayer bead technology (Aptensio XR). In May 2015, the FDA approved a new formulation of an ER methylphenidate known as Aptensio XR. The capsules contain multilayer beads designed to provide both a rapid onset and a long duration of action. This formulation of methylphenidate has been available in Canada as Biphentin since 2006. The recommended starting dosage in patients older than 6 years is 10 mg every morning with or without food. The dosage can be increased in weekly increments of 10 mg up to a maximum of 60 mg taken once daily. The capsules may be swallowed whole or, alternatively, opened, sprinkled on applesauce, and taken immediately. In a randomized, double-blind, placebo-controlled trial, 221 patients had significantly lower DSM-IV ADHD-RS scores with Aptensio XR versus placebo in the double-blind phase as well as an 11-week open-label phase (Wigal et al. 2015). No studies are available comparing Aptensio XR directly with other LA methylphenidate formulations, and this lack of comparison studies limits any conclusion about clinical advantage over existing preparations at this time.

More Palatable Methylphenidate Preparations

Methylin Chewable Tablets and Methylin Oral Solution are two forms of a short-duration branded methylphenidate generic formulated for young children who have difficulty swallowing pills or capsules. Methylin Chewable Tablets show peak plasma methylphenidate concentrations in 1–2 hours, with a mean peak concentration of 10 ng/mL after a 20-mg chewable tablet is taken. High-fat meals delay the peak by 1 hour (1.5 hours fasted, and 2.4 hours fed), which is similar to that seen with an IR methylphenidate tablet. Methylin Chewable Tablets are available in doses of 2.5 mg, 5 mg, and 10 mg. Methylin Oral Solution is available in 5 mg/mL and 10 mg/mL strengths. No large-scale clinical trials published that used Methylin Chewable Tablets or Methylin Oral Solution have been published.

In January 2013, the first ER liquid methylphenidate preparation, Quillivant XR, was released. It is available as a liquid (25 mg/5 mL suspension), which must be reconstituted before administration, and has a duration of action of 12 hours. In one randomized, double-blind, placebo-controlled crossover study of 45 children ages 6–12 years, Quillivant significantly reduced ADHD symptoms compared with placebo (Cortese et al. 2017). The same manufacturer also produces a chewable version of Quillivant called QuilliChew. QuilliChew significantly improved ADHD symptoms compared with placebo in one randomized, double-blind, placebo-controlled study of 90 children ages 6–12 years (Cortese et al. 2017).

Transdermal Methylphenidate Preparations

Methylphenidate is available in a transdermal patch (Daytrana). It is steadily absorbed through the skin, with no noticeable reduction in ADHD symptoms for the first 2 hours. This delivery method bypasses the first-pass effect, so blood levels of *l*-methylphenidate are higher than those obtained from the oral route. Steady dosing with the patch results in higher peak methylphenidate levels than does equivalent doses of OROS methylphenidate, suggesting increased absorption. Duration of action for a 9-hour wear period is about 11.5 hours. A double-blind, placebo-controlled crossover study conducted in a laboratory classroom showed significantly lower ADHD symptom scores and higher mathematics test scores for participants receiving the active versus placebo patch for postdose hours 2–9 (McGough et al. 2006). Transdermal methylphenidate appears to be as effective as other long-duration preparations, but adverse effects, including anorexia, insomnia, and tics, occur more frequently with the patch, and mild skin reactions are common. There has been a single report of possible Stevens-Johnson syndrome occurring in a child treated with the transdermal patch.

Amphetamines

Pharmacokinetics. As with methylphenidate, amphetamines are manufactured in the single dextro isomer (e.g., dextroamphetamine [Dexedrine] and lisdexamfetamine [Vyvanse]) or in a racemic version, with mixtures of *d*- and *l*-amphetamine (e.g., Adderall, Adderall XR, and Evekeo). The efficacy of these amphetamine products matches that of methylphenidate products in controlling overactivity, inattention, and impulsivity in patients with ADHD. Some children who experience severe adverse events associated with taking methylphenidate may achieve response without such problems when taking amphetamine products. Absorption of amphetamines is rapid, and the plasma levels of the drug peak 3 hours after oral administration. All of the amphetamines are metabolized hepatically. Urine acidification increases urinary output of amphetamines (Greenhill et al. 2002). Taking the medication with ascorbic acid or fruit juice decreases absorption, whereas taking it with alkalinizing agents such as sodium bicarbonate increases it (Vitiello 2007).

Effects of dextroamphetamine can be seen within 1 hour of ingestion, and the duration of action is up to 5 hours, which is somewhat longer than that of methylphenidate. Nevertheless, at least twice-daily administration is needed to extend the IR preparation treatment throughout the school day.

Racemic Adderall and Adderall XR. Adderall uses a mixture of the various salts of amphetamine. Adderall XR is a dual-pulse capsule preparation that includes both IR and ER beads. These mixed amphetamine salts have not been shown to offer any advantage over similarly designed long-duration methylphenidate products, but some patients' symptoms may respond better to one and not to another.

Lisdexamfetamine dimesylate (Vyvanse) is the first formulation of amphetamine available for the treatment of ADHD in a prodrug formulation intended for a single, long-duration, daily-dose regimen. The preparation is inactive parenterally because the *d*-amphetamine molecule is covalently bonded to L-lysine, an essential amino acid. The pharmacologically active *d*-amphetamine is released after digestion when the covalent bond is cleaved. This bond is an amide bond, which means that a proteolytic enzyme or enzymes in the digestive tract or in red blood cells release the amphetamine. Prodrugs were originally employed to reduce a medication's potential for abuse, diversion, or overdose toxicity (Jasinski and Krishnan 2009).

Two double-blind, placebo-controlled RCTs involving a total of 342 children with ADHD found that those receiving lisdexamfetamine at dosages of 30–50 mg for 3 or 4 weeks showed more improvement in DSM-IV ADHD-RS scores than those receiving placebo. The first study—a Phase II, double-blind, placebo-controlled, randomized crossover trial involving 52 children with ADHD (Biederman et al. 2007a)—showed significant reductions of ADHD behaviors with lisdexamfetamine compared with placebo according to trained but observer-blind ratings across eight hourly sessions of a 12-hour day. The second study—a multisite, Phase III RCT of 290 children with ADHD ages 6–12 years, with a parallel design (Biederman et al. 2007b)—showed significant decreases in ADHD behaviors reported by parents for morning, afternoon, and early evening on the Conners' Parent Rating Scale.

Maintenance of efficacy with lisdexamfetamine has been demonstrated. In a Phase III extension randomized-withdrawal, placebo-controlled study, 157 children ages 6–17 years with ADHD who completed the 26-week open-label trial period were randomly assigned to either their optimized dosage of lisdexamfetamine dimesylate (30 mg/day, 50 mg/day, or 70 mg/day) or placebo for a 6-week withdrawal period (Coghill et al. 2014). Significantly fewer patients who continued taking the stimulant compared with those receiving placebo met the criteria for treatment failure, which was defined as an at least 50% increase in DSM-IV ADHD-RS total score and at least a two-point increase in Clinical Global Impression–Severity score.

More palatable preparations. Multiple amphetamine options are available for those who cannot swallow pills. Vyvanse can be dissolved in juice or water; it is also available as a chewable tablet. Orally disintegrating tablets are available as Evekeo ODT and Adzenys XR-ODT. Adzenys ER, Dyanavel XR, and ProCentra are liquids. Additionally, Adderall XR and Mydayis capsules can be opened and sprinkled on a small amount of food such as applesauce.

Adverse Events and Effects

The most common adverse effects associated with stimulants include delay in sleep onset, appetite loss, weight decrease, headache, and abdominal pain. Infrequent adverse events include tics, nausea, dry throat, dizziness, tachycardia, and palpitations. Rare but serious adverse events include angina, tactile and visual hallucinations, urticaria, fever, arthralgia, exfoliative dermatitis, erythema multiforme, and thrombocytopenic purpura. Also rare are priapism, peripheral vasculopathy, visual disturbance, insect phobias, leukopenia, anemia, eosinophilia, transient depression, hair loss, and reports of sudden unexpected death. One case of neuroleptic malignant syndrome has been reported in an individual treated with a combination of methylphenidate and venlafaxine.

Standard Warnings

All stimulant products carry a black box warning in the package insert that the product should be used with care in patients with a history of drug dependence or alcoholism. In addition, there is a warning about the extremely rare adverse event of sudden death that may be associated with preexisting cardiac abnormalities or other serious heart problems. For adults, the warning extends to stroke and myocardial infarction.

The package insert text warns adults that they should be cautious about taking stimulants if they have preexisting hypertension, heart failure, recent myocardial infarction, or ventricular arrhythmia. Patients with preexisting psychotic and bipolar psychiatric illness are cautioned against taking stimulants because of the psychotomimetic properties of these agents at high doses. Additionally, there is a warning about stimulants' ability to slow growth rates and lower the convulsive threshold in children. However, in ADHD patients without epilepsy, stimulant treatment did not increase the incidence of seizures compared with placebo, and even in those with well-controlled epilepsy, methylphenidate was effective for ADHD and had a low seizure risk (Cortese et al. 2013).

These concerns arose from an FDA review of the cardiovascular and psychiatric adverse events associated with approved stimulant medications. On June 30, 2005, FDA began this review by examining the passive surveillance reports associated with OROS methylphenidate (Concerta; U.S. Food and Drug Administration 2017). The review uncovered 135 adverse events, including 36 psychiatric and 20 cardiovascular events. In particular, the reports included 12 instances of tactile and visual hallucinations (classified under "psychosis") during OROS methylphenidate use. These OROS methylphenidate adverse event reports are rare, representing 135 of 1.3 million cases. Patients with active psychosis, mania, substance abuse disorders, and/or eating disorders should not be treated with stimulants until their symptoms stabilize.

More worrisome were the reports of 20 cases of sudden unexpected death (14 children and 6 adults) and 12 cases of stroke in patients taking mixed amphetamine salts (Adderall XR). This led to Health Canada suspending the sales of Adderall XR (Center for Drug Evaluation and Research 2011). Five patients who died had preexisting structural heart defects. The rest had "family histories of ventricular tachycardia, association of death with heat exhaustion, fatty liver, heart attack, and Type 1 diabetes."

Pliszka and AACAP Work Group on Quality Issues (2007) noted that the rate of sudden, unexpected death is estimated to be 0.5 per 100,000 patient-years in patients taking mixed amphetamine salts and 0.19 per 100,000 patient-years in patients taking methylphenidate, whereas the rate of sudden, unexpected death in the general population has been estimated at 1.3–1.6 per 100,000 patient-years (Liberthson 1996), which is higher than the risk associated with stimulant treatment. Even so, patients with preexisting heart disease should be referred to a cardiologist before stimulant treatment is initiated. Some more recent studies (Cooper et al. 2011) have shown no significant differences in risks of vascular events or symptoms with stimulant use. However, a case-control study in the United States and a nationwide prospective cohort study of children born in Denmark did show that, although rare, cardiovascular events were about twice as likely in stimulant users as they were in those who did not use stimulants (Dalsgaard et al. 2014; Gould et al. 2009).

In summary, serious unexpected cardiac or psychiatric adverse events associated with taking stimulants are extremely rare. The rates are too low to prove a causal association with stimulants in patients with no history of previous heart disease. Routine electrocardiograms and echocardiograms are not indicated prior to starting stimulant treatment in patients with unremarkable medical histories and physical examinations. Physicians prescribing stimulants should first ask the patient and their family for a history of structural heart disease and whether they have previously consulted with a cardiologist. Known cardiac problems that raise concern about using stimulants include tetralogy of Fallot, cardiac artery abnormalities, and obstructive subaortic stenosis. Clinicians should be alert if the patient has hypertension or complains of syncope, arrhythmias, or chest pain because these may indicate hypertrophic cardiomyopathy, which has been associated with sudden, unexpected death.

Other Rare Adverse Events: Growth Slowdown

Growth slowdown is another infrequent psychostimulant adverse reaction that has been controversial since it was first observed in a publication in 1972 (Safer et al. 1972). Myriad methodological difficulties prevent an easy interpretation of studies showing growth slowdown. Few studies employ the optimal controls, which include untreated children with ADHD, a psychiatric control group, and an ADHD group receiving treatment with a class of medications other than stimulants. Studies differ in the quality of compliance measures used and whether the children were using the stimulants on weekends or during the summer.

Most recently, growth slowdown for height and weight was reported for children with ADHD ages 7–10 years who were treated with methylphenidate at a mean dosage of 30 mg/kg/day in the MTA study (MTA Cooperative Group 2004). School-age children grew 1.0 cm less and gained 2.5 kg less than predicted from CDC growth charts. Similar effects were observed for preschool children, who grew 1.5 cm less in height and gained 2.5 kg less weight than predicted while being treated with methylphenidate at a mean dosage of 14 mg/kg/day. Spencer et al. (1996) detected similar differential growth for children with ADHD that could be associated with the disorder itself and not only with stimulant treatment.

Interestingly, a longitudinal study of BMI trajectories from electronic health records of 163,820 children ages 3–18 years from January 2001 to February 2012 found that age at first stimulant use and longer duration of stimulant use were each associated with slower BMI growth earlier in childhood but with a more rapid rebound to higher BMIs compared with control subjects in late adolescence (Schwartz et al. 2014).

The psychostimulant mechanism for any growth slowdown is unknown. Exposure to oral methylphenidate in clinical doses in young monkeys led to a 6-month delay in the onset of puberty but no loss of weight or height (Mattison et al. 2011). Early theories blamed the medication's putative growth-suppressant action on its effects on growth hormone or prolactin, but research studies failed to confirm this effect. The most parsimonious explanation for this drug effect is the medication's suppression of appetite, leading to reduced caloric intake. No study, however, has collected the standardized diet diaries necessary to track calories consumed by children with ADHD who are taking psychostimulants.

Data regarding long-term growth effects of stimulants are mixed. A prospective adult follow-up study of 5,718 subjects found no association between differences in height or significant changes in growth over a 2-year period of treatment with stimulants (Harstad et al. 2014). During naturalistic follow-up of participants in the MTA study at age 25 years, the subgroup that self-selected to consistently take stimulants was significantly shorter than participants with ADHD who did not take stimulants (by 4.06 cm) and those who inconsistently took stimulants (by 2.74 cm) (Greenhill et al. 2020). The consistent and inconsistent subgroups initially had decreased weight compared with the negligible subgroup. Weights converged during adolescence; by age 25 years, the consistent and inconsistent subgroups weighed more than the negligible group.

Height and weight should be measured at 6-month intervals during stimulant treatment and recorded on age-adjusted growth forms to determine the presence of a drug-related reduction in height or weight velocity. If such a decrement is discovered during maintenance therapy with psychostimulants, a reduction in dosage or change to another class of medication can be carried out, as shown in reports of growth changes in the MTA study and the PATS (Biederman et al. 2010; Faraone et al. 2008; Swanson et al. 2007).

Stimulants and Tics

Although FDA labels include a warning that stimulants may exacerbate tics, this has not been supported by more recent studies. A meta-analysis of 22 studies involving 2,385 children found no difference in the risk of new-onset or worsening tics in those receiving stimulant treatment versus those receiving placebo. Type of stimulant, dosage, age, or duration of treatment did not change the risk of tics (Cohen et al. 2015).

Stimulants and Anxiety

Stimulant side effects were originally thought to be exacerbated by the presence of comorbid anxiety symptoms; this led to a warning against using methylphenidate in youth with comorbid anxiety disorders. Other concerns were that anxiety disorders interfered with a stimulant's ability to lower ADHD symptoms. Tannock et al. (1995a) reported findings from a treatment study involving 40 children with ADHD, some with ($n=18$) and some without ($n=22$) comorbid anxiety symptoms, in a double-blind, randomized, crossover design with three methylphenidate doses (0.3, 0.6, and 0.9 mg/kg). The two groups showed equal decreases in motor activity, but the group with comorbid anxiety did more poorly on a serial addition task and had a differential heart-rate response to methylphenidate. DuPaul et al. (1994) found that 40 children with ADHD and comorbid anxiety were less likely to achieve response to methylphenidate and experienced more side effects for three methylphenidate dosages (5 mg, 10 mg, and 15 mg) and placebo than children with ADHD and no comorbid anxiety. However, the study did not collect ratings for anxiety symptoms, so the direct effect of methylphenidate on such symptoms was not recorded.

Subsequent studies failed to support these early impressions. One controlled study (Gadow et al. 1995) that tested the effects of methylphenidate in children with comorbid anxiety symptoms found equally good response for those with and those without anxiety disorder. Results of a meta-analysis of 23 studies involving 2,959 children with ADHD found that risk of anxiety was significantly reduced in participants receiving stimulants compared with those receiving placebo, perhaps because of a secondary effect of improved ADHD symptoms (Coughlin et al. 2015). It therefore appears appropriate to conclude that stimulants may improve anxiety symptoms and that a comorbid anxiety disorder does not predict a poor response to treatment.

Stimulant Medication Use in the Treatment of ADHD in the United States

Outpatient visits for ADHD have been increasing since the early 1990s (Jensen et al. 1999). Rates of ADHD diagnosis have likewise increased. The National Survey of Children's Health found that American parents' report of their child ever being diagnosed with ADHD increased from 7.8% in 2003 to 11% in 2011 (Visser et al. 2014). In the 1990s, methylphenidate-based products dominated the types of prescriptions for ADHD for children (Vitiello and Jensen 1997). However, since the early 2000s, amphetamine products have shown a 40-fold increase in rates of prescriptions, surpassing methylphenidate products, which increased 8-fold (Safer 2016). This has led to concerns about potentially overmedicating patients for ADHD, but data on this are mixed. An analysis of data from the Great Smoky Mountain Study found that although 72% of children meeting DSM-III-R criteria (American Psychiatric Association 1987) for ADHD received stimulants, an additional 22% of subjects received stimulants even though they did not meet criteria for ADHD (Angold et al. 2000). However, another epidemiologically based survey in the United States found that only 12.5% of children diagnosed with ADHD received adequate stimulant treatment (Jensen et al. 1999). More recently, annual rates of stimulant prescribing in the United States have continued to rise, from 5.6 per 100 persons in 2014 to 6.1 per 100 persons in 2019 (Board et al. 2020). Notably, this rise is due to increased rates of prescribing for adults, with rates for those age 19 years or younger actually decreasing from 2014 to 2019.

Predicting Responses to Stimulant Medications

Predicting drug response in the a child with ADHD is difficult. Although pretreatment patient characteristics (young age, low rates of anxiety, low severity of disorder, high IQ) may influence response to methylphenidate on global rating scales (Buitelaar et al. 1995), most research shows that neurological, physiological, or psychological measures of functioning are not reliable predictors of response to psychostimulants (Pelham and Milich 1991). In the NIMH MTA study, participants with comorbid anxiety disorders experienced a better response to behavioral treatments than the overall study population, with behavioral treatment being superior to community care and no longer inferior to medication or combined treatment. The frequency of physician visits mediated the benefits of stimulant treatment, with more frequent visits associated with more effective medication treatment (MTA Cooperative Group 1999a).

Determining How Much Improvement Constitutes a Meaningful Clinical Response

Once a child's symptoms respond to medication, there has been no universally agreed-upon criterion for how much the symptoms must change before the clinician stops increasing the dosage, and there is no standard for the outcome measure. Some have advocated a 25% reduction of ADHD symptoms as a threshold, whereas others suggest that the dosage should continue to be adjusted until the child's behavior and classroom performance are normalized.

The concept of *normalization* has helped standardize the definition of a categorical responder across domains and studies. Studies now use classroom control subjects instead of just statistical significance to determine whether the improvement from treatment is clinically meaningful. Further advances occurred when investigators used statistically derived definitions of clinically meaningful change during psychotherapeutic treatment (Jacobson and Truax 1991). Rapport et al. (1994) used this technique to calculate reliable change and normalization on the Conners' Abbreviated Teacher Rating Scale using national norms. The researchers determined that a child's behavior would be considered normalized when their Conners' Abbreviated Teacher Rating Scale score fell closer to the mean of the general population (matched with children without ADHD) than to the mean of the ADHD population. Using this technique in a controlled trial of four methylphenidate doses in children with ADHD, Rapport et al. (1994) found that methylphenidate normalized behavior and, to a lesser extent, academic performance (94% and 53%, respectively). Similarly, DuPaul and Rapport (1993) found that methylphenidate normalized behavior for all children with ADHD who were treated, but only 75% of the children showed normalized academic performance. In another study, DuPaul et al. (1994) reported that normalization in behavior and academic performance occurred less often when ADHD subjects had high levels of comorbid internalizing disorders. Swanson et al. (2001) applied this approach to the cumulative distribution curves on the SNAP-IV parent and teacher behavior ratings at the end of the MTA study. They found that 88% of children without ADHD, 68% of children with ADHD treated with medication plus behavior therapy, and 56% of children with ADHD treated with medication alone achieved symptom scores of 1 or less, which represented a *normal* response on those scales.

Limitations of Stimulant Treatment for ADHD

Although there is good evidence showing stimulants are effective through 14 months of treatment, there is less evidence for longer-term efficacy. Following 14 months of randomized treatment, the MTA sample transitioned to care in their communities. These data were reported in a series of publications that describe responses of the MTA sample (n=515) versus 289 classroom control subjects (the local normative comparative group) during an uncontrolled long-term follow-up period that extended to 16 years after the MTA's baseline (Swanson et al. 2017). By 22 months after the end of assigned treatment, there were no longer significant differences in ADHD symptoms between the treatment groups. This lack of significant differences between the original treatment groups continued in the 6- to 8-year follow-up report, with the ADHD group presenting as having more ADHD symptoms and poorer functioning than the control group (Molina et al. 2009). By 16 years after the MTA's baseline, when participants were age 25 years on average, the ADHD group continued to have significantly more ADHD symptoms (Swanson et al. 2017) and poorer functioning (Hechtman et al. 2016) than the control group. There were no significant differences in ADHD symptoms between three naturalistic subgroups of consistent, inconsistent, or negligible stimulant treatment during the follow-up period (Swanson et al. 2017). Although clear conclusions cannot be drawn, these findings highlight the need for longer-term RCTs to better understand the long-term efficacy of stimulants.

Other caveats have been expressed about using psychostimulants to treat ADHD in children. Approximately 25% of children with ADHD are not helped by the first psychostimulant given or experience side effects so bothersome that meaningful dosage adjustments cannot be made (DuPaul and Barkley 1990). Stimulants cannot be given too late in the day because delayed sleep onset and insomnia may result, so they are less helpful for nighttime homework and behavioral challenges. Second, indications for choosing a particular psychostimulant and the best methods for adjusting the dosage remain unclear, and these factors may prove confusing to the clinician and family. Some practitioners use the child's weight as a guideline (dose-by-weight method), and others titrate each child's response through the approved dosage range until clinical response occurs or side effects limit further dosage increases (stepwise titration method). Studies have shown no consistent relationship between weight-adjusted methylphenidate doses and behavioral responses, calling into question this practice. Third, the credibility of many treatment studies is limited by methodological problems, including failure to control for prior medication treatment and inappropriately short washout periods.

In addition, a few studies have reported problems with dissociation of cognitive and behavioral responses to methylphenidate, showing an inverted-U dose-response curve with an optimal cognitive response at 0.3 mg/kg and an optimal behavioral response at 1.0 mg/kg. Parents worry about stigmatization, dependence, growth delays, and blunted emotional responses in their children from long-term exposure to stimulant treatment.

Role of Nonstimulant Medication in the Treatment of ADHD

Because nonstimulants have a smaller effect size than stimulants for lowering ADHD symptoms, they are not first-line medications for ADHD treatment (Hirota et al. 2014; Newcorn et al. 2008). Nonstimulants may be used when there is an unsatisfactory response to or significant adverse effects from two different stimulants. In addition, some families have concerns about stimulants being classified by the Drug Enforcement Administration as drugs of abuse and controlled substances; nonstimulant options do not have this problem. This approach has been supported by the Texas Children's Medication Algorithm Project (TCMAP), which recommends that atomoxetine be used when two different stimulants fail to be effective because of nonresponse, unwanted side effects, or parental preference (Pliszka et al. 2006). The α_2 agonists guanfacine and clonidine are also good second-line options (Table 2–3).

Atomoxetine and Viloxazine

Atomoxetine and viloxazine are selective norepinephrine reuptake inhibitors. Atomoxetine was approved by the FDA in 2002 and was the first nonstimulant and first adult treatment approved for ADHD (Rosack 2002). Per the TCMAP, atomoxetine represents the first nonstimulant medication option after a patient has demonstrated partial response or nonresponse to two stimulants (Pliszka et al. 2006).

Table 2–3. Nonstimulant medications approved by the FDA for the treatment of ADHD

		Pediatric dosage[a]		Adult dosage	
Medication	**Duration of action, *hours***	**Starting**	**Typical**	**Starting**	**Typical**
α_2 Agonists					
Intuniv (Shire); guanfacine ER generic[b,c]	8–24	1 mg/day	1–7 mg/day	1 mg/day	1–6 mg/day
Kapvay (Concordia); clonidine ER generic[b]	12	0.1 mg qPM	0.1–0.2 mg bid	No adult data	No adult data
Selective norepinephrine reuptake inhibitors					
Strattera (Lilly); atomoxetine generic	24	0.5 mg/kg/day or divided bid	1.2 mg/kg/day	20 mg bid or 40 mg/day	80 mg/day
Qelbree (Supernus); viloxazine[b,d]	12; dual pulse	6–11 years: 100 mg/day 12–17 years: 200 mg/day	100–400 mg/day	200 mg/day	200–600 mg/day

[a]Dosage for children age 6 years or older.
[b]FDA approved only for use in children ages 6–17 years.
[c]See Ota et al. 2021 for adult dosing information.
[d]Contents of capsule can be sprinkled on small amount of applesauce or ice cream to disguise bitter taste and be given immediately. See Supernus 2021a for additional information.

Atomoxetine

Atomoxetine is not a controlled substance. It is rapidly absorbed, and peak serum concentrations occur in 1 hour without food and in 3 hours with food. The drug undergoes hepatic metabolism with the cytochrome P450 2D6 isozyme (CYP2D6) and is then glucuronidated and excreted in urine. Plasma elimination half-life averages 5 hours for most patients. However, 5%–10% of patients have a loss-of-function polymorphism for the allele that codes for CYP2D6; for them, the half-life of atomoxetine can be as long as 24 hours. If a patient is a known poor metabolizer, the FDA label recommends lower doses; however, genetic testing is not needed prior to starting atomoxetine (de Leon 2015).

Atomoxetine's pharmacodynamics differs from its pharmacokinetics in that the duration of action in reducing symptoms of ADHD is much longer than the pharmacokinetic half-life. ADHD symptoms can be managed with once-daily dosing. Atomoxetine also can be given in the evening, whereas stimulants cannot. Atomoxetine is valued as a treatment for patients whose symptoms have not responded to or who cannot tolerate stimulants or for those who do not want treatment with a Schedule II medication (Abramowicz 2003).

Efficacy. Atomoxetine's effect size in reducing symptoms of ADHD was calculated to be 0.64, which indicates a medium effect size. This calculation was borne out in a meta-analysis (Schwartz and Correll 2014) that examined 25 double-blind RCTs (N=3,928). In practice, some clinicians have been concerned by the low numbers of children with ADHD responding to atomoxetine.

Dosage and administration. Atomoxetine is available in capsule strengths of 10 mg, 18 mg, 25 mg, 40 mg, 60 mg, 80 mg, and 100 mg. To limit adverse events, youth weighing 70 kg or less should have the medication started at 0.5 mg/kg/day in divided doses, with the dosage increased after 1 week to a target of 1.2 mg/kg/day. The maximum total daily dose is 1.4 mg/kg or 100 mg, whichever is less. Patients with hepatic dysfunction should take half the usual dosage.

Drug interactions. Atomoxetine and monoamine oxidase inhibitors should not be used together or within 2 weeks of each other. The initial dosage of atomoxetine should not be increased rapidly if the patient is taking a potent CYP2D6 inhibitor such as fluoxetine (Prozac).

Adverse events. Somnolence, nausea, decreased appetite, weight loss, vomiting, and headache have occurred in children starting atomoxetine, particularly when the dosage is increased from the initial to top levels within 3 days. Slow metabolizers displayed higher rates of decreased appetite. Starting with twice-daily dosing can minimize side effects (Greenhill et al. 2007).

The FDA has added two warnings to the atomoxetine package insert instructions. The first warning, added on December 17, 2004, was based on reports of severe liver injury and jaundice in two patients (one adult and one child). The FDA warned that atomoxetine should be discontinued in patients who develop jaundice, have dark urine, or have laboratory evidence of liver injury. A second warning, added in September 29, 2005, was based on the report by Eli Lilly stating that 5 of 1,800 youth in atomoxetine trials spontaneously reported suicidal ideation, whereas none of the youth randomly assigned to placebo made such reports. The FDA required that atomoxetine's label carry a black box warning about its possible association with suicidality. It is noteworthy that both warnings are based on spontaneous reports, not systematically elicited adverse events. A 2014 meta-analysis examined this warning further and found that although there was one pediatric attempted suicide (N=3,883 pediatric patients), there were no completed suicides, and the risk compared with placebo was not significant (Bangs et al. 2014). The meta-analysis concluded that there was no evidence of increased risk for suicidal behavior in atomoxetine-treated pediatric or adult patients (Bangs et al. 2014). Treatment of children with ADHD using the nonstimulant atomoxetine has also been associated with transient growth suppression (Spencer et al. 2007a).

Viloxazine

In 2021, viloxazine was approved by the FDA for the treatment of ADHD based on four double-blind, placebo-controlled randomized, multicenter, parallel trials including 1,354 patients ages 6–17 years (Johnson et al. 2020; Nasser et al. 2021; Supernus 2021b). Treatment with viloxazine led to significant improvement in DSM-IV ADHD-RS scores (total, inattentive symptoms, and hyperactive symptoms) by 2 weeks, with more improvement by 6 weeks, and an effect size of about 0.6. The most common adverse reactions included somnolence, decreased appetite, nausea, vomiting, insomnia, and irritability. Viloxazine also had a black box warning of possible association with suicidality based on reports of suicidal thoughts in 0.9% of those taking viloxazine compared with 0.4% of those taking placebo (Supernus 2021b). No completed suicides occurred in these studies.

Viloxazine is metabolized by CYP2D6 and is then glucuronidated and excreted in urine. It is a strong CYP1A2 inhibitor and should not be administered with CYP1A2 substrates such as duloxetine or with monoamine oxidase inhibitors. Viloxazine is dosed once daily and reaches steady state after 2 days. Children ages 6–11 years start with 100 mg/day, which can be increased by 100 mg/week to a maximum dosage of 400 mg/day, depending on response and tolerability. Youth ages 12–17 years start with 200 mg/day and can increase to a maximum dosage of 400 mg/day after 1 week (Table 2–3). Unlike atomoxetine, which must be swallowed whole, viloxazine can be swallowed or the capsule can be opened and the contents sprinkled on a teaspoonful of food such as applesauce (Supernus 2021b).

Clonidine and Guanfacine

ER clonidine (Kapvay) and guanfacine (Intuniv) were FDA approved for the treatment of ADHD in youth ages 6–17 years in 2009. These agents are approved both as a monotherapy and as an adjunct to stimulants. They are presynaptic α_2-adrenergic agonists and are also called *norepinephrine receptor agonists*. Clonidine binds to α_{2A}, α_{2B}, and α_{2C} receptors, whereas guanfacine binds specifically to α_{2A} receptors. These agents were originally developed for the treatment of hypertension.

Efficacy

A meta-analysis of 12 pediatric studies (N=2,276) determined that α_2 agonists significantly reduced overall ADHD symptoms, inattention, hyperactivity/impulsivity, and oppositionality, with an overall effect size of 0.59 (Hirota et al. 2014). However, no significant differences in efficacy between different α_2 agonists were found. Although clonidine ER and guanfacine ER were each significantly superior to placebo, neither IR formulation separated from placebo. The α_2 agonists also significantly improved ADHD symptoms compared with placebo when added to ongoing psychostimulant treatment.

Adverse Events

The α_2 agonists are well tolerated overall, with rates of discontinuation due to adverse effects comparable with placebo. Sedation is the most common side effect. Less common side effects include headache, dizziness, nausea, and hypotension (Hirota et al. 2014). Rare adverse effects include hallucinations with guanfacine. There is one case report of sudden death in a patient taking clonidine and methylphenidate, but it is not clear that the medication caused the death. Many clinicians feel that side effects such as sedation and hypotension are less common with guanfacine than with clonidine, although head-to-head trials of these medications in children with ADHD are absent. These agents are not associated with significant changes in body weight, making them a good choice for patients who struggle with the appetite suppression or weight-loss effects of stimulants.

Dosage and Administration

The starting dosage for clonidine ER is 0.1 mg at bedtime. It can be increased by 0.1 mg/week based on response and tolerability up to 0.4 mg/day, with the dosage divided twice daily (Table 2–3). Guanfacine ER is started at 1 mg/day and can be increased by 1 mg/week based on response and tolerability up to a maximum of 4 mg/day for children ages 6–12 years and 7 mg/day for adolescents ages 13–17 years. Guanfacine is primarily metabolized by CYP3A4. Dosage adjustments are recommended when administering guanfacine with CYP3A4 inhibitors or inducers. Clonidine is mostly metabolized by CYP2D6. These agents should be tapered gradually (clonidine by 0.1 mg and guanfacine by 1 mg every 3–7 days) because rebound hypertension following abrupt discontinuation has been reported.

Bupropion

Bupropion is an atypical antidepressant with noradrenergic activity and has been reported effective for some ADHD symptoms in placebo-controlled trials. It is FDA approved for the treatment of depression in adults but not for ADHD. A systematic review of bupropion use in children with ADHD found six clinical trials (Ng et al. 2017) showing that bupropion reduced ADHD symptoms. Three of the trials compared bupropion with methylphenidate and found no significant differences between the medications. However, in the largest trial, although bupropion was superior to placebo, effect sizes were smaller than for stimulants (Conners et al. 1996; Ng 2017). In contrast, a 2018 meta-analysis of 133 double-blind RCTs of medication for ADHD in youth and adults, including three bupropion trials in children, found that bupropion was superior to placebo, with a large effect size of 0.96 in clinician-rated overall ADHD symptoms in youth, which was comparable with stimulants (Cortese et al. 2018). Bupropion is a third-line treatment for ADHD and should be considered for individuals with poor symptom responses to stimulants, α_2 agonists, and atomoxetine. It is also reasonable to consider bupropion for adolescents with ADHD and depression who may benefit from its effects on both disorders.

Modafinil

Modafinil is a dopamine reuptake inhibitor that is FDA approved for the treatment of narcolepsy in adults. The meta-analysis by Cortese et al. (2018) of ADHD medications included seven trials of modafinil in children; the researchers found that modafinil was superior to placebo, with a medium effect size of 0.62 for clinician-rated overall ADHD symptoms. One study compared modafinil with methylphenidate and showed no significant difference between the two treatments on parent and teacher ADHD rating scales (Amiri et al. 2008). In trials of modafinil for ADHD, 8 of 933 youth treated with modafinil stopped the drug due to concerns for rash, including one case of possible Stevens-Johnson syndrome (Rugino 2007). As a result, the FDA advisory committee did not recommend approval of modafinil for ADHD in children and adolescents and requested additional studies to better understand the potential risk.

Monitoring Treatment

The AACAP practice parameter for ADHD (Pliszka and AACAP Work Group on Quality Issues 2007) recommends that patients be monitored for treatment-emergent side effects during psychopharmacological intervention for ADHD. The effectiveness of regular monthly visits and dosage adjustments based on tolerability and lingering ADHD symptoms was shown in the MTA study (MTA Cooperative Group 1999a, 1999b). Those children assigned to medication management based on the NIMH protocol had significantly lower ADHD symptom scores than those followed by community providers, even though 67% of this group also received medication. When compared, children in the medication treatment arm had five times the rate of appointments, more often had dosage adjustments based on teacher feedback, and had higher mean methylphenidate total daily dosages than those in the community control group.

Monitoring can be done through direct patient-provider visits, by phone calls with the patient and family, or even by electronic messaging. Teacher input should be sought at least once a semester for patients with ADHD attending primary, middle, or high school. Monitoring should follow a predetermined plan that is worked out with the patient and, if the patient is a child, with the parents. Generally, the schedule of monitoring visits is weekly during the initial dosage-adjustment phase, then monthly for the first few months of maintenance. After that, the visits can be regularly scheduled but less frequent. During the monitoring visit, the clinician should collect information on the exact dosage used and the schedule according to which the stimulants were administered, including times of day and skipped doses. The clinician should ask about possible side effects. The family and clinician should then decide whether the patient should continue taking the stimulant at the same dosage or the dosage should be changed. The patient should leave the visit with a prescription, a plan for administration, possibly a schedule for intervisit phone or message contact, and the next appointment date.

The practitioner and family should agree on the frequency of stimulant treatment during the day and the week. One choice is between the daily administration of stimulant medications or treatment only for school days, with the patient not taking the drug on weekends and holidays, versus daily administration. Those patients with more impairing ADHD symptoms will benefit from treatment with stimulants daily. Nonstimulants should be consistently taken daily. Patients should have their need for continued treatment with stimulant medication verified once per year through a brief period of medication discontinuation. The discontinuation period should be planned for a part of the school year when testing is not in progress.

Strategies for maintaining adherence to treatment are a key monitoring component. These include the option to adjust stimulant dosages to reduce treatment-emergent adverse events. When a treatment-emergent adverse event occurs, the practitioner would do well to assess the impairment induced by the event. Some adverse events may not interfere with the child's health or cause significant interruption of routine. If the adverse event worsens, then dosage reduction is indicated. If the dosage reduction alleviates the adverse event but leads to worsening of the ADHD symptoms, the clinician may want to consider switching the patient to another stimulant or augmenting with an α_2 agonist.

The AACAP practice parameter (Pliszka and AACAP Work Group on Quality Issues 2007) suggests that adjunctive pharmacotherapy can be used to address a troublesome adverse event during stimulant treatment. Patients with stimulant-induced delay of sleep onset may benefit from the addition of antihistamines, clonidine, or a bedtime dose (3 mg) of melatonin (Tjon Pian Gi et al. 2003).

Choice of Medication

An international consensus statement (Kutcher et al. 2004), the AACAP practice parameter for ADHD, the TCMAP (Pliszka et al. 2006), and the AAP clinical practice guideline (Wolraich et al. 2019) all recommend stimulant medications as the first line of treatment for school-age children with ADHD. Direct comparisons of methylphenidate and atomoxetine in a double-blind, randomized, multisite trial (Newcorn et al. 2008) have shown a decided benefit for methylphenidate and confirm the meta-analysis by Faraone et al. (2003) that suggested methylphenidate had a larger effect size (0.91) than atomoxetine (0.62). Although no direct comparisons of stimulants and α-agonists have been published, multiple meta-analyses indicate a larger effect size for stimulants than clonidine or guanfacine (Catalá-López et al. 2017; Cortese et al. 2018).

According to the AACAP practice parameter (Pliszka and AACAP Work Group on Quality Issues 2007), treatment should commence with either an amphetamine-based or methylphenidate-based stimulant in a long-duration formulation. The specific medication used can be chosen based on its rapidity of onset, duration of action, and effectiveness for the specific patient in treatment. Short-acting stimulants can be used at first for small children or preschoolers if there is no long-acting preparation available in a low-enough dosage. Dual-pulse methylphenidate and amphetamine products (see Table

2–1) have strong effects in the morning and early afternoon, but these effects wear off by late afternoon. These medications work best for children who have academic problems at the beginning and middle of the school day, for those whose appetite is strongly suppressed, or for those whose sleep onset is delayed during stimulant treatment. Because transdermal stimulants are reported to have a higher-than-average number of adverse events, orally administered stimulants should be tried first. Atomoxetine or an α_2 agonist should be employed if the full-dosage-range trials of both a long-duration methylphenidate and a long-duration amphetamine formulation fail, if the family does not want treatment with a controlled substance, or if the patient has a relative contraindication for stimulants (e.g., an untreated eating disorder, mania, or a stimulant use disorder). Although pharmacogenetic tests for genetic markers that may affect the pharmacokinetics or pharmacodynamics of stimulants have been developed, evidence of their clinical utility to support their regular use in clinical practice is insufficient (Wolraich et al. 2019).

The AACAP practice parameter for ADHD (Pliszka and AACAP Work Group on Quality Issues 2007) wisely points out that none of the extant practice guidelines should be interpreted as justification for requiring that a patient experience treatment failure (or adverse events) with one agent before allowing the trial of another.

Conclusion

Psychostimulant medications are a mainstay in the treatment of ADHD based on their proven efficacy during controlled studies. Although the long-term response of children with ADHD to psychostimulants has not been examined in an RCT much longer than 24 months, reports suggest that children experience a relapse when their medication is withdrawn, and their symptoms respond when it is restarted. The MTA open, uncontrolled follow-up study (MTA Cooperative Group 2004), with reports at 3 years, 6 years, 9 years, and 16 years, has suggested that treatments in the community involve either psychotherapy or low-dose stimulant medication. The results include a low response rate in terms of ADHD symptom reduction, with only 10% of patients continuing medication treatment after 10 years. More research is needed on the barriers to maintaining effective stimulant treatment among adolescents and young adults.

The initial effects of psychostimulants are rapid, dramatic, and normalizing, especially during the first 2 years of treatment. The risk of long-term side effects remains low, and no substantial impairments have emerged to lessen the remarkable therapeutic benefit-risk ratio of these medications. More expensive and demanding treatments, including behavior modification and cognitive-behavioral therapies, have only equaled psychostimulant treatment at best. The combination of behavioral and medication therapies is more effective than medication alone in reducing symptoms associated with ADHD (MTA Cooperative Group 1999a). For those whose symptoms do not respond well to stimulants, other FDA-approved pharmacological treatments include atomoxetine, viloxazine, clonidine ER, or guanfacine ER.

Psychostimulant treatment research has continued support from the pharmaceutical industry. However, there is ample opportunity for more studies of nonstimulant medications. Not all patients experience a response to psychostimulants, and this is particularly true in patients with comorbid psychiatric disorders. More psychopharmacological studies with patients with ADHD and comorbid disorders to examine differential responses to new medications are needed. In addition, continued research on the underlying mechanisms of ADHD, as well as its diagnosis, pharmacogenetics, and treatment combinations, will further refine approaches to treating ADHD over time.

Clinical Pearls

- ADHD is characterized by a persistent, developmentally inappropriate pattern of gross motor overactivity, inattention, and impulsivity that impairs academic, social, and family functioning. Symptoms must start in childhood and have a chronic course.
- Two-thirds of young children with ADHD also meet criteria for other childhood psychiatric disorders, including anxiety, depressive, oppositional defiant, conduct, learning, and mood disorders.
- Because of its high prevalence, screening for ADHD should be included in routine mental health assessments. This can be accomplished by asking questions about inattention, impulsivity, and hyperactivity and about whether such symptoms cause impairment.

- ADHD symptoms are rapidly reduced by treatment with stimulant medications. Medication treatment can begin with either an amphetamine or a methylphenidate stimulant in a long-duration formulation chosen based on its rapidity of onset, duration of action, and effectiveness in the specific patient under treatment.
- Immediate-release stimulant preparations can be used at first for small children and/or preschoolers if there is no long-acting preparation available in a low-enough dose.
- Optimizing each child's dosing based on the child's response has become the standard method of initiating treatment (*stepwise titration* method).
- Stimulants come in numerous forms, including capsule (which can be swallowed or sprinkled), chewable, liquid, oral dissolvable tablet, and transdermal patch formulations.
- Short- and long-duration stimulants result in the same adverse effects, including delay in sleep onset, appetite loss, weight loss, headache, abdominal pain, and potential growth slowdown. Several clinical conditions can be worsened by stimulant treatment, including florid psychosis, mania, stimulant abuse, and eating disorders.
- Stimulants carry a warning about sudden death that may be associated with preexisting cardiac abnormalities or other serious heart problems. Clinicians should ask the patient and family about a history of structural heart disease and be alert if the patient has hypertension or complains of syncope, arrhythmias, or chest pain. Routine electrocardiograms and echocardiograms are not indicated prior to starting treatment in patients with an unremarkable medical history and physical examination.
- If a patient's symptoms fail to respond to trials of two stimulants, second-line options include atomoxetine, viloxazine, extended-release guanfacine, and extended-release clonidine.

- Optimal treatment involves initial titration to optimize the dosage, followed by regular appointments. Patients should be monitored for treatment-emergent side effects. Teacher input should be sought at least once a semester.

References

Abramowicz M: Atomoxetine (Strattera) for ADHD. Med Lett Drugs Ther 45(1149):11–12, 2003 12571539

Achenbach TM, Ruffle TM: The Child Behavior Checklist and related forms for assessing behavioral/emotional problems and competencies. Pediatr Rev 21(8):265–271, 2000 10922023

American Psychiatric Association: Diagnostic and Statistical Manual of Mental Disorders, 3rd Edition Revised. Washington, DC, American Psychiatric Association, 1987

American Psychiatric Association: Diagnostic and Statistical Manual of Mental Disorders, 4th Edition. Washington, DC, American Psychiatric Association, 1994

American Psychiatric Association: Diagnostic and Statistical Manual of Mental Disorders, 4th Edition, Text Revision. Washington, DC, American Psychiatric Association, 2000

American Psychiatric Association: Diagnostic and Statistical Manual of Mental Disorders, 5th Edition. Arlington, VA, American Psychiatric Association, 2013

American Psychiatric Association: Diagnostic and Statistical Manual of Mental Disorders, 5th Edition, Text Revision. Washington, DC, American Psychiatric Association, 2022

Amiri S, Mohammadi M-R, Mohammadi M, et al: Modafinil as a treatment for attention-deficit/hyperactivity disorder in children and adolescents: a double blind, randomized clinical trial. Prog Neuropsychopharmacol Biol Psychiatry 32(1):145–149, 2008 17765380

Angold A, Erkanli A, Egger HL, Costello EJ: Stimulant treatment for children: a community perspective. J Am Acad Child Adolesc Psychiatry 39(8):975–984, discussion 984–994, 2000 10939226

Bangs ME, Wietecha LA, Wang S, et al: Meta-analysis of suicide-related behavior or ideation in child, adolescent, and adult patients treated with atomoxetine. J Child Adolesc Psychopharmacol 24(8):426–434, 2014 25019647

Biederman J, Quinn D, Weiss M, et al: Efficacy and safety of Ritalin LA, a new, once daily, extended-release dosage form of methylphenidate, in children with attention deficit hyperactivity disorder. Paediatr Drugs 5(12):833–841, 2003 14658924

Biederman J, Boellner SW, Childress A, et al: Lisdexamfetamine dimesylate and mixed amphetamine salts extended-release in children with ADHD: a double-blind, placebo-controlled, crossover analog classroom study. Biol Psychiatry 62(9):970–976, 2007a 17631866

Biederman J, Krishnan S, Zhang Y, et al: Efficacy and tolerability of lisdexamfetamine dimesylate (NRP-104) in children with attention-deficit/hyperactivity disorder: a phase III, multicenter, randomized, double-blind, forced-dose, parallel-group study. Clin Ther 29(3):450–463, 2007b 17577466

Biederman J, Spencer TJ, Monuteaux MC, Faraone SV: A naturalistic 10-year prospective study of height and weight in children with attention-deficit hyperactivity disorder grown up: sex and treatment effects. J Pediatr 157(4):635–640, 640.e1, 2010 20605163

Board AR, Guy G, Jones CM, Hoots B: Trends in stimulant dispensing by age, sex, state of residence, and prescriber specialty—United States, 2014–2019. Drug Alcohol Depend 217:108297, 2020 32961454

Buitelaar JK, Van der Gaag RJ, Swaab-Barneveld H, Kuiper M: Prediction of clinical response to methylphenidate in children with attention-deficit hyperactivity disorder. J Am Acad Child Adolesc Psychiatry 34(8):1025–1032, 1995 7665441

Castellanos FX, Giedd JN, Elia J, et al: Controlled stimulant treatment of ADHD and comorbid Tourette's syndrome: effects of stimulant and dose. J Am Acad Child Adolesc Psychiatry 36(5):589–596, 1997 9136492

Catalá-López F, Hutton B, Núñez-Beltrán A, et al: The pharmacological and non-pharmacological treatment of attention deficit hyperactivity disorder in children and adolescents: a systematic review with network meta-analyses of randomised trials. PLoS One 12(7):e0180355, 2017 28700715

Center for Drug Evaluation and Research: Addendum: Statistical Safety Review and Evaluation. Washington, DC, Center for Drug Evaluation and Research, 2011. Available at: http://wayback.archive-it.org/7993/20170113112122/http:/www.fda.gov/downloads/Drugs/DrugSafety/UCM278891.pdf. Accessed April 26, 2023.

Childress AC, Brams M, Cutler AJ, et al: The efficacy and safety of Evekeo, racemic amphetamine sulfate, for treatment of attention-deficit/hyperactivity disorder symptoms: a multicenter, dose-optimized, double-blind, randomized, placebo-controlled crossover laboratory classroom study. J Child Adolesc Psychopharmacol 25(5):402–414, 2015 25692608

Chou WJ, Chen SJ, Chen YS, et al: Remission in children and adolescents diagnosed with attention-deficit/hyperactivity disorder via an effective and tolerable titration scheme for osmotic release oral system methylphenidate. J Child Adolesc Psychopharmacol 22(3):215–225, 2012 22537358

Coghill DR, Banaschewski T, Lecendreux M, et al: Maintenance of efficacy of lisdexamfetamine dimesylate in children and adolescents with attention-deficit/hyperactivity disorder: randomized-withdrawal study design. J Am Acad Child Adolesc Psychiatry 53(6):647–657.e1, 2014 24839883

Cohen SC, Mulqueen JM, Ferracioli-Oda E, et al: Meta-analysis: risk of tics associated with psychostimulant use in randomized, placebo-controlled trials. J Am Acad Child Adolesc Psychiatry 54(9):728–736, 2015 26299294

Conners CK, Casat CD, Gualtieri CT, et al: Bupropion hydrochloride in attention deficit disorder with hyperactivity. J Am Acad Child Adolesc Psychiatry 35(10):1314–1321, 1996 8885585

Cooper WO, Habel LA, Sox CM, et al: ADHD drugs and serious cardiovascular events in children and young adults. N Engl J Med 365(20):1896–1904, 2011 22043968

Cortese S, Kelly C, Chabernaud C, et al: Toward systems neuroscience of ADHD: a meta-analysis of 55 fMRI studies. Am J Psychiatry 169(10):1038–1055, 2012 22983386

Cortese S, Holtmann M, Banaschewski T, et al: Practitioner review: current best practice in the management of adverse events during treatment with ADHD medications in children and adolescents. J Child Psychol Psychiatry 54(3):227–246, 2013 23294014

Cortese S, D'Acunto G, Konofal E, et al: New formulations of methylphenidate for the treatment of attention-deficit/hyperactivity disorder: pharmacokinetics, efficacy, and tolerability. CNS Drugs 31(2):149–160, 2017 28130762

Cortese S, Adamo N, Del Giovane C, et al: Comparative efficacy and tolerability of medications for attention-deficit hyperactivity disorder in children, adolescents, and adults: a systematic review and network meta-analysis. Lancet Psychiatry 5(9):727–738, 2018 30097390

Coughlin CG, Cohen SC, Mulqueen JM, et al: Meta-analysis: reduced risk of anxiety with psychostimulant treatment in children with attention-deficit/hyperactivity disorder. J Child Adolesc Psychopharmacol 25(8):611–617, 2015 26402485

Cox DJ, Merkel RL, Penberthy JK, et al: Impact of methylphenidate delivery profiles on driving performance of adolescents with attention-deficit/hyperactivity disorder: a pilot study. J Am Acad Child Adolesc Psychiatry 43(3):269–275, 2004 15076259

Dalsgaard S, Kvist AP, Leckman JF, et al: Cardiovascular safety of stimulants in children with attention-deficit/hyperactivity disorder: a nationwide prospective cohort study. J Child Adolesc Psychopharmacol 24(6):302–310, 2014 24956171

Danielson ML, Bitsko RH, Ghandour RM, et al: Prevalence of parent-reported ADHD diagnosis and associated treatment among U.S. children and adolescents, 2016. J Clin Child Adolesc Psychol 47(2):199–212, 2018 29363986

de Leon J: Translating pharmacogenetics to clinical practice: do cytochrome P450 2D6 ultrarapid metabolizers need higher atomoxetine doses? J Am Acad Child Adolesc Psychiatry 54(7):532–534, 2015 26088654

Doshi JA, Hodgkins P, Kahle J, et al: Economic impact of childhood and adult attention-deficit/hyperactivity disorder in the United States. J Am Acad Child Adolesc Psychiatry 51(10):990–1002.e2, 2012 23021476

Douglas VI, Barr RG, Desilets J, Sherman E: Do high doses of stimulants impair flexible thinking in attention-deficit hyperactivity disorder? J Am Acad Child Adolesc Psychiatry 34(7):877–885, 1995 7649958

DuPaul GJ, Barkley RA: Medication therapy, in Attention-Deficit Hyperactivity Disorder: A Handbook for Diagnosis and Treatment, 2nd Edition. Edited by Barkley RA. New York, Guilford, 1990, pp 573–612

DuPaul GJ, Rapport MD: Does methylphenidate normalize the classroom performance of children with attention deficit disorder? J Am Acad Child Adolesc Psychiatry 32(1):190–198, 1993 8428871

DuPaul GJ, Barkley RA, McMurray MB: Response of children with ADHD to methylphenidate: interaction with internalizing symptoms. J Am Acad Child Adolesc Psychiatry 33(6):894–903, 1994 8083147

Elia J, Borcherding BG, Rapoport JL, Keysor CS: Methylphenidate and dextroamphetamine treatments of hyperactivity: are there true nonresponders? Psychiatry Res 36(2):141–155, 1991 2017529

Ernst M, Zametkin A: The interface of genetics, neuroimaging, and neurochemistry in attention-deficit hyperactivity disorder, in Psychopharmacology: The Fourth Generation of Progress, 4th Edition. Edited by Bloom F, Kupfer D. New York, Raven, 1995, pp 1643–1652

Faraone SV, Spender T, Aleardi M, et al: Comparing the efficacy of medications used for ADHD using meta-analysis. Presented at the annual meeting of the American Psychiatric Association, San Francisco, CA, May 17–22, 2003

Faraone SV, Biederman J, Morley CP, Spencer TJ: Effect of stimulants on height and weight: a review of the literature. J Am Acad Child Adolesc Psychiatry 47(9):994–1009, 2008 18580502

Fernández de la Cruz L, Simonoff E, McGough JJ, et al: Treatment of children with attention-deficit/hyperactivity disorder (ADHD) and irritability: results from the Multimodal Treatment Study of Children With ADHD (MTA). J Am Acad Child Adolesc Psychiatry 54(1):62–70, 2015 25524791

Findling RL, Cutler AJ, Saylor K, et al: A long-term open-label safety and effectiveness trial of lisdexamfetamine dimesylate in adolescents with attention-deficit/hyperactivity disorder. J Child Adolesc Psychopharmacol 23(1):11–21, 2013 23410138

Findling RL, McBurnett K, White C, Youcha S: Guanfacine extended release adjunctive to a psychostimulant in the treatment of comorbid oppositional symptoms in children and adolescents with attention-deficit/hyperactivity disorder. J Child Adolesc Psychopharmacol 24(5):245–252, 2014 24945085

Gadow KD, Sverd J, Sprafkin J, et al: Efficacy of methylphenidate for attention-deficit hyperactivity disorder in children with tic disorder. Arch Gen Psychiatry 52(6):444–455, 1995 7771914

Gillberg C, Melander H, von Knorring AL, et al: Long-term stimulant treatment of children with attention-deficit hyperactivity disorder symptoms: a randomized, double-blind, placebo-controlled trial. Arch Gen Psychiatry 54(9):857–864, 1997 9294377

Gould MS, Walsh BT, Munfakh JL, et al: Sudden death and use of stimulant medications in youths. Am J Psychiatry 166(9):992–1001, 2009 19528194

Greenhill L, Swanson JM, Vitiello B, et al: Impairment and deportment responses to different methylphenidate doses in children with ADHD: the MTA titration trial. J Am Acad Child Adolesc Psychiatry 40(2):180–187, 2001 11211366

Greenhill L, Pliszka S, Dulcan MK, et al: Practice parameter for the use of stimulant medications in the treatment of children, adolescents, and adults. J Am Acad Child Adolesc Psychiatry 41(2 Suppl):26S–49S, 2002 11833633

Greenhill L, Kollins S, Abikoff H, et al: Efficacy and safety of immediate-release methylphenidate treatment for preschoolers with ADHD. J Am Acad Child Adolesc Psychiatry 45(11):1284–1293, 2006a 17023867

Greenhill L, Biederman J, Boellner SW, et al: A randomized, double-blind, placebo-controlled study of modafinil film-coated tablets in children and adolescents with attention-deficit/hyperactivity disorder. J Am Acad Child Adolesc Psychiatry 45(5):503–511, 2006b 16601402

Greenhill L, Muniz R, Ball RR, et al: Efficacy and safety of dexmethylphenidate extended-release capsules in children with attention-deficit/hyperactivity disorder. J Am Acad Child Adolesc Psychiatry 45(7):817–823, 2006c 16832318

Greenhill L, Newcorn JH, Gao H, Feldman PD: Effect of two different methods of initiating atomoxetine on the adverse event profile of atomoxetine. J Am Acad Child Adolesc Psychiatry 46(5):566–572, 2007 17450047

Greenhill L, Swanson JM, Hechtman L, et al: Trajectories of growth associated with long-term stimulant medication in the multimodal treatment study of attention-deficit/hyperactivity disorder. J Am Acad Child Adolesc Psychiatry 59(8):978–989, 2020 31421233

Harstad EB, Weaver AL, Katusic SK, et al: ADHD, stimulant treatment, and growth: a longitudinal study. Pediatrics 134(4):e935–e944, 2014 25180281

Hart H, Marquand AF, Smith A, et al: Predictive neurofunctional markers of attention-deficit/hyperactivity disorder based on pattern classification of temporal processing. J Am Acad Child Adolesc Psychiatry 53(5):569–78, 2014 24745956

Hechtman L, Swanson JM, Sibley MH, et al: Functional adult outcomes 16 years after childhood diagnosis of attention-deficit/hyperactivity disorder: MTA results. J Am Acad Child Adolesc Psychiatry 55(11):945–952, 2016

Hinshaw SP, Heller T, McHale JP: Covert antisocial behavior in boys with attention-deficit hyperactivity disorder: external validation and effects of methylphenidate. J Consult Clin Psychol 60(2):274–281, 1992 1592958

Hirota T, Schwartz S, Correll CU: Alpha-2 agonists for attention-deficit/hyperactivity disorder in youth: a systematic review and meta-analysis of monotherapy and add-on trials to stimulant therapy. J Am Acad Child Adolesc Psychiatry 53(2):153–173, 2014 24472251

Hodgkins P, Shaw M, Coghill D, Hechtman L: Amfetamine and methylphenidate medications for attention-deficit/hyperactivity disorder: complementary treatment options. Eur Child Adolesc Psychiatry 21(9):477–492, 2012 22763750

Jacobson NS, Truax P: Clinical significance: a statistical approach to defining meaningful change in psychotherapy research. J Consult Clin Psychol 59(1):12–19, 1991 2002127

Jasinski DR, Krishnan S: Abuse liability and safety of oral lisdexamfetamine dimesylate in individuals with a history of stimulant abuse. J Psychopharmacol 23(4):419–427, 2009 19329547

Jensen PS, Kettle L, Roper MT, et al: Are stimulants overprescribed? Treatment of ADHD in four U.S. communities. J Am Acad Child Adolesc Psychiatry 38(7):797–804, 1999 10405496

Johnson JK, Liranso T, Saylor K, et al: A phase II double-blind, placebo-controlled, efficacy and safety study of SPN-812 (extended-release viloxazine) in children with ADHD. J Atten Disord 24(2):348–358, 2020 30924702

Keating GM, Figgitt DP: Dexmethylphenidate. Drugs 62(13):1899–1904, discussion 1905–1908, 2002 12215063

Kessler RC, Adler L, Barkley R, et al: The prevalence and correlates of adult ADHD in the United States: results from the National Comorbidity Survey Replication. Am J Psychiatry 163(4):716–723, 2006 16585449

Kieling C, Kieling RR, Rohde LA, et al: The age at onset of attention deficit hyperactivity disorder. Am J Psychiatry 167(1):14–16, 2010 20068122

Klein RG, Abikoff H, Klass E, et al: Clinical efficacy of methylphenidate in conduct disorder with and without attention deficit hyperactivity disorder. Arch Gen Psychiatry 54(12):1073–1080, 1997 9400342

Kutcher S, Aman M, Brooks SJ, et al: International consensus statement on attention-deficit/hyperactivity disorder (ADHD) and disruptive behaviour disorders (DBDs): clinical implications and treatment practice suggestions. Eur Neuropsychopharmacol 14(1):11–28, 2004 14659983

Lahey BB, Willcutt EG: Predictive validity of a continuous alternative to nominal subtypes of attention-deficit/hyperactivity disorder for DSM-5. J Clin Child Adolesc Psychol 39(6):761–775, 2010 21058124

Levin FR, Mariani JJ, Specker S, et al: Extended-release mixed amphetamine salts vs placebo for comorbid adult attention-deficit/hyperactivity disorder and cocaine use disorder: a randomized clinical trial. JAMA Psychiatry 72(6):593–602, 2015 25887096

Liberthson RR: Sudden death from cardiac causes in children and young adults. N Engl J Med 334(16):1039–1044, 1996 8598843

Manor I, Magen A, Keidar D, et al: The effect of phosphatidylserine containing omega3 fatty-acids on attention-deficit hyperactivity disorder symptoms in children: a double-blind placebo-controlled trial, followed by an open-label extension. Eur Psychiatry 27(5):335–342, 2012 21807480

Matochik JA, Liebenauer LL, King AC, et al: Cerebral glucose metabolism in adults with attention deficit hyperactivity disorder after chronic stimulant treatment. Am J Psychiatry 151(5):658–664, 1994 8166305

Mattison DR, Plant TM, Lin HM, et al: Pubertal delay in male nonhuman primates (Macaca mulatta) treated with methylphenidate. Proc Natl Acad Sci USA 108(39):16301–16306, 2011 21930929

McElroy SL, Hudson JI, Mitchell JE, et al: Efficacy and safety of lisdexamfetamine for treatment of adults with moderate to severe binge-eating disorder: a randomized clinical trial. JAMA Psychiatry 72(3):235–246, 2015 25587645

McGough JJ, Wigal SB, Abikoff H, et al: A randomized, double-blind, placebo-controlled, laboratory classroom assessment of methylphenidate transdermal system in children with ADHD. J Atten Disord 9(3):476–485, 2006 16481664

McKeown RE, Holbrook JR, Danielson ML, et al: The impact of case definition on attention-deficit/hyperactivity disorder prevalence estimates in community-based samples of school-aged children. J Am Acad Child Adolesc Psychiatry 54(1):53–61, 2015 25524790

Modi NB, Wang B, Noveck RJ, Gupta SK: Dose-proportional and stereospecific pharmacokinetics of methylphenidate delivered using an osmotic, controlled-release oral delivery system. J Clin Pharmacol 40(10):1141–1149, 2000 11028253

Molina BSG, Hinshaw SP, Swanson JM, et al: The MTA at 8 years: prospective follow-up of children treated for combined-type ADHD in a multisite study. J Am Acad Child Adolesc Psychiatry 48(5):484–500, 2009 19318991

MTA Cooperative Group: Moderators and mediators of treatment response for children with attention-deficit/hyperactivity disorders. Arch Gen Psychiatry 56(12):1088–1096, 1999a 10591284

MTA Cooperative Group: Multimodal Treatment Study of Children With ADHD: a 14-month randomized clinical trial of treatment strategies for attention-deficit/hyperactivity disorder. Arch Gen Psychiatry 56(12):1073–1086, 1999b 10591283

MTA Cooperative Group: National Institute of Mental Health Multimodal Treatment Study of ADHD follow-up: changes in effectiveness and growth after the end of treatment. Pediatrics 113(4):762–769, 2004 15060225

Musten LM, Firestone P, Pisterman S, et al: Effects of methylphenidate on preschool children with ADHD: cognitive and behavioral functions. J Am Acad Child Adolesc Psychiatry 36(10):1407–1415, 1997 9334554

Nasser A, Kosheleff AR, Hull JT, et al: Evaluating the likelihood to be helped or harmed after treatment with viloxazine extended-release in children and adolescents with attention-deficit/hyperactivity disorder. Int J Clin Pract 75(8):e14330, 2021 33971070

Newcorn JH, Kratochvil CJ, Allen AJ, et al: Atomoxetine and osmotically released methylphenidate for the treatment of attention deficit hyperactivity disorder: acute comparison and differential response. Am J Psychiatry 165(6):721–730, 2008 18281409

Newcorn JH, Stein MA, Childress AC, et al: Randomized, double-blind trial of guanfacine extended release in children with attention-deficit/hyperactivity disorder: morning or evening administration. J Am Acad Child Adolesc Psychiatry 52(9):921–930, 2013 23972694

Ng QX: A systematic review of the use of bupropion for attention-deficit/hyperactivity disorder in children and adolescents. J Child Adolesc Psychopharmacol 27(2):112–116, 2017

Ota T, Yamamuro K, Okazaki K, Kishimoto T: Evaluating guanfacine hydrochloride in the treatment of attention deficit hyperactivity disorder (ADHD) in adult patients: design, development and place in therapy. Drug Des Devel Ther 15:1965–1969, 2021 34007156

Pelham WE, Milich R: Individual differences in response to Ritalin in classwork and social behavior, in Ritalin: Theory and Patient Management. Edited by Greenhill LL, Osman B. New York, Mary Ann Liebert, 1991, pp 203–222

Peterson BS, Potenza MN, Wang Z, et al: An fMRI study of the effects of psychostimulants on default-mode processing during Stroop task performance in youths with ADHD. Am J Psychiatry 166(11):1286–1294, 2009 19755575

Philipsen A, Jans T, Graf E, et al: Effects of group psychotherapy, individual counseling, methylphenidate, and placebo in the treatment of adult attention-deficit/hyperactivity disorder: a randomized clinical trial. JAMA Psychiatry 72(12):1199–1210, 2015 26536057

Pliszka SR, AACAP Work Group on Quality Issues: Practice parameter for the assessment and treatment of attention-deficit/hyperactivity disorder. J Am Acad Child Adolesc Psychiatry 46(7):894–921, 2007 17581453

Pliszka SR, Crismon ML, Hughes CW, et al: The Texas Children's Medication Algorithm Project: revision of the algorithm for pharmacotherapy of attention-deficit/hyperactivity disorder. J Am Acad Child Adolesc Psychiatry 45(6):642–657, 2006 16721314

Posner J, Maia TV, Fair D, et al: The attenuation of dysfunctional emotional processing with stimulant medication: an fMRI study of adolescents with ADHD. Psychiatry Res 193(3):151–160, 2011a 21778039

Posner J, Nagel BJ, Maia TV, et al: Abnormal amygdalar activation and connectivity in adolescents with attention-deficit/hyperactivity disorder. J Am Acad Child Adolesc Psychiatry 50(8):828–37.e3, 2011b 21784302

Quinn D, Wigal S, Swanson J, et al: Comparative pharmacodynamics and plasma concentrations of d-threo-methylphenidate hydrochloride after single doses of d-threo-methylphenidate hydrochloride and d,l-threo-methylphenidate hydrochloride in a double-blind, placebo-controlled, crossover laboratory school study in children with attention-deficit/hyperactivity disorder. J Am Acad Child Adolesc Psychiatry 43(11):1422–1429, 2004 15502602

Rapport MD, Denney C, DuPaul GJ, Gardner MJ: Attention deficit disorder and methylphenidate: normalization rates, clinical effectiveness, and response prediction in 76 children. J Am Acad Child Adolesc Psychiatry 33(6):882–893, 1994 8083146

Reale L, Bartoli B, Cartabia M, et al: Comorbidity prevalence and treatment outcome in children and adolescents with ADHD. Eur Child Adolesc Psychiatry 26(12):1443–1457, 2017 28527021

Rommel AS, Lichtenstein P, Rydell M, et al: Is physical activity causally associated with symptoms of attention-deficit/hyperactivity disorder? J Am Acad Child Adolesc Psychiatry 54(7):565–570, 2015 26088661

Rosack J: FDA approves first nonstimulant medication for ADHD treatment. Psychiatric News, December 20, 2002

Rugino T: A review of modafinil film-coated tablets for attention-deficit/hyperactivity disorder in children and adolescents. Neuropsychiatr Dis Treat 3(3):293–301, 2007

Safer DJ: Recent trends in stimulant usage. J Atten Disord 20(6):471–477, 2016 26486603

Safer D, Allen R, Barr E: Depression of growth in hyperactive children on stimulant drugs. N Engl J Med 287(5):217–220, 1972 4556640

Scahill L, McCracken JT, King BH, et al: Extended-release guanfacine for hyperactivity in children with autism spectrum disorder. Am J Psychiatry 172(12):1197–1206, 2015 26315981

Scassellati C, Bonvicini C, Faraone SV, Gennarelli M: Biomarkers and attention-deficit/hyperactivity disorder: a systematic review and meta-analyses. J Am Acad Child Adolesc Psychiatry 51(10):1003–1019.e20, 2012 23021477

Schachar RJ, Tannock R, Cunningham C, Corkum PV: Behavioral, situational, and temporal effects of treatment of ADHD with methylphenidate. J Am Acad Child Adolesc Psychiatry 36(6):754–763, 1997 9183129

Schachter HM, Pham B, King J, et al: How efficacious and safe is short-acting methylphenidate for the treatment of attention-deficit disorder in children and adolescents? A meta-analysis. CMAJ 165(11):1475–1488, 2001 11762571

Schwartz BS, Bailey-Davis L, Bandeen-Roche K, et al: Attention deficit disorder, stimulant use, and childhood body mass index trajectory. Pediatrics 133(4):668–676, 2014 24639278

Schwartz S, Correll CU: Efficacy and safety of atomoxetine in children and adolescents with attention-deficit/hyperactivity disorder: results from a comprehensive meta-analysis and metaregression. J Am Acad Child Adolesc Psychiatry 53(2):174–187, 2014 24472252

Sonuga-Barke EJ, Castellanos FX: Spontaneous attentional fluctuations in impaired states and pathological conditions: a neurobiological hypothesis. Neurosci Biobehav Rev 31(7):977–986, 2007 17445893

Spencer T, Wilens T, Biederman J, et al: A double-blind, crossover comparison of methylphenidate and placebo in adults with childhood-onset attention-deficit hyperactivity disorder. Arch Gen Psychiatry 52(6):434–443, 1995 7771913

Spencer TJ, Biederman J, Harding M, et al: Growth deficits in ADHD children revisited: evidence for disorder-associated growth delays? J Am Acad Child Adolesc Psychiatry 35(11):1460–1469, 1996 8936912

Spencer TJ, Kratochvil CJ, Sangal RB, et al: Effects of atomoxetine on growth in children with attention-deficit/hyperactivity disorder following up to five years of treatment. J Child Adolesc Psychopharmacol 17(5):689–700, 2007a 17979588

Spencer TJ, Adler LA, McGough JJ, et al: Efficacy and safety of dexmethylphenidate extended-release capsules in adults with attention-deficit/hyperactivity disorder. Biol Psychiatry 61(12):1380–1387, 2007b 17137560

Supernus: Supernus announces Qelbree sNDA for adult indication accepted for review by FDA. Rockville, MD, Supernus Pharmaceuticals, September 2, 2021a. Available at: https://ir.supernus.com/news-releases/news-release-details/supernus-announces-qelbreetm-snda-adult-indication-accepted. Accessed February 25, 2022.

Supernus: Viloxazine. Rockville, MD, Supernus Pharmaceuticals, 2021b. Available at: https://www.accessdata.fda.gov/drugsatfda_docs/label/2021/211964s000lbl.pdf. Accessed August 17, 2021.

Swanson JM: School-Based Assessments and Interventions for ADD Students. Irvine, CA, KC Publishing, 1992

Swanson JM, Wigal S, Greenhill LL, et al: Analog classroom assessment of Adderall in children with ADHD. J Am Acad Child Adolesc Psychiatry 37(5):519–526, 1998 9585654

Swanson JM, Kraemer HC, Hinshaw SP, et al: Clinical relevance of the primary findings of the MTA: success rates based on severity of ADHD and ODD symptoms at the end of treatment. J Am Acad Child Adolesc Psychiatry 40(2):168–179, 2001 11211365

Swanson J, Gupta S, Lam A, et al: Development of a new once-a-day formulation of methylphenidate for the treatment of attention-deficit/hyperactivity disorder: proof-of-concept and proof-of-product studies. Arch Gen Psychiatry 60(2):204–211, 2003 12578439

Swanson JM, Wigal SB, Wigal T, et al: A comparison of once-daily extended-release methylphenidate formulations in children with attention-deficit/hyperactivity disorder in the laboratory school (the COMACS Study). Pediatrics 113(3 Pt 1):e206–e216, 2004 14993578

Swanson JM, Elliott GR, Greenhill LL, et al: Effects of stimulant medication on growth rates across 3 years in the MTA follow-up. J Am Acad Child Adolesc Psychiatry 46(8):1015–1027, 2007 17667480

Swanson JM, Arnold LE, Molina BSG, et al: Young adult outcomes in the follow-up of the multimodal treatment study of attention-deficit/hyperactivity disorder: symptom persistence, source discrepancy, and height suppression. J Child Psychol Psychiatry 58(6):663–678, 2017 28295312

Tannock R, Ickowicz A, Schachar R: Differential effects of methylphenidate on working memory in ADHD children with and without comorbid anxiety. J Am Acad Child Adolesc Psychiatry 34(7):886–896, 1995a 7649959

Tannock R, Schachar R, Logan G: Methylphenidate and cognitive flexibility: dissociated dose effects in hyperactive children. J Abnorm Child Psychol 23(2):235–266, 1995b 7642836

Thomas R, Sanders S, Doust J, et al: Prevalence of attention-deficit/hyperactivity disorder: a systematic review and meta-analysis. Pediatrics 135(4):e994–e1001, 2015 25733754

Tjon Pian Gi CV, Broeren JPA, Starreveld JS, A Versteegh FG: Melatonin for treatment of sleeping disorders in children with attention deficit/hyperactivity disorder: a preliminary open label study. Eur J Pediatr 162(7–8):554–555, 2003 12783318

U.S. Food and Drug Administration: Label for Concerta (methylphenidate HCl) Extended-Release Tablets. Washington, DC, U.S. Food and Drug Adminstration, 2017. Available at: https://www.accessdata.fda.gov/drugsatfda_docs/label/2017/021121s038lbl.pdf. Accessed April 26, 2023.

Vande Voort JL, He JP, Jameson ND, Merikangas KR: Impact of the DSM-5 attention-deficit/hyperactivity disorder age-of-onset criterion in the US adolescent population. J Am Acad Child Adolesc Psychiatry 53(7):736–744, 2014 24954823

Visser SN, Danielson ML, Bitsko RH, et al: Trends in the parent-report of health care provider-diagnosed and medicated attention-deficit/hyperactivity disorder: United States, 2003–2011. J Am Acad Child Adolesc Psychiatry 53(1):34–46, 2014 24342384

Vitiello B: Research in child and adolescent psychopharmacology: recent accomplishments and new challenges. Psychopharmacology (Berl) 191(1):5–13, 2007 16718480

Vitiello B, Jensen PS: Medication development and testing in children and adolescents: current problems, future directions. Arch Gen Psychiatry 54(9):871–876, 1997 9294379

Vitiello B, Elliott GR, Swanson JM, et al: Blood pressure and heart rate over 10 years in the Multimodal Treatment Study of Children With ADHD. Am J Psychiatry 169(2):167–177, 2012 21890793

Vitiello B, Lazzaretto D, Yershova K, et al: Pharmacotherapy of the Preschool ADHD Treatment Study (PATS) children growing up. J Am Acad Child Adolesc Psychiatry 54(7):550–556, 2015 26088659

Volkow ND, Ding YS, Fowler JS, et al: Is methylphenidate like cocaine? Studies on their pharmacokinetics and distribution in the human brain. Arch Gen Psychiatry 52(6):456–463, 1995 7771915

Volkow ND, Wang G, Fowler JS, et al: Therapeutic doses of oral methylphenidate significantly increase extracellular dopamine in the human brain. J Neurosci 21(2):RC121, 2001 11160455

Wang LJ, Chen CK, Huang YS: Neurocognitive performance and behavioral symptoms in patients with attention-deficit/hyperactivity disorder during twenty-four months of treatment with methylphenidate. J Child Adolesc Psychopharmacol 25(3):246–253, 2015 25574708

Weissman DH, Roberts KC, Visscher KM, Woldorff MG: The neural bases of momentary lapses in attention. Nat Neurosci 9(7):971–978, 2006 16767087

Wigal S, Swanson JM, Feifel D, et al: A double-blind, placebo-controlled trial of dexmethylphenidate hydrochloride and d,l-threo-methylphenidate hydrochloride in children with attention-deficit/hyperactivity disorder. J Am Acad Child Adolesc Psychiatry 43(11):1406–1414, 2004 15502600

Wigal SB, Nordbrock E, Adjei AL, et al: Efficacy of methylphenidate hydrochloride extended-release capsules (Aptensio XR) in children and adolescents with attention-deficit/hyperactivity disorder: a phase III, randomized, double-blind study. CNS Drugs 29(4):331–340, 2015 25877989

Wilens TE, McBurnett K, Bukstein O, et al: Multisite controlled study of OROS methylphenidate in the treatment of adolescents with attention-deficit/hyperactivity disorder. Arch Pediatr Adolesc Med 160(1):82–90, 2006 16389216

Wilens TE, Robertson B, Sikirica V, et al: A randomized, placebo-controlled trial of guanfacine extended release in adolescents with attention-deficit/hyperactivity disorder. J Am Acad Child Adolesc Psychiatry 54(11):916–25.e2, 2015 26506582

Wolraich ML, Lambert W, Doffing MA, et al: Psychometric properties of the Vanderbilt ADHD diagnostic parent rating scale in a referred population. J Pediatr Psychol 28(8):559–567, 2003 14602846

Wolraich ML, Hagan JF Jr, Allan C, et al: Clinical practice guideline for the diagnosis, evaluation, and treatment of attention-deficit/hyperactivity disorder in children and adolescents. Pediatrics 144(4):e20192528, 2019 31570648

3

Disruptive Behavior Disorders and Aggression

Ekaterina Stepanova, M.D, Ph.D.

Solomon G. Zaraa, D.O.

Peter S. Jensen, M.D.

Disruptive behavior disorders (DBDs), which include disruptive, impulse-control, and conduct disorders (American Psychiatric Association 2022), are associated with increased risk of psychopathology later in life, substance abuse, and incarceration (Bambauer and Connor 2005; Kazdin 1995; Tremblay et al. 2004). Aggressive behaviors that frequently occur in youth with DBDs are one of the most common reasons children and their families seek mental health services (Connor 2002). Such behaviors can manifest in the context of oppositional defiant disorder (ODD), conduct disorder (CD), and intermittent explosive disorder (IED). However, symptoms of aggression are seen in youth with diagnoses other than DBDs. Aggression can be present in children with ADHD, mood disorders, PTSD, autism spectrum disorder (ASD), and other psychiatric illnesses. Although aggression co-occurs with several psychiatric conditions, it is a distinct construct. For example, aggression with impulsivity and reactivity can be distinguished from attention problems, rule-breaking behaviors, and mood disorders (Young et al. 2020; Youngstrom et al. 2023). Given the public health importance of aggression, it is helpful to understand the nosology of aggressive behaviors as it relates to DBDs.

Different classifications of aggression have been described in the literature. Most commonly, aggression is divided into two subtypes: proactive and reactive (Connor 2002; Dodge and Coie 1987). *Proactive aggression* (PA), also referred to as instrumental or deliberate, often occurs without provocation. *Reactive aggression*, on the other hand, often happens in response to a trigger. It is also called *impulsive aggression* (IA), or "hot" or "hostile" aggression (Vitiello and Stoff 1997).

These two forms of aggression and their relationship to the DBDs are yet to be fully understood. This conceptual gap has been largely a result of the limited number of clinical trials studying aggression in youth. In addition, many clinical trials are not evaluating aggression in this way. It is often difficult to separate aggression into reactive/impulsive and proactive because many youth exhibit both. Nevertheless, the type of aggression may affect the prognosis and treatment response. For example, PA is more likely to be associated with callous and unemotional traits (Kimonis et al. 2006) and may have poorer long-term outcomes compared with IA (Fontaine et al. 2011; Pardini and Fite 2010; Pardini and Loeber 2008). However, one trial of youth with DBDs and aggressive behavior reported that callous and unemotional traits and PA improved when optimized ADHD treatment was provided (Blader et al. 2013). Conversely, Malone et al. (1998) found preferential response to lithium in youth with IA but not in those with PA. Many trials, however, do not discriminate between PA and IA; therefore, potential clinical benefits of management of different forms of aggression have not yet been fully addressed (Pappadopulos et al. 2006). Some investigators have suggested that the response to pharmacological intervention differs based on the aggression subtype (Gillberg and Hellgren 1986; Malone et al. 1998; Padhy et al. 2011; Steiner et al. 2011). As we discuss further in this chapter, youth with CD and IA may greatly benefit from pharmacotherapy (Connor et al. 2004; Jensen et al. 2007; Steiner et al. 2003b; Vitiello and Stoff 1997; Vitiello et al. 1990).

Similarly, IA in children with ADHD may also respond to medication management (Jensen et al. 2007). However, data are limited as to whether psychopharmacological agents ameliorate symptoms of PA in CD (Jensen et al. 2007). Therefore, future randomized controlled trials (RCTs) may benefit from including a reliable measure of aggression that distinguishes between the aggressive subtypes (Brown et al. 1996). In this chapter, we address what is currently known about the treatment of DBDs and aggression.

Epidemiology

Oppositional Defiant Disorder and Aggression

Diagnosis of ODD requires the presence of a frequent and consistent pattern of angry/irritable mood, argumentative/defiant behavior, or vindictiveness that persists for at least 6 months (American Psychiatric Association 2022). For the diagnostic criteria for ODD to be met, the patient must exhibit at least four of the following behaviors: often losing their temper, being easily annoyed by others, being angry or resentful, arguing with adults, refusing to comply with authority figures, deliberately doing things to annoy other people, blaming others for their mistakes or behavior, and being spiteful or vindictive. Although none of the symptoms required for the diagnosis of ODD describes aggressive behaviors, many youth with ODD also exhibit IA. Symptoms of ODD can be conceptualized as falling into three dimensions: irritable, headstrong, and/or hurtful (Stringaris and Goodman 2009). Approximately 1%–11% of children in the United States have a pattern of behaviors that meets the ODD criteria (Canino et al. 2010). Prevalence is even higher in children who are also diagnosed with ADHD, up to 19% (Mitchison and Njardvik 2019).

ODD appears to precede the development of CD but is only marginally predictive of PA (Lahey et al. 1998; Rowe et al. 2010). Whereas most youth with ODD do not subsequently develop CD, the *spiteful/vindictive* symptoms that fall into the hurtful dimension of ODD carry the most risk for development of CD (Stringaris and Goodman 2009). On the other hand, many features of ODD may be indicative of verbal forms of IA, such as losing one's temper, being easily annoyed by others, arguing with adults, and being angry or resentful. However, the relationship between different subtypes of ODD and IA should be explored in future research.

Conduct Disorder

CD occurs in 2%–9% of children and adolescents worldwide (Costello et al. 2005; INSERM Collective Expertise Centre 2005). The definition of CD has transformed drastically over the past several decades. Earlier descriptions of childhood-onset CD characterized explosive and aggressive children, suggesting a significant role of impulsivity underlying the aggressive behaviors (Campbell et al. 1984). However, with each consecutive iteration of CD in DSM, the role of PA was emphasized more and more, along with a stronger emphasis on the callous-unemotional traits (DSM-III, American Psychiatric Association 1987; DSM-IV, American Psychiatric Association 1994). CD is currently defined as a repetitive and persistent pattern of behavior in which the rights of others and/or major societal norms or rules are violated (American Psychiatric Association 2022). These behaviors fall into four main categories: aggression toward people and animals, destruction of property, deceitfulness or theft, and serious violations of rules. As with ODD, it is possible that the features of this behavior disorder may correspond to either IA or PA. Emerging evidence suggests that PA, rather than IA, is a significant predictor of CD (Fite et al. 2009; Pardini and Fite 2010; Stringaris and Goodman 2009; Vitaro et al. 1998), but this area needs further study.

Intermittent Explosive Disorder

IED is another diagnosis that may describe youth with aggressive and disruptive behaviors. The current definition of IED includes individuals with recurrent behavioral outbursts representing failure to control aggressive impulses (American Psychiatric Association 2022). The symptoms of IED are verbal and physical aggression. Physical aggression can involve property damage or physical injury to people and animals. Compared with past iterations, DSM-5 specifies more frequent presence of aggressive behaviors, up to three times a week. However, it is still unclear whether IED appropriately describes youth with aggression who have multiple outbursts on an almost daily basis. Additionally, the research available to date shows that the age at onset of IED is around adolescence, despite the DSM criterion of starting at age 6 years (Coccaro et al. 2005; Galbraith et al. 2018). More data are needed to clarify these important distinctions.

Differential Diagnosis

In addition to ODD, CD, and IED, aggressive behaviors occur in the context of other disorders, such as ADHD, mood disorders, psychotic disorders, anxiety, PTSD, ASD, and others (Burke et al. 2010; Jensen et al. 2007). Therefore, aggression co-occurs with many diagnoses. In particular, IA is a distinct construct and is not specific to any particular disorder (Jensen et al. 2007; Young et al. 2020; Youngstrom et al. 2023). Whether IA represents a separate diagnosis remains to be determined.

Course and Outcome

The occurrence of a DBD in youth may lead to the subsequent development of other mental disorders. For example, ODD may precede a CD diagnosis (Burke et al. 2010; Pardini et al. 2010). Loeber et al. (1993) found that youth who were diagnosed with ODD had a 43% chance of eventually developing CD. However, the emergence of CD does not necessarily mitigate or supersede a diagnosis of ODD; in fact, it is more common for ODD symptoms to persist even after full CD symptoms emerge. Furthermore, studies indicate that a number of youth with CD may also develop antisocial personality disorder in adulthood (Loeber et al. 2002, 2003, 2009). The diagnosis of ODD confers an increased risk of emotional disorders in adulthood, including anxiety, depression, substance abuse, impulse-control problems, and antisocial behavior (Burke et al. 2014; Kim-Cohen et al. 2003; Nock et al. 2007; Rowe et al. 2010). Individuals with IED have psychosocial impairments and worse quality of life, as well as legal problems (Rynar and Coccaro 2018). However, no studies have evaluated children with IED prospectively, and little is known about their prognosis.

In general, the prognosis for DBDs is especially poor if the youth's symptoms fail to respond to behavioral interventions, which are often considered the first line of treatment for behavior disorders and symptoms of aggression. A significant predictor of nonresponse is the presence of PA, compared with IA (Malone et al. 1998; Masi et al. 2011). However, the response to treatment also may depend on the underlying disorder. For example, in children with ADHD and a combination of IA and PA, the presence of baseline PA did not reduce the effectiveness of stimulant therapy on aggressive behavior (Blader et al. 2013).

Because of the limitations of current psychotherapeutic interventions, however, a growing body of literature has focused on the outcomes of psychopharmacological treatment of aggressive symptoms in youth with DBDs (Connor et al. 1999, 2002, 2019; dosReis et al. 2003; Pappadopulos et al. 2003; Schur et al. 2003; Steiner et al. 2003b), which our focus in this chapter.

Rationale and Justification for Psychopharmacological Treatment

The first line of treatment for DBDs is evidence-based psychotherapeutic interventions, such as parent management training, family therapy, and others. However, when those interventions are not sufficiently effective, providers may consider pharmacological options. As with treating any illness, pharmacotherapy should target the underlying diagnosis. Unfortunately, treating disruptive behaviors is more complicated than that, largely due to the fact that youth with aggressive or disruptive behaviors often do not fit a single diagnostic category. As discussed previously, aggression frequently co-occurs with multiple diagnoses. To identify potential medications that could help children with disruptive behaviors, many clinical trials were designed to target aggression as a symptom rather than as a particular diagnosis. What makes it even more complicated for clinicians is that comorbid diagnoses differ greatly among different studies and may include ADHD, CD, ODD or a combination of DBDs. Nevertheless, the research available to date offers some insight into effective pharmacotherapy of aggressive behaviors in youth.

Review of Treatment Studies

Atypical Antipsychotics

Risperidone

Risperidone is currently the most extensively studied medication in the treatment of aggression in youth (Loy et al. 2017), with RCTs testing short- and long-term benefits of this agent. These studies include larger-scale, multisite trials and small-scale RCTs.

Short-term efficacy. One of the largest studies of risperidone in this population is the National Institute of Mental Health (NIMH)–funded Treatment of Severe Child Aggression (TOSCA) study, which included 168 children ages 6–12 years with ADHD and co-occurring DBDs (Farmer et al. 2011). Children initially received a 3-week open titration of a stimulant. Those who did not show an adequate clinical response were randomly assigned to two groups. Both groups received parent training and stimulant treatment. Of these, one group received risperidone in addition to the stimulant and parent training, while the other group received placebo instead of risperidone for 9 weeks. Participants in the risperidone group showed lower aggression scores (measured with the Nisonger Child Behavior Rating Form [NCBRF]), compared with those in the placebo group (Aman et al. 2014). No serious adverse events were reported in the study. Prolactin elevation was noted in the augmented group, whereas trouble falling asleep was more common in the placebo group.

Post hoc analysis also suggests that children with more severe ADHD and callous and unemotional symptoms demonstrate a more robust and faster treatment response, regardless of the treatment received (Farmer et al. 2015). Several other trials suggest that children receiving a stimulant and risperidone whose parents also received parent training reported a greater reduction in symptom-related impairment, aggression, ADHD, and ODD severity compared with children who were given a stimulant and a placebo whose parents also received parent training (Aman et al. 2014; Gadow et al. 2014).

Two industry-sponsored, multisite RCTs were conducted to test the efficacy of risperidone in the treatment of aggressive symptoms and/or DBDs in youth with low to normal or subaverage intelligence. The first RCT evaluated 118 children (ages 5–12) with subaverage intelligence and a primary diagnosis of DBD, including ODD, CD, or DBD not otherwise specified (Aman et al. 2002). Compared with subjects receiving placebo, those receiving risperidone experienced a significant reduction in aggressive symptoms as measured by the Conduct Problem subscale of the NCBRF. The second study achieved comparable results in a similarly designed RCT (Snyder et al. 2002).

Several smaller trials have yielded comparable results. For example, Findling et al. (2000) demonstrated significant reductions in aggressive behaviors as measured by the Rating of Aggression Against People and/or Property Scale in a sample of 20 youth with CD (ages 5–15) who were receiving outpatient treatment. Similar reductions were noted in an RCT that specifically targeted symptoms of severe aggression during a 6-week trial of 38 inpatient adolescents with subaverage intelligence and DBDs (Buitelaar et al. 2001). Their aggressive symptoms were measured by the Clinical Global Impression (CGI) Severity of Illness subscale and the Aberrant Behavior Checklist (ABC). Moreover, during the 2-week washout trial following the 6 weeks of treatment, the risperidone group experienced a statistically significant worsening of aggressive behaviors as measured by the CGI Severity of Illness subscale, the ABC, and the Overt Aggression Scale (OAS)–Modified.

The efficacy of risperidone in the treatment of aggressive symptoms was also documented in an 8-week, double-blind RCT of 101 youth with autism (McCracken et al. 2002). Risperidone treatment was associated with significant reductions in aggression as indicated by scores on the ABC and the CGI within 4 weeks of receiving treatment. Additionally, a significant treatment-by-time interaction effect indicated that the risperidone group continued to improve through weeks 4–8, whereas the placebo group deteriorated. Currently, risperidone is one of the two antipsychotics that are FDA approved for the management of irritability associated with ASD (autistic disorder).

Although the aforementioned trials offer some guidance in the acute management of aggressive behaviors, they do not evaluate comorbidity, treatment in various settings, effects of childhood adversity, and other factors. In addition, these trials offer information on short-term outcomes and adverse events. Longer-term studies are discussed later in this chapter. Despite these limitations, available data suggest that risperidone appears to be effective in the short-term treatment of aggressive symptoms and/or behavior disorders in youth. For specific dosage information pertaining to the effective use of risperidone in the treatment of aggression in youth, see Table 3–1.

Long-term and maintenance efficacy. In addition to evidence of the short-term efficacy of risperidone for symptoms of aggression and DBDs, emerging evidence suggests risperidone may be beneficial for the long-term maintenance of treatment gains. In one study of long-term efficacy (Reyes et al. 2006a), 335 youth ages 5–17 whose symptoms had responded to open-label risperidone treatment over 12 weeks were then blindly and randomly assigned to an additional 6 months of either a continuation of risperidone or placebo. The NCBRF was used to assess both PA and IA. On average, symptom recurrence was slower in the risperidone group. Significant aggressive symptoms re-

Table 3–1. Selected agents prescribed for the treatment of aggressive youth with disruptive behavior disorders (DBDs)

Class	Generic (trade)	Dosing for DBDs[a,b]	FDA dosing[a,c]
Antipsychotics, atypical	Aripiprazole (Abilify)	2.5–30	2–30
	Clozapine (Clozaril)	150–600	NA
	Olanzapine (Zyprexa)	2.5–20	2.5–10
	Paliperidone (Invega)	3–12	3–12
	Quetiapine (Seroquel)	100–600	400–600
	Risperidone (Risperdal)	0.25–1.5	0.5–6
	Ziprasidone (Geodon)	40–160	NA
Antipsychotics, typical	Haloperidol (Haldol)	1–16	0.5–15
	Thioridazine (Mellaril)	1.75 mg/kg/day	0.5–3 mg/kg/day
Stimulants	Dexmethylphenidate (Focalin, Focalin XR)		5–30
	Dextroamphetamine (Dexedrine, ProCentra, Zenzedi)		2.5–40
	Lisdexamfetamine (Vyvanse)		20–70
	Methylphenidate (Ritalin, Ritalin LA, Metadate, Metadate CD, Methylin, Quillivant XR)	5–60	5–60
	Methylphenidate (Concerta)		18–72
	Methylphenidate transdermal (Daytrana)		10–30 mg/9 hours
	Mixed amphetamine salts (Adderall, Adderall XR, Evekeo)		2.5–40
Norepinephrine reuptake inhibitor	Atomoxetine (Strattera)		40–100

Table 3–1. Selected agents prescribed for the treatment of aggressive youth with disruptive behavior disorders (DBDs) *(continued)*

Class	Generic (trade)	Dosing for DBDs[a,b]	FDA dosing[a,c]
Mood stabilizers	Carbamazepine (Tegretol)	600–800	10–20 mg/kg/day[d]
	Lithium, lithium carbonate (Eskalith, Lithobid)	1,800 mean	10–30 mg/kg/day[e]
	Valproic acid (Depakene, Depakote, Depakote ER, Depakote Sprinkle Capsules)	250–1,500	15–60 mg/kg/day[f]
α_2-Agonists	Clonidine (Catapres, Kapvay)	0.1–0.2	0.1–0.4
	Guanfacine (Tenex, Intuniv)	1–4	1–4
β-Blockers	Nadolol (Corgard)	30–220	20–200

Note. See Jensen et al. (2004) and Martin et al. (2003) for additional information.
[a]Dosages are mg/day unless otherwise noted.
[b]Dosing is based on randomized controlled trials of DBDs.
[c]FDA-approved dosing for other indications in youth.
[d]Carbamazepine dosages optimally adjusted based on blood levels, 4–14 μg/L.
[e]Lithium doses optimally adjusted based on blood levels, 0.6–1.1 mEq/L.
[f]Valproic acid doses optimally adjusted based on blood levels, 50–125 μg/L.

occurred after 119 days in 25% of patients in the risperidone group and in 47.1% of patients in the placebo group. Notably, the results indicated that more than half of the placebo group did not experience a recurrence of symptoms. Therefore, psychopharmacological discontinuation may be a plausible option for some youth with resolved symptoms of aggression or DBD. Reyes et al. (2006a) also reported significant treatment gains in hyperactive, compliant, and adaptive social behaviors in the risperidone group compared with the placebo group. After the completion of this yearlong study, an additional 1-year open-label expansion study was conducted involving 48 responders, and maintenance of the original treatment gains was again demonstrated (Reyes et al. 2006b). Overall, these studies suggest that risperidone may be efficacious in the treatment of DBDs or aggression in children for a cumulative period up to 2 years.

The TOSCA postacute efficacy and maintenance studies showed similar results. In a 12-week postacute trial, the augmented group's symptoms remained improved (Findling et al. 2017); at a 12-month follow-up, the groups did not separate on primary outcome measures, but the augmented group had lower illness severity scores (Gadow et al. 2016). Of note, more than half of the participants in both groups failed to adhere to the prescribed regimen at 12 months, which could affect the overall results of the study.

Similar results are also supported by other yearlong, open-label trials assessing the sustained safety and efficacy of risperidone in youth of subaverage intelligence with symptoms of aggression and other disruptive behaviors (Aman et al. 2004; Croonenberghs et al. 2005; Turgay et al. 2002). In general, across these extension studies of initial RCTs, youth maintained treatment gains reported in the initial waves of the study (see subsection "Short-Term Efficacy" for risperidone). Of particular interest within the aggressive subtype literature, a highly significant decrease was seen in scores on the secondary outcome measure (the Vineland Adaptive Behavior Scales) used to assess physical aggression and emotional outbursts (Turgay et al. 2002). Therefore, preliminary evidence appears to indicate the utility of risperidone in the treatment of IA.

Furthermore, risperidone showed effectiveness in the long-term treatment of aggressive youth with a primary diagnosis of ASD or other pervasive developmental disorders. In the Research Units on Pediatric Psychopharmacology (RUPP) follow-up study, two-thirds of patients maintained behavioral improvements for 6 months following the initial risperidone treatment, after being reassigned to either risperidone or placebo (Research Units on Pediatric Psychopharmacology Autism Network 2005). Symptoms did not relapse in 37.5% of youth who had taken risperidone in the original study, even while they were taking placebo in the follow-up. Furthermore, youth with different subtypes of aggression reported comparable benefits with risperidone treatment (Carroll et al. 2014). Similarly, Troost et al. (2005) studied 36 children ages 5–17 with ASD who had symptoms of severe aggression or self-injurious behavior. These youth initially received an 8-week, open-label trial of risperidone. Those whose symptoms responded continued treatment for another 16 weeks, and then a double-blind discontinuation ($n=24$) was carried out, consisting of either 3 weeks of tapering and 5 weeks of placebo or continued use of risperidone. Only 25% of patients who continued risperidone experienced relapse, compared with 66.67% of youth who were switched to placebo. Thus, both studies suggest that continuing treatment with risperidone was more efficacious than placebo in preventing relapse. Findings from both studies also imply that at least a subset of initially treated children may not experience relapse when their risperidone is switched to placebo, suggesting that consideration of medication discontinuation may be appropriate for some children who have done well for a substantial period of time.

Overall, there is increasing evidence to suggest that risperidone may be efficacious in the long-term treatment of aggressive symptoms and/or behavior disorders in youth.

Paliperidone

There are low-evidence data on the use of paliperidone in treating aggressive behaviors in youth. An 8-week open-label study of youth and young adults with ASD (autistic disorder) reported that paliperidone was well tolerated and associated with improvement of irritability symptoms (Stigler et al. 2012). In another open-label study, paliperidone was noted to reduce aggressive behaviors in youth with developmental disorders or ADHD whose symptoms had inadequate response to risperidone (Fernández-Mayoralas et al. 2012). Further evaluation of paliperidone in the treatment of DBDs is warranted.

Olanzapine

Several small studies of olanzapine appear promising in the treatment of aggressive disorders in children and adolescents (see Table 3–1 for dosage information). In a study by Stephens et al. (2004), 10 children with Tourette's disorder and aggression were treated in single-blind fashion (after a 2-week placebo run-in) with olanzapine over 8 weeks. The study participants demonstrated significant reductions in both aggressive symptoms and tic severity, as assessed with standard rating scales. In one open-label trial of olanzapine in children, adolescents, and adults with pervasive developmental disorders, significant behavioral improvement was documented within the first several weeks of treatment (Potenza et al. 1999). Similarly, a case report by Horrigan et al. (1997) concluded that olanzapine was associated with decreased aggression toward people and property and fewer explosive outbursts in youth. A 10-week open-label study reported reduced ADHD and aggression symptoms with the combination of olanzapine and atomoxetine given to youth with

ADHD and comorbid DBDs (Holzer et al. 2013). Although these reports suggest that olanzapine may have a role in treating aggression and DBDs, firm conclusions about its potential efficacy cannot be reached without further studies.

Quetiapine

A 7-week RCT of quetiapine involving 19 adolescents with CD showed benefit in the treatment of aggressive behaviors in CD (Connor et al. 2008). Findings from an 8-week open-label trial involving 16 youth with CD suggested that quetiapine may be effective in the treatment of aggression in that population (Findling et al. 2006). In the 26-week open-label extension of that trial, the benefit of quetiapine was found to be sustained, and medications were well tolerated (Findling et al. 2007). One open-label trial of quetiapine and methylphenidate found a reduction in aggression and ADHD symptoms in youth with severe aggression whose symptoms did not respond to methylphenidate monotherapy (Kronenberger et al. 2007). An open-label trial of low-dose quetiapine in youth with ASD reported decreased severity of aggressive behavior (Golubchik et al. 2011). Quetiapine had similar efficacy compared with risperidone in reducing aggression in adolescents with bipolar II disorder and comorbid CD in a 12-week, open-label, flexible-dose trial (Masi et al. 2015). At this time, further research on quetiapine in the treatment of aggression and DBDs is needed (see Table 3–1 for dosage information).

Aripiprazole

Aripiprazole is FDA-approved for the management of irritability associated with ASD in children, based on two short-term RCTs that support its efficacy (Marcus et al. 2009; Owen et al. 2009). Findings from a 52-week open-label study of aripiprazole in youth with ASD support the medication's efficacy in long-term reduction of irritable symptoms (Marcus et al. 2011). However, one RCT reported no statistical significance between aripiprazole and placebo in preventing relapse of irritable symptoms in youth with ASD during a 16-week period of maintenance therapy (Findling et al. 2014b). In an open-label study of youth with CD, aripiprazole was well tolerated and was associated with improvements in aggressive behaviors. The authors also found that lower starting dosages of aripiprazole improved tolerability and reduced side effects in youth (Findling et al. 2009). Another open-label study of children and adolescents with ADHD and CD reported that aripiprazole reduced symptoms of both disorders (Ercan et al. 2012). Further evaluation of aripiprazole in the treatment of DBDs is warranted (see Table 3–1 for dosage information).

Clozapine

To date, no RCTs have evaluated the efficacy of clozapine in the treatment of aggressive symptoms in children or adults. However, several case studies have suggested that clozapine is an effective treatment for aggression in adults (Rabinowitz et al. 1996; Volavka and Citrome 1999). Significant reductions in physical and verbal aggression were seen in 75 adults with schizophrenia over 6 months of clozapine treatment (Rabinowitz et al. 1996). Few studies have evaluated clozapine's effectiveness in the treatment of aggression in youth (Chalasani et al. 2001; Kranzler et al. 2005). In a chart review of six children and adolescents with schizophrenia spectrum disorders treated with clozapine, violent episodes reduced significantly and global function improved significantly (Chalasani et al. 2001). Similarly, an open-label study by Kranzler et al. (2005) indicated that clozapine yielded significant pre-to-post benefits in patients with treatment-refractory schizophrenia and aggression. An open, naturalistic, observational study reported that treatment with clozapine led to reductions in aggression over a 26-week period in youth with CD (Teixeira et al. 2013). Finally, findings from a retrospective cohort study of patients with ASD and severe DBDs suggest that clozapine may decrease aggressiveness in patients whose symptoms are treatment resistant (Beherec et al. 2011). Nonetheless, additional research is needed to assess the efficacy of clozapine in the treatment of aggression and DBDs in youth (see Table 3–1 for dosage information).

Other Atypical Antipsychotics

Available data have not demonstrated efficacy of ziprasidone in the management of aggressive symptoms in youth with DBDs. One RCT of low-dose ziprasidone in youth with DBDs found no significant difference between the treatment and placebo groups (Fleischhaker et al. 2011). Therefore, additional research is needed to further assess the comparative efficacy of other atypical antipsychotics. This research may be especially beneficial in treatment planning for youth with DBDs and/or aggression in light of the reported efficacy of the other atypical antipsychotics (principally risperidone) that have been extensively studied. Moreover, it would be of great clinical relevance for assessing the different side effect profiles of the various atypical antipsychotics to meet the need for a wider array of safe and effective therapeutic agents in the management of aggressive symptoms and DBDs in youth (see Table 3–1 for dosage information).

Risks and Benefits of Atypical Antipsychotics

Overall, atypical antipsychotics have demonstrated efficacy in reducing aggressive behaviors in youth. To date, risperidone and aripiprazole have the most evidence to support their use in the treatment of aggression.

Similar to many other medications, atypical antipsychotics are associated with mild to moderate side effects, including extrapyramidal symptoms, somnolence, headache, increases in prolactin levels, gynecomastia, and weight gain (Aman et al. 2004; Peuskens et al. 2014; Rosenbloom 2010; Snyder et al. 2002). Of particular importance to pediatric care providers, youth treated with these agents appear to experience significantly greater weight gain than adults using atypical antipsychotics, even at low dosages (Sikich et al. 2004). Less commonly reported problems in youth may include type 2 diabetes and cardiac rhythm abnormalities, but more studies may be needed to address concerns about these possible side effects (Schur et al. 2003). Data on a retrospective cohort of more than 9,000 children and adolescents suggest a significant increase in the incidence of diabetes mellitus in those treated with atypical antipsychotics (Andrade et al. 2011). In children and adolescents, long-term risks typically associated with atypical antipsychotic use also include withdrawal symptoms, tardive dyskinesia, parkinsonism, and neuroleptic malignant syndrome. Table 3–2 provides additional information on the potential side effects of atypical antipsychotics.

Because atypical antipsychotics are associated with an array of serious side effects, the FDA has required that these medications carry warning labels to specifically indicate their potential risk for increased weight gain and disruption of metabolic functioning (Stigler et al. 2004; U.S. Food and Drug Administration 2005). Given the concerns about side effects and the increasing rates at which atypical antipsychotics are being prescribed to youth with symptoms of aggression (Olfson et al. 2006), additional studies are necessary to examine the safety of these agents in the treatment of aggression in this population.

Table 3–2. Common and serious side effects for various classes of psychopharmacological agents

Class	Common side effects	Serious or uncommon side effects
Atypical antipsychotics	Insomnia, agitation, extrapyramidal symptoms, headache, anxiety, rhinitis, constipation, nausea/vomiting, dyspepsia, dizziness, dyslipidemia, tachycardia, somnolence, increased dream activity, dry mouth, diarrhea, weight gain, visual disturbance, sexual dysfunction, hyperprolactinemia, gynecomastia, menstrual irregularities	Hypotension, severe syncope (rare), severe tardive dyskinesia, neuroleptic malignant syndrome, hyperglycemia, severe diabetes mellitus, seizures (rare), priapism (rare), stroke, transient ischemic attack
Typical antipsychotics	Extrapyramidal symptoms, tardive dyskinesia, akathisia, dystonia, insomnia, anxiety, drowsiness, lethargy, weight changes, anticholinergic effects, gynecomastia, breast tenderness, galactorrhea, menstrual irregularities, injection-site reaction (depot), elevated prolactin levels	Neuroleptic malignant syndrome, pneumonia, arrhythmia, hypotension, hypertension, seizures, jaundice, hyperpyrexia, heat stroke
Stimulants	Nervousness, insomnia, abdominal pain, nausea, anorexia, motor tics, headache, palpitations, dizziness, blurred vision, tachycardia, weight loss, fever, depression, transient drowsiness, dyskinesia, angina, rash, urticaria, blood pressure changes	Growth suppression (long term), seizures, dependence, abuse, arrhythmia, leukopenia (rare), thrombocytopenic purpura (rare), toxic psychosis (rare), Tourette's disorder (rare), exfoliative dermatitis (rare), erythema multiforme (rare), neuroleptic malignant syndrome (rare), cerebral arteritis (rare), hepatotoxicity (rare)

Table 3–2. Common and serious side effects for various classes of psychopharmacological agents *(continued)*

Class	Common side effects	Serious or uncommon side effects
Norepinephrine reuptake inhibitor	Nausea, vomiting, fatigue, decreased appetite, abdominal pain, somnolence, insomnia, constipation, dry mouth, dizziness, sexual dysfunction, urinary hesitancy	Suicidal ideation (rare), severe hepatic injury (rare), sudden death (rare), stroke (rare), myocardial infarction (rare), dysphoria (rare), irritability (rare), severe mood lability (rare), hallucinations (rare), mania (rare), aggressive behavior
Mood stabilizers	Enuresis, fatigue, ataxia, increased thirst, nausea, vomiting, urinary frequency, gastrointestinal upset, sleepiness, weight gain	Disruption in hepatic, hematological, and metabolic functioning
α_2 Agonists	Drowsiness and dizziness, dry mouth, irritability, dysphoria, rebound hypertension, abdominal pain, headache, agitation	Syncope (rare), hypotension (rare)
β-Blockers	Sedation, mild hypotension, lowered heart rate, bronchoconstriction, dizziness, sleep disruption	Hypoglycemia (in patients with diabetes), growth-hormone regulation issues

Note. Side effects for specific medications may vary within classes; specific details of differences among specific agents can be found elsewhere (Connor et al. 2001; Pappadopulos et al. 2003; Weiner 1996).

Source. Center for the Advancement of Children's Mental Health, Office of Mental Health: "10 Tips: Navigating Child and Adolescent Inpatient and Residential Services in New York State." Unpublished document.

Typical Antipsychotics

Haloperidol

Prior to the emergence of atypical antipsychotics, conventional antipsychotics were considered first-line agents in the treatment of aggression and DBDs in youth (see Campbell et al. 1999). Haloperidol may be an effective means to treat aggression; for example, during a double-blind study of inpatient youth (ages 5.2–12.9) with treatment-resistant CD, a significant reduction in aggressive symptoms was seen in those given haloperidol compared with those given placebo (Campbell et al. 1984). However, a double-blind, placebo-controlled study of haloperidol in the treatment of aggression in adolescents with subaverage intelligence found that the treatment led to only moderate behavioral improvements (Aman et al. 1989). See Table 3–1 for dosage information.

Other Typical Antipsychotics

Several early studies of thioridazine suggest its efficacy in managing aggressive symptoms in youth. For example, an RCT of thioridazine in children with subaverage intelligence showed modest clinical improvements in symptoms of aggression (Aman et al. 1991), with thioridazine leading to a reduction in hyperactivity and conduct problems. A meta-analysis of three RCTs of antipsychotics suggested a lower effect size for thioridazine (0.35) versus haloperidol (0.8) in the management of aggression in youth. Chlorpromazine was associated with reduction in aggressive symptoms in youth with CD; however, this agent was difficult to tolerate due to sedation (Campbell et al. 1972).

Risks and Benefits of Typical Antipsychotics

Early studies suggested that low dosages of typical antipsychotics were effective for managing aggressive behaviors in youth. However, typical antipsychotics can be associated with adverse events (see Table 3–2), including an increased occurrence of extrapyramidal symptoms and tardive dyskinesia (Connor et al. 2001; McConville and Sorter 2004). Therefore, the risks and benefits of treatment with this drug class in a given patient should be evaluated before initiating therapy. It is often wise to consider the patient's personal and family history of medication response, current medical comorbidities (diabetes, cardiac and neurological problems), weight, psychiatric diagnoses, and other factors when making a decision to start medications treatment.

Stimulants

Methylphenidate

Short-term efficacy. To date, a growing number of short-term RCTs have provided evidence for the efficacy of methylphenidate and other stimulants in the treatment of aggression and DBDs in youth. In fact, treatment with methylphenidate was shown to improve emotional impulsivity and self-regulation in about half of youth with ADHD (Connor et al. 2002). The effect size of stimulants in the management of symptoms in aggressive youth is medium to large, ranging from 0.69 to 0.84 (Faraone et al. 2020). Moreover, the use of methylphenidate and other stimulants to treat aggression appears to have a substantial treatment effect that is independent from effects on core ADHD symptoms in youth with ADHD and aggressive behavior. For example, an RCT testing the efficacy of methylphenidate in 84 children with CD with or without ADHD found significant reductions in core behaviors associated with CD, independent of the effects on the children's ADHD symptoms (Klein et al. 1997). Another RCT of methylphenidate in 31 children with ADHD and comorbid tic disorder found improvement of oppositional behavior and peer aggression (Gadow et al. 2008).

Long-term and maintenance efficacy. Several reports from the NIMH's Multimodal Treatment of ADHD (MTA) study have explored longer-term treatment for youth experiencing comorbid IA and ADHD. For example, the MTA study's 14-month follow-up indicated that stimulants (principally methylphenidate) not only alleviated the core symptoms of ADHD but also reduced the secondary symptoms of ODD and aggression (MTA Cooperative Group 1999) as rated on the revised Swanson, Nolan, and Pelham rating scale (SNAP-IV; Swanson et al. 2001). However, symptoms of aggression and oppositionality that are present along with internalizing disorders such as depression or anxiety may improve most with psychopharmacological treatment used in combination with a behavioral intervention (Jensen et al. 2001). Despite promising results with stimulants in treating aggressive behaviors in some youth, about 44% of children with aggression remain aggressive after a stimulant trial (Jensen et al. 2007). Overall, the evidence suggests that methylphenidate may be efficacious in treating aggressive symptoms associated with DBDs and ADHD.

Other Stimulants

Although methylphenidate is the most common stimulant used in RCTs for the treatment of ADHD and co-occurring aggressive symptoms, some evidence suggests that other stimulants may also be efficacious (see also Chapter 2, "Attention-Deficit/Hyperactivity Disorder"). One open-label study of lisdexamfetamine found improvement of ADHD symptoms and emotional control functioning as rated on the Behavior Rating Inventory of Executive Function (BRIEF; Katic et al. 2013). Given the small number of studies currently available for evaluation, however, more research on stimulants other than methylphenidate is required to determine whether they are comparable with methylphenidate for the treatment of aggression (see Table 3–1 for dosage information).

Benefits of Stimulants

Stimulants are recommended as a first-line treatment for youth with comorbid ADHD and aggression (Pappadopulos et al. 2006). The rationale for stimulant use in the management of aggressive symptoms of ADHD or behavior disorder is based on the number of controlled trials demonstrating its efficacy and its large overall effect size (Connor et al. 2002; Pappadopulos et al. 2006). In contrast to earlier concerns regarding stimulant usage, MTA data also suggest that stimulant use is effective in treating ADHD, even among youth who present with co-occurring symptoms of mania and aggression (Galanter et al. 2003). Youth with comorbid ADHD and aggression may be more likely than nonaggressive youth to experience an insufficient response to stimulant monotherapy and may require more rigorous dosing for symptom remission (Blader et al. 2010). Stimulant treatment also appears to yield improvements in global functioning and social interaction (Bukstein and Kolko 1998; MTA Cooperative Group 1999; Swanson et al. 2001).

Risks of Stimulants

Despite their efficacy, stimulants are associated with several adverse effects, including insomnia, reduced appetite, stomachache, headache, and dizziness. In addition, the FDA has recommended that stimulants be labeled with a black box warning indicating their potential for adverse cardiac effects in children (U.S. Food and Drug Administration 2022). Please refer to Chapter 2 for further details on the risks of stimulant medications.

Mood Stabilizers

Lithium

Most existing literature on the efficacy of mood stabilizers in the treatment of aggression in children and adolescents has focused on the use of lithium in patients with CD. Overall, these results suggest that lithium is associated with a reduction in aggressive behavior (Campbell et al. 1992, 1995; Malone et al. 2000). For example, in one RCT, inpatient youth with a primary diagnosis of CD received either lithium or placebo (Campbell et al. 1995). Lithium was associated with a reduction in aggressive behaviors across a number of standardized measures, including the Children's Psychiatric Symptom Rating Scale (CPRS). An RCT comparing lithium and placebo in 40 children with CD demonstrated improvements in aggressive behaviors, as measured by the OAS, for those who received lithium (Malone et al. 2000).

Overall, lithium has been shown to reduce temper outbursts in severely aggressive, inpatient children and adolescents with CD (Campbell et al. 1984, 1995; Carlson et al. 1992; Malone et al. 2000). This evidence implies that lithium may have an important role in the treatment of IA in youth. However, the necessity of frequent monitoring and blood draws associated with this treatment may render it a second-line choice after pharmacological agents such as the atypical antipsychotics (Pappadopulos et al. 2003) (see Table 3–1 for dosage information).

Divalproex

Some evidence indicates that divalproex is effective in reducing aggressive symptoms and DBDs in youth. For example, in one RCT, improvement in impulse control was observed in incarcerated male youth who were treated with high doses of divalproex; moreover, global improvements among the patients, as measured by the CGI scale (Steiner et al. 2003a), were also noted. Similarly, another trial found that divalproex was associated with a reduction in aggressive symptoms in youth with CD (Donovan et al. 2000, 2003). Evidence also suggests that divalproex may be especially beneficial for treating children and adolescents who present with severe IA (Donovan et al. 1997) as well as for treating IA symptoms in those with pervasive developmental disorders (Hollander et al. 2001). Another RCT found that when administered adjunctive treatment with a stimulant and divalproex, 30 youth with ADHD and chronic aggression refractory to stimulant monotherapy had higher rates of remission of aggressive behavior compared with placebo (Blader et al. 2009).

An RCT involving 58 male subjects with severe CD in the juvenile justice system found significantly higher response to divalproex among male youth with IA than among those with PA (Padhy et al. 2011). Another RCT directly compared adjunct divalproex, risperidone, and placebo when added to optimized stimulant therapy in children ages 6–12 years (Blader et al. 2021). Both the divalproex and risperidone groups demonstrated significant reductions in aggressive behavior when compared with placebo, although the participants given risperidone gained more weight. Therefore, evidence suggests that divalproex may be efficacious in treating youth with an array of psychiatric disorders, including CD, ADHD, and bipolar disorder, whose behavior includes severe IA (see Table 3–1 for dosage information).

Carbamazepine

The use of carbamazepine and other mood stabilizers/anticonvulsants in the treatment of aggressive disorders has increased twofold over the past decade and a half (Hunkeler et al. 2005). Data on the efficacy of carbamazepine in the management of aggression in youth are limited and mixed. Preliminary research indicates that carbamazepine may lead to decreases in aggressiveness and explosiveness, with a moderate effect size (Evans et al. 1987; Kafantaris et al. 1992; Pappadopulos et al. 2006). On the other hand, countervailing evidence suggests that carbamazepine does not differ from placebo in reducing aggression (Cueva et al. 1996). Thus, the results are inconclusive with regard to the efficacy of carbamazepine (see Table 3–1 for dosage information).

Benefits of Mood Stabilizers

In general, some mood stabilizers appear to be beneficial in the treatment of aggression in youth with behavior disorders. A mood stabilizer such as lithium may be a suitable alternative to atypical antipsychotics or stimulants. Overall, the current evidence largely supports the efficacy of lithium and divalproex in the treatment of IA in youth with CD. However, because many of the symptoms of CD correspond to PA, more research is needed to determine whether either subtype of aggression responds differentially to mood stabilizers.

Risks of Mood Stabilizers

To date, studies pertaining to mood stabilizers in the treatment of aggression in youth have been limited in that they have measured only short-term treatment outcomes. Therefore, certain adverse effects may not become evident during the limited duration of these studies but may appear in trials spanning longer periods. Additional research is needed to measure the risks, benefits, and efficacy of mood stabilizers in aggressive youth in an array of settings (e.g., outpatient and emergency care).

Mood stabilizers are associated with a variety of adverse side effects (see Table 3–2). Common side effects of lithium include enuresis, fatigue, ataxia, increased thirst, nausea, vomiting, urinary frequency, and weight gain (Bassarath 2003; Malone et al. 2000). Moreover, frequent blood draws for dosage monitoring are required; thus, lithium may be less suitable for children who have difficulty tolerating blood draws (Malone et al. 2000). Side effects associated with divalproex include gastrointestinal upset and sleepiness (Steiner et al. 2003b). Carbamazepine may carry the greatest risk for adverse side effects among the mood stabilizers and has been linked to disruption in hepatic, hematological, and metabolic functioning (Cummings and Miller 2004). In 2008, the FDA found that patients treated with anticonvulsants had nearly twice the risk of suicidal ideation or behavior compared with those given placebo and therefore mandated warning labeling for anticonvulsant medications (U.S. Food and Drug Administration 2008).

Other Agents

α_2 Agonists

Clonidine. Some evidence supports the use of α_2 agonists in the treatment of aggressive symptoms and DBDs among children and adolescents. Specifically, clonidine has demonstrated efficacy in the treatment of aggression in youth, according to a meta-analysis of 11 double-blind RCTs (Connor et al. 1999). Hazell and Stuart (2003) reported gains in a 6-week randomized, double-blind, placebo-controlled trial of a combined clonidine-plus-stimulant treatment. Specifically, conduct problems were improved in youth with ADHD and comorbid ODD or CD. Further research on clonidine in the treatment of aggression and DBDs is needed (see Table 3–1 for dosage information).

Guanfacine. Guanfacine demonstrated efficacy in the treatment of aggressive symptoms in an 8-week RCT involving 34 youth ages 7–15 with ADHD and a tic disorder (Scahill et al. 2001). A 9-week RCT of extended-release guanfacine in 217 youth with ADHD and oppositional symptoms resulted in a significant reduction in both oppositional and ADHD symptoms (Connor et al. 2010). Furthermore, one RCT (Findling et al. 2014a) involving youth with ADHD whose symptoms responded suboptimally to stimulant monotherapy demonstrated reductions in oppositional symptoms after the participants received extended-release guanfacine. Thus, it appears that guanfacine may be beneficial in the treatment of oppositional symptoms in youth with comorbid ADHD; however, further research is needed to provide conclusive support for the use of this agent in the treatment of DBDs in this population (see Table 3–1 for dosage information).

Risks and benefits of α_2 agonists. Overall, α_2 agonists have shown promise when added to stimulants in the treatment of aggression in children with ADHD. Additional research is needed to compare the efficacy of α_2 agonists with that of other psychotropic agents in the treatment of aggressive symptoms in youth with behavior disorders.

The α_2 agonists are associated with several adverse side effects, including drowsiness, dizziness, headache, abdominal pain, and changes in blood pressure and heart rate (Cantwell et al. 1997; Connor et al. 2010). Earlier reports warned against the risk of syncopal episodes, whereas more recent studies did not find a high risk of serious adverse events. Nevertheless, caution should be executed in administering α_2 agonists to youth, and their vital signs should be frequently checked. (See Table 3–2 for additional details on the potential adverse effects associated with α_2 agonists.)

β-Blockers

Current literature on the efficacy of β-blockers in the treatment of aggression in youth is sparse. Connor et al. (1997) reported treatment gains for more than 80% of children and adults with developmental disabilities who were prescribed β-blockers to manage symptoms of aggression (see Table 3–1 for dosage information). To date, no RCTs on the use of β-blockers in the treatment of youth have been conducted. Therefore, firm conclusions about the efficacy of these agents cannot be drawn. Some of the adverse effects associated with β-blockers include sedation, mild hypotension, lowered heart rate, bronchoconstriction, hypoglycemia (in patients with diabetes), dizziness, sleep disruption, and potential growth-hormone regulation disturbances (see Table 3–2) (Riddle et al. 1999). Further research is needed on the benefits and risks associated with using β-blockers to treat youth with aggressive symptoms.

Norepinephrine Reuptake Inhibitors

Atomoxetine. In an RCT evaluating atomoxetine treatment of comorbid ADHD and ODD, Newcorn et al. (2005) found that atomoxetine improves ADHD and ODD symptoms and suggested that higher dosages may be needed to treat youth who meet criteria for both conditions. However, a meta-analysis of aggression in RCTs of atomoxetine found that the risk of aggressive or hostile events in patients taking atomoxetine was not statistically significant from that in those given placebo (Polzer et al. 2007). Despite the fact that atomoxetine did not improve aggressive symptoms, it may be beneficial in the treatment of ODD, as seen in a randomized, placebo-controlled, double-blind study of 180 youth with ADHD and comorbid ODD (Dittmann et al. 2011). The group receiving atomoxetine had significant reductions in symptoms of ADHD and ODD after 9 weeks of treatment. A meta-analysis of 25 RCTs reported that atomoxetine had a medium effect size of 0.33 in treating ODD symptoms in youth with ADHD (Schwartz and Correll 2014). Finally, an RCT of 97 patients with ADHD and ASD reported significant improvement in ADHD symptoms but no difference from placebo in oppositional subscale measures (Harfterkamp et al. 2012). Further research on the long-term benefits and risks associated with using atomoxetine to treat youth with DBDs is needed.

Risks of norepinephrine reuptake inhibitors. Children and adolescents who take atomoxetine may experience dry mouth, fatigue, irritability, nausea, appetite change, constipation, dizziness, sweating, dysuria, urinary retention or hesitancy, priapism, increased obsessive behaviors, weight changes, palpitations, suicidal ideation, hepatic injury, increased heart rate, and increased blood pressure. Six cases of drug-induced liver injury were reported between 2005 and 2008 (U.S. Food and Drug Administration 2009). The FDA has mandated a black box warning for atomoxetine because of increased risk of suicidal ideation in children and adolescents (Gephart 2005).

Safety Issues

Monitoring

Antipsychotics

Height and weight should be thoroughly monitored during treatment with antipsychotic agents. If weight gain is identified in a patient taking these agents, the physician should implement a diet and exercise plan. Vital signs, with particular attention to cardiac function, should also be routinely assessed in patients taking antipsychotics (Schur et al. 2003). If cardiac symptoms emerge, the physician should consider consulting with a cardiology specialist.

In youth taking typical or atypical antipsychotics, physicians should carefully monitor for extrapyramidal symptoms such as akathisia, akinesia, tremor, dystonia, and emergent tardive dyskinesia (Connor et al. 2001; McConville and Sorter 2004). Furthermore, youth should be routinely screened for abnormalities in liver function and lipid production, particularly in the presence of weight gain. Monitoring of glucose metabolism is important, given that certain agents may be linked to juvenile diabetes (Clark and Burge 2003). Furthermore, prolactin levels should be monitored if endocrine abnormalities are suspected (Wudarsky et al. 1999). Patients should be monitored for rare but life-threatening side effects, including neuroleptic malignant syndrome, seizures, and heat stroke. Finally, one cohort study of 153 youth with DBDs, Tourette's disorder, and ASD reported that combining stimulant treatment with atypical antipsychotics did not significantly reduce the risk for weight gain and metabolic changes caused by atypical antipsychotics (Penzner et al. 2009).

Stimulants

Children and adolescents who are prescribed stimulants should be routinely monitored for adverse symptoms, including insomnia, reduced appetite, stomachache, headache, and dizziness (Lisska and Rivkees 2003; MTA Cooperative Group 1999). Stimulant use has been linked to long-term adverse effects, including height and weight suppression; therefore, it is important for vital signs, height and weight, and abnormalities in metabolic function to be thoroughly monitored throughout the course of treatment. If the stimulant is being taken concurrently with another psychopharmacological agent, such as clonidine, additional caution is recommended (Fenichel and Lipicky 1994).

Mood Stabilizers

Certain mood-stabilizing agents such as lithium require frequent blood draws for dosage monitoring and therefore may be less suitable in the treatment of children who have difficulty tolerating blood draws (Bassarath 2003; Malone et al. 2000). In addition, common side effects associated with mood stabilizers include enuresis, fatigue, ataxia, increased thirst, nausea, vomiting, and urinary frequency. Therefore, careful monitoring of these symptoms is required. Moreover, because weight gain is associated with the use of mood stabilizers, height and weight should be monitored during the treatment course. Importantly, because carbamazepine has been linked to serious adverse effects, including hepatotoxic, hematological, and metabolic reactions, comprehensive assessment of these systems is important (Cummings and Miller 2004).

α_2 *Agonists*

Careful thought is needed before prescribing α_2 agonists to youth with aggression. Concerns about the safety of these agents have been raised following reports of harmful and potentially life-threatening side effects in several children treated with clonidine (Cantwell et al. 1997). Careful monitoring of vital signs and educating patients and families about the risks of rebound hypertension with abrupt discontinuation of α_2 agonists should minimize safety concerns. Moreover, clonidine can produce drowsiness and dizziness, and patients should be routinely monitored for these symptoms (Hazell and Stuart 2003).

Preventing Adverse Effects

Conservative dosing procedures may prevent the possible occurrence of adverse effects in youth taking psychopharmacological agents. The general rule of thumb is to "start low, go slow, and taper slowly" (Pappadopulos et al. 2003). Potential side effects should be monitored on a systematic basis with rating scales or structured assessment methods (Pappadopulos et al. 2003). It is best to avoid polypharmacy whenever possible to prevent adverse effects. Youth who remain aggressive may require medication changes rather than the addition of other agents. In addition, if aggressive symptoms remit for a significant period of time, providers may consider initiating a slow taper of medications. If the treatment response is maintained during the taper, it may be possible to eventually discontinue the medications.

Interventions to Address Adverse Effects of Psychotropic Agents

The side effects of pharmacological interventions range in severity from life-threatening, irreversible, and acutely distressing to merely uncomfortable. In Table 3–2, we separate the potential side effects of various psychotropic agents into two categories: common and uncommon but serious. As a general rule of thumb, if the side effect is considered serious, the medication must be discontinued. In some cases, consultation with a specialist is appropriate to address adverse events. Once the serious adverse event is resolved, a different psychopharmacological intervention may be a suitable next step.

Practical Management Strategies

Treatment Guidelines

As discussed earlier, several studies suggest the efficacy of some psychopharmacological agents for the treatment of aggression associated with DBDs. However, these trials have limitations that make it difficult for clinicians to choose specific medications for their patients. Some of the problems discussed earlier in this chapter involve the different inclusion diagnoses used to enroll participants into the studies. In addition, several versions of DSM have been published since the first trials of aggression were conducted; therefore, it is often difficult to compare the results of those studies. For example, as discussed previously, the criteria for the CD changed dramatically over the past 20 years, and the results of the earlier studies on CD may not be comparable with more recent studies on CD. In addition, very few trials have offered head-to-head comparisons of the medications used; therefore, the possibility of comparing their efficacy is lacking.

Practice parameters offer some insight to help clinicians make decisions on evidence-based psychopharmacology. Unfortunately, the American Academy of Child and Adolescent Psychiatry practice parameters are outdated and therefore are not discussed in this chapter (see www.jaacap.org). However, specific clinical guidelines have been developed by other sources for the management and treatment of maladaptive aggression in youth (Knapp et al. 2012; Pappadopulos et al. 2003; Scotto Rosato et al. 2012). Jensen et al. (2004) created Treatment Recommendations for the Use of Antipsychotic

Medications for Aggressive Youth using evidence and consensus-based methodologies. The Centers for Education and Research on (Mental Health) Therapeutics (CERT) Treatment of Maladaptive Aggression in Youth (T-MAY) was created to identify specific practice guidelines for outpatient management of youth with severe and persistent behavioral issues (Pappadopulos et al. 2011). These guidelines suggest starting treatment with family engagement, performing a full assessment, and establishing a diagnosis. Further recommendations include engaging in family skills training, targeting underlying psychiatric disorders with evidence-based guidelines, avoiding polypharmacy, and monitoring for treatment response and side effects (Scotto Rosato et al. 2012).

The T-MAY recommendations can be briefly summarized as follows. Patients and families should be engaged during an initial evaluation (preferably using a standardized assessment tool) before starting psychosocial treatment to manage aggressive symptoms. The provider should obtain collateral information, provide psychoeducation, and monitor aggressive symptoms with the child and their parents in order to develop an appropriate plan and establish community supports. If at any time the patient presents with significant aggression risk factors, they should be referred to a mental health clinician (or to the emergency department) for acute management. Typically, an evidence-based psychosocial intervention is a first-line method of treatment in an aggressive youth. If psychotherapy is not successful in reducing the aggressive behaviors, evidence-based psychopharmacological treatment of the underlying condition may be warranted. If the youth's symptoms fail to improve with the agent best suited for their primary disorder, adding an atypical antipsychotic is recommended. Regardless of the psychopharmacological approach, it is wise to use a conservative dosing strategy. During the course of treatment, the physician should routinely and systematically assess the youth for potential adverse effects and ensure an adequate trial of the agent before modifying the treatment plan. (For additional information about the T-MAY and the CERT guidelines, see Knapp et al. 2012; Pappadopulos et al. 2003; Scotto Rosato et al. 2012.)

Role of Nonmedication Interventions

Regardless of whether a psychopharmacological intervention is ultimately used, psychoeducation is a critical component of the successful treatment of aggressive disorders in youth. Psychoeducation enables the patient and family to understand and identify triggers for aggressive behaviors as well as to figure out which coping skills and other interventions are most successful. Moreover, it helps them learn about plausible treatment options, including psychopharmacological treatments and behavioral interventions.

As noted in the T-MAY guidelines, empirically supported behavioral interventions should typically constitute the first-line treatment approach for aggressive youth (Knapp et al. 2012; Scotto Rosato et al. 2012). Evidence-based psychosocial interventions for aggression in youth include cognitive-behavioral therapy for aggressive disorders and parent management training. These evidence-based treatments work to increase positive time that the youth and family members spend together, help set rules and consequences, and provide training on problem-solving and social skills. Other psychosocial interventions have been considered for addressing DBDs (Waddell et al. 2018); however, a review of behavioral interventions is beyond the scope of this chapter. It is important to note that moderate to severe aggressive symptoms in youth typically require a combination of psychoeducation, cognitive and behavioral management strategies, and pharmacological agents.

Involvement of Others

It is often necessary to involve community supports to help the child and family deal with aggressive behaviors. These may include teachers, youth leaders, sports coaches, and other important adults in the child's life. Parents often benefit from attending support groups themselves. Many such groups are offered online and thus are accessible even to people living in remote areas. Organizations offering such groups include the National Alliance on Mental Illness (www.nami.org), Children and Adults with Attention-Deficit/Hyperactivity Disorder (www.chadd.org), the Depression and Bipolar Support Alliance (www.dbsalliance.org), the National Federation of Families for Children's Mental Health (www.ffcmh.org), and Mental Health America (formerly the National Mental Health Association; www.mentalhealthamerica.net).

It is important to provide evidence-based psychotherapeutic support for children and families. Various psychosocial interventions have been developed for treating aggression and related conduct problems, including parent management training (Brestan and Eyberg 1998; Burke et al. 2002; Kazdin et al. 1989, 1992), parent-child interaction therapy (Schuhmann et al. 1998), some school and community-based programs (Farmer et al. 2004), and some individual cognitive-behavioral treatments, including anger management training and problem-solving skills training (Brestan and Eyberg 1998; Lochman and Curry 1986; Lochman and Lampron 1988).

Conclusion

Several medications have shown promise in RCTs in addressing aggressive behaviors. However, further studies are needed to establish the short- and long-term efficacy, safety, and tolerability of psychotropic agents in managing the symptoms of aggression and DBDs in youth. More data comparing the efficacy of various agents are needed.

Additional research in systematically assessing and treating symptoms of PA and IA in youth is also needed. Because these two forms of aggression may have different etiological pathways, they may respond differently to various forms of treatment. Thus far, some, albeit limited, evidence suggests that certain psychopharmacological agents may be best suited to manage IA in youth. Moreover, the development of a standardized measure of aggression subtypes would assist in the goal of understanding and subsequently successfully treating the subtypes of aggression.

Clinical Pearls

- Carefully consider using and following the currently available evidence- and consensus-based guidelines to achieve the best possible outcomes.
- Treat the underlying condition first.
- Whenever possible, avoid polypharmacy. Consider adjusting the dosage of the current medication until either the maximum allowed dosage is reached or side effects develop.
- Always start low, go slow, and taper slowly.
- Assess and address compliance and adherence.
- Encourage youth and their parents to actively participate in psychosocial interventions.

References

Aman MG, Teehan CJ, White AJ, et al: Haloperidol treatment with chronically medicated residents: dose effects on clinical behavior and reinforcement contingencies. Am J Ment Retard 93(4):452–460, 1989 2649118

Aman MG, Marks RE, Turbott SH, et al: Clinical effects of methylphenidate and thioridazine in intellectually subaverage children. J Am Acad Child Adolesc Psychiatry 30(2):246–256, 1991 2016229

Aman MG, De Smedt G, Derivan A, et al: Double-blind, placebo-controlled study of risperidone for the treatment of disruptive behaviors in children with subaverage intelligence. Am J Psychiatry 159(8):1337–1346, 2002 12153826

Aman MG, Binder C, Turgay A: Risperidone effects in the presence/absence of psychostimulant medicine in children with ADHD, other disruptive behavior disorders, and subaverage IQ. J Child Adolesc Psychopharmacol 14(2):243–254, 2004 15319021

Aman MG, Bukstein OG, Gadow KD, et al: What does risperidone add to parent training and stimulant for severe aggression in child attention-deficit/hyperactivity disorder? J Am Acad Child Adolesc Psychiatry 53(1):47–60, 2014 24342385

American Psychiatric Association. Diagnostic and Statistical Manual of Mental Disorders, 3rd Edition, Revised. Washington, DC, 1987

American Psychiatric Association: Diagnostic and Statistical Manual of Mental Disorders, 4th Edition. Washington, DC, American Psychiatric Association, 1994

American Psychiatric Association: Diagnostic and Statistical Manual of Mental Disorders, 5th Edition, Text Revision. Washington, DC, American Psychiatric Association, 2022

Andrade SE, Lo JC, Roblin D, et al: Antipsychotic medication use among children and risk of diabetes mellitus. Pediatrics 128(6):1135–1141, 2011 22106077

Bambauer KZ, Connor DF: Characteristics of aggression in clinically referred children. CNS Spectr 10(9):709–718, 2005 16142211

Bassarath L: Medication strategies in childhood aggression: a review. Can J Psychiatry 48(6):367–373, 2003 12894610

Beherec L, Lambrey S, Quilici G, et al: Retrospective review of clozapine in the treatment of patients with autism spectrum disorder and severe disruptive behaviors. J Clin Psychopharmacol 31(3):341–344, 2011 21508854

Blader JC, Schooler NR, Jensen PS, et al: Adjunctive divalproex versus placebo for children with ADHD and aggression refractory to stimulant monotherapy. Am J Psychiatry 166(12):1392–1401, 2009 19884222

Blader JC, Pliszka SR, Jensen PS, et al: Stimulant-responsive and stimulant-refractory aggressive behavior among children with ADHD. Pediatrics 126(4):e796–e806, 2010 20837589

Blader JC, Pliszka SR, Kafantaris V, et al: Callous-unemotional traits, proactive aggression, and treatment outcomes of aggressive children with attention-deficit/hyperactivity disorder. J Am Acad Child Adolesc Psychiatry 52(12):1281–1293, 2013 24290461

Blader JC, Pliszka SR, Kafantaris V, et al: Stepped treatment for attention-deficit/hyperactivity disorder and aggressive behavior: a randomized, controlled trial of adjunctive risperidone, divalproex sodium, or placebo after stimulant medication optimization. J Am Acad Child Adolesc Psychiatry 60(2):236–251, 2021 32007604

Brestan EV, Eyberg SM: Effective psychosocial treatments of conduct-disordered children and adolescents: 29 years, 82 studies, and 5,272 kids. J Clin Child Psychol 27(2):180–189, 1998 9648035

Brown K, Atkins MS, Osborne ML, Milnamow M: A revised teacher rating scale for reactive and proactive aggression. J Abnorm Child Psychol 24(4):473–480, 1996 8886943

Buitelaar JK, van der Gaag RJ, Cohen-Kettenis P, Melman CT: A randomized controlled trial of risperidone in the treatment of aggression in hospitalized adolescents with subaverage cognitive abilities. J Clin Psychiatry 62(4):239–248, 2001 11379837

Bukstein OG, Kolko DJ: Effects of methylphenidate on aggressive urban children with attention deficit hyperactivity disorder. J Clin Child Psychol 27(3):340–351, 1998 9789193

Burke JD, Loeber R, Birmaher B: Oppositional defiant disorder and conduct disorder: a review of the past 10 years, part II. J Am Acad Child Adolesc Psychiatry 41(11):1275–1293, 2002 12410070

Burke JD, Waldman I, Lahey BB: Predictive validity of childhood oppositional defiant disorder and conduct disorder: implications for the DSM-5. J Abnorm Psychol 119(4):739–751, 2010 20853919

Burke JD, Rowe R, Boylan K: Functional outcomes of child and adolescent oppositional defiant disorder symptoms in young adult men. J Child Psychol Psychiatry 55(3):264–272, 2014 24117754

Campbell M, Fish B, Korein J, et al: Lithium and chlorpromazine: a controlled crossover study of hyperactive severely disturbed young children. J Autism Child Schizophr 2(3):234–263, 1972 4567547

Campbell M, Small AM, Green WH, et al: Behavioral efficacy of haloperidol and lithium carbonate: a comparison in hospitalized aggressive children with conduct disorder. Arch Gen Psychiatry 41(7):650–656, 1984 6428371

Campbell M, Gonzalez NM, Silva RR: The pharmacologic treatment of conduct disorders and rage outbursts. Psychiatr Clin North Am 15(1):69–85, 1992 1549549

Campbell M, Adams PB, Small AM, et al: Lithium in hospitalized aggressive children with conduct disorder: a double-blind and placebo-controlled study. J Am Acad Child Adolesc Psychiatry 34(4):445–453, 1995 7751258

Campbell M, Rapoport JL, Simpson GM: Antipsychotics in children and adolescents. J Am Acad Child Adolesc Psychiatry 38(5):537–545, 1999 10230185

Canino G, Polanczyk G, Bauermeister JJ, et al: Does the prevalence of CD and ODD vary across cultures? Soc Psychiatry Psychiatr Epidemiol 45(7):695–704, 2010 20532864

Cantwell DP, Swanson J, Connor DF: Case study: adverse response to clonidine. J Am Acad Child Adolesc Psychiatry 36(4):539–544, 1997 9100429

Carlson GA, Rapport MD, Pataki CS, Kelly KL: Lithium in hospitalized children at 4 and 8 weeks: mood, behavior and cognitive effects. J Child Psychol Psychiatry 33(2):411–425, 1992 1564083

Carroll D, Hallett V, McDougle CJ, et al: Examination of aggression and self-injury in children with autism spectrum disorders and serious behavioral problems. Child Adolesc Psychiatr Clin N Am 23(1):57–72, 2014 24231167

Chalasani L, Kant R, Chengappa KN: Clozapine impact on clinical outcomes and aggression in severely ill adolescents with childhood-onset schizophrenia. Can J Psychiatry 46(10):965–968, 2001 11816319

Clark C, Burge MR: Diabetes mellitus associated with atypical anti-psychotic medications. Diabetes Technol Ther 5(4):669–683, 2003 14511422

Coccaro EF, Posternak MA, Zimmerman M: Prevalence and features of intermittent explosive disorder in a clinical setting. J Clin Psychiatry 66(10):1221–1227, 2005 16259534

Connor DF: Aggression and Antisocial Behavior in Children and Adolescents: Research and Treatment. New York, Guilford, 2002

Connor DF, Ozbayrak KR, Benjamin S, et al: A pilot study of nadolol for overt aggression in developmentally delayed individuals. J Am Acad Child Adolesc Psychiatry 36(6):826–834, 1997 9183139

Connor DF, Fletcher KE, Swanson JM: A meta-analysis of clonidine for symptoms of attention-deficit hyperactivity disorder. J Am Acad Child Adolesc Psychiatry 38(12):1551–1559, 1999 10596256

Connor DF, Fletcher KE, Wood JS: Neuroleptic-related dyskinesias in children and adolescents. J Clin Psychiatry 62(12):967–974, 2001 11780878

Connor DF, Glatt SJ, Lopez ID, et al: Psychopharmacology and aggression I: a meta-analysis of stimulant effects on overt/covert aggression-related behaviors in ADHD. J Am Acad Child Adolesc Psychiatry 41(3):253–261, 2002 11886019

Connor DF, Steingard RJ, Cunningham JA, et al: Proactive and reactive aggression in referred children and adolescents. Am J Orthopsychiatry 74(2):129–136, 2004 15113242

Connor DF, McLaughlin TJ, Jeffers-Terry M: Randomized controlled pilot study of quetiapine in the treatment of adolescent conduct disorder. J Child Adolesc Psychopharmacol 18(2):140–156, 2008 18439112

Connor DF, Findling RL, Kollins SH, et al: Effects of guanfacine extended release on oppositional symptoms in children aged 6–12 years with attention-deficit hyperactivity disorder and oppositional symptoms: a randomized, double-blind, placebo-controlled trial. CNS Drugs 24(9):755–768, 2010 20806988

Connor DF, Newcorn JH, Saylor KE, et al: Maladaptive aggression: with a focus on impulsive aggression in children and adolescents. J Child Adolesc Psychopharmacol 29(8):576–591, 2019 31453715

Costello EJ, Egger H, Angold A: 10-year research update review: the epidemiology of child and adolescent psychiatric disorders: I. Methods and public health burden. J Am Acad Child Adolesc Psychiatry 44(10):972–986, 2005 16175102

Croonenberghs J, Fegert JM, Findling RL, et al: Risperidone in children with disruptive behavior disorders and subaverage intelligence: a 1-year, open-label study of 504 patients. J Am Acad Child Adolesc Psychiatry 44(1):64–72, 2005 15608545

Cueva JE, Overall JE, Small AM, et al: Carbamazepine in aggressive children with conduct disorder: a double-blind and placebo-controlled study. J Am Acad Child Adolesc Psychiatry 35(4):480–490, 1996 8919710

Cummings MR, Miller BD: Pharmacologic management of behavioral instability in medically ill pediatric patients. Curr Opin Pediatr 16(5):516–522, 2004 15367845

Dittmann RW, Schacht A, Helsberg K, et al: Atomoxetine versus placebo in children and adolescents with attention-deficit/hyperactivity disorder and comorbid oppositional defiant disorder: a double-blind, randomized, multicenter trial in Germany. J Child Adolesc Psychopharmacol 21(2):97–110, 2011 21488751

Dodge KA, Coie JD: Social-information-processing factors in reactive and proactive aggression in children's peer groups. J Pers Soc Psychol 53(6):1146–1158, 1987 3694454

Donovan SJ, Susser ES, Nunes EV, et al: Divalproex treatment of disruptive adolescents: a report of 10 cases. J Clin Psychiatry 58(1):12–15, 1997 9055831

Donovan SJ, Stewart JW, Nunes EV, et al: Divalproex treatment for youth with explosive temper and mood lability: a double-blind, placebo-controlled crossover design. Am J Psychiatry 157(5):818–820, 2000 10784478

Donovan SJ, Nunes EV, Stewart JW, et al: "Outer-directed irritability": a distinct mood syndrome in explosive youth with a disruptive behavior disorder? J Clin Psychiatry 64(6):698–701, 2003 12823085

dosReis S, Barnett S, Love RC, Riddle MA: A guide for managing acute aggressive behavior of youths in residential and inpatient treatment facilities. Psychiatr Serv 54(10):1357–1363, 2003 14557521

Ercan ES, Uysal T, Ercan E, Akyol Ardic U: Aripiprazole in children and adolescents with conduct disorder: a single-center, open-label study. Pharmacopsychiatry 45(1):13–19, 2012 21993869

Evans RW, Clay TH, Gualtieri CT: Carbamazepine in pediatric psychiatry. J Am Acad Child Adolesc Psychiatry 26(1):2–8, 1987 3583995

Faraone SV, Rostain AL, Montano CB, et al: Systematic review: nonmedical use of prescription stimulants: risk factors, outcomes, and risk reduction strategies. J Am Acad Child Adolesc Psychiatry 59(1):100–112, 2020 31326580

Farmer CA, Arnold LE, Bukstein OG, et al: The treatment of severe child aggression (TOSCA) study: design challenges. Child Adolesc Psychiatry Ment Health 5(1):36, 2011 22074813

Farmer CA, Brown NV, Gadow KD, et al: Comorbid symptomatology moderates response to risperidone, stimulant, and parent training in children with severe aggression, disruptive behavior disorder, and attention-deficit/hyperactivity disorder. J Child Adolesc Psychopharmacol 25(3):213–224, 2015 25885011

Farmer EM, Dorsey S, Mustillo SA: Intensive home and community interventions. Child Adolesc Psychiatr Clin N Am 13(4):857–884, vi, 2004 15380786

Fenichel RR, Lipicky RJ: Combination products as first-line pharmacotherapy. Arch Intern Med 154(13):1429–1430, 1994 7880229

Fernández-Mayoralas DM, Fernández-Jaén A, Muñoz-Jareño N, et al: Treatment with paliperidone in children with behavior disorders previously treated with risperidone: an open-label trial. Clin Neuropharmacol 35(5):227–230, 2012 22935606

Findling RL, McNamara NK, Branicky LA, et al: A double-blind pilot study of risperidone in the treatment of conduct disorder. J Am Acad Child Adolesc Psychiatry 39(4):509–516, 2000 10761354

Findling RL, Reed MD, O'Riordan MA, et al: Effectiveness, safety, and pharmacokinetics of quetiapine in aggressive children with conduct disorder. J Am Acad Child Adolesc Psychiatry 45(7):792–800, 2006 16832315

Findling RL, Reed MD, O'Riordan MA, et al: A 26-week open-label study of quetiapine in children with conduct disorder. J Child Adolesc Psychopharmacol 17(1):1–9, 2007 17343549

Findling RL, Kauffman R, Sallee FR, et al: An open-label study of aripiprazole: pharmacokinetics, tolerability, and effectiveness in children and adolescents with conduct disorder. J Child Adolesc Psychopharmacol 19(4):431–439, 2009 19702495

Findling RL, McBurnett K, White C, Youcha S: Guanfacine extended release adjunctive to a psychostimulant in the treatment of comorbid oppositional symptoms in children and adolescents with attention-deficit/hyperactivity disorder. J Child Adolesc Psychopharmacol 24(5):245–252, 2014a 24945085

Findling RL, Mankoski R, Timko K, et al: A randomized controlled trial investigating the safety and efficacy of aripiprazole in the long-term maintenance treatment of pediatric patients with irritability associated with autistic disorder. J Clin Psychiatry 75(1):22–30, 2014b 24502859

Findling RL, Townsend L, Brown NV, et al: The Treatment of Severe Childhood Aggression Study: 12 weeks of extended, blinded treatment in clinical responders. J Child Adolesc Psychopharmacol 27(1):52–65, 2017 28212067

Fite PJ, Raine A, Stouthamer-Loeber M, et al: Reactive and proactive aggression in adolescent males: examining differential outcomes 10 years later in early adulthood. Crim Justice Behav 37(2):141–157, 2009 20589225

Fleischhaker C, Hennighausen K, Schneider-Momm K, et al: Ziprasidone for severe conduct and other disruptive behavior disorders in children and adolescents: a placebo-controlled, randomized, double-blind clinical trial. Poster presented at the joint annual meeting of the American Academy of Child and Adolescent Psychiatry and the Canadian Academy of Child and Adolescent Psychiatry, Toronto, ON, Canada, October 2011

Fontaine NMG, McCrory EJP, Boivin M, et al: Predictors and outcomes of joint trajectories of callous-unemotional traits and conduct problems in childhood. J Abnorm Psychol 120(3):730–742, 2011 21341879

Gadow KD, Nolan EE, Sverd J, et al: Methylphenidate in children with oppositional defiant disorder and both comorbid chronic multiple tic disorder and ADHD. J Child Neurol 23(9):981–990, 2008 18474932

Gadow KD, Arnold LE, Molina BS, et al: Risperidone added to parent training and stimulant medication: effects on attention-deficit/hyperactivity disorder, oppositional defiant disorder, conduct disorder, and peer aggression. J Am Acad Child Adolesc Psychiatry 53(9):948–959, 2014 25151418

Gadow KD, Brown NV, Arnold LE, et al: Severely aggressive children receiving stimulant medication versus stimulant and risperidone: 12-month follow-up of the TOSCA Trial. J Am Acad Child Adolesc Psychiatry 55(6):469–478, 2016 27238065

Galanter CA, Carlson GA, Jensen PS, et al: Response to methylphenidate in children with attention deficit hyperactivity disorder and manic symptoms in the multimodal treatment study of children with attention deficit hyperactivity disorder titration trial. J Child Adolesc Psychopharmacol 13(2):123–136, 2003 12880507

Galbraith T, Carliner H, Keyes KM, et al: The co-occurrence and correlates of anxiety disorders among adolescents with intermittent explosive disorder. Aggress Behav 44(6):581–590, 2018 30040122

Gephart HR: FDA Public Health Advisory: Atomoxetine (Strattera) and Suicidal Thinking in Children and Adolescents. Rockville, MD, U.S. Food and Drug Administration. November 4, 2005. Available at: https://www.jwatch.org/pa200511040000009/2005/11/04/fda-public-health-advisory-atomoxetine-strattera. Accessed March 17, 2023.

Gillberg C, Hellgren L: Mental disturbances in adolescents: a knowledge review [in Swedish]. Nord Med 101(2):49–53, 1986 3951982

Golubchik P, Sever J, Weizman A: Low-dose quetiapine for adolescents with autistic spectrum disorder and aggressive behavior: open-label trial. Clin Neuropharmacol 34(6):216–219, 2011 21996644

Harfterkamp M, van de Loo-Neus G, Minderaa RB, et al: A randomized double-blind study of atomoxetine versus placebo for attention-deficit/hyperactivity disorder symptoms in children with autism spectrum disorder. J Am Acad Child Adolesc Psychiatry 51(7):733–741, 2012 22721596

Hazell PL, Stuart JE: A randomized controlled trial of clonidine added to psychostimulant medication for hyperactive and aggressive children. J Am Acad Child Adolesc Psychiatry 42(8):886–894, 2003 12874489

Hollander E, Dolgoff-Kaspar R, Cartwright C, et al: An open trial of divalproex sodium in autism spectrum disorders. J Clin Psychiatry 62(7):530–534, 2001 11488363

Holzer B, Lopes V, Lehman R: Combination use of atomoxetine hydrochloride and olanzapine in the treatment of attention-deficit/hyperactivity disorder with comorbid disruptive behavior disorder in children and adolescents 10–18 years of age. J Child Adolesc Psychopharmacol 23(6):415–418, 2013 23952189

Horrigan JP, Barnhill LJ, Courvoisie HE: Olanzapine in PDD. J Am Acad Child Adolesc Psychiatry 36(9):1166–1167, 1997 9291716

Hunkeler EM, Fireman B, Lee J, et al: Trends in use of antidepressants, lithium, and anticonvulsants in Kaiser Permanente-insured youths, 1994–2003. J Child Adolesc Psychopharmacol 15(1):26–37, 2005 15741783

INSERM Collective Expertise Centre: Conduct Disorder in Children and Adolescents. Paris, Institut National de la Santé et de la Recherche Médicale, 2005. Available at: https://www.ncbi.nlm.nih.gov/books/NBK7133. Accessed March 17, 2023.

Jensen PS, Hinshaw SP, Kraemer HC, et al: ADHD comorbidity findings from the MTA study: comparing comorbid subgroups. J Am Acad Child Adolesc Psychiatry 40(2):147–158, 2001 11211363

Jensen PS, MacIntyre JC, Pappadopulos EA (eds): Treatment Recommendations for the Use of Antipsychotic Medications for Aggressive Youth (TRAAY): Pocket Reference Guide for Clinicians in Child and Adolescent Psychiatry. New York, New York State Office of Mental Health and Center for the Advancement of Children's Mental Health at Columbia University, 2004

Jensen PS, Youngstrom EA, Steiner H, et al: Consensus report on impulsive aggression as a symptom across diagnostic categories in child psychiatry: implications for medication studies. J Am Acad Child Adolesc Psychiatry 46(3):309–322, 2007 17314717

Kafantaris V, Campbell M, Padron-Gayol MV, et al: Carbamazepine in hospitalized aggressive conduct disorder children: an open pilot study. Psychopharmacol Bull 28(2):193–199, 1992 1513924

Katic A, Dirks B, Babcock T, et al: Treatment outcomes with lisdexamfetamine dimesylate in children who have attention-deficit/hyperactivity disorder with emotional control impairments. J Child Adolesc Psychopharmacol 23(6):386–393, 2013 23952185

Kazdin AE: Child, parent and family dysfunction as predictors of outcome in cognitive-behavioral treatment of antisocial children. Behav Res Ther 33(3):271–281, 1995 7726803

Kazdin AE, Bass D, Siegel T, Thomas C: Cognitive-behavioral therapy and relationship therapy in the treatment of children referred for antisocial behavior. J Consult Clin Psychol 57(4):522–535, 1989 2768614

Kazdin AE, Siegel TC, Bass D: Cognitive problem-solving skills training and parent management training in the treatment of antisocial behavior in children. J Consult Clin Psychol 60(5):733–747, 1992 1401389

Kim-Cohen J, Caspi A, Moffitt TE, et al: Prior juvenile diagnoses in adults with mental disorder: developmental follow-back of a prospective-longitudinal cohort. Arch Gen Psychiatry 60(7):709–717, 2003 12860775

Kimonis ER, Frick PJ, Boris NW, et al: Callous-unemotional features, behavioral inhibition, and parenting: independent predictors of aggression in a high-risk preschool sample. J Child Fam Stud 15(6):745–756, 2006

Klein RG, Abikoff H, Klass E, et al: Clinical efficacy of methylphenidate in conduct disorder with and without attention deficit hyperactivity disorder. Arch Gen Psychiatry 54(12):1073–1080, 1997 9400342

Knapp P, Chait A, Pappadopulos E, et al: Treatment of maladaptive aggression in youth: CERT guidelines, I: engagement, assessment, and management. Pediatrics 129(6):e1562–e1576, 2012 22641762

Kranzler H, Roofeh D, Gerbino-Rosen G, et al: Clozapine: its impact on aggressive behavior among children and adolescents with schizophrenia. J Am Acad Child Adolesc Psychiatry 44(1):55–63, 2005 15608544

Kronenberger WG, Giauque AL, Lafata DE, et al: Quetiapine addition in methylphenidate treatment-resistant adolescents with comorbid ADHD, conduct/oppositional-defiant disorder, and aggression: a prospective, open-label study. J Child Adolesc Psychopharmacol 17(3):334–347, 2007 17630867

Lahey BB, Loeber R, Quay HC, et al: Validity of DSM-IV subtypes of conduct disorder based on age of onset. J Am Acad Child Adolesc Psychiatry 37(4):435–442, 1998 9549965

Lisska MC, Rivkees SA: Daily methylphenidate use slows the growth of children: a community based study. J Pediatr Endocrinol Metab 16(5):711–718, 2003 12880120

Lochman JE, Curry JF: Effects of social problem-solving training and self-instruction training with aggressive boys. J Clin Child Psychol 15(2):159–164, 1986

Lochman JE, Lampron LB: Cognitive-behavioral interventions for aggressive boys: seven months follow-up effects. J Child Adolesc Psychother 5(1):15–23, 1988

Loeber R, Keenan K, Lahey BB, et al: Evidence for developmentally based diagnoses of oppositional defiant disorder and conduct disorder. J Abnorm Child Psychol 21(4):377–410, 1993 8408986

Loeber R, Burke JD, Lahey BB: What are adolescent antecedents to antisocial personality disorder? Crim Behav Ment Health 12(1):24–36, 2002 12357255

Loeber R, Green SM, Lahey BB: Risk factors for antisocial personality, in Early Prevention of Adult Antisocial Behaviour. Edited by Coid J, Farrington DP. Cambridge, UK, Cambridge University Press, 2003, pp 79–108

Loeber R, Burke J, Pardini DA: Perspectives on oppositional defiant disorder, conduct disorder, and psychopathic features. J Child Psychol Psychiatry 50(1–2):133–142, 2009 19220596

Loy JH, Merry SN, Hetrick SE, Stasiak K: Atypical antipsychotics for disruptive behaviour disorders in children and youths. Cochrane Database Syst Rev (8):CD008559, 2017 28791693

Malone RP, Bennett DS, Luebbert JF, et al: Aggression classification and treatment response. Psychopharmacol Bull 34(1):41–45, 1998 9564197

Malone RP, Delaney MA, Luebbert JF, et al: A double-blind placebo-controlled study of lithium in hospitalized aggressive children and adolescents with conduct disorder. Arch Gen Psychiatry 57(7):649–654, 2000 10891035

Marcus RN, Owen R, Kamen L, et al: A placebo-controlled, fixed-dose study of aripiprazole in children and adolescents with irritability associated with autistic disorder. J Am Acad Child Adolesc Psychiatry 48(11):1110–1119, 2009 19797985

Marcus RN, Owen R, Manos G, et al: Aripiprazole in the treatment of irritability in pediatric patients (aged 6–17 years) with autistic disorder: results from a 52-week, open-label study. J Child Adolesc Psychopharmacol 21(3):229–236, 2011 21663425

Martin A, Scahill L, Charney DS, et al (eds): Pediatric Psychopharmacology: Principles and Practice. Oxford, UK, Oxford University Press, 2003

Masi G, Manfredi A, Milone A, et al: Predictors of nonresponse to psychosocial treatment in children and adolescents with disruptive behavior disorders. J Child Adolesc Psychopharmacol 21(1):51–55, 2011 21309697

Masi G, Milone A, Stawinoga A, et al: Efficacy and safety of risperidone and quetiapine in adolescents with bipolar II disorder comorbid with conduct disorder. J Clin Psychopharmacol 35(5):587–590, 2015 26226481

McConville BJ, Sorter MT: Treatment challenges and safety considerations for antipsychotic use in children and adolescents with psychoses. J Clin Psychiatry 65(Suppl 6):20–29, 2004 15104523

McCracken JT, McGough J, Shah B, et al: Risperidone in children with autism and serious behavioral problems. N Engl J Med 347(5):314–321, 2002 12151468

Mitchison GM, Njardvik U: Prevalence and gender differences of ODD, anxiety, and depression in a sample of children with ADHD. J Atten Disord 23(11):1339–1345, 2019 26443719

MTA Cooperative Group: Multimodal Treatment Study of Children with ADHD: a 14-month randomized clinical trial of treatment strategies for attention-deficit/hyperactivity disorder. Arch Gen Psychiatry 56(12):1073–1086, 1999 10591283

Newcorn JH, Spencer TJ, Biederman J, et al: Atomoxetine treatment in children and adolescents with attention-deficit/hyperactivity disorder and comorbid oppositional defiant disorder. J Am Acad Child Adolesc Psychiatry 44(3):240–248, 2005 15725968

Nock MK, Kazdin AE, Hiripi E, Kessler RC: Lifetime prevalence, correlates, and persistence of oppositional defiant disorder: results from the National Comorbidity Survey Replication. J Child Psychol Psychiatry 48(7):703–713, 2007 17593151

Olfson M, Blanco C, Liu L, et al: National trends in the outpatient treatment of children and adolescents with antipsychotic drugs. Arch Gen Psychiatry 63(6):679–685, 2006 16754841

Owen R, Sikich L, Marcus RN, et al: Aripiprazole in the treatment of irritability in children and adolescents with autistic disorder. Pediatrics 124(6):1533–1540, 2009 19948625

Padhy R, Saxena K, Remsing L, et al: Symptomatic response to divalproex in subtypes of conduct disorder. Child Psychiatry Hum Dev 42(5):584–593, 2011 21706221

Pappadopulos E, Macintyre Ii JC, Crismon ML, et al: Treatment recommendations for the use of antipsychotics for aggressive youth (TRAAY): part II. J Am Acad Child Adolesc Psychiatry 42(2):145–161, 2003 12544174

Pappadopulos E, Woolston S, Chait A, et al: Pharmacotherapy of aggression in children and adolescents: efficacy and effect size. J Can Acad Child Adolesc Psychiatry 15(1):27–39, 2006 18392193

Pappadopulos E, Scotto Rosato N, Correll CU, et al: Experts' recommendations for treating maladaptive aggression in youth. J Child Adolesc Psychopharmacol 21(6):505–515, 2011 22196314

Pardini DA, Fite PJ: Symptoms of conduct disorder, oppositional defiant disorder, and callous-unemotional traits as unique predictors of psychosocial maladjustment in boys: advancing an evidence base for DSM-5. J Am Acad Child Adolesc Psychiatry 49:1134–1144, 2010 20970701

Pardini DA, Loeber R: Interpersonal callousness trajectories across adolescence: early social influences and adult outcomes. Crim Justice Behav 35(2):173–196, 2008 21394215

Pardini DA, Frick PJ, Moffitt TE: Building an evidence base for DSM-5 conceptualizations of oppositional defiant disorder and conduct disorder: introduction to the special section. J Abnorm Psychol 119(4):683–688, 2010 21090874

Penzner JB, Dudas M, Saito E, et al: Lack of effect of stimulant combination with second-generation antipsychotics on weight gain, metabolic changes, prolactin levels, and sedation in youth with clinically relevant aggression or oppositionality. J Child Adolesc Psychopharmacol 19(5):563–573, 2009 19877981

Peuskens J, Pani L, Detraux J, De Hert M: The effects of novel and newly approved antipsychotics on serum prolactin levels: a comprehensive review. CNS Drugs 28(5):421–453, 2014 24677189

Polzer J, Bangs ME, Zhang S, et al: Meta-analysis of aggression or hostility events in randomized, controlled clinical trials of atomoxetine for ADHD. Biol Psychiatry 61(5):713–719, 2007 16996485

Potenza MN, Holmes JP, Kanes SJ, McDougle CJ: Olanzapine treatment of children, adolescents, and adults with pervasive developmental disorders: an open-label pilot study. J Clin Psychopharmacol 19(1):37–44, 1999 9934941

Rabinowitz J, Avnon M, Rosenberg V: Effect of clozapine on physical and verbal aggression. Schizophr Res 22(3):249–255, 1996 9000322

Research Units on Pediatric Psychopharmacology Autism Network: Risperidone treatment of autistic disorder: longer-term benefits and blinded discontinuation after 6 months. Am J Psychiatry 162(7):1361–1369, 2005 15994720

Reyes M, Buitelaar J, Toren P, et al: A randomized, double-blind, placebo-controlled study of risperidone maintenance treatment in children and adolescents with disruptive behavior disorders. Am J Psychiatry 163(3):402–410, 2006a 16513860

Reyes M, Croonenberghs J, Augustyns I, Eerdekens M: Long-term use of risperidone in children with disruptive behavior disorders and subaverage intelligence: efficacy, safety, and tolerability. J Child Adolesc Psychopharmacol 16(3):260–272, 2006b 16768634

Riddle MA, Bernstein GA, Cook EH, et al: Anxiolytics, adrenergic agents, and naltrexone. J Am Acad Child Adolesc Psychiatry 38(5):546–556, 1999 10230186

Rosenbloom AL: Hyperprolactinemia with antipsychotic drugs in children and adolescents. Int J Pediatr Endocrinol 2010:159402, 2010 20871665

Rowe R, Costello EJ, Angold A, et al: Developmental pathways in oppositional defiant disorder and conduct disorder. J Abnorm Psychol 119(4):726–738, 2010 21090876

Rynar L, Coccaro EF: Psychosocial impairment in DSM-5 intermittent explosive disorder. Psychiatry Res 264:91–95, 2018 29627702

Scahill L, Chappell PB, Kim YS, et al: A placebo-controlled study of guanfacine in the treatment of children with tic disorders and attention deficit hyperactivity disorder. Am J Psychiatry 158(7):1067–1074, 2001 11431228

Scotto Rosato N, Correll CU, Pappadopulos E, et al: Treatment of maladaptive aggression in youth: CERT guidelines II: treatments and ongoing management. Pediatrics 129(6):e1577–e1586, 2012 22641763

Schuhmann EM, Foote RC, Eyberg SM, et al: Efficacy of parent-child interaction therapy: interim report of a randomized trial with short-term maintenance. J Clin Child Psychol 27(1):34–45, 1998 9561935

Schur SB, Sikich L, Findling RL, et al: Treatment recommendations for the use of antipsychotics for aggressive youth (TRAAY) part I: a review. J Am Acad Child Adolesc Psychiatry 42(2):132–144, 2003 12544173

Schwartz S, Correll CU: Efficacy and safety of atomoxetine in children and adolescents with attention-deficit/hyperactivity disorder: results from a comprehensive meta-analysis and metaregression. J Am Acad Child Adolesc Psychiatry 53(2):174–187, 2014 24472252

Sikich L, Hamer RM, Bashford RA, et al: A pilot study of risperidone, olanzapine, and haloperidol in psychotic youth: a double-blind, randomized, 8-week trial. Neuropsychopharmacology 29(1):133–145, 2004 14583740

Snyder R, Turgay A, Aman M, et al: Effects of risperidone on conduct and disruptive behavior disorders in children with subaverage IQs. J Am Acad Child Adolesc Psychiatry 41(9):1026–1036, 2002 12218423

Steiner H, Petersen ML, Saxena K, et al: Divalproex sodium for the treatment of conduct disorder: a randomized controlled clinical trial. J Clin Psychiatry 64(10):1183–1191, 2003a 14658966

Steiner H, Saxena K, Chang K: Psychopharmacologic strategies for the treatment of aggression in juveniles. CNS Spectr 8(4):298–308, 2003b 12679744

Steiner H, Silverman M, Karnik NS, et al: Psychopathology, trauma and delinquency: subtypes of aggression and their relevance for understanding young offenders. Child Adolesc Psychiatry Ment Health 5:21, 2011 21714905

Stephens RJ, Bassel C, Sandor P: Olanzapine in the treatment of aggression and tics in children with Tourette's syndrome: a pilot study. J Child Adolesc Psychopharmacol 14(2):255–266, 2004 15319022

Stigler KA, Potenza MN, Posey DJ, McDougle CJ: Weight gain associated with atypical antipsychotic use in children and adolescents: prevalence, clinical relevance, and management. Paediatr Drugs 6(1):33–44, 2004 14969568

Stigler KA, Mullett JE, Erickson CA, et al: Paliperidone for irritability in adolescents and young adults with autistic disorder. Psychopharmacology (Berl) 223(2):237–245, 2012 22549762

Stringaris A, Goodman R: Longitudinal outcome of youth oppositionality: irritable, headstrong, and hurtful behaviors have distinctive predictions. J Am Acad Child Adolesc Psychiatry 48(4):404–412, 2009 19318881

Swanson JM, Kraemer HC, Hinshaw SP, et al: Clinical relevance of the primary findings of the MTA: success rates based on severity of ADHD and ODD symptoms at the end of treatment. J Am Acad Child Adolesc Psychiatry 40(2):168–179, 2001 11211365

Teixeira EH, Celeri EV, Jacintho AC, Dalgalarrondo P: Clozapine in severe conduct disorder. J Child Adolesc Psychopharmacol 23(1):44–48, 2013 23347126

Tremblay RE, Nagin DS, Séguin JR, et al: Physical aggression during early childhood: trajectories and predictors. Pediatrics 114(1):e43–50, 2004 15231972

Troost PW, Lahuis BE, Steenhuis MP, et al: Long-term effects of risperidone in children with autism spectrum disorders: a placebo discontinuation study. J Am Acad Child Adolesc Psychiatry 44(11):1137–1144, 2005 16239862

Turgay A, Binder C, Snyder R, Fisman S: Long-term safety and efficacy of risperidone for the treatment of disruptive behavior disorders in children with subaverage IQs. Pediatrics 110(3):e34, 2002 12205284

U.S. Food and Drug Administration: Antidepressant Use in Children, Adolescents, and Adults. Rockville, MD, U.S. Food and Drug Administration, 2005

U.S. Food and Drug Administration: Statistical Review and Evaluation: Antiepileptic Drugs and Suicidality. Rockville, MD, U.S. Food and Drug Administration, 2008

U.S. Food and Drug Administration: Drug Safety Newsletter, Vol 2. Rockville, MD, Center for Drug Evaluation and Research, U.S Food and Drug Administration, 2009

U.S. Food and Drug Administration: Drug Safety and Risk Management Advisory Committee (DSaRM). Rockville, MD, Center for Drug Evaluation and Research, U.S. Food and Drug Administration, Department of Health and Human Services, 2022. Available at: https://www.fda.gov/advisory-committees/human-drug-advisory-committees/drug-safety-and-risk-management-advisory-committee. Accessed March 17, 202e.

Vitaro F, Gendreau PL, Tremblay RE, Oligny P: Reactive and proactive aggression differentially predict later conduct problems. J Child Psychol Psychiatry 39(3):377–385, 1998 9670093

Vitiello B, Stoff DM: Subtypes of aggression and their relevance to child psychiatry. J Am Acad Child Adolesc Psychiatry 36(3):307–315, 1997 9055510

Vitiello B, Behar D, Hunt J, et al: Subtyping aggression in children and adolescents. J Neuropsychiatry Clin Neurosci 2(2):189–192, 1990 2136074

Volavka J, Citrome L: Atypical antipsychotics in the treatment of the persistently aggressive psychotic patient: methodological concerns. Schizophr Res 35(Suppl):S23–S33, 1999 10190223

Waddell C, Schwartz C, Andres C, et al: Fifty years of preventing and treating childhood behaviour disorders: a systematic review to inform policy and practice. Evid Based Ment Health 21(2):45–52, 2018 29703717

Weiner B (ed): Physician's Desk Reference Generics, 2nd Edition. Montvale, NJ, Medical Economics, 1996

Wudarsky M, Nicolson R, Hamburger SD, et al: Elevated prolactin in pediatric patients on typical and atypical antipsychotics. J Child Adolesc Psychopharmacol 9(4):239–245, 1999 10630453

Young AS, Youngstrom EA, Findling RL, et al: Developing and validating a definition of impulsive/reactive aggression in youth. J Clin Child Adolesc Psychol 49(6):787–803, 2020 31343896

Youngstrom EA, Young AS, Van Eck K, et al: Developing empirical latent profiles of impulsive aggression and mood in youths across three outpatient samples. J Clin Child Adolesc Psychol 52(2):196–211, 2023 34125637

4

Anxiety Disorders

Moira A. Rynn, M.D.
Paula K. Yanes-Lukin, Ph.D.
Pablo H. Goldberg, M.D.

Anxiety disorders begin in childhood and often evolve well into adulthood, resulting in lifelong impairment in multiple areas, such as school achievement, work, relationships, and health. Anxiety disorders are insidious in nature; if not identified and treated, they can lead to a person experiencing chronic symptoms, typically with a waxing and waning course, and often without relief. This lack of acknowledgment—and, consequently, treatment—is partly due to patient and clinician belief that symptoms of anxiety are an expected part of normal life. A bias exists among health care providers that having an anxiety disorder is not as serious as having other psychiatric disorders, such as major depressive disorder (MDD). In fact, an analysis of the data from the National Comorbidity Survey–Adolescent Supplement (NCS-A) found that among adolescents with psychiatric disorders, those with any anxiety disorder or a specific phobia were the least likely to receive treatment within a 12-month period (Costello et al. 2014), and anxiety was estimated to be the most prevalent mental health disorder worldwide at 6.5% (Polanczyk et al. 2015).

The evolution of anxiety disorders as a diagnostic entity is reflected in the diagnostic definitions given in editions of DSM revisions. Initially, the anxiety disorders were all classified as *psychoneurotic disorders* (reactions) in DSM-I (American Psychiatric Association 1952) and as neuroses in DSM-II (American Psychiatric Association 1968). It was not until DSM-III (American Psychiatric Association 1980) that the anxiety disorders diagnosis began to take shape, with delineated criteria for both adults and children, and separation anxiety disorder was specified and included. In DSM-IV and DSM-IV-TR (American Psychiatric Association 1994, 2000), most of the childhood anxiety disorders were subsumed under the adult definitions for generalized anxiety disorder (GAD), OCD, PTSD, social anxiety disorder (social phobia), and panic disorder (Rickels and Rynn 2001). For example, children who in the past may have been diagnosed with overanxious disorder in childhood would now receive the diagnosis of GAD on the basis of contemporary psychiatric nosology. This trend continued in DSM-5 (American Psychiatric Association 2013, 2022). The chapter on disorders usually first diagnosed in infancy, childhood, or adolescence that separated childhood-related disorders was eliminated in DSM-5, and previously childhood-specific disorders (e.g., separation anxiety disorder) can now be diagnosed in adulthood. OCD and PTSD are presented in different chapters in DSM-5; however, they are still related to the anxiety disorders. The exception to this trend is the inclusion of a new subtype of PTSD in DSM-5 for preschool-age children 6 years or younger, which adapts the criteria in order to be developmentally sensitive and appropriate.

Epidemiology

Anxiety disorders such as GAD (earlier known as overanxious disorder) and social anxiety disorder are among the most common diagnoses reported in epidemiological studies of child and adolescent populations (Feehan et al. 1994; Lewinsohn et al. 1993; McGee et al. 1990). Beesdo et al. (2009) found that the lifetime prevalence rate of a child or adolescent having symptoms that meet criteria for any anxiety disorder is about 15%–20%. In community epidemiological studies, the prevalence rates for overanxious disorder ranged from 2.9% to 4.6%, and the rates for separation anxiety disorder ranged from 2.4% to 4.1% (Anderson et al. 1987; Bowen et al. 1990; Costello 1989). In one general pediatric clinical sample, 8%–10% of patients had symptoms that met the criteria for any anxiety disorder (Costello et al. 1988; Egger and Angold 2006). The NCS-A, which used a DSM-IV in-person survey of 10,123 adolescents (ages 13–18) in the United States, found that anxiety disorders were the most common, at 31.9% (Merikangas et al. 2010b).

In addition, social avoidance that interferes with functioning and is manifested in worry, isolation, hypersensitivity, sadness, and self-consciousness has been reported in 10%–20% of school-age children (Orvaschel and Weissman 1986). Prevalence rates for internalizing disorders are also greater in clinical samples, with 14% of patients being diagnosed with an anxiety disorder (Keller et al. 1992).

For specific anxiety disorders, the reported prevalence rates are variable (for a review, see Costello et al. 2005). GAD/overanxious disorder is the most common, and separation anxiety disorder is the second most common. The prevalence rate of PTSD is 5% for adolescents (Merikangas et al. 2010a) but is thought to be rare for children, at less than 0.5% (Copeland et al. 2007). The prevalence of OCD is 1%–2%, and the prevalence of panic disorder approaches 1% in population studies (Geller et al. 1998; Rasmussen and Eisen 1992). However, these reported rates vary depending on whether the level of functional impairment is included in the definition. A child with some impaired functioning may not exhibit every symptom to satisfy the full diagnostic criteria and, unfortunately, may not be recommended for treatment.

Prevalence rates among young males and females do not differ significantly, but a difference in rates becomes noticeable in adolescence, as females become two to three times more likely to experience an anxiety disorder (Costello et al. 2003; Rockhill et al. 2010).

Course and Outcome

Children with anxiety disorders often experience low self-esteem and social isolation, which fosters inadequate social skills (Strauss 1988). These children also report higher rates of physical symptoms, such as headaches, stomachaches, and irritable bowel syndrome (Livingston et al. 1988). These symptoms can then increase visits to the pediatrician, leading to an increase in medical costs. Furthermore, there is concern that the presence of anxiety disorders early in childhood provides a pathway for the development of subsequent mood and substance abuse disorders (Weissman et al. 1999). Pine and Grun (1998) reported that children with a history of long-term anxiety disorder exhibited increased rates of other psychiatric disorders, psychiatric hospitalizations, and suicide attempts as adults.

Anxiety disorders and symptoms are not simply transitory but persist over time (Beidel et al. 1996; Cantwell and Baker 1989; Keller et al. 1992). Dadds et al. (1997) performed a school-based prevention study in which untreated anxious children were identified by self-report or teachers' ratings as having features of an anxiety disorder but not meeting the full diagnostic criteria. The results revealed that 54% of the children developed a full anxiety disorder over the remaining 6 months of the study. Children with GAD/overanxious disorder were also found to be at a higher risk for concurrent additional anxiety disorders (Last et al. 1987a). A prospective 3- to 4-year follow-up study by Last et al. (1996) showed that children with anxiety disorders, although free from their initial anxiety diagnosis at follow-up, were more likely than control subjects to develop new psychiatric disorders, usually a different anxiety disorder, over the time course.

There also appears to be an association between childhood disorders and the presence of adult anxiety disorders. A large number of adults who receive an anxiety diagnosis report childhood histories of separation anxiety or overanxious disorders (Aronson and Logue 1987; Last et al. 1987b, 1987c). One of the few prospective studies to assess anxious children's adjustment to early adulthood found that those with anxiety, especially those with comorbid depression, were less likely than control subjects with no history of psychiatric illness to be living independently, working, or attending school (Last et al. 1997). In an outpatient setting, approximately 30% of children with an anxiety disorder have comorbid depression (for a review, see Brady and Kendall 1992).

The Great Smoky Mountains Study, a longitudinal study examining the development of emotional and behavioral disorders and the need for mental health treatment in North Carolina, has also provided valuable data regarding outcome predictions (Costello et al. 1996). Bittner et al. (2007) reported that within this sample, childhood separation anxiety was associated with subsequent separation anxiety in adolescence; childhood overanxious disorder was associated with the development of overanxious disorder, panic attacks, depression, and conduct disorder in adolescence; GAD was associated with conduct disorder; and social anxiety in childhood was related to social anxiety, overanxious disorder, and ADHD in adolescence. Furthermore, the presence of comorbid anxiety and depression increased the chance of high-risk behaviors such as substance use and suicidality (Federman et al. 1997; Foley et al. 2006).

In addition, there is some evidence that as many as 41% of children or adolescents who experience MDD had or have an anxiety disorder that preceded their depression (Brady and Kendall 1992; Kovacs et al. 1989). The presence of an anxiety disorder was found to predict a worse prognosis for the depression and, at times, had an effect on the length of, or recovery from, the depressive episode. Furthermore, after treatment of and recovery from depression, the anxiety disorder usually persisted (Kovacs et al. 1989). Similar results have been found for bipolar disorder; 42% of adults diagnosed with bipolar disorder reported having a childhood anxiety disorder (separation anxiety and overanxious disorder) compared with 5% of adults without a diagnosis of bipolar disorder (Henin et al. 2007). Early treatment intervention for anxiety disorders may prevent and alter the course of developing depression and other psychiatric disorders, leading to an improved opportunity for a successful adulthood.

Rationale and Justification for Psychopharmacological Treatment

Strong evidence suggests that antidepressants, particularly the selective serotonin reuptake inhibitor (SSRI) class of medications, are safe and efficacious for treating childhood anxiety disorders. In addition to medication treatment, there is an extensive literature supporting the use of cognitive-behavioral therapy (CBT) for the treatment of these disorders as well. The American Academy of Child and Adolescent Psychiatry (AACAP) practice parameter for OCD recommends, when possible, to treat first with CBT for patients with symptoms of mild to moderate severity and to use a combination of CBT plus an SSRI for patients with more severe symptoms (American Academy of Child and Adolescent Psychiatry 2012; Walter et al. 2020). For anxiety disorders, the AACAP practice parameter recommends considering an SSRI + CBT combination first for moderate to severe cases, given that remission rates were found to be greater for children receiving combination treatment than for those receiving monotherapy with either approach (Walter et al. 2020). This is supported by the results from the largest anxiety clinical trial to date, the Child/Adolescent Anxiety Multimodal Study (CAMS), which supported the effectiveness of combined treatment of CBT with medication (Walkup et al. 2008). Unfortunately, one of the challenges of recommending CBT for patients is its limited availability in many communities. This may necessitate the use of medication treatment as the first-line approach with supportive therapy.

Another issue concerning the use of medication treatment is a consideration of the risk-benefit profile. The available safety data from completed randomized controlled trials (RCTs) demonstrate that the adverse effect profiles of SSRIs in children resemble those in adults and that, overall, these medications are safe and well tolerated. However, the FDA has required a boxed warning on all antidepressants, as well as on medications for adjunctive treatment of MDD (e.g., aripiprazole), because of concern for a potentially increased risk of suicidal ideation or behaviors for children taking these medications (U.S. Food and Drug Administration 2005). In contrast to the pediatric depression RCTs, most pediatric anxiety studies did not show evidence of increased suicidal thinking or behaviors for children given medications compared with those given placebo.

Medications for Pediatric Anxiety Disorders: Review of Treatment Studies

Selective Serotonin Reuptake Inhibitors

To date, the most widely studied pharmacological treatments for pediatric anxiety disorders are SSRIs (Table 4–1), which include fluvoxamine (Luvox), sertraline (Zoloft), fluoxetine (Prozac), citalopram (Celexa), escitalopram (Lexapro), and paroxetine (Paxil), among others. Although SSRIs are characterized as antidepressants, they are unique in that they specifically inhibit the reuptake of the neurotransmitter serotonin, therefore resulting in increased amounts of serotonin in the synapses of the brain. Decreased serotonin levels are attributed to various disorders, including depression (Roy et al. 1989) and anxiety disorders (Nutt and Lawson 1992; Pigott 1996; Tancer 1993). Exten-

Table 4–1. Selected medications for pediatric anxiety disorders

Drug	Total daily dosage	Dosing schedule	Main indications	Side effects / Recommended action
Antidepressants				
Tricyclic antidepressants				
Tertiary amines				
Clomipramine	2–5 mg/kg	qd or bid	OCD, school refusal	Anticholinergic effects (e.g., dizziness, drowsiness, dry mouth)
Imipramine	2–5 mg/kg	qd or bid	GAD, PD	Requires ECG monitoring
Secondary amines				
Desipramine	2–5 mg/kg	qd or bid	OCD	Potential for cardiac toxicity
Selective serotonin reuptake inhibitors				GI side effects, weight gain and loss, sweating, dry mouth, headache, irritability, insomnia, fatigue, hypersomnia, restlessness, increased hyperactivity, tremor, increased risk for self-injury and SIBs, mania, withdrawal effects, sexual side effects

Table 4–1. Selected medications for pediatric anxiety disorders *(continued)*

Drug	Total daily dosage	Dosing schedule	Main indications	Side effects / Recommended action
Selective serotonin reuptake inhibitors (continued)				
Citalopram	20–40 mg	qAM	SOC	Due to risk of QTc prolongation, dosage should not be increased above total of 40 mg
Children ages 7–11 years	Initial 2.5–10 mg qd; titrate every 1–2 weeks to target of 10–20 mg/day			
Children/adolescents age ≥ 12 years	Initial 10 mg qd; titrate every 1–2 weeks to target of 20–40 mg/day			
Escitalopram				
Children/adolescents age ≥ 12 years	Initial range 5–10 mg qd; may be increased to 20 mg after at least 3 weeks	qd		Due to risk of QTc prolongation, dosage should not be increased above total of 40 mg
Fluoxetine	10–60 mg	qAM	OCD, GAD, SAD, SOC	
Fluvoxamine	50–300 mg	qAM	OCD, GAD, SAD, SOC	
Paroxetine	10–40 mg	qAM	SAD, SOC	
Sertraline	25–200 mg	qAM	PD	

Table 4–1. Selected medications for pediatric anxiety disorders *(continued)*

Drug	Total daily dosage	Dosing schedule	Main indications	Side effects / Recommended action
Serotonin-norepinephrine reuptake inhibitors				
Atomoxetine	Starting at 40 mg/day, may increase after 3 days to 80 mg/day; single daily dose qAM or two divided doses, one qAM and one qPM. Depending on clinical response, may increase to 100 mg/day after another 2–4 weeks	qd or bid	ADHD and may reduce comorbid anxiety symptoms	Monitor for mania and serotonin syndrome
Venlafaxine XR	37.5–225 mg	qd	GAD, SAD, SOC	GI side effects, headache, weight loss, fatigue, insomnia, irritability, hypersomnia Monitor blood pressure
Duloxetine	30–120 mg	qd	GAD	GI side effects, oropharyngeal pain, dizziness, cough, and palpitations

Table 4–1. Selected medications for pediatric anxiety disorders *(continued)*

Drug	Total daily dosage	Dosing schedule	Main indications	Side effects / Recommended action
Benzodiazepines				
Long-acting				
Clonazepam*	0.25–2 mg	qd, bid, tid	GAD, PD	Sedation, drowsiness, decreased alertness, disinhibition; taper
Short- to intermediate-acting				
Alprazolam*	0.25–4 mg	prn, qd, bid, tid	GAD, PD	Sedation, drowsiness, decreased alertness, disinhibition; taper
Lorazepam*	0.25–6 mg	prn, qd, bid, tid	GAD, PD	Sedation, drowsiness, decreased alertness, disinhibition; taper
Nonbenzodiazepines				
Buspirone	0.2–0.6 mg/kg	bid or tid	OCD, GAD, SOC	Light-headedness, dizziness, nausea, sedation

Note. ECG=electrocardiogram; GAD=generalized anxiety disorder; GI=gastrointestinal; PD=panic disorder; SAD=separation anxiety disorder; SIB=self-injurious behavior; SOC=social anxiety disorder.

*Adjunct treatment.

sive empirical literature supports the efficacy of SSRIs in treating adult anxiety disorders (Katzelnick et al. 1995; Liebowitz et al. 2002; Pohl et al. 1998; Pollack et al. 2001).

Acute Treatment

The use of SSRIs and other, newer antidepressants in the U.S. population younger than age 18 years increased significantly from 1.3% in 2005 to 1.6% in 2012 (Bachmann et al. 2016), with the SSRI class of antidepressants being the most common. Owing to the evidence presented in the current literature and their relatively minimal side effects, SSRIs are presently considered the first-line pharmacotherapy choice for childhood anxiety disorders. The field began with numerous promising open-label and limited sample studies (Birmaher et al. 1994; Compton et al. 2001), which paved the way for the subsequent RCTs discussed in the following sections and, taken together, demonstrated the most compelling evidence for the acute treatment of anxiety disorders with SSRIs.

Fluoxetine (Prozac). To date, several well-designed fluoxetine studies for the treatment of pediatric anxiety disorders have been published. Black and Uhde (1994) conducted a double-blind, placebo-controlled trial to examine the efficacy of fluoxetine in treating children (ages 5–16) with the primary diagnosis of selective mutism. Sixteen children were given a placebo run-in for 2 weeks (Phase I). Nonresponders were then randomly assigned to either placebo ($n=9$) or to fluoxetine ($n=6$; mean maximum dosage, 21.4 mg/day; range, 12–27 mg/day) for another 12 weeks (Phase II).

By the end of the trial, although the participants in the fluoxetine group showed improvement over time on all parent, patient, and clinician ratings, an analysis of variance (ANOVA) indicated few significant results (Black and Uhde 1994). The fluoxetine group, compared with the placebo group, had significantly greater improvement in one symptom—mutism—as reflected by a change in ratings on two of the nine parent scales, the mutism Clinical Global Impression (CGI) Scale ($P<0.0003$) and global CGI ($P<0.04$), and on one teacher rating, the Conners' Anxiety Scale ($P<0.02$). The proportion of children rated as treatment responders based on their parent's rating of mutism change ($P<0.03$) and global change ($P<0.03$) was also significantly greater in the fluoxetine group. Side effects were minimal and did not differ significantly between treatment groups.

Several reasons may account for the lack of significant results in the study by Black and Uhde (1994). The sample size was relatively small, and the length of the trial may not have been long enough to show the effects of fluoxetine, given that treatment response did not increase markedly until weeks 8–12. In addition, the investigators noted that timing may have affected treatment response. Clinical response in an earlier case report (Black and Uhde 1992), in which treatment began before the start of the school year, was more striking than in their 1994 study, which was carried out in the last half of the school year, when children with selective mutism may have already known what to expect from their teachers and peers and were less motivated to improve.

In a later, double-blind, placebo-controlled trial, Geller et al. (2001) studied response to fluoxetine in children and adolescents diagnosed with OCD. Participants were randomly assigned to fluoxetine (n=71; mean total dosage, 24.6 mg/day) or placebo (n=32) for 13 weeks. The fluoxetine was initiated at 10 mg/day for the first 2 weeks and then increased to 20 mg/day. If subjects' symptoms were unresponsive after 4 weeks of treatment, as indicated by no change or worsening on the CGI Severity of Illness subscale (CGI-S), the medication dosage could be titrated to 40 mg/day and again to 60 mg/day at week 7.

In an intent-to-treat analysis, Geller et al. (2001) found that participants randomly assigned to fluoxetine showed a greater reduction in OCD severity on the primary efficacy measure, the total Children's Yale-Brown Obsessive Compulsive Scale (CY-BOCS) score (P=0.026). The reduction trended toward significance at week 5 (P=0.086) and reached significance thereafter (P<0.05). Almost half of the youth (49%) in the fluoxetine group were considered responders (defined as a ≥40% reduction in symptoms on the CY-BOCS) compared with 25% in the placebo group (P=0.030, Mantel-Haenszel exact test). In addition, significantly more participants in the fluoxetine group were rated as being "much improved" or "very much improved" on the CGI Improvement subscale (CGI-I) (55% vs. 18.8% placebo; P<0.001). Patient and parent improvement ratings also reflected this trend (P<0.001). Fluoxetine was well tolerated in this trial, with no adverse effects occurring significantly more often in the fluoxetine group than in the placebo group.

Although the results of this study do support the efficacy of fluoxetine in treating children and adolescents with OCD, these findings have are some notable limitations. The investigators indicated that the week in which treatment differences became significant occurred slightly later in this trial than in similar trials using different SSRIs. Also, the study design did not allow for a comparison of efficacy between fixed doses of fluoxetine, so it is difficult to determine whether the higher dosage caused treatment effects or whether participants would have improved at a later point in the study while taking the fluoxetine at a lower dosage. These results are supported by a similar crossover trial (Riddle et al. 1992).

Birmaher et al. (2003) completed a fluoxetine treatment study involving children and adolescents diagnosed with separation anxiety disorder, social phobia, and/or GAD. Seventy-four individuals (ages 7–17) were randomly assigned to placebo or fluoxetine (maximum dose, 20 mg/day) for a period of 12 weeks. The investigators found that at treatment end, the fluoxetine group showed significantly more improvement in CGI-I scores, the primary outcome variable (61% vs. 35% placebo; $\chi^2=4.93$). Fluoxetine-treated subjects diagnosed with social phobia seemed to have the best outcome, with significantly improved scores on the CGI-I ($\chi^2=12.13$) and the Children's Global Assessment Scale (CGAS; $\chi^2=6.01$) compared with those receiving placebo. Side effects in this study were minimal for the most part but included occasional headaches, drowsiness, abdominal pain, nausea, and agitation. The investigators noted that approximately half of the subjects remained symptomatic by the end of the trial, and they suggested that some subjects may have required a higher dosage or may have fared better with concurrent psychotherapy.

Sertraline (Zoloft). RCTs using sertraline as treatment have focused on pediatric populations diagnosed with OCD, GAD, and PTSD. In a double-blind, placebo-controlled trial, March et al. (1998) tested the efficacy of sertraline for children ($n=107$, ages 6–12) and adolescents ($n=80$, ages 13–17) with OCD. Subjects were randomly assigned to placebo ($n=95$) or sertraline ($n=92$) for 12 weeks, with the dosage starting at 25 mg/day for children and 50 mg/day for adolescents. The dosage was then titrated upward (in a forced design) by 50 mg/week to a maximum of 200 mg/day (mean total dosage, 167 mg/day). Efficacy analyses revealed that by the end of week 2, subjects treated with sertraline showed significantly greater improvement on the primary outcome variable—CY-BOCS ($P=0.005$) and National Institute of Mental Health Global Obsessive-Compulsive Scale (NIMH-GOCS; $P=0.002$) scores—compared with those given placebo. In addition, 53% of the sertraline group was considered responders compared with 37% of the placebo group ($P=0.03$), as indicated by their CY-BOCS scores. The results were similar on the NIMH-GOCS (42% vs. 26%; $P=0.02$). Side effects reported in the trial by March et al. (1998) were generally mild to moderate, with sertraline-treated subjects reporting significantly more incidences of insomnia, nausea, agitation, and tremor ($P<0.05$). The results of this study indicate that sertraline is efficacious in treating children and adolescents with OCD in the short term. As with other studies, some subjects continued to exhibit symptoms at the end of the trial, which may indicate the need for concurrent psychotherapy.

Rynn et al. (2001) conducted a double-blind, placebo-controlled trial to assess the efficacy of a lower daily dosage of sertraline (50 mg/day) in youth diagnosed with GAD ($N=22$, ages 5–17). An analysis of covariance (ANCOVA) on the primary outcome variables revealed that significant treatment differences were apparent by week 4 and continued until the end of the study. At the end of week 9, subjects receiving sertraline were rated as endorsing fewer symptoms on all Hamilton Anxiety Scale scores than subjects receiving placebo, including Total ($F=15.3$; $P<0.001$), Psychic Factor ($F=22.6$; $P<0.001$), and Somatic Factor ($F=8.91$; $P<0.01$); measuring less severity on the CGI-S ($F=30.5$; $P<0.001$); and showing greater improvement in CGI-I scores ($F=14.9$; $P<0.001$). At treatment end point, 90% of sertraline-treated subjects were considered to have improved symptoms based on CGI-I scores (1 = very much improved or 2 = much improved), as opposed to 10% of subjects given placebo ($P<0.001$, Fisher exact test). Yet only 18% of subjects in the improved sertraline group were rated as markedly improved, which represents a small remission rate. Side effects did not differ significantly between the sertraline and placebo groups. This trial suggests that sertraline 50 mg/day may be an effective, safe dosage for short-term use in young patients diagnosed with GAD, reducing both psychic and somatic symptoms of anxiety with mild side effects. However, given the low rate of markedly improved ratings, these findings suggest that a higher dosage may be needed to achieve remission.

Evidence of the efficacy of SSRIs and other medications in treating PTSD in children and adolescents is limited. Robb et al. (2010) conducted one of the few existing RCTs on the treatment of pediatric PTSD, comparing sertraline (50–200 mg/day) with placebo ($N=131$, ages 6–17) over 10 weeks. The study failed to find any significant effects for sertraline and, in fact, provided evidence for the superiority of placebo on some of the secondary outcome measures, although sertraline has demonstrated efficacy in treating PTSD in adults.

Fluvoxamine (Luvox). In a multisite, randomized, placebo-controlled trial, Riddle et al. (2001) studied the effects of fluvoxamine in pediatric OCD. Following a 1- to 2-week, single-blind screening period, eligible patients ($N=120$, ages 8–17) were randomly assigned to placebo or fluvoxamine (maximum dosage, 200 mg/day) for 10 weeks. The investigators found that fluvoxamine was significantly more effective than placebo in ameliorating OCD symptoms on all measures. A two-way ANOVA on the CY-BOCS total score revealed significant treatment effects at weeks 1, 2, 3, 4, 6, and 10. At the end of the study, 42% of subjects given fluvoxamine were defined as treatment responders, with a 25% reduction of symptoms based on CY-BOCS scores since baseline, versus 25% of those given placebo ($P=0.065$, Cochran-Mantel-Haenszel test). Responder analysis on the CGI-I also revealed that significantly more subjects treated with fluvoxamine had a meaningful response to treatment ("much" or "very much" improved) at the end of 10 weeks (29.8% vs. 17.5% placebo; $P=0.078$, Cochran-Mantel-Haenszel test). Adverse effects that were significantly more prevalent in the fluvoxamine group included asthenia (fatigue, loss of energy, or weakness) and insomnia.

Riddle et al. (2001) demonstrated that fluvoxamine is both fast acting and effective as a short-term pediatric OCD treatment. A limitation of the study is that most subjects did not have comorbid diagnoses—a sample that is less typical of the OCD population, in which psychiatric comorbidity is high.

In another large-scale study, the Research Units on Pediatric Psychopharmacology (RUPP) Anxiety Study Group (2001) assessed the efficacy of fluvoxamine treatment in children and adolescents ($N=128$, ages 6–17) whose signs and symptoms met criteria for social phobia, separation anxiety disorder, or GAD. Subjects were randomly assigned to fluvoxamine ($n=63$) or placebo ($n=65$) for 8 weeks. The fluvoxamine dosage was titrated upward 50 mg/week to a maximum of 300 mg/day for adolescents and 250 mg/day for children (age 12 years or younger). From an intent-to-treat analysis, the investigators found that participants receiving fluvoxamine had a greater reduction in anxiety symptoms and higher rates of clinical response than did those given placebo. Treatment differences on one primary outcome variable, the Pediatric Anxiety Rating Scale (PARS), reached significance by week 3 and increased through week 6. By the end of the study, the fluvoxamine group had significantly lower PARS scores, indicating mild symptoms of anxiety ($P<0.001$). The CGI-I score, which defines meaningful clinical response to treatment as scores of 3 (improved), 2 (much improved), or 1 (free of symptoms), revealed that at study end point, significantly more subjects treated with fluvoxamine received scores less than 4 (76% vs. 29% placebo; $P<0.001$). They also reported significantly more abdominal discomfort ($P=0.02$) and showed a trend for increased motor activity ($P=0.06$).

Following the acute trial, the RUPP group investigated possible moderators and mediators of pharmacological treatment in children and adolescents with anxiety disorders (RUPP Anxiety Study Group 2002; Walkup et al. 2003). Although no significant moderators were found, analyses revealed that subjects presenting with social phobia ($P<0.05$) and a greater severity of baseline illness ($P<0.001$) were less likely to improve, regardless of treatment group.

Paroxetine (Paxil). In a placebo-controlled multicenter trial, Wagner et al. (2004) evaluated the effects of treatment with paroxetine in children and adolescents ($N=319$, ages 8–17) diagnosed with social anxiety disorder. Participants were randomly assigned to either paroxetine ($n=163$; mean dosage, 24.8 mg/day) or placebo ($n=156$) for a 16-week trial.

Results at week 16 demonstrated that 77.6% of paroxetine-treated subjects were defined as treatment responders, having a score of "improved" or "much improved" on the CGI-I, compared with 38.3% of subjects given placebo ($P<0.001$). This trend appeared even within the first 4 weeks of treatment. Adverse effects were rated from mild to moderate in severity, with insomnia ($P=0.02$), decreased appetite ($P=0.11$), and vomiting ($P=0.07$) considered treatment emergent. Because paroxetine treatment exhibited a greater response rate than placebo, and treatment differences reached significance on all five secondary outcome variables, Wagner et al. (2004) supported the use of paroxetine in treating pediatric social anxiety disorder. Another interesting finding is that the children and adolescents in this study (77.6%) demonstrated a greater response to treatment than did socially anxious adults treated with paroxetine (55%; Stein et al. 1998). The investigators acknowledged that commonly occurring comorbid disorders such as MDD were identified as exclusions and that their findings, therefore, cannot be generalized to a broader population. Similar findings were presented in another large-scale, multisite trial (Geller et al. 2004).

Citalopram (Celexa) and escitalopram (Lexapro). Limited data are available examining the effectiveness of citalopram and escitalopram, which is the pharmacologically active *S*-enantiomer of citalopram. Escitalopram received FDA approval for the treatment of adolescent depression (ages 12–17) (Wagner et al. 2006). Strawn et al. (2020) conducted an 8-week randomized placebo-controlled double-blind study in adolescents ($n=51$; ages 12–17) with the primary diagnosis of GAD in which they examined the efficacy and safety of escitalopram with a dosage titration based on response to the maximum of 20 mg/day. The study found that escitalopram led to significant clinical improvement compared with placebo as measured by the primary outcome measure, the PARS ($P<0.001$). Additionally, this study examined the impact of phenotype variations of CYP2C19, which leads to individual differences in pharmacokinetics that may impact treatment effectiveness.

In an open-label study evaluating the treatment impact of escitalopram for children and adolescents (age 10–17 years) diagnosed with primary social phobia, Isolan et al. (2007) showed that 65% of the sample (13 of 20) experienced greater improvement at the end of 12 weeks of treatment with a maximum dose of 20 mg/day. In another open-label study of citalopram treatment for children and adolescents (ages 9–18) diagnosed with primary OCD, participants received flexible dosing for 10 weeks; results suggested that this treatment was effective and safe (Thomsen 1997). As reported on ClinicalTrials.gov, in September 2021 the pharmaceutical company Allergan Inc. completed a randomized, double-blind, flexible-dose study of escitalopram (10–20 mg) versus placebo for the efficacy and safety in children and adolescents ($n=256$, ages 7–17) with the primary diagnosis of GAD. At this time, the results have not been posted (ClinicalTrials.gov identifier NCT03924323).

Meta-Analytic Data

A meta-analysis of pediatric OCD trials conducted by Geller et al. (2003) revealed a highly significant pooled effect for each SSRI and clomipramine versus placebo ($P<0.001$). There were no significant pooled mean differences between one SSRI and another, indicating that no one SSRI was more efficacious than another in treating pediatric OCD. There was, however, a significant pooled mean difference favoring clomipramine over the SSRIs (P=0.002, χ^2 test), indicating that clomipramine was more effective in reducing OCD symptoms across studies.

Although this analysis showed clomipramine as superior to the SSRIs, Geller et al. (2003) did not recommend using clomipramine as a first-line pharmacological agent because of its side effect profile and association with cardiac toxicity. In less severe cases, the investigators suggest that SSRIs should be the first-choice medication, specifying that the choice of individual SSRI should be based more on adverse effect profiles and pharmacokinetic properties such as half-life than on efficacy.

The meta-analysis for non-OCD anxiety studies involved nine studies (N=1,673) and six medications (SSRIs/serotonin-norepinephrine reuptake inhibitors [SNRIs]) (Strawn et al. 2015b). The medications studied showed efficacy of moderate magnitude (Cohen's d=0.62, 95% CI 0.34–0.89; P=0.009). Regarding adverse events, activation appeared more likely with antidepressant treatment (OR 1.86, 95% CI 0.98–3.53; P=0.054). However, the study investigators found no increased risk for nausea/abdominal symptoms (P=0.262), discontinuation due to an adverse event (P=0.132), or presence of suicidality (OR 1.3, 95% CI 0.53–3.2; P=0.514).

Risks of SSRIs

Currently, the FDA has approved only fluoxetine, sertraline, and fluvoxamine for the treatment of pediatric OCD. The consensus is that, in most cases, the benefits of SSRIs outweigh their risks. However, the use of psychopharmaceuticals, including SSRIs, for anxiety disorders in children and adolescents is not without risk. SSRI-related side effects include nausea, diarrhea, gastrointestinal distress, headaches, lack of energy, sexual dysfunction, sweating, dry mouth, restlessness, initial insomnia, sleepiness, increased hyperactivity, vivid dreams, and tremor. These problems are usually short-lived and dose related and tend to resolve with time. Potentially more serious side effects include the development of hypomania, mania, serotonin syndrome, seizures, and abnormal bleeding (AACAP anxiety practice parameter; Walter et al. 2020). However, discontinuation symptoms are possible with some SSRIs, such as paroxetine, sertraline, and fluvoxamine, which have increasingly been associated with a withdrawal syndrome on discontinuation (Leonard et al. 1997; Rosenbaum et al. 1998). Withdrawal symptoms do not generally occur with fluoxetine because of its long half-life, and there is somewhat less concern with sertraline because of the presence of its one weak metabolite. Some trials (Geller et al. 2001; Riddle et al. 2001) have also reported cases of participants who showed abnormal vital signs—an unsurprising finding, given that the medication has been associated with changes in weight and decreases in blood pressure. As with any medication, there is always a risk of allergic reaction.

In addition to these issues, the FDA issued an advisory to physicians that the use of antidepressants may lead to suicidal thinking/suicide attempts in youth (U.S. Food and Drug Administration 2005). This warning highlights the need for close observation for signs of worsening symptoms and the emergence of suicidality in children treated with these medications.

Long-Term Treatment

Benefits. Following their acute trial (described in the "Fluvoxamine [Luvox]" section), the RUPP group conducted a 6-month, open-label extension study (Walkup et al. 2002) to examine the effects of continuing treatment with fluvoxamine or with a second SSRI in the remaining subjects. The study design was such that active treatment responders from the acute trial continued with fluvoxamine (group I, $n=35$), active nonresponders switched to fluoxetine (group II, $n=14$), and placebo nonresponders began fluvoxamine (group III, $n=48$), with dosage schedules that varied according to treatment group.

This study was not controlled; therefore, data analyses are suggestive and pertain more to clinical functioning (Walkup et al. 2002). Using the CGI-I as a primary outcome measure, the investigators found that 94% of subjects who continued receiving open-label fluvoxamine (mean final dosage, 131 mg/day) were considered responders (scores ≤ 3 on the CGI-I) after 24 weeks and maintained response. After 24 weeks, 71% of subjects to whom fluoxetine was administered (mean final dosage, 24 mg/day) met the criteria for response. Finally, 56% of placebo nonresponders who began receiving open-label fluvoxamine (135 mg/day) were considered responders at week 24. Side effects were mild and generally transient. Data from this extension study suggest that relapse rates for anxious children maintained on SSRI treatment are low and that extended SSRI treatment is generally safe.

In addition to the RUPP extension study, data from long-term OCD trials can provide some indication of the efficacy and safety of maintenance treatment with SSRIs. Following a 12-week double-blind study (March et al. 1998),

Cook et al. (2001) conducted a 52-week sertraline extension trial for subjects who completed the acute phase. Dosages for subjects (*N*=137, ages 6–18) were titrated to and maintained at the level at which satisfactory clinical response was exhibited (not to exceed 200 mg/day). Data analysis was performed according to age, with a mean dosage of 108 mg/day for children (*n*=72) and 132 mg/day for adolescents (*n*=65). Response rates, with response defined as a greater than 25% decrease in baseline CY-BOCS score and a CGI-I score of 1 or 2 at trial end point, were 67% for the combined age groups, 72% for children, and 61% for adolescents. Significant improvements over the course of treatment were evident on all outcome measures ($P<0.05$). By the end of the study, 85% of active treatment responders who completed the full 52 weeks maintained responder status compared with 43% of nonresponders. Side effects were common, with an incidence of 77% among all subjects, and included headache, insomnia, nausea, diarrhea, somnolence, abdominal pain, hyperkinesia, nervousness, dyspepsia, and vomiting.

These results provide support for long-term sertraline treatment in youth with OCD. The most striking feature of the analyses is that of participants who did not respond to sertraline in the acute phase, 43% were considered responders by the end of the extension trial. Although side effects generally improved as treatment continued, the percentage of participants withdrawing because of adverse events (12%) seems somewhat high in comparison with other trials.

A smaller trial assessing the long-term effects of citalopram concurrent with CBT on adolescents with OCD (Thomsen et al. 2001) revealed similar results. Following a 10-week open-label trial (*N*=23) of citalopram (maximum dosage, 40 mg/day) (Thomsen 1997), subjects given citalopram (*N*=30, ages 13–18) continued in an open trial (mean dosage, 46.5 mg/day; range, 20–80 mg/day) for a 6-month to 2-year period. Although 28 of the subjects continued taking citalopram for a year, only 14 completed the 2-year study. Analyzing the data from baseline to the 2-year end point, investigators found that the decrease in Yale-Brown Obsessive Compulsive Scale (Y-BOCS)/CY-BOCS scores was statistically significant for each time period (baseline to 10 weeks, 10 weeks to 6 months, 6 months to 1 year, and baseline to 2 years; $P<0.001$), except for the time from the 1-year end point to the 2-year end point. This finding indicated that subjects maintaining citalopram treatment for 4.5 months following the acute trial continued to exhibit a reduction of symptoms on the Y-BOCS/CY-BOCS, with an even greater reduction over the next 6 months, but that symptom reduction did not continue in the second year of treatment. Side effects, similar to those reported in other SSRI trials, were generally mild and decreased with continued treatment. Only sexual dysfunction and sedation were reported as persistent, causing two subjects to drop out of the trial.

In addition to these trials, review articles provide guidance on the long-term SSRI use in children and adolescents. In his review of acute-anxiety trials and adult and animal studies, Pine (2002) argued that children who have shown satisfactory response to SSRI treatment should be given a medication-free trial instead of having long-term treatment maintained, and they should be promptly returned to medication if their symptoms relapse. Longitudinal data suggest that mood and anxiety disorders evident in childhood carry a significant risk for mood and anxiety disorders later in life. If left untreated, these disorders may have considerable harmful effects on development, with possible long-term implications. Pine (2002) stated that this finding must be weighed against potential risks in using SSRI medication long term. Evidence from animal studies also provides an interesting dilemma. Although serotonin plays a role in neural plasticity, and long-term SSRI use may adversely affect cellular processes that involve serotonin, stress and impairing anxiety symptoms in early life can also greatly impact brain development. Currently, the AACAP anxiety practice parameter recommendation regarding treatment length is to continue the antidepressant treatment at the best tolerated dosage for 12 months, beginning at remission, and then carefully monitor for any return of symptoms over the following several months (Walter et al. 2020).

Risks of long-term treatment. Side effects reported in long-term studies were similar to those reported in acute trials, which included gastrointestinal disturbance, headache, and insomnia. These effects were often mild in nature and decreased with continued treatment. Overall, adverse effects did not typically lead to study withdrawal, and most trials reported relatively low dropout rates. However, there were reports of hyperkinesia (Cook et al. 2001) that was severe enough to warrant study withdrawal, as well as persistent complaints of sexual dysfunction and sedation (Thomsen et al. 2001) in some long-term studies. Reports have also documented a decrease in growth rate among youth treated with various SSRIs over a period ranging from 6 months to 5 years (dosage, 20–100 mg/day) (Weintrob et al. 2002).

Serotonin-Norepinephrine Reuptake Inhibitors

Pharmacological treatments tend to focus on several neurotransmitter systems believed to form the biological foundation of anxiety disorders, such as serotonin and GABA. Another class of medications that shows promise in the treatment of pediatric anxiety disorders is the SNRIs, which target both the serotonergic and noradrenergic systems. The SNRI venlafaxine XR (extended release) has been shown to be effective in adult GAD at total daily doses between 75 and 225 mg in several large, double-blind, placebo-controlled trials (Davidson et al. 1999; Gelenberg et al. 2000; Rickels et al. 2000). As has been the case with SSRI use, children with anxiety disorders appear to respond to venlafaxine XR in the same manner as adults (Rynn et al. 2004). Duloxetine, another SNRI considered effective for adult MDD and possibly for adult GAD (Rynn et al. 2007), was also shown to be effective for youth with GAD at total daily doses between 30 mg and 120 mg (Strawn et al. 2015a). Duloxetine has been FDA approved for pediatric GAD.

Acute Treatment

Benefits. Rynn et al. (2007) reported on the results of a pooled analysis of two combined multisite, 8-week studies examining the efficacy and safety of venlafaxine XR (n=154) compared with placebo (n=159) in the treatment of childhood GAD (ages 6–17; P<0.001). Exclusions included concurrent psychiatric disorders such as MDD, social anxiety disorder, and separation anxiety disorder. Dosing for venlafaxine XR began with 37.5 mg/day, and the total daily dose was increased on the basis of body weight (37.5–112.5 mg for children weighing 25–39 kg; minimum dosage range of 75–150 mg for those weighing 40–49 kg; and a maximum dosage of 225 mg for those weighing ≥50 kg). In an analysis of the two studies, one showed statistically significant improvement favoring venlafaxine XR on both primary (P<0.001) and secondary (P<0.01) outcome measures. The other study showed significant improvement for venlafaxine XR on some secondary outcome measures but not on the primary measure (P=0.06). Pooled analysis indicated a greater mean decrease on the primary outcome for venlafaxine XR versus placebo (–17.4 vs. –12.7; P<0.001). Response rates, with response defined as a CGI-I score less than 3, were also significantly greater for venlafaxine XR (69% vs. 48%; P=0.004).

Tourian et al. (2004) found similar results when comparing venlafaxine XR (n=137) and placebo (n=148) in children and adolescents (ages 8–17) with social anxiety disorder (P<0.001) over 16 weeks. Subjects with scores of 50 or more on the Social Anxiety Scale (SAS), 4 or more in the CGI-S, and no concurrent psychiatric disorder were eligible. Results showed that baseline-to-end point improvement in total SAS scores was significantly higher for the venlafaxine XR group compared with the placebo group (22.5 vs. 14.9 points, adjusted change; P<0.001).

Examining the treatment effects of duloxetine on pediatric GAD, Strawn et al. (2015a) conducted a randomized, double-blind, placebo-controlled study in which children and adolescents (ages 7–17) were assigned to either duloxetine (n=135) or placebo (n=137) over 10 weeks. Duloxetine dosing was flexible, beginning at 30 mg once daily for 2 weeks before titration and continuing up to 120 mg based on tolerability and response. The results suggested a significant treatment effect of duloxetine compared with placebo on the main outcome measure—severity of GAD based on PARS score (mean change, 9.7 vs. 7.1; P<0.001)—as well as greater symptom response and functional remission (P<0.05).

Risks of SNRIs. In the study by Rynn et al. (2007), the incidence of asthenia, pain, anorexia, and somnolence in subjects treated with venlafaxine XR was twice that (≥5%) in the placebo group. Only the development of anorexia differed significantly between treatment groups (13% for venlafaxine XR vs. 3% for placebo); also, two medication-treated subjects displayed suicidal ideation and behavior, leading to their removal from the study. In addition, there were statistically significant mean increases from baseline cholesterol serum levels for children treated with venlafaxine XR and statistically significant mean changes from baseline in subjects' vital signs, with a difference in pulse rate of approximately 4 beats per minute (bpm) and a difference in blood pressure (supine diastolic and systolic) of approximately 2 mm Hg for children treated with venlafaxine XR. The group treated with venlafaxine XR had a height increase of 0.3 cm from baseline (P<0.05) compared with 1.0 cm (P<0.001) in children given placebo (difference between groups: P=0.041).

In the study by Tourian et al. (2004), the most common adverse effects among venlafaxine XR–treated patients were influenza, anorexia, asthenia, weight loss, nausea, and pharyngitis. Three adolescents in the medication group also displayed suicidal ideation, as opposed to none in the placebo arm. As found in the GAD study, patients treated with venlafaxine XR experienced significant mean weight loss compared with the placebo group ($P<0.001$); in several cases ($n=8$), the weight loss was considered clinically significant.

In the study of duloxetine by Strawn et al. (2015a), children and adolescents who were randomly assigned to the duloxetine group were more likely to experience nausea, vomiting, decreased appetite, oropharyngeal pain, dizziness, cough, and palpitations those randomly assigned to placebo ($P<0.05$). The proportion of patients who experienced at least one adverse event was significantly greater for the duloxetine group (106 of 135 [78.5%] vs. 90 of 137 [65.7%]; $P=0.022$). The investigators also found significant differences in mean change in pulse (increase of 6.5 bpm in the duloxetine group compared with 2.0 bpm in the placebo group) and weight loss of 0.1 kg in the duloxetine group compared with weight gain of 1.1 kg in the placebo group ($P<0.01$).

Long-Term Treatment

In the Strawn et al. (2015a) study of duloxetine for pediatric GAD, following the 10-week acute trial, participants in both the duloxetine and placebo groups were treated with open-label duloxetine for an additional 18 weeks. All participants demonstrated mean score improvement in PARS severity for GAD at 28 weeks (3.96 for participants initially randomly assigned to duloxetine vs. 4.68 for participants initially randomly assigned to placebo). The probability of achieving remission based on PARS severity for GAD was roughly the same for both groups at week 28 (84% for those initially randomly assigned to duloxetine vs. 87% for those initially randomly assigned to placebo).

Two adult studies (Allgulander et al. 2001; Gelenberg et al. 2000) were conducted to assess response to 6 months of treatment with venlafaxine XR compared with placebo. The results indicated no decrease in the efficacy of venlafaxine XR over the 6-month treatment period. Although neither adult study was designed to assess relapse rates following treatment discontinuation as a function of long-term treatment, both suggested that patients with GAD may benefit from at least 6 months of continuous treatment. Presently, very limited data exist evaluating the long-term use of this class of compound for pediatric anxiety disorders.

Benzodiazepines

Benzodiazepines have been used as effective anxiolytics and sedatives in adults since they first appeared in clinical practice in the early 1960s, before their mechanism of action was understood. It was not until almost two decades later that researchers discovered specific benzodiazepine receptors on the neurons of the brain and began to understand how benzodiazepines produce their varying effects. Following this discovery, they posited that benzodiazepines function by activating GABA, an inhibitory neurotransmitter, which slows the response of neural activity in the brain and produces an overall sedating effect.

Although the exact chemical process by which benzodiazepines produce anxiolytic effects is yet to be completely determined, their effect is strongly linked to the relationship between benzodiazepines and the GABAergic system. Bernstein et al. (1993) hypothesized that because abnormalities in norepinephrine and GABA levels in the brain are thought to underlie anxiety disorders, correcting these levels with agents such as benzodiazepines should lead to a reduction of anxiety symptoms.

Benzodiazepines vary widely in terms of what are considered to be their effective daily dose and *half-life*, which represents how fast the drug is metabolized by the body. According to the cited literature, some benzodiazepines, such as clonazepam, can be effective in adults at a total daily dose of 0.5–3.0 mg; others, such as lorazepam, are effective at a dose of 1–6 mg/day (Witek et al. 2005). Clonazepam also has a much longer half-life than lorazepam (18–50 hours compared with 10–20 hours), indicating that clonazepam remains in the body for a longer period of time. This means that clonazepam is long-acting, and although it may be useful in relieving long-term anxiety, it may also lengthen the incidence for side effects.

Justification for using benzodiazepines in clinical practice for the treatment of anxious children is provided by adult studies on GAD and panic disorder. In a large, multisite, placebo-controlled study, Ballenger et al. (1988) examined the effects of alprazolam on 481 adults diagnosed with panic disorder in an 8-week trial. According to the end-point analysis, subjects in the alprazolam group were judged to have significantly higher physician- and patient-rated global improvement scores ($P<0.0001$) and fewer phobic ($P<0.0001$) and anxiety ($P<0.0001$) symptoms on the Overall Phobia Rating Scale and clinician-rated Hamilton Anxiety Scale, respectively, and they reported significantly fewer panic attacks.

Benzodiazepines have also been effective in treating adults with GAD. Rickels et al. (1983) found that anxious adults (N=151) randomly assigned to alprazolam or diazepam greatly improved compared with those assigned to placebo during the 4-week trial. More patients dropped out of the placebo group; subjects in the medication groups had significantly more improvement on patient and physician ratings as early as 1 week into the study (mean alprazolam dosage 1.2 mg/day; mean diazepam dosage 20 mg/day). Significance between active treatment and placebo was also apparent on many of the ratings scales at end-point analysis, indicating that effects were maintained throughout the trial. Alprazolam is the only benzodiazepine approved by the FDA for the treatment of GAD.

Acute Treatment

Benefits. Unlike the substantial literature available about treatment with SSRIs, relatively few structured investigations assessing the efficacy of benzodiazepines for pediatric anxiety disorders have been published.

In one of the earliest RCTs measuring the efficacy of benzodiazepines in children with anxiety disorders, Bernstein et al. (1990) examined the effect of alprazolam and imipramine for the treatment of young school refusers. Encouraged by the positive results of an open-label trial, in which 67% of patients randomly assigned to alprazolam showed marked or moderate improvement and 55% returned to school, the investigators created a double-blind crossover study. Subjects were randomly assigned to alprazolam, imipramine, or placebo for 8 weeks, and then the medication was tapered for 1–2 weeks and discontinued. The investigators discovered that the treatments produced statistically significant differences at week 8 on the Anxiety Rating for Children measure, with subjects randomly assigned to alprazolam (maximum dosage, 3 mg/day) showing the most improvement. However, these results failed to reach significance once the baseline scores were factored in as covariates in the ANCOVA.

Simeon et al. (1992) conducted an RCT following the results of their open study (Simeon and Ferguson 1987). As in the Bernstein et al. (1990) trial, the follow-up, placebo-controlled, double-blind study failed to corroborate the earlier findings. Subjects (N=30) were children with presentations meeting DSM-III criteria for anxiety and avoidance who were given placebo for

1 week and then randomly assigned to alprazolam or placebo for 4 weeks (mean maximum dosage 1.57 mg/day; range, 0.5–3.5 mg/day). The medication was tapered for 2 additional weeks and then replaced with placebo. Subjects either received the replacement placebo or continued receiving the original placebo, respectively. Although their evaluations, administered after the double-blind trial (day 28), seemed to indicate symptom improvement among the children given alprazolam, Simeon and colleagues found that differences in clinical global ratings were not statistically significant.

Following the Simeon et al. (1992) trial, Graae et al. (1994) performed a double-blind, crossover pilot study involving children with similar anxiety diagnoses (N=15). All but one of the children were diagnosed with separation anxiety disorder according to DSM-III criteria, and all but two presented with comorbid anxiety disorders. In this study, unlike in the Simeon et al. (1992) study, subjects were immediately randomly assigned to either clonazepam (maximum dosage, 2 mg/day) or placebo for a 4-week, double-blind trial. Although at the end of the study, half the children no longer had symptoms that met the criteria for an anxiety disorder, treatment-effect comparisons did not reach significant levels. No significant treatment differences were found related to the frequency and severity of anxiety symptoms identified by the other measures, the Diagnostic Interview Schedule for Children and the Children's Manifest Anxiety Scale. The authors did not support using clonazepam at the dosing schedule of 2 mg/day in children and adolescents with anxiety disorders.

Risks of benzodiazepines. Side effects for most benzodiazepines have been reported as infrequent and mild, although they vary in severity across studies. The most common side effects were dry mouth and drowsiness. Simeon et al. (1992) also reported that sedation and disinhibition, manifested by aggressivity, irritability, and incoordination, were common. In addition, 71% of participants in the Bernstein et al. (1990) trial presented with abdominal pain, dizziness, and headaches.

Graae et al. (1994), in their study, reported the most severe side effects. Disinhibition, irritability, and oppositionality were notable in their sample; in three cases, these side effects were severe enough to cause the subjects to drop out of the study during Phase I. Benzodiazepines can lead to dependence with chronic use, usually defined as longer than 8 weeks of treatment (Nishino et al. 1995). Although none of the reviewed studies indicated withdrawal symptoms during the tapering period, it would be wise to monitor children closely during this period and to not administer benzodiazepines on a long-term basis. Although the review findings indicate that benzodiazepine treatment offers some benefits for anxious children and adolescents, there have not been enough well-designed clinical trials with large sample sizes to clearly evaluate the safety and efficacy of this class of compounds.

Long-Term Treatment

Because of concern that dependence will develop as a result of long-term treatment with benzodiazepines, many of the published RCTs have been acute studies, and no long-term studies have evaluated treatment for anxious children and adolescents. However, many long-term studies have used benzodiazepines in adults diagnosed with anxiety disorders, especially panic disorder, because the chronic nature of panic disorder tends to require longer treatment duration. For example, in a large, placebo-controlled study, Schweizer et al. (1993) studied the treatment effect of long-term alprazolam (mean dosage, 5.7 mg/day) and imipramine (mean dosage, 175 mg/day) use in adults with panic disorder, with or without agoraphobia (N= 106, ages 18–65). Following an acute trial, participants who experienced symptom improvement were randomly assigned to alprazolam (n=27), imipramine (n= 13), or placebo (n= 11) for 6 months of maintenance treatment. Monthly assessments included measures of panic attack frequency and severity, generalized anxiety, and phobias.

The results indicated that following maintenance treatment, panic attack frequency declined for all patients except one in the placebo group. At week 32, only 9% of the alprazolam group, 0% of the imipramine group, and 22% of the placebo group still reported experiencing minor symptom attacks. Subjects receiving maintenance treatment with alprazolam who showed tolerance to adverse events such as sedation, a common side effect for benzodiazepines, had a decrease in incidence from 49% during the acute trial to 7%.

Although this study had a high attrition rate from the acute trial to the maintenance phase, with significantly more subjects remaining in the alprazolam group, the results are striking. Alprazolam-treated patients showed significantly more difficulty than imipramine- or placebo-treated subjects in discontinuing medication. In addition, the investigators noted that after 1-year follow-up, patients who had originally been treated with imipramine or placebo did just as well on clinical measures as those who had been treated with alprazolam but without exhibiting any of the physical dependence or withdrawal symptoms. This finding indicates that the sustained treatment effects of long-term therapy with benzodiazepines might not be worth the risk, especially in the pediatric population.

Tricyclic Antidepressants

Tricyclic antidepressants (TCAs), named for their three-ring structure, are known for their mood-elevating effects. For this reason, they have been used as a front-line pharmacological treatment for adults with depression and anxiety since the mid-1960s (Potter et al. 1995). Precursors to the safer SSRIs, TCAs bind to presynaptic transporter proteins in the brain and inhibit the reuptake of norepinephrine and serotonin in the presynaptic terminal. Although all TCAs are equally effective in inhibiting both norepinephrine and serotonin, some are more preferential to one or the other, causing them to be referred to as "noradrenergic" or "serotonergic," respectively (Meyer and Quenzer 2005). TCAs may be helpful for long-term treatment of anxiety because inhibition of norepinephrine and serotonin extends the duration of the transmitter action at the synapse and changes both the presynaptic and postsynaptic receptors. This adaptation over time may increase the potential for clinical improvement, but it also extends the potential for side effects. In terms of half-life, most TCAs remain in the body for approximately 24 hours, allowing for once-daily dosing (Potter et al. 1995). In adults, TCAs are used for the treatment of MDD, anxiety disorders (GAD, panic disorder, OCD), and pain syndromes.

Acute Treatment

Benefits. Although some RCTs (Bernstein et al. 2000; Gittelman-Klein and Klein 1971) indicated significant treatment differences between TCAs and placebo, a number of studies were unable to replicate and support these findings (Berney et al. 1981; Bernstein et al. 1990; Klein et al. 1992). Additionally, investigators have reported serious side effects in children taking TCAs, suggesting that the risk involved may outweigh the potential benefits.

Gittelman-Klein and Klein (1971) performed the first RCT evaluating the effect of TCAs on children with school phobia. In a double-blind, placebo-controlled study, they randomly assigned children with school phobia (N=35) to either imipramine or placebo (mean dosage, 152 mg/day; range,

100–200 mg/day) for 6 weeks. Assessments included measures of global improvement on a seven-point scale, school attendance, and psychiatric ratings of symptoms. At the end of the 6-week trial, the investigators found that imipramine was significantly more effective than placebo in increasing school attendance, and greater improvement on all other measures was indicated. Of children given medication, 81% returned to school, as opposed to 47% of those given placebo (P<0.05), a significantly greater frequency of improvement in the imipramine group.

Berney et al. (1981) followed the Gittelman-Klein and Klein (1971) study with a 12-week trial assessing the efficacy of clomipramine in child and adolescent school refusers (N=46). Subjects were randomly selected to receive clomipramine or placebo, prescribed according to age (40 mg/day for ages 9–10; 50 mg/day for ages 11–12; 75 mg/day for ages 13–14). Although the investigators discovered a significant shift toward improvement on global scores within both the placebo and the medication groups, they found that this significance disappeared when the groups were compared in an ANCOVA. By the end of the study, more than one-third of the sample still had serious difficulty returning to school.

In a double-blind, placebo-controlled study comparing the use of alprazolam and imipramine in treating children and adolescents who refused to attend school (N=24), Bernstein et al. (1990) found similar effects. An ANOVA showed that subjects randomly assigned to imipramine (n=9; mean total daily dose, 164.29 mg) for the full 8 weeks showed significantly less improvement in Anxiety Rating for Children scores compared with those in the alprazolam group (n=7; mean total daily dose, 1.82 mg) but demonstrated significantly more improvement than those given placebo (n=7; P=0.03). However, these results were no longer significant after ANCOVAs were performed.

Following this trial, Klein et al. (1992) conducted another RCT comparing imipramine and placebo in children with separation anxiety disorder (N=20). If subjects' symptoms did not respond to a 4-week behavioral treatment, they were randomly assigned to placebo or imipramine (mean dosage, 153 mg/day; range, 75–275 mg/day) for a 6-week trial. By the end of the study, the results were not significant on any of the ratings, which included parent and child self-reports, teacher and psychiatrist ratings, and global improvement scores. Although half of the subjects reported improved symptoms, these results do not appear to support the use of TCAs as a monotherapy for pediatric anxiety disorders. The targeted sample had pure separation anxiety without comorbid depression, not school phobia, yet the medication did not prove to be any more effective than placebo. Also, children in the imipramine group reported some severe side effects and were still receiving psychotherapy as an adjunctive treatment.

Studies assessing the efficacy of the serotonergic TCA clomipramine in children with OCD also give some insight into the overall efficacy of TCAs for anxiety disorders. In a 10-week, double-blind crossover trial (N=48), Leonard et al. (1989) compared two TCAs: clomipramine, which has been shown to be effective in children with OCD, and desipramine, which is less potent in inhibiting serotonin reuptake (Ross and Renyi 1975). Following a 2-week, single-blind placebo phase to assess efficacy, subjects were randomly assigned to either clomipramine or desipramine for the first 5 weeks (Phase A), with their medication switched to the alternate medication for another 5 weeks (Phase B). Doses were on a fixed schedule, with a target total daily dose of 3 mg/kg, and were based on weight (mean dosage for clomipramine, 150 mg/day; for desipramine, 153 mg/day; range, 50–250 mg/day). An ANCOVA showed that clomipramine, but not desipramine, produced a significant decrease in all obsessive-compulsive rating (NIMH-GOCS; P=0.0002) and depression ratings (Hamilton Rating Scale for Depression, P=0.006; NIMH depression scales, P=0.0001) and an increase in a measure of global functioning (P=0.001).

Drug order was also shown to have a significant effect. Of the subjects who were switched from clomipramine in Phase A to desipramine in Phase B, 64% showed signs of relapse, defined as at least a 1-point decline on the NIMH-GOCS by the fifth week of Phase B. This would indicate that desipramine did not produce the same positive clinical effects as clomipramine and could not sustain those effects following clomipramine treatment. DeVeaugh-Geiss et al. (1992) found similar results in their 8-week multisite study assessing clomipramine use in children and adolescents with OCD (N=60). Subjects were randomly assigned to clomipramine (maximum dosage by body weight: 25–30 kg, 75 mg/day; 31–45 kg, 100 mg/day; 46–60 kg, 150 mg/day; and >60 kg, 200 mg/day) or to continue with placebo. Those in the clomipramine group had a 37% mean reduction of symptoms on the Y-BOCS compared with 8% in those receiving placebo and had a 34% mean reduction on the NIMH-GOCS compared with 6% for the placebo group. Both findings were significant after an ANCOVA was performed (P<0.05).

Risks of TCAs. Side effects for TCAs ranged in severity across studies. Gittelman-Klein and Klein (1971) found that most side effects disappeared without requiring a dosage change. The most common were drowsiness, dizziness, dry mouth, and constipation. Similarly, Berney et al. (1981) argued that although side effects were reported, they were usually not severe. No subject in the Bernstein et al. (1990) study had side effects that were rated higher than mild, the most common being headache, dizziness, dry mouth, abdominal pain, and nausea.

Klein et al. (1992) reported the most severe cases, with the most frequent side effects being irritability or angry outbursts and dry mouth. Children in the imipramine group experienced considerably more side effects than those in the placebo group ($\chi^2=5.05$; $P<0.03$), with all complaints lasting at least 3 days, and two-thirds of those reported being in the moderate to severe range. This is troubling because the mean daily dosage in this trial was similar to that administered by Gittelman-Klein and Klein (1971), although their sample was significantly smaller. Side effects in studies using clomipramine and desipramine to treat children with OCD were similar. Leonard et al. (1989) reported dry mouth, tiredness, and dizziness as the most common adverse effects. However, participants who received clomipramine experienced more tremor and other side effects, such as chest pain, hot flashes, heartburn, rash, and acne.

Beyond these side effects, some case studies have reported sudden, unexplained death in children taking TCA medications (Biederman 1991; Riddle et al. 1993; Varley and McClellan 1997). In many of the reported cases, the children were being treated with desipramine at varying but therapeutic or even subtherapeutic levels for attention-deficit disorder or ADHD. Monitoring seems to have been inconsistent among the cases, but the cause of death was usually linked to adverse cardiac events. Because of the possibility of cardiac toxicity in young children, clinicians are advised to monitor the effects of TCA levels on their subjects very closely and to follow serial electrocardiograms (ECGs) over the course of treatment to ensure that plasma levels are not above the therapeutic threshold.

Overall, there does not yet appear to be enough evidence to support the frequent use of TCAs as a monotherapy for children and adolescents with anxiety disorders, with the exception of OCD and clomipramine treatment.

Long-Term Treatment

Although long-term studies with small sample sizes assessing the efficacy of TCAs in children with pure anxiety disorders are very limited, evidence from long-term OCD trials provides some indication of effects. Following their short-term, placebo-controlled trial, DeVeaugh-Geiss et al. (1992) continued with an open-label extension study for 1 year. They found that efficacy was maintained in subjects who elected to participate and completed the whole year (n=25). By the end of the year, the mean Y-BOCS score was 9.5, compared with 23 at the beginning of the extension. The investigators reported that clomipramine was still well tolerated.

Leonard et al. (1991) also performed an 8-month trial similar in design to their previous short-term crossover trial. Children and adolescents from the previous trial receiving maintenance clomipramine treatment (N=26) entered into the study and continued to receive clomipramine (mean dosage, 143 mg/day) for 3 months. At month 4, subjects were randomly assigned to desipramine substitution (mean dosage, 123 mg/day) or to continue with clomipramine for 2 months. For the final 3-month phase, all subjects continued to receive clomipramine treatment. For subjects completing the entire trial (N=20), results revealed that during the months of the substitution, those randomly assigned to desipramine showed greater impairment across ratings than those continuing with clomipramine. These results were only significant, however, on the NIMH-GOCS scale once the investigators controlled for the error rate. This study would seem to indicate that efficacy was maintained in subjects receiving long-term TCA treatment, given that few subjects in the clomipramine group experienced symptom relapse. However, even those subjects receiving clomipramine for the full 8 months still experienced OCD symptoms, which varied in severity over time. Thus, long-term clomipramine treatment for children and adolescents with OCD seems to be effective in decreasing symptoms but does not completely eliminate troubling symptoms.

Buspirone

Two randomized, placebo-controlled trials have examined the efficacy of buspirone in pediatric patients with GAD. In these studies, patients ages 6–17 (N=559) received 15–60 mg of buspirone daily (Bristol-Myers Squibb 2010). There were no unexpected safety findings associated with buspirone. The studies did not find significant differences in patients' GAD symptoms between buspirone and placebo. However, pharmacokinetic studies of buspirone have shown that plasma exposure to buspirone—and to its active metabolite, 1-(2-pyrimidinyl)-piperazine—is equivalent or greater in pediatric patients compared with adults. Much of the other available information on this agent stems from case reports, case series, and open-label trials. Although individual case reports seem to indicate some usefulness of buspirone in relieving anxiety symptoms, they also do not provide evidence of its efficacy (Alessi and Bos 1991; Balon 1994; Kranzler 1988).

Two controlled trials and one open-label study have assessed the efficacy of buspirone in treating pediatric anxiety disorders. The two controlled trials (one flexibly dosed and one fixed dose), which were sponsored by Bristol-Myers Squibb, examined the efficacy of buspirone versus placebo for the treatment of GAD in the pediatric population. Both studies found no separation between buspirone and placebo. Adverse events occurred more frequently in the patients receiving the active treatment (Strawn et al. 2018). In a small open-label study, Pfeffer et al. (1997) investigated the treatment effects of buspirone in child psychiatric inpatients ages 5–12 ($N=25$) who exhibited symptoms of anxiety and moderate aggression. Subjects who received high scores on the Revised Children's Manifest Anxiety Scale (RCMAS) and the Measure of Aggression, Violence, and Rage in Children (MAVRIC) were eligible to receive buspirone treatment. The total daily dosage was titrated up 5–10 mg every 3 days (maximum dosage, 50 mg) for 3 weeks (Phase II), after which the medication was kept at the optimum dosage for a 6-week maintenance period (Phase III). The results indicated that by the end of the 9-week trial, subjects had a significant reduction in symptoms on the Social Anxiety factor of the RCMAS ($P<0.04$) but not on the total RCMAS score. There was also a significant reduction in overall aggression, as measured by the MAVRIC ($P<0.02$), and in the number of seclusions and daily physical restraints used ($P<0.01$). Some children ($n=6$) had to discontinue use of buspirone because of severe side effects, including agitation, increased aggressivity, euphoric symptoms, increased impulsivity, and out-of-control behavior.

Although the results of this study are limited by its open-label design, they do demonstrate some efficacy in treating pediatric social anxiety disorder with buspirone. The 19 participants who completed the trial tolerated buspirone (mean dosage, 28 mg/day) well, reporting few side effects other than headache. However, as the investigators noted, it is troubling that almost 25% of the sample had to discontinue treatment because of interfering adverse events.

A later case series (Thomsen and Mikkelsen 1999) also seemed to support the addition of buspirone to SSRI treatment in adolescents diagnosed with OCD (*N*=6, ages 15–19). If patients did not show improvement following previous SSRI treatment or an SSRI+CBT combination, they were treated with buspirone (mean dosage, 20 mg/day). Although cases varied in severity, the investigators reported that buspirone in combination with continuing SSRI treatment showed a positive reduction effect on obsessive-compulsive symptoms, especially anxiety and distress. In addition, dramatic clinical improvement, as measured by the Y-BOCS, was seen in three of the six cases. Buspirone was well tolerated, inasmuch as no patients reported severe side effects or had to discontinue combined treatment.

Other Potential Compounds

Guanfacine

Guanfacine is another medication that has also been used to treat anxiety disorders in pediatric populations. Guanfacine and other α_2 agonists, such as clonidine, were initially developed to manage hypertension. Guanfacine XR, which is sometimes prescribed to address impulsive or disruptive behavior, is FDA approved for the treatment of ADHD in patients ages 6–17 years. Guanfacine is less sedating than clonidine and yet should be carefully managed in relation to cardiovascular side effects (e.g., hypotension, bradycardia); guanfacine XR is a longer-acting and potentially more tolerable formulation.

Evidence for the use of guanfacine in the treatment of pediatric anxiety disorders is limited. In an RCT, Strawn et al. (2016) examined the safety and tolerability of guanfacine XR in children and adolescents ages 6–17 with GAD, separation anxiety disorder, or social anxiety disorder. In the trial, patients (*N*=83) received flexibly dosed guanfacine XR (1–6 mg/day) or placebo for a period of 12 weeks. The medication was well tolerated, but the study lacked the power to detect treatment-related differences in efficacy between guanfacine XR and placebo.

An open-label study by Connor et al. (2013) found support for the use of guanfacine XR in treating PTSD in pediatric patients ages 6–18 (*N*=17). Participants in the study were prescribed 1–4 mg/day. Of the 13 patients who completed the 8-week open-label trial, 70.6% were rated as having very much improved or much improved symptoms on the CGI-I. Specifically, guanfacine XR may be effective in decreasing PTSD Cluster B (reexperiencing), Cluster C (avoidant), and Cluster D (overarousal) symptoms.

Atomoxetine

Atomoxetine is a highly selective SNRI and currently is FDA approved for the treatment of pediatric ADHD. However, a study completed by Geller et al. (2007) evaluated the treatment effectiveness of atomoxetine for children and adolescents diagnosed with both ADHD and an anxiety disorder such as GAD, social phobia, or separation anxiety disorder. In their double-blind, placebo-controlled 12-week trial, a total of 176 participants (ages 8–17) were randomly assigned to treatment, and dosing was based on weight, not to exceed a dosage of 120 mg/day. On both of the primary outcome measures (Attention-Deficit/Hyperactivity Disorder Rating Scale IV–Parent Version and the PARS), total scores in the treatment groups improved significantly at the end of the study as compared with the placebo group, with *P* values of 0.001 and 0.011, respectively. The only statistically significant adverse event in the atomoxetine group compared with the placebo group was decreased appetite.

Safety Issues

Monitoring

Prior to initiating medication treatment, it is important to review the family's medical and psychiatric history as well as the patient's laboratory results and previous medical evaluations. When prescribing a medication, the clinician should document the child's baseline weight, height, and vital signs and then monitor them over time, as well as consult with the child's primary care physician in order to obtain additional medical information (e.g., concomitant medication history, last physical examination) and to establish a collaborative treatment relationship. Informed consent and assent should be obtained from the parent and child following a full explanation of the risks and benefits of the selected medication treatment. It is helpful to identify for the child and parent a list of the most impairing anxiety symptoms to track over time, with the expectation that the medication will lead to improvement in these symptoms.

No laboratory tests are required for the use of SSRIs. SSRIs are well tolerated by children and adolescents, and the pediatric side effect profile is similar to that seen in adult clinical studies. The main side effects of concern are gastrointestinal discomfort, drowsiness, headache, insomnia, nervousness, hyperkinesia, and hostility (Waslick 2006). There are reports of withdrawal symptoms accompanying the discontinuation of SSRIs; patients may experience gastric distress, headache, dizziness, irritability, and agitation (Labellarte et al. 1998). Given this possibility, it is recommended that these medications not be abruptly discontinued.

Recent acute-treatment studies showed that children receiving venlafaxine XR had statistically significant changes in blood pressure, heart rate, weight, height, and total cholesterol. From these results, it is unclear what impact long-term exposure to this medication would have on these clinical parameters. When using this agent, clinicians should monitor vital signs, weight, and height and conduct a periodic laboratory assessment of cholesterol with acute and long-term treatment.

TCA use in children has the potential for cardiac risk. When a TCA is prescribed, the child's baseline vital signs, including sitting and standing blood pressure with pulse, and a baseline ECG should be obtained. Once the clinician has titrated the medication to the therapeutic dosage, another ECG should be performed when the serum level of the medication has been reached. This process should be repeated with each dosage adjustment and with periodic monitoring for long-term use. Another concern with this class of medication is the risk of lethal overdose.

In 2004, the FDA issued a directive to add a black box warning for all antidepressant medications after examining the outcome of all pediatric placebo-controlled trials of antidepressant medications and finding an increased incidence of suicidal thoughts and behaviors in the medication group (4%) compared with the placebo group (2%) (Leslie et al. 2005; U.S. Food and Drug Administration 2005). More recently, a meta-analysis by Bridge et al. (2007), which involved a larger number of pediatric clinical trials, showed—in terms of suicidality and behaviors—a number needed to harm (NNH) of 143 for all conditions and specifically an NNH of 140 for non-OCD anxiety disorders and an NNH of 200 for OCD. Clinicians should review this information with the parents and stress the need to contact them if the child experiences changes in behaviors, sleep patterns, and activity levels.

Prevention and Intervention of Adverse Effects

The best prevention and intervention for the management of medication adverse effects is educating the parent and child about what to expect in terms of adverse effects and how the clinician plans to manage these if they occur. As part of this education, it must be stressed that although there may be mild side effects initially, most will usually resolve in the first several weeks of treatment. The clinician should also document the child's baseline physical symptoms and levels of severity prior to starting medication and review these with the child and family at treatment initiation and at each medication visit to assess changes in severity or identify the development of a new symptom. Children with anxiety disorders have somatic symptoms that may be confused with adverse medication effects. Documenting the presence of somatic symptoms at baseline will assist in delineating the development of new adverse events or the worsening of previous symptoms.

For all medications, treatment should be initiated at a low dosage for the first 7 days, with the dosage slowly increased over subsequent weeks, depending on the child's clinical response and tolerability of the medication. Unfortunately, there is a dearth of information about dosing guidelines for these medications in treating specific anxiety disorders. Once a clinically efficacious dosage is achieved, it should be maintained for 8–12 weeks and later reevaluated to gauge successful treatment of the primary anxiety target symptoms and tolerability of the medication.

Practical Management Strategies: Treatment Approaches, Algorithms, and Guidelines

Psychotherapy

Several clinical trials have clearly demonstrated that 10- to 16-week cognitive-behavioral treatments (with in vivo exposure) lead to a significant reduction in anxiety symptoms in children (Barrett et al. 1996; Kendall et al. 1997). Given this information, it is reasonable for clinicians to initially recommend treatment with CBT. However, some families may find it difficult to obtain CBT treatment because of the limited availability of pediatric therapists proficient in this modality. If CBT is tried initially, it should be noted that a significant percentage of children remain symptomatic following CBT treatment. Another consideration is the presence of comorbid diagnoses, such as MDD, and the severity of illness, for which the prudent approach would be to treat with a combination of CBT and an SSRI.

Medication

In general, medication is often considered for treating pediatric anxiety disorders either when a psychosocial intervention trial has failed or when anxiety symptoms are considered to be in the moderate to severe range, leading to functional impairment such as poor school performance, school refusal, insomnia, and the development of comorbid diagnoses (e.g., MDD).

Combination Treatment

The scientific evidence demonstrates that both CBT and medications (SSRIs) are efficacious treatments, and recent research has been focused on the effects of combining these two treatments at onset. For example, Bernstein et al. (2000) investigated the efficacy of imipramine plus CBT in treating adolescents with school phobia (N=47) who were diagnosed with comorbid anxiety and MDD in an 8-week trial. Subjects were randomly assigned to imipramine (mean total daily dose, 182.3 mg) or placebo, in combination with CBT. The results of this study indicated that school attendance improved significantly only in the imipramine+CBT group (z=4.36; P<0.001) and that that group improved at a faster rate than did the placebo+CBT group (3.6% vs. 0.9%; z=2.39; P=0.017), even when comparisons were made with baseline. Anxiety and depression symptoms on various measures decreased significantly for both imipramine and placebo groups, with only one measure—the Children's Depression Rating Scale, Revised—favoring imipramine (z=2.08; P=0.037). Additionally, remission on clinical measures significantly favored imipramine + CBT only on the school attendance variable (χ^2=7.38; P=0.007).

Bernstein et al. (2000) provided data on the use of TCAs in combination with CBT for youth with a combination of anxiety and depression symptoms who refuse to attend school. As with many previous studies, a comorbidity factor precludes recommending TCAs for pure anxiety disorders; nevertheless, school attendance did improve significantly.

Another study (Neziroglu et al. 2000) investigated the possible additional benefits of treating children and adolescents ages 10–17 with OCD (N=10) using a combination of fluvoxamine and behavior therapy compared with using fluvoxamine alone. Subjects were eligible if they had previously failed a trial of behavior therapy lasting at least 10 sessions by not complying either inside or outside of treatment sessions. Following randomization, all subjects received 10 weeks of fluvoxamine (maximum dosage, 200 mg/day) until week 5, when 5 of the subjects were assigned to receive 20 sessions of behavior therapy. Results showed that 8 of the 10 total subjects had improved scores on the primary outcome variable, the CY-BOCS, following the initial 10 weeks of fluvoxamine treatment. At week 43, 3 of the 5 subjects in the fluvoxamine + behavior therapy group had significantly improved CY-BOCS scores, and 2 subjects remained stable; 1 of the 5 subjects in the fluvoxamine-only group experienced significant symptom improvement, 2 remained stable, and 2 deteriorated significantly. At week 52, the pattern was similar; by 2-year follow-up, subjects in both treatment groups all continued to report improved symptoms or remained stable.

The Pediatric OCD Treatment Study (POTS) Team (2004) later conducted a multisite, placebo-controlled, double-blind study assessing the efficacy of sertraline, CBT, and their combination for children and adolescents ages 7–17 diagnosed with OCD (N= 122). During Phase I, subjects were randomly assigned to sertraline (target dosage, 200 mg/day), CBT, combination therapy, or placebo for 12 weeks. Results from intent-to-treat random regression analyses revealed that all active treatments were significantly more effective than placebo, based on change in CY-BOCS score (CBT: P=0.003; sertraline: P=0.007; combination: P=0.001), and that combined treatment was superior to CBT alone (P=0.008) and to sertraline alone (P=0.006). The results for the CBT-alone and sertraline-alone groups did not differ significantly from each other. Furthermore, the rate of clinical remission, defined as a CY-BOCS score of 10 or less in the combined treatment group, differed significantly from that of the sertraline-only (P=0.03) and placebo groups (P<0.001) but did not differ significantly from that of the CBT-only group. Side effects included decreased appetite, diarrhea, enuresis, motor activity, nausea, and stomachache. Despite these reports, there were no serious adverse events or reports of suicidality. The POTS showed that sertraline, CBT, and their combination are effective treatments for pediatric OCD. However, because the combination and CBT-only groups showed both a higher reduction of symptoms on the CY-BOCS and a higher rate of clinical remission, the investigators recommended combination treatment or CBT alone as first-line treatment approaches.

Beidel et al. (2007) conducted a study comparing fluoxetine, pill placebo, and Social Effectiveness Therapy for Children (SET-C), a behavioral therapy combining group sessions and individualized exposure sessions for treating social phobia in children and adolescents. Their findings indicate that both SET-C and fluoxetine were more effective than placebo in reducing the symptoms of social phobia, with 79% of the SET-C group and 36.4% of the fluoxetine group having a significant improvement in CGI-I scores versus 6.3% of the placebo group.

The largest NIMH-funded anxiety multisite study examining combination treatment to date, the CAMS, provided strong evidence in favor of combining CBT and an SSRI when treating non-OCD pediatric anxiety disorders. The trial compared the outcomes of children ages 7–17 (N=488) with primary diagnoses of GAD, separation anxiety disorder, and social anxiety disorder who were randomly assigned to CBT alone, CBT in combination with sertraline (up to 200 mg/day), or sertraline alone versus placebo for 12 weeks (Walkup et al. 2008). The results showed that 80.7% of the children who were assigned to the combination treatment group experienced symptom improvement (P<0.001) compared with the 59.7% assigned to CBT (P<0.001) and the 54.9% assigned to sertraline (P<0.001), as measured by the CGI-I scale (Walkup et al. 2008). All of the active treatments were statistically superior to placebo (P<0.001), which led to only 23.7% improvement in participants. There were no significant differences in the frequency of adverse events in the sertraline versus the placebo groups, although there were fewer reports of physical symptoms with the CBT group compared with the sertraline group. A secondary analysis examining adverse events from the CAMS (Rynn et al. 2015) found that the rate of psychiatric adverse events was higher in children younger than 12 years across all study arms, leading to the recommendation for additional adverse monitoring when medication treatment is initiated in this younger population.

These findings demonstrate that both pharmacological treatment and psychotherapy are effective in treating pediatric anxiety disorders but that their combination is the most effective approach.

Conclusion

Empirical evidence supports the use of pharmacological and psychotherapy (specifically CBT) treatments for pediatric anxiety disorders. The data suggest that several classes of medications can be used safely and lead to an efficacious outcome and that the SSRIs should be considered first-line treatment. For pediatric OCD, evidence supports using a combination treatment approach, but CBT alone should be considered first. Additional long-term medication studies are warranted to examine both safety and treatment outcomes.

Clinical Pearls

- Before initiating medication treatment, develop a list of target anxiety symptoms to be tracked during treatment in order to determine response.
- Carefully assess for comorbid diagnoses and the severity of the anxiety symptoms. Greater severity may indicate the need for combination treatment with medication and cognitive-behavioral therapy.
- To prevent early termination from a medication trial, spend an adequate amount of time educating the child and their guardian on what to expect from medication treatment and about potential adverse events.
- Maintaining a suboptimal dosage of medication will frustrate the child and family, leading to treatment nonadherence and a prematurely failed treatment trial.
- As their symptoms respond positively to treatment, the child's behavior may change, which may be interpreted by the parent as a possible adverse event. For example, a child who is ordinarily compliant may begin to challenge their guardian. However, if the behavior change is unusual and is thought to be a significant change from baseline, a careful assessment should be made to evaluate whether the medication is the cause.

References

Alessi N, Bos T: Buspirone augmentation of fluoxetine in a depressed child with obsessive-compulsive disorder. Am J Psychiatry 148(11):1605–1606, 1991 1928487

Allgulander C, Hackett D, Salinas E: Venlafaxine extended release (ER) in the treatment of generalised anxiety disorder: twenty-four-week placebo-controlled dose-ranging study. Br J Psychiatry 179:15–22, 2001 11435263

American Academy of Child and Adolescent Psychiatry: Practice parameter for the assessment and treatment of children and adolescents with obsessive-compulsive disorder. J Am Acad Child Adolesc Psychiatry 51(1):98–113, 2012 22176943

American Psychiatric Association: Diagnostic and Statistical Manual: Mental Disorders. Washington, DC, American Psychiatric Association, 1952

American Psychiatric Association: Diagnostic and Statistical Manual of Mental Disorders, 2nd Edition. Washington, DC, American Psychiatric Association, 1968

American Psychiatric Association: Diagnostic and Statistical Manual of Mental Disorders, 3rd Edition. Washington, DC, American Psychiatric Association, 1980

American Psychiatric Association: Diagnostic and Statistical Manual of Mental Disorders, 4th Edition. Washington, DC, American Psychiatric Association, 1994

American Psychiatric Association: Diagnostic and Statistical Manual of Mental Disorders, 4th Edition, Text Revision. Washington, DC, American Psychiatric Association, 2000

American Psychiatric Association: Diagnostic and Statistical Manual of Mental Disorders, 5th Edition. Arlington, VA, American Psychiatric Association, 2013

American Psychiatric Association: Diagnostic and Statistical Manual of Mental Disorders, 5th Edition, Text Revision. Washington, DC, American Psychiatric Association, 2022

Anderson JC, Williams S, McGee R, Silva PA: DSM-III disorders in preadolescent children: prevalence in a large sample from the general population. Arch Gen Psychiatry 44(1):69–76, 1987 2432848

Aronson TA, Logue CM: On the longitudinal course of panic disorder: development history and predictors of phobic complications. Compr Psychiatry 28(4):344–355, 1987 3608468

Bachmann CJ, Aagaard L, Burcu M, et al: Trends and patterns of antidepressant use in children and adolescents from five Western countries, 2005–2012. Eur Neuropsychopharmacol 26(3): 411–419, 2016 26970020

Ballenger JC, Burrows GD, DuPont RL Jr, et al: Alprazolam in panic disorder and agoraphobia: results from a multicenter trial I: efficacy in short-term treatment. Arch Gen Psychiatry 45(5):413–422, 1988 3282478

Balon R: Buspirone in the treatment of separation anxiety in an adolescent boy. Can J Psychiatry 39(9):581–582, 1994 7874664

Barrett PM, Dadds MR, Rapee RM: Family treatment of childhood anxiety: a controlled trial. J Consult Clin Psychol 64(2):333–342, 1996 8871418

Beesdo K, Knappe S, Pine DS: Anxiety and anxiety disorders in children and adolescents: developmental issues and implications for DSM-5. Psychiatr Clin North Am 32(3):483–524, 2009 19716988

Beidel DC, Fink CM, Turner SM: Stability of anxious symptomatology in children. J Abnorm Child Psychol 24(3):257–269, 1996 8836801

Beidel DC, Turner SM, Sallee FR, et al: SET-C versus fluoxetine in the treatment of childhood social phobia. J Am Acad Child Adolesc Psychiatry 46(12):1622–1632, 2007 18030084

Berney T, Kolvin I, Bhate SR, et al: School phobia: a therapeutic trial with clomipramine and short-term outcome. Br J Psychiatry 138:110–118, 1981 7020816

Bernstein GA, Garfinkel BD, Borchardt CM: Comparative studies of pharmacotherapy for school refusal. J Am Acad Child Adolesc Psychiatry 29(5):773–781, 1990 2228932

Bernstein GA, Shaw K, American Academy of Child and Adolescent Psychiatry: Practice parameters for the assessment and treatment of anxiety disorders. J Am Acad Child Adolesc Psychiatry 32(5):1089–1098, 1993 8175638

Bernstein GA, Borchardt CM, Perwien AR, et al: Imipramine plus cognitive-behavioral therapy in the treatment of school refusal. J Am Acad Child Adolesc Psychiatry 39(3):276–283, 2000 10714046

Biederman J: Sudden death in children treated with a tricyclic antidepressant. J Am Acad Child Adolesc Psychiatry 30(3):495–498, 1991 2055889

Birmaher B, Waterman GS, Ryan N, et al: Fluoxetine for childhood anxiety disorders. J Am Acad Child Adolesc Psychiatry 33(7):993–999, 1994 7961355

Birmaher B, Axelson DA, Monk K, et al: Fluoxetine for the treatment of childhood anxiety disorders. J Am Acad Child Adolesc Psychiatry 42(4):415–423, 2003 12649628

Bittner A, Egger HL, Erkanli A, et al: What do childhood anxiety disorders predict? J Child Psychol Psychiatry 48(12):1174–1183, 2007 18093022

Black B, Uhde TW: Elective mutism as a variant of social phobia. J Am Acad Child Adolesc Psychiatry 31(6):1090–1094, 1992 1342579

Black B, Uhde TW: Treatment of elective mutism with fluoxetine: a double-blind, placebo-controlled study. J Am Acad Child Adolesc Psychiatry 33(7):1000–1006, 1994 7961338

Bowen RC, Offord DR, Boyle MH: The prevalence of overanxious disorder and separation anxiety disorder: results from the Ontario Child Health Study. J Am Acad Child Adolesc Psychiatry 29(5):753–758, 1990 2228929

Brady EU, Kendall PC: Comorbidity of anxiety and depression in children and adolescents. Psychol Bull 111(2):244–255, 1992 1557475

Bridge JA, Iyengar S, Salary CB, et al: Clinical response and risk for reported suicidal ideation and suicide attempts in pediatric antidepressant treatment: a meta-analysis of randomized controlled trials. JAMA 297(15):1683–1696, 2007 17440145

Bristol-Myers Squibb: Buspirone package insert. Princeton, NJ, Bristol-Myers Squibb, 2010

Cantwell DP, Baker L: Stability and natural history of DSM-III childhood diagnoses. J Am Acad Child Adolesc Psychiatry 28(5):691–700, 1989 2793796

Compton SN, Grant PJ, Chrisman AK, et al: Sertraline in children and adolescents with social anxiety disorder: an open trial. J Am Acad Child Adolesc Psychiatry 40(5):564–571, 2001 11349701

Connor DF, Grasso DJ, Slivinsky MD, et al: An open-label study of guanfacine extended release for traumatic stress related symptoms in children and adolescents. J Child Adolesc Psychopharmacol 23(4):244–251, 2013 23683139

Cook EH, Wagner KD, March JS, et al: Long-term sertraline treatment of children and adolescents with obsessive-compulsive disorder. J Am Acad Child Adolesc Psychiatry 40(10):1175–1181, 2001 11589530

Copeland WE, Keeler G, Angold A, Costello EJ: Traumatic events and posttraumatic stress in childhood. Arch Gen Psychiatry 64(5):577–584, 2007 17485609

Costello EJ: Child psychiatric disorders and their correlates: a primary care pediatric sample. J Am Acad Child Adolesc Psychiatry 28(6):851–855, 1989 2808254

Costello EJ, Costello AJ, Edelbrock C, et al: Psychiatric disorders in pediatric primary care: prevalence and risk factors. Arch Gen Psychiatry 45(12):1107–1116, 1988 3264146

Costello EJ, Angold A, Burns BJ, et al: The Great Smoky Mountains Study of Youth: functional impairment and serious emotional disturbance. Arch Gen Psychiatry 53(12):1137–1143, 1996 8956680

Costello EJ, Mustillo S, Erkanli A, et al: Prevalence and development of psychiatric disorders in childhood and adolescence. Arch Gen Psychiatry 60(8):837–844, 2003 12912767

Costello EJ, Egger HL, Angold A: The developmental epidemiology of anxiety disorders: phenomenology, prevalence, and comorbidity. Child Adolesc Psychiatr Clin N Am 14(4):631–648, vii, 2005 16171696

Costello EJ, He JP, Sampson NA, et al: Services for adolescents with psychiatric disorders: 12-month data from the National Comorbidity Survey–Adolescent. Psychiatr Serv 65(3):359–366, 2014 24233052

Dadds MR, Spence SH, Holland DE, et al: Prevention and early intervention for anxiety disorders: a controlled trial. J Consult Clin Psychol 65(4):627–635, 1997 9256564

Davidson JRT, DuPont RL, Hedges D, Haskins JT: Efficacy, safety, and tolerability of venlafaxine extended release and buspirone in outpatients with generalized anxiety disorder. J Clin Psychiatry 60(8):528–535, 1999 10485635

DeVeaugh-Geiss J, Moroz G, Biederman J, et al: Clomipramine hydrochloride in childhood and adolescent obsessive-compulsive disorder: a multicenter trial. J Am Acad Child Adolesc Psychiatry 31(1):45–49, 1992 1537780

Egger HL, Angold A: Common emotional and behavioral disorders in preschool children: presentation, nosology, and epidemiology. J Child Psychol Psychiatry 47(3–4):313–337, 2006 16492262

Federman EB, Costello EJ, Angold A, et al: Development of substance use and psychiatric comorbidity in an epidemiologic study of white and American Indian young adolescents the Great Smoky Mountains Study. Drug Alcohol Depend 44(2–3):69–78, 1997 9088778

Feehan M, McGee R, Raja SN, Williams SM: DSM-III-R disorders in New Zealand 18-year-olds. Aust N Z J Psychiatry 28(1):87–99, 1994 8067973

Foley DL, Goldston DB, Costello EJ, Angold A: Proximal psychiatric risk factors for suicidality in youth: the Great Smoky Mountains Study. Arch Gen Psychiatry 63(9):1017–1024, 2006 16953004

Gelenberg AJ, Lydiard RB, Rudolph RL, et al: Efficacy of venlafaxine extended-release capsules in nondepressed outpatients with generalized anxiety disorder: a 6-month randomized controlled trial. JAMA 283(23):3082–3088, 2000 10865302

Geller DA, Biederman J, Jones J, et al: Obsessive-compulsive disorder in children and adolescents: a review. Harv Rev Psychiatry 5(5):260–273, 1998 9493948

Geller DA, Hoog SL, Heiligenstein JH, et al: Fluoxetine treatment for obsessive-compulsive disorder in children and adolescents: a placebo-controlled clinical trial. J Am Acad Child Adolesc Psychiatry 40(7):773–779, 2001 11437015

Geller DA, Biederman J, Stewart SE, et al: Which SSRI? A meta-analysis of pharmacotherapy trials in pediatric obsessive-compulsive disorder. Am J Psychiatry 160(11):1919–1928, 2003 14594734

Geller DA, Wagner KD, Emslie G, et al: Paroxetine treatment in children and adolescents with obsessive-compulsive disorder: a randomized, multicenter, double-blind, placebo-controlled trial. J Am Acad Child Adolesc Psychiatry 43(11):1387–1396, 2004 15502598

Geller D, Donnelly C, Lopez F, et al: Atomoxetine treatment for pediatric patients with attention-deficit/hyperactivity disorder with comorbid anxiety disorder. J Am Acad Child Adolesc Psychiatry 46(9):1119–1127, 2007 17712235

Gittelman-Klein R, Klein DF: Controlled imipramine treatment of school phobia. Arch Gen Psychiatry 25:204–207, 1971 18730587

Graae F, Milner J, Rizzotto L, Klein RG: Clonazepam in childhood anxiety disorders. J Am Acad Child Adolesc Psychiatry 33(3):372–376, 1994 8169182

Henin A, Biederman J, Mick E, et al: Childhood antecedent disorders to bipolar disorder in adults: a controlled study. J Affect Disord 99(1–3):51–57, 2007 17045657

Isolan L, Pheula G, Salum GA Jr, et al: An open-label trial of escitalopram in children and adolescents with social anxiety disorder. J Child Adolesc Psychopharmacol 17(6):751–760, 2007 18315447

Katzelnick DJ, Kobak KA, Greist JH, et al: Sertraline for social phobia: a double-blind, placebo-controlled crossover study. Am J Psychiatry 152(9):1368–1371, 1995 7653696

Keller MB, Lavori PW, Wunder J, et al: Chronic course of anxiety disorders in children and adolescents. J Am Acad Child Adolesc Psychiatry 31(4):595–599, 1992 1644719

Kendall PC, Flannery-Schroeder E, Panichelli-Mindel SM, et al: Therapy for youths with anxiety disorders: a second randomized clinical trial. J Consult Clin Psychol 65(3):366–380, 1997 9170760

Klein RG, Koplewicz HS, Kanner A: Imipramine treatment of children with separation anxiety disorder. J Am Acad Child Adolesc Psychiatry 31(1):21–28, 1992 1347039

Kovacs M, Gatsonis C, Paulauskas SL, Richards C: Depressive disorders in childhood IV: a longitudinal study of comorbidity with and risk for anxiety disorders. Arch Gen Psychiatry 46(9):776–782, 1989 2774847

Kranzler HR: Use of buspirone in an adolescent with overanxious disorder. J Am Acad Child Adolesc Psychiatry 27(6):789–790, 1988 3198569

Labellarte MJ, Walkup JT, Riddle MA: The new antidepressants: selective serotonin reuptake inhibitors. Pediatr Clin North Am 45(5): 1137–1155, ix, 1998

Last CG, Hersen M, Kazdin AE, et al: Comparison of DSM-III separation anxiety and overanxious disorders: demographic characteristics and patterns of comorbidity. J Am Acad Child Adolesc Psychiatry 26(4):527–531, 1987a 3654505

Last CG, Hersen M, Kazdin AE, et al: Psychiatric illness in the mothers of anxious children. Am J Psychiatry 144(12):1580–1583, 1987b 3688283

Last CG, Phillips JE, Statfeld A: Childhood anxiety disorders in mothers and their children. Child Psychiatry Hum Dev 18(2):103–112, 1987c 3436173

Last CG, Perrin S, Hersen M, Kazdin AE: A prospective study of childhood anxiety disorders. J Am Acad Child Adolesc Psychiatry 35(11):1502–1510, 1996 8936917

Last CG, Hansen C, Franco N: Anxious children in adulthood: a prospective study of adjustment. J Am Acad Child Adolesc Psychiatry 36(5):645–652, 1997 9136499

Leonard HL, Swedo SE, Rapoport JL, et al: Treatment of obsessive-compulsive disorder with clomipramine and desipramine in children and adolescents: a double-blind crossover comparison. Arch Gen Psychiatry 46(12):1088–1092, 1989 2686576

Leonard HL, Swedo SE, Lenane MC, et al: A double-blind desipramine substitution during long-term clomipramine treatment in children and adolescents with obsessive-compulsive disorder. Arch Gen Psychiatry 48(10):922–927, 1991 1929762

Leonard HL, March J, Rickler KC, Allen AJ: Pharmacology of the selective serotonin reuptake inhibitors in children and adolescents. J Am Acad Child Adolesc Psychiatry 36(6):725–736, 1997 9183126

Leslie LK, Newman TB, Chesney PJ, Perrin JM: The Food and Drug Administration's deliberations on antidepressant use in pediatric patients. Pediatrics 116(1):195–204, 2005 15995053

Lewinsohn PM, Hops H, Roberts RE, et al: Adolescent psychopathology I: prevalence and incidence of depression and other DSM-III-R disorders in high school students. J Abnorm Psychol 102(1):133–144, 1993 8436689

Liebowitz MR, Stein MB, Tancer M, et al: A randomized, double-blind, fixed-dose comparison of paroxetine and placebo in the treatment of generalized social anxiety disorder. J Clin Psychiatry 63(1):66–74, 2002 11838629

Livingston R, Taylor JL, Crawford SL: A study of somatic complaints and psychiatric diagnosis in children. J Am Acad Child Adolesc Psychiatry 27(2):185–187, 1988 3360721

March JS, Biederman J, Wolkow R, et al: Sertraline in children and adolescents with obsessive-compulsive disorder: a multicenter randomized controlled trial. JAMA 280(20):1752–1756, 1998 9842950

McGee R, Feehan M, Williams S, et al: DSM-III disorders in a large sample of adolescents. J Am Acad Child Adolesc Psychiatry 29(4):611–619, 1990 2387797

Merikangas KR, He JP, Brody D, et al: Prevalence and treatment of mental disorders among US children in the 2001–2004 NHANES. Pediatrics 125(1):75–81, 2010a 20008426

Merikangas KR, He JP, Burstein M, et al: Lifetime prevalence of mental disorders in U.S. adolescents: results from the National Comorbidity Survey Replication—Adolescent Supplement (NCS-A). J Am Acad Child Adolesc Psychiatry 49(10):980–989, 2010b 20855043

Meyer JS, Quenzer LQ: Psychopharmacology: Drugs, the Brain, and Behavior. Sunderland, MA, Sinauer Associates, 2005, pp 412–438

Neziroglu F, Yaryura-Tobias JA, Walz J, McKay D: The effect of fluvoxamine and behavior therapy on children and adolescents with obsessive-compulsive disorder. J Child Adolesc Psychopharmacol 10(4):295–306, 2000 11191690

Nishino S, Mignot E, Dement WC: Sedative-hypnotics, in The American Psychiatric Press Textbook of Psychopharmacology. Edited by Schatzberg AF, Nemeroff CB. Washington, DC, American Psychiatric Press, 1995, pp 405–416

Nutt D, Lawson C: Panic attacks: a neurochemical overview of models and mechanisms. Br J Psychiatry 160:165–178, 1992 1540756

Orvaschel H, Weissman M: Epidemiology of anxiety in children, in Anxiety Disorders of Childhood. Edited by Gittelman R. New York, Guilford, 1986

Pediatric OCD Treatment Study (POTS) Team: Cognitive-behavior therapy, sertraline, and their combination for children and adolescents with obsessive-compulsive disorder: the Pediatric OCD Treatment Study (POTS) randomized controlled trial. JAMA 292(16):1969–1976, 2004 15507582

Pfeffer CR, Jiang H, Domeshek LJ: Buspirone treatment of psychiatrically hospitalized prepubertal children with symptoms of anxiety and moderately severe aggression. J Child Adolesc Psychopharmacol 7(3):145–155, 1997 9466232

Pigott TA: OCD: where the serotonin selectivity story begins. J Clin Psychiatry 57(Suppl 6):11–20, 1996 8647793

Pine DS: Treating children and adolescents with selective serotonin reuptake inhibitors: how long is appropriate? J Child Adolesc Psychopharmacol 12(3):189–203, 2002 12427293

Pine DS, Grun J: Anxiety disorders, in Child Psychopharmacology. Edited by Walsh TB (Review of Psychiatry Series, Vol 17; Oldham JM and Riba MB, series eds). Washington, DC, American Psychiatric Press, 1998, pp 115–148

Pohl RB, Wolkow RM, Clary CM: Sertraline in the treatment of panic disorder: a double-blind multicenter trial. Am J Psychiatry 155(9):1189–1195, 1998 9734541

Polanczyk GV, Salum GA, Sugaya LS, et al: Annual research review: a meta-analysis of the worldwide prevalence of mental disorders in children and adolescents. J Child Psychol Psychiatry 56(3):345–365, 2015 25649325

Pollack MH, Zaninelli R, Goddard A, et al: Paroxetine in the treatment of generalized anxiety disorder: results of a placebo-controlled, flexible-dosage trial. J Clin Psychiatry 62(5):350–357, 2001 11411817

Potter WZ, Manji HK, Rudorfer MV: Tricyclic and tetracyclics, in The American Psychiatric Press Textbook of Psychopharmacology. Edited by Schatzberg AF, Nemeroff CB. Washington, DC, American Psychiatric Press, 1995, pp 141–160

Rasmussen SA, Eisen JL: The epidemiology and clinical features of obsessive compulsive disorder. Psychiatr Clin North Am 15(4):743–758, 1992 1461792

Research Units on Pediatric Psychopharmacology (RUPP) Anxiety Study Group: Fluvoxamine for the treatment of anxiety disorders in children and adolescents. N Engl J Med 344(17):1279–1285, 2001 11323729

Research Units on Pediatric Psychopharmacology (RUPP) Anxiety Study Group: The Pediatric Anxiety Rating Scale (PARS): development and psychometric properties. J Am Acad Child Adolesc Psychiatry 41(9):1061–1069, 2002 12218427

Rickels K, Rynn MA: What is generalized anxiety disorder? J Clin Psychiatry 62(Suppl 11):4–12, discussion 13–14, 2001 11414550

Rickels K, Csanalosi I, Greisman P, et al: A controlled clinical trial of alprazolam for the treatment of anxiety. Am J Psychiatry 140(1):82–85, 1983 6128927

Rickels K, Pollack MH, Sheehan DV, Haskins JT: Efficacy of extended-release venlafaxine in nondepressed outpatients with generalized anxiety disorder. Am J Psychiatry 157(6):968–974, 2000 10831478

Riddle MA, Scahill L, King RA, et al: Double-blind, crossover trial of fluoxetine and placebo in children and adolescents with obsessive-compulsive disorder. J Am Acad Child Adolesc Psychiatry 31(6):1062–1069, 1992 1429406

Riddle MA, Geller B, Ryan N: Another sudden death in a child treated with desipramine. J Am Acad Child Adolesc Psychiatry 32(4):792–797, 1993 8340300

Riddle MA, Reeve EA, Yaryura-Tobias JA, et al: Fluvoxamine for children and adolescents with obsessive-compulsive disorder: a randomized, controlled, multicenter trial. J Am Acad Child Adolesc Psychiatry 40(2):222–229, 2001 11211371

Robb AS, Cueva JE, Sporn J, et al: Sertraline treatment of children and adolescents with posttraumatic stress disorder: a double-blind, placebo-controlled trial. J Child Adolesc Psychopharmacol 20(6):463–471, 2010 21186964

Rockhill C, Kodish I, DiBattisto C, et al: Anxiety disorders in children and adolescents. Curr Probl Pediatr Adolesc Health Care 40(4):66–99, 2010 20381781

Rosenbaum JF, Fava M, Hoog SL, et al: Selective serotonin reuptake inhibitor discontinuation syndrome: a randomized clinical trial. Biol Psychiatry 44(2):77–87, 1998 9646889

Ross SB, Renyi AL: Tricyclic antidepressant agents I: comparison of the inhibition of the uptake of 3-H-noradrenaline and 14-C-5-hydroxytryptamine in slices and crude synaptosome preparations of the midbrain-hypothalamus region of the rat brain. Acta Pharmacol Toxicol (Copenh) 36(Suppl 5):382–394, 1975 1173528

Roy A, De Jong J, Linnoila M: Cerebrospinal fluid monoamine metabolites and suicidal behavior in depressed patients: a 5-year follow-up study. Arch Gen Psychiatry 46(7):609–612, 1989 2472124

Rynn MA, Siqueland L, Rickels K: Placebo-controlled trial of sertraline in the treatment of children with generalized anxiety disorder. Am J Psychiatry 158(12):2008–2014, 2001 11729017

Rynn M, Yeung PP, Riddle MA, et al: Venlafaxine ER as a treatment for GAD in children and adolescents. Presented at the 157th Annual Meeting of the American Psychiatric Association, New York, May 1–6, 2004

Rynn MA, Riddle MA, Yeung PP, Kunz NR: Efficacy and safety of extended-release venlafaxine in the treatment of generalized anxiety disorder in children and adolescents: two placebo-controlled trials. Am J Psychiatry 164(2):290–300, 2007 17267793

Rynn MA, Walkup JT, Compton SN, et al: Child/adolescent anxiety multimodal study: evaluating safety. J Am Acad Child Adolesc Psychiatry 54(3):180–190, 2015

Schweizer F., Rickels K, Weiss S, Zavodnick S: Maintenance drug treatment of panic disorder I: results of a prospective, placebo-controlled comparison of alprazolam and imipramine. Arch Gen Psychiatry 50(1):51–60, 1993 8422222

Simeon JG, Ferguson HB: Alprazolam effects in children with anxiety disorders. Can J Psychiatry 32(7):570–574, 1987 3315169

Simeon JG, Ferguson HB, Knott V, et al: Clinical, cognitive, and neurophysiological effects of alprazolam in children and adolescents with overanxious and avoidant disorders. J Am Acad Child Adolesc Psychiatry 31(1):29–33, 1992 1537778

Stein MB, Liebowitz MR, Lydiard RB, et al: Paroxetine treatment of generalized social phobia (social anxiety disorder): a randomized controlled trial. JAMA 280(8):708–713, 1998 9728642

Strauss CC: Behavioral assessment and treatment of overanxious disorder in children and adolescents. Behav Modif 12(2):234–251, 1988 3069094

Strawn JR, Prakash A, Zhang Q, et al: A randomized, placebo-controlled study of duloxetine for the treatment of children and adolescents with generalized anxiety disorder. J Am Acad Child Adolesc Psychiatry 54(4):283–293, 2015a 25791145

Strawn JR, Welge JA, Wehry AM, et al: Efficacy and tolerability of antidepressants in pediatric anxiety disorders: a systematic review and meta-analysis. Depress Anxiety 32(3):149–157, 2015b 25449861

Strawn J, Compton S, Robertson B, et al: Guanfacine extended-release in pediatric anxiety disorders: a randomized, placebo-controlled trial. Poster session presented at the annual meeting of the Anxiety and Depression Association of America, Philadelphia, PA, March 31 to April 3, 2016

Strawn JR, Mills JA, Cornwall GJ, et al: Buspirone in children and adolescents with anxiety: a review and Bayesian analysis of abandoned randomized controlled trials. J Child Adolesc Psychopharmacol 28(1):2–9, 2018 28846022

Strawn JR, Mills JA, Schroeder H, et al. Escitalopram in adolescents with generalized anxiety disorder: a double-blind, randomized, placebo-controlled study. J Clin Psychiatry 81(5):20m13396, 2020 32857933

Tancer ME: Neurobiology of social phobia. J Clin Psychiatry 54(Suppl):26–30, 1993 8276747

Thomsen PH: Child and adolescent obsessive-compulsive disorder treated with citalopram: findings from an open trial of 23 cases. J Child Adolesc Psychopharmacol 7(3):157–166, 1997 9466233

Thomsen PH, Mikkelsen HU: The addition of buspirone to SSRI in the treatment of adolescent obsessive-compulsive disorder: a study of six cases. Eur Child Adolesc Psychiatry 8(2):143–148, 1999 10435463

Thomsen PH, Ebbesen C, Persson C: Long-term experience with citalopram in the treatment of adolescent OCD. J Am Acad Child Adolesc Psychiatry 40(8):895–902, 2001 11501688

Tourian KA, March JS, Mangano R: Venlafaxine extended release in children and adolescents with social anxiety disorder. Presented at the annual meeting of the American Psychiatric Association, New York, May 1–6, 2004

U.S. Food and Drug Administration: Medication guide about using antidepressants in children and adolescents. Washington, DC, U.S. Food and Drug Administration, 2005

Varley CK, McClellan J: Case study: two additional sudden deaths with tricyclic antidepressants. J Am Acad Child Adolesc Psychiatry 36(3):390–394, 1997 9055520

Wagner KD, Berard R, Stein MB, et al: A multicenter, randomized, double-blind, placebo-controlled trial of paroxetine in children and adolescents with social anxiety disorder. Arch Gen Psychiatry 61(11):1153–1162, 2004 15520363

Wagner KD, Jonas J, Findling RL, et al: A double-blind, randomized, placebo-controlled trial of escitalopram in the treatment of pediatric depression. J Am Acad Child Adolesc Psychiatry 45(3):280–288, 2006 16540812

Walkup J, Labellarte M, Riddle MA, et al: Treatment of pediatric anxiety disorders: an open-label extension of the Research Units on Pediatric Psychopharmacology anxiety study. J Child Adolesc Psychopharmacol 12(3):175–188, 2002 12427292

Walkup JT, Labellarte MJ, Riddle MA, et al: Searching for moderators and mediators of pharmacological treatment effects in children and adolescents with anxiety disorders. J Am Acad Child Adolesc Psychiatry 42(1):13–21, 2003 12500072

Walkup JT, Albano AM, Piacentini J, et al: Cognitive behavioral therapy, sertraline, or a combination in childhood anxiety. N Engl J Med 359(26):2753–2766, 2008 18974308

Walter HJ, Bukstein OG, Abright AR, et al: Clinical practice guideline for the assessment and treatment of children and adolescents with anxiety disorders. J Am Acad Child Adolesc Psychiatry 59(10):1107–1124, 2020 32439401

Waslick B: Psychopharmacology interventions for pediatric anxiety disorders: a research update. Child Adolesc Psychiatr Clin N Am 15(1):51–71, 2006 16321725

Weintrob N, Cohen D, Klipper-Aurbach Y, et al: Decreased growth during therapy with selective serotonin reuptake inhibitors. Arch Pediatr Adolesc Med 156(7):696–701, 2002 12090838

Weissman MM, Wolk S, Wickramaratne P, et al: Children with prepubertal-onset major depressive disorder and anxiety grown up. Arch Gen Psychiatry 56(9):794–801, 1999 12884885

Witek MW, Rojas V, Alonso C, et al: Review of benzodiazepine use in children and adolescents. Psychiatr Q 76(3):283–296, 2005 16080423

5

Major Depressive Disorder

Boris Birmaher, M.D.
Manivel Rengasamy, M.D.

Pediatric major depressive disorder (MDD) is a familial recurrent illness associated with poor psychosocial functioning; academic, substance abuse, anxiety, and psychosocial difficulties; and an increased risk of suicide and suicide attempts (Birmaher et al. 1996b, 2002; Lewinsohn et al. 1999; Pine et al. 1998). The prevalence of MDD in children and adolescents is approximately 2% and 6%, respectively (Birmaher et al. 1996b). Because pediatric MDD is continuous into adulthood, early identification and prompt treatment at its early stages are critical.

Our primary aim in this chapter is to review the current pharmacological treatments for children and adolescents with MDD. Although psychotherapy interventions, including cognitive-behavioral therapy (CBT)—either alone (Brent et al. 1997) or in combination with antidepressants (Brent et al. 2009; Kennard et al. 2014; March et al. 2004)—and interpersonal psychotherapy (Mufson et al. 2004), are also found to be efficacious for the acute treatment

Table 5–1. Definitions of treatment outcome

Response	No symptoms or a significant reduction in depressive symptoms for at least 2 weeks
Remission	A period of at least 2 weeks and less than 2 months with no or very few depressive symptoms
Recovery	Absence of symptoms of major depressive disorder for 2 months or more (e.g., can have no more than two symptoms to be considered in recovery)
Relapse	A major depressive episode during the period of remission
Recurrence	A new major depressive episode during the period of recovery

of pediatric MDD, particularly for adolescents, treatment using only these interventions is not reviewed in this chapter.

Five terms—*response*, *remission*, *recovery*, *relapse*, and *recurrence*—are useful for understanding treatment outcomes. Their current definitions (Birmaher et al. 2000; Emslie et al. 1997, 2002, 2008) are presented in Table 5–1.

Assessment of Treatment Response

Understanding the research definition of treatment response can aid clinicians in interpreting the research-based evidence for the effectiveness of each antidepressant in day-to-day practice. Treatment response has traditionally been determined by the absence of MDD criteria (e.g., no more than one DSM symptom) or, more frequently, by a significant reduction in symptom severity (usually 50%). However, when the latter criterion is used, patients (deemed *responders*) may still have considerable residual depressive symptoms. Therefore, an absolute final score of 9 or lower on the Beck Depression Inventory (Beck 1967), 7 or less on the 17-item Hamilton Rating Scale for Depression (Hamilton 1960), o r28 or lower on the Children's Depression Rating Scale–Revised (CDRS-R; Poznanski et al. 1985), together with persistent improvement in the patient's functioning for at least 2 weeks, may better reflect a satisfactory response. *Overall improvement* has also been measured with the Clinical Global Impression–Improvement (CGI-I; Guy 1976) subscale, with scores of 1 and 2 indicating "very much" and "much improvement," respectively. *Func-*

tional improvement can be measured using several rating scales, such as the Global Assessment Scale (American Psychiatric Association 1994) or the Children's Global Assessment Scale (Shaffer et al. 1983).

Treatment Phases

Treatment of MDD is divided into three phases: acute, continuation, and maintenance (American Academy of Child and Adolescent Psychiatry 1998; American Psychiatric Association 2010). The main goal during the *acute phase* is to achieve response and, more importantly, remission of the depressive symptoms. This phase usually lasts 6–12 weeks. The *continuation phase* usually lasts 4–12 months, during which remission is consolidated to prevent relapses. The *maintenance phase* lasts 1 year or longer, and its main objective is the prevention of depression recurrences. Almost all studies of children and adolescents have evaluated treatments during the acute phase, and few have been continuation studies (Clarke et al. 2005; Emslie et al. 2008; Goodyer et al. 2007; Kennard et al. 2014). No maintenance treatment studies have been reported to date. Therefore, recommendations regarding maintenance treatments are extrapolated from the adult research literature. However, caution is warranted because youth may respond differently to interventions that thus far have been tested only on adults with MDD (Birmaher et al. 1996a).

Treatment of MDD With Selective Serotonin Reuptake Inhibitors and Other Novel Antidepressants

Psychoeducation and Supportive Therapy

The optimal pharmacological management of MDD in children and adolescents should involve educative and supportive psychotherapy. In fact, at least for youth with mild to moderate depression, supportive management and education may be sufficient to ameliorate the symptoms of depression (Goodyer et al. 2007; Mufson et al. 2004; Renaud et al. 1998). Education of the patient and family about the illness, nature of treatment, and prognosis is critical to engagement in treatment and enhancement of compliance (Brent et al. 1993).

During and after the depression remission, psychosocial scars or complications (e.g., family conflict, poor self-esteem and social skills, academic difficulties, problems with peers) must be addressed with psychotherapy (Birmaher et al. 2000; Kovacs and Goldston 1991; Puig-Antich et al. 1985; Rao et al. 1995; Stein et al. 2000; Strober et al. 1993).

Parents of depressed youth may also be experiencing depression and other psychiatric disorders (Klein et al. 2001), and this depression may lead to adverse outcomes in their children. In fact, successful treatment of the parents may ameliorate or even prevent the development of psychopathology in their children (Birmaher 2011; Pilowsky et al. 2014). Thus, to treat the child successfully, the clinician should assess the parents and refer them for their own treatment.

Acute Phase

Studies on the acute treatment of children and adolescents with MDD have focused on the effects of tricyclic antidepressants (TCAs), selective serotonin reuptake inhibitors (SSRIs), and serotonin-norepinephrine reuptake inhibitors (SNRIs; e.g., venlafaxine, duloxetine). Agomelatine also demonstrated modest efficacy for the treatment of pediatric MDD in one randomized controlled trial (RCT) (Arango et al. 2021). Preliminary open-label studies or RCTs have suggested that bupropion (Kim et al. 2012) and the monoamine oxidase inhibitors (MAOIs) can be used safely in children and adolescents (Ryan et al. 1988b), although noncompliance with the dietary requirements may present a significant problem for these patients. Other antidepressants, including the heterocyclics (e.g., amoxapine), intranasal esketamine, and intravenous ketamine, have been found to be efficacious for the treatment of depressed adults (American Psychiatric Association 2010), but they have not been well studied for the treatment of MDD in children and adolescents (e.g., only one existing small open-label trial exists for ketamine; Zheng et al. 2020). Large failed/negative trials have been noted for specific SSRIs (paroxetine, vilazodone, vortioxetine) and specific SNRIs (duloxetine, desvenlafaxine). The TCAs have not been found to be better than placebo (Hazell et al. 2002) and are associated with significant side effects and a high risk for lethality in the event of an overdose. Therefore, we mainly describe the use of SSRIs and SNRIs for youth with MDD. Table 5–2 summarizes data on RCTs examining SSRIs in pediatric depression.

Table 5–2. Selected data on SSRIs and SNRIs in pediatric MDD

	Randomized controlled trials			
Medication	**Study**	**Dosage, *mg/day***	**Outcome and sample size[a]**	**FDA approval**
Citalopram	Wagner et al. 2004	20–40	Citalopram > placebo (n=174)	No
	von Knorring et al. 2006	10–40	Did not separate from placebo (n=233)	
Desvenlafaxine	Atkinson et al. 2018	20–50 (weight-based)	Did not separate from placebo (n=363)	No
	Weihs et al. 2018	25–50 (weight-based)	Did not separate from placebo (n=227); fluoxetine also did not separate from placebo	
Duloxetine	Atkinson et al. 2014	30–120	Did not separate from placebo in adolescents (n=220); also no separation between fluoxetine (20–40 mg/day) and placebo	No
	Emslie et al. 2014	30–60	Did not separate from placebo in children (n=346); also no separation between fluoxetine (20 mg/day) and placebo	No
Escitalopram	Wagner et al. 2006	10–20	Did not separate from placebo in general population; escitalopram > placebo in adolescents (n=261)	Yes: MDD ages 12–17 years
	Emslie et al. 2009	10–20	Escitalopram > placebo (n=311)	

Table 5–2. Selected data on SSRIs and SNRIs in pediatric MDD *(continued)*

	Randomized controlled trials			
Medication	**Study**	**Dosage, *mg/day***	**Outcome and sample size[a]**	**FDA approval**
Fluoxetine	Simeon et al. 1990	20–60	Did not separate from placebo (n=32)	Yes; MDD ages 8–18 years
	Emslie et al. 1997	20	Fluoxetine > placebo (n=96)	
	Emslie et al. 2002	20	Fluoxetine > placebo (n=219)	
	March et al. 2004	10–40	Fluoxetine > placebo (n=221)	
Paroxetine	Keller et al. 2001	20–40	Paroxetine > placebo (n=180)	No
	Berard et al. 2006	20–40	Did not separate from placebo (n=275)	
	Emslie et al. 2006	10–50	Did not separate from placebo (n=206)	
Sertraline	Wagner et al. 2003[b]	50–200	Sertraline > placebo (n=364)	No
	Donnelly et al. 2006	50–200	Did not separate from placebo in children; sertraline > placebo in adolescents (n=199)	
Vilazodone	Durgam et al. 2018	15–30	Did not separate from placebo (n=529)	No

Table 5–2. Selected data on SSRIs and SNRIs in pediatric MDD *(continued)*

	Randomized controlled trials			
Medication	**Study**	**Dosage, *mg/day***	**Outcome and sample size[a]**	**FDA approval**
Venlafaxine[c]	Mandoki et al. 1997	Children: 37.5 Adolescents: 75	Did not separate from placebo in adolescents ($n=33$, very low dosages)	No
	Emslie et al. 2007[b]	37.5–225 (weight-based)	Did not separate from placebo overall ($n=334$); venlafaxine > placebo in adolescents ($n=197$)	
Vortioxetine	Findling et al. 2022	10–20	Did not separate from placebo at either 10 mg ($n=147$) or 20 mg ($n=161$) dosages; fluoxetine 20 mg ($n=153$) separated from placebo ($n=154$)	No

Note. MDD=major depressive disorder; SNRI=serotonin-norepinephrine reuptake inhibitor; SSRI=selective serotonin reuptake inhibitor.
[a]Sample size refers to combined sample size of participants receiving antidepressant described and placebo unless otherwise specified.
[b]Data pooled from two controlled trials.
[c]An unpublished study was also negative, but a reanalysis showed that venlafaxine was only positive for adolescents (cited by Bridge et al. 2009).

Using CGI-I scores of 2 ("much improved" to "very much improved") as indicating a positive outcome, in general, RCTs using the SSRIs have shown that children and adolescents with MDD had significantly better symptom response to acute treatment with these antidepressants (50%–60%) than to placebo (30%–50%) (Bridge et al. 2009). Of these SSRIs, fluoxetine showed the largest effect sizes, in part because of a low placebo response rate. In contrast, other antidepressants showed small effect sizes (e.g., sertraline, citalopram, escitalopram) or no effects (e.g., duloxetine, paroxetine), particularly when the studies were done in large multicenter studies (see Table 5–2). Moreover, despite the significant rates of response with some antidepressants, a smaller proportion of patients (30%–40%) achieved full remission (usually defined as a score of 28 or less on the CDRS-R) (Emslie et al. 1997, 2008; March et al. 2004; Wagner et al. 2004).

A possible explanation for the low rate of remission is that optimal pharmacological treatment may involve a higher dosage or a longer duration of treatment or that the ideal treatment for some individuals may involve a combination of pharmacological and psychosocial interventions, as suggested by the Treatment for Adolescents with Depression Study (TADS; March et al. 2004). However, in the TADS, although the rate of remission was higher with combination treatment (37% for the combination vs. 23% for medication alone), particularly for less severely depressed subjects, it was not optimal. Moreover, other studies did not show an advantage to adding CBT to regular SSRI treatment (Clarke et al. 2005; Goodyer et al. 2007).

As noted earlier, several published or unpublished industry-sponsored studies with SSRIs and SNRIs found small or no differences between active medication and placebo (for review, see Atkinson et al. 2014; Bridge et al. 2009; Emslie et al. 2014; Mandoki et al. 1997; Mann et al. 2006). Overall, participants responded to SSRIs (46%–63%), but the placebo response was also high (about 50%). The placebo response was associated with less depressive severity at intake and a large number of centers involved in the trial (Bridge et al. 2009).

Except in a large fluoxetine study in which no age differences were found (Emslie et al. 1997), younger subjects overall have higher placebo responses than older adolescents. Mild to moderate depressive symptoms may have responded to supportive management offered in these studies. Also, other methodological issues may have been responsible for the lack of difference between medication and placebo. (For a review of the limitations of pharmacological RCTs, see Cheung et al. 2005.)

A clinically meaningful way to understand the effect of treatment is through the concept of the *number needed to treat* (NNT), which refers to the number of patients who must be treated to observe one response that is attributable to active treatment and not placebo. Across all of the published and unpublished SSRI RCTs, patients with depression treated with SSRIs had relatively good response rates (50%–70% clinically improved), but the placebo response rates were also high (30%–60%), resulting in an overall NNT of 9 (Bridge et al. 2009; Cheung et al. 2005). Fluoxetine was the first medication to receive FDA approval for the treatment of pediatric depression, and studies show a larger difference between fluoxetine and placebo than other antidepressants, with an overall NNT of 4. It is not clear whether this difference is attributable to actual differences in the medication's effect, to other related properties of the medication (long half-life may lessen the impact of poor adherence to treatment), or to better design and performance of the fluoxetine studies, which may have included more severely depressed patients. Interestingly, in contrast to MDD, for pediatric anxiety the NNT is 3, even in large multicenter studies, which is mainly accounted for by lower placebo response in the anxiety studies.

In addition to fluoxetine, which was approved for youth ages 8–18 years with depression, escitalopram has been approved to treat MDD in adolescents ages 12–17. Data from several trials of escitalopram, in addition to safety data from studies of citalopram, led to FDA approval of escitalopram. In the trials of escitalopram, differences in response between children younger than 12 and adolescents led to the 12–17 age range associated with FDA approval (Emslie et al. 2009; Wagner et al. 2004, 2006).

Few RCTs have evaluated the effects of other classes of antidepressants for the treatment of depressed youth. Two unpublished, industry-sponsored RCTs with mirtazapine (pooled $N=250$) were negative (cited by Bridge et al. 2009; Mann et al. 2006). Although bupropion is being used clinically for the treatment of youth with MDD, no placebo-controlled RCTs have been conducted, although a few smaller open-label studies (Ns<25) and a larger chart review ($N=127$) suggest its potential efficacy (Kim et al. 2012). A recent large multicenter RCT compared a flexible dose of selegiline transdermal system (an MAOI) and placebo in a sample of adolescents with moderate to severe MDD ($n=308$) (DelBello et al. 2014). Results showed that the selegiline transdermal system was safe and well tolerated; both groups had a decline from baseline in depressive symptoms over the length of the study, without statistical superiority by either group. One study showed better response in most measurements between nefazodone and placebo for adolescents with MDD (Bridge et al. 2007), but a second study including depressed children and adolescents was negative (Cheung et al. 2005). Although the generic form of this medication is still available, nefazodone is largely not used in the United States, with several brand-name forms withdrawn previously because of a rare but serious side effect—liver damage resulting in hepatic failure.

Several medications available in Europe but not in the United States may also be beneficial for youth with MDD. In a recent placebo-controlled RCT (Arango et al. 2021), youth receiving agomelatine ($n=94$) dosed at 25 mg/day demonstrated greater improvement in depressive symptoms than youth receiving placebo ($n=99$). Open-label trials of mianserin (a tetracyclic antidepressant; $n=110$), reboxetine ($n=14$), and tianeptine ($n=60$) suggest that further research may be useful for understanding the benefit of these antidepressants for children and youth (Dugas et al. 1985; Graovac 2009; Toren et al. 2019).

Side Effects

Overall, SSRIs, SNRIs, and other novel antidepressants have been well tolerated by both children and adolescents, with only a few short-term side effects commonly reported. It appears that the side effects of SSRIs and SNRIs are similar and dose dependent and may subside with time (Cheung et al. 2005; Emslie et al. 1999; Leonard et al. 1997; Safer and Zito 2006). The most common side effects include gastrointestinal symptoms, restlessness, diaphoresis, headache, akathisia, changes in appetite (increase or decrease), sleep changes (e.g., vivid dreams, nightmares, impaired sleep), and impaired sexual functioning. Approximately 3%–8% of children and adolescents taking antidepressants may show increased impulsivity, agitation, irritability, silliness, and behavioral activation (Hammad et al. 2006; Martin et al. 2004; Wilens et al. 1998). These symptoms must be differentiated from the mania or hypomania that may appear in children and adolescents with bipolar disorder or in those predisposed to develop bipolar disorder (Wilens et al. 1998).

More rarely, the use of antidepressants has been associated with serotonin syndrome (Boyer and Shannon 2005) (see "Interactions With Other Medications" later in this section), with increased suicidal behaviors (see "Suicidal Behaviors" later), and with bruising (Lake et al. 2000). Citalopram was found to be associated with arrhythmias and prolonged QTc interval, particularly at dosages higher than 40 mg/day (www.fda.gov), but this finding has been questioned. Because of the risk of bruising, patients treated with SSRIs and SNRIs who will undergo surgery should inform their physicians, and they may wish to discontinue treatment during the preoperative period. Venlafaxine and perhaps other SNRIs may elevate blood pressure and cause tachycardia (e.g., typically <5 mm Hg for systolic blood pressure/diastolic blood pressure and <10 beats per minute), but not all studies have indicated this effect (Brent et al. 2009; Findling et al. 2014). Mirtazapine, a serotonin and α_2-adrenergic receptor blocker, may increase appetite, weight, and somnolence. Trazodone, a serotonin-2A ($5\text{-}HT_{2A}$) receptor blocker and weak serotonin reuptake inhibitor, and mirtazapine are mainly used as adjunctive and transient treatments for insomnia. Trazodone must be used with caution in males because it can induce priapism. Serzone, the branded form of nefazodone, a $5\text{-}HT_{2A}$ receptor blocker and weak serotonin reuptake inhibitor, was taken off the market by major manufacturers because it may induce liver problems.

The long-term side effects of antidepressants have not been systematically evaluated. Bupropion has been associated with headache, tremor, and seizure. Risk of seizures can be minimized by titrating the dosage slowly and avoiding high dosages (no more than 450 mg/day). It seems that bupropion cannot be used for patients with eating disorders with potential electrolyte abnormalities because of the high risk for seizures (American Psychiatric Association 2010).

Suicidal Behaviors

There are two ways to ascertain side effects. The first relies on spontaneous reporting of side effects by patients or their families (i.e., adverse events). The second uses side effects questionnaires. Compared with pediatric patients given placebo, those taking antidepressants appear to have a small but statistically significant increase in *spontaneous* self-harm behavior and suicidal ideation (suicide-related events [SREs]). In an FDA-sponsored meta-analysis conducted in collaboration with Columbia University (Hammad et al. 2006) that included 24 RCTs (16 studies of MDD, 4 of OCD, 2 of generalized anxiety disorder, 1 of social anxiety disorder, and 1 of ADHD) comparing several antidepressants with placebo, the overall risk ratio for SREs was 1.95 (95% CI, 1.28–2.98). For only MDD studies, the overall risk ratio was 1.66 (95% CI, 1.02–2.68). Only the TADS showed a significant difference between active treatment and placebo; among the antidepressants, only venlafaxine showed a statistically significant association with suicidality (March et al. 2004). In general, these results translate to 2 emergent or worsened SREs for every 100 youth treated with one of the antidepressants included in the FDA meta-analysis. The study authors reported very few suicide attempts and no completions.

In contrast to the SRE analyses, evaluation of the suicidality ascertained through rating scales in 17 studies did not show significant onset or worsening of suicidality (RR 0.92–0.93) (Hammad et al. 2006). It is not clear why the FDA meta-analysis had increased rates of spontaneously reported SREs for subjects taking medication versus placebo but no differences in suicidality on regularly assessed clinical measures. It is possible that in a subgroup of patients treated with antidepressants, particularly those already agitated or suicidal, treatment causes a disinhibition that leads to worsening of ideation or a greater tendency to make suicidal threats. Because suicidal ideation usually leads to removal of the subject from the study and a change in treatment, analyses that look at the slope of suicidal ideation will not find an effect (although the TADS found greater reduction of suicidal ideation in the fluoxetine+CBT arm, which was not found in the fluoxetine-only or CBT-only arm). In addition, as measured on rating scales, suicidal ideation is highly correlated with the severity of depression, which is more likely to decline in those given the study drug than in those given placebo.

These results must be viewed in the context of the FDA study's limitations, which include use of the metric of relative risk (limited to trials with at least one event), inability to generalize the results to populations not included in RCTs, short-term data, failure to include all available RCTs, and multiple comparisons (Hammad et al. 2006). As stated by the FDA (Hammad et al. 2006), the implications and clinical significance of these findings are uncertain, given that with the increase in SSRI use, rates of adolescent suicide have declined dramatically (Olfson et al. 2003). Moreover, pharmacoepidemiological studies, which are correlative rather than causal, support a positive relationship between SSRI use and the reduction in the rate of adolescent and young adult suicides (Gibbons et al. 2005; Olfson et al. 2003; Valuck et al. 2004). Finally, one study showed increased suicide attempts only immediately *before* the SSRIs were administered (Simon et al. 2006), and later studies in several countries showed that after the FDA's black box warning for SSRIs was implemented, a surge occurred in the number of suicides (e.g., Katz et al. 2008; Libby et al. 2009).

A thorough meta-analysis extended the FDA analyses by including all of the existing published and unpublished antidepressant studies (13 of MDD, 6 of OCD, and 6 of anxiety disorders) (Bridge et al. 2009). This meta-analysis found comparable *overall* findings when similar statistical methods (relative risk) were used rather than the methods used in the FDA study (Bridge et al. 2009)—namely, a significantly increased relative risk for spontaneously reported suicidality *only* for subjects with MDD. However, in pooled random-effects analyses of risk differences, which make possible an analysis of *all* existing RCTs, a nonsignificant risk difference (drug minus placebo) was found for MDD (0.8%; 95% CI –0.2% to 1.8%) and other disorders. The overall *number needed to harm* (NNH; i.e., number of subjects needed to treat in order to observe one adverse event that can be attributed to the active treatment) for MDD was 125 (Bridge et al. 2009). As stated earlier in the "Acute Phase" discussion, the overall NNT for antidepressants in pediatric depression is 9. Thus, nearly 14 times more depressed patients will respond favorably to antidepressants than will spontaneously report suicidality (although one must keep in mind the limitations of meta-analyses). The benefit-risk ratio was larger for the SSRIs (10) than for non-SSRI antidepressants (5).

In conclusion, SREs appear to be more common with antidepressant treatment than with placebo. Nevertheless, given the greater number of patients who benefit from antidepressant treatment (particularly the SSRIs) than who experience these SREs, as well as the decline in overall suicidal ideation on rating scales, the risk-benefit ratio for SSRI use in pediatric depression appears to be favorable, with careful monitoring. Additional work is required to determine whether the risk-benefit ratio is indeed less favorable for children than for adolescents. Also, it remains to be clarified whether certain factors are related to increased risk for suicidality (Apter et al. 2006; Brent 2004; Hammad et al. 2006; Safer and Zito 2006), such as gender or biological sex, subject or family history of suicidality, disorder type (the effects of disorder type appear to be more obvious in depressed youth), severity of depressive symptoms at intake, medication dosages, medication half-life (in terms of efficacy), type of antidepressants administered, treatment duration, poor adherence to treatment, withdrawal side effects (due to noncompliance or short medication half-life), susceptibility to side effects (e.g., slow metabolizers or variations in genetic polymorphisms), and/or induction of agitation, activation, or hypomania.

Pharmacokinetic Studies

Aside from fluoxetine, which has a half-life of 24–72 hours in children (whereas norfluoxetine, the active metabolite of fluoxetine, has an a half-life of 7 days), the half-lives of most of the SSRIs (including paroxetine, sertraline, citalopram, and sustained-release bupropion) are between 14 and 16 hours (Axelson et al. 2000a, 2000b; Clein and Riddle 1995; Daviss et al. 2005; Findling et al. 1999, 2000, 2006). One study suggested that sertraline at a dosage of 200 mg/day can be prescribed once daily (Alderman et al. 1998). The results of previously mentioned studies suggest that SSRIs, particularly when prescribed at lower dosages, may need to be given twice daily. However, since this may be impractical, and adherence to treatment, which usually is low, may be worse with twice-daily regimens, it is recommended to first administer the SSRI once daily and to carefully evaluate the child for withdrawal side effects. If withdrawal side effects occur, twice-daily dosing is necessary. Otherwise, children and adolescents may experience withdrawal side effects during the evening, and these symptoms can be confused with lack of response or medication side effects. More pharmacokinetic studies conducted on the other antidepressants (i.e., SNRIs, atypical antidepressants) are necessary, because it appears that youth metabolize these medications faster than adult populations do.

Interactions With Other Medications

Careful attention to possible medication interactions is recommended, given that the antidepressants and their metabolites are metabolized in different degrees by the hepatic cytochrome P450 (CYP) enzymes. Of the five major CYP enzymes mediating known oxidative drug metabolism, CYP3A3/4 and CYP2D6 are responsible for approximately 50% and 30%, respectively. Except for citalopram/escitalopram and sertraline, the currently available SSRIs are mainly metabolized by CYP3A3/4 and/or CYP2D6 enzymes. One notable interaction is fluvoxamine and fluoxetine's inhibition of CYP2D6 (which also metabolizes aripiprazole and several TCAs). Bupropion is mainly metabolized by the CYP2B6 enzyme, but it also inhibits the enzyme CYP2D6. Venlafaxine is metabolized by the CYP2D6 enzyme. Substantial inhibition of these enzymes converts a normal metabolizer into a slow metabolizer, with regard to this specific pathway. Therefore, clinicians should be aware that toxicity could result in patients who are also taking other medications metabolized by the CYP system, including the TCAs, neuroleptics, antipsychotics, antiarrhythmics, antihypertensives, theophylline, atomoxetine, benzodiazepines, carbamazepine, and warfarin. It is impossible to memorize all interactions, but, fortunately, several websites and mobile applications provide up-to-date information about medication metabolism and interaction, including Medscape (https://reference.medscape.com), Epocrates (https://online.epocrates.com), Micromedex (www.micromedexsolutions.com), and UpToDate (www.uptodate.com).

Interactions of antidepressants with other serotonergic medications, particularly MAOIs, may induce the serotonin syndrome, which is marked by agitation, confusion, and hyperthermia (Boyer and Shannon 2005). MAOIs should not be given within 5 weeks of stopping fluoxetine and at least 2 weeks of stopping other SSRIs due to the possibility of inducing this syndrome.

Some antidepressants also have a high rate of protein binding, which can lead to increased therapeutic or toxic effects when taken with other protein-bound medications.

Discontinuation

Sudden or rapid cessation, especially for antidepressants with shorter half-lives (e.g., paroxetine and SNRIs), may induce withdrawal symptoms that can mimic a relapse or recurrence of a depressive episode (e.g., tiredness, irritability). Furthermore, rapid discontinuation of antidepressants may induce relapses or recurrences of depression. Therefore, if these medications must be discontinued, they should be tapered progressively.

Summary and Recommendations for Acute Treatment

Given that 30%–60% of children and adolescents with MDD respond to placebo (Bridge et al. 2009; Cheung et al. 2005; Mann et al. 2006) or very brief or supportive psychotherapy treatments (Goodyer et al. 2007; Mufson et al. 2004; Renaud et al. 1998), it is reasonable, when treating a patient with a mild depression or mild psychosocial impairment, to offer psychoeducation, support, and case management related to possible environmental stressors in the family and school. If the symptoms of mild depression worsen or the child has not responded after 4–6 weeks of supportive therapy, more specific forms of psychotherapy or antidepressants are warranted.

In contrast, youth who present with chronic or recurrent depression, moderate to severe psychosocial impairment, comorbid disorder, suicidal ideation, or a significant family history of depression will initially require more specific types of psychotherapies or antidepressants.

Independent of the treatment administered, the patient and their family will require education about the nature and treatment of depression, support, and management of daily problems. Problems at school, academic issues, school refusal, abuse of drugs, exposure to negative events (e.g., abuse, conflict with parents), and peer issues must be addressed. For example, family discord is associated with slower recovery and a greater chance of recurrence (Birmaher et al. 2000), and ongoing disappointments have been associated with chronic depression (Goodyer et al. 1998). Therefore, addressing family discord and improving the patient's coping skills are likely to improve outcomes with either psychosocial or psychopharmacological treatment. Moreover, a high incidence of parental mental health problems indicates the need for evaluation and appropriate referral of the parents and siblings of depressed youth, particularly because several studies have demonstrated that a mother's depression is associated with an increased risk for psychopathology in her children (Birmaher 2011). Finally, a high degree of comorbidity also emphasizes the importance of a multimodal pharmacological and psychosocial treatment approach (Hughes et al. 1999). For example, a child with MDD and ADHD may not experience symptom response to treatment with an SSRI alone and may require either combined treatment with a stimulant plus an SSRI or an alternative medication such as a TCA, bupropion, or venlafaxine (Daviss et al. 2001; Pliszka 2000).

Currently, SSRIs are the antidepressants of choice to treat children and adolescents with MDD. Fluoxetine has the most consistent data showing separation from placebo, but in clinical practice, other antidepressants may also be useful. Other important factors to consider when selecting the appropriate antidepressants include prior response to a specific antidepressant, patient and family preference, costs, safety or tolerably of side effects for the individual patient, pharmacological properties of the antidepressants (e.g., potential interactions with other medications, metabolism, half-life), and co-occurring psychiatric and medical illnesses (American Academy of Child and Adolescent Psychiatry 1998; American Psychiatric Association 2002). Patients should be treated with adequate dosages for at least 6 weeks before the clinician declares

Table 5–3. Dosages of antidepressants usually administered to youth with MDD

Medication group	Medication	Starting dosage, *mg/day*[a]	Dosage range, *mg/day*
SSRIs	Citalopram	10	20–60[b]
	Escitalopram	10	10–40
	Fluoxetine	10	20–80
	Fluvoxamine	25	50–150
	Paroxetine	10	20–60
	Sertraline	25	50–300
SSRI/serotonin modulators	Vilazodone	10	10–40
	Vortioxetine	5	5–20
SNRIs	Desvenlafaxine	25	50–100
	Duloxetine	20	60–120
	Venlafaxine XR	37.5	75–375
Others	Bupropion SR	100	150–450
	Bupropion XL	150	150–450
	Mirtazapine	7.5	7.5–30

Note. MDD=major depressive disorder; SNRI=serotonin-norepinephrine reuptake inhibitor; SR=sustained release; SSRI=selective serotonin reuptake inhibitor; XL=extended release; XR=extended release.
[a]For children, consider using lower dosages.
[b]For citalopram dosages above 40 mg, an electrocardiogram should be done both prior to and following dosage increase, given concerns of QT prolongation.

a lack of response to treatment (the treatment of nonresponders is described in subsection "Treatment-Resistant Depression" later in this chapter).

The dosages of SSRIs and SNRIs prescribed for children and adolescents usually are similar to those used for adult patients (American Psychiatric Association 2010; Birmaher et al. 2007; Leonard et al. 1997) (Table 5–3), except that lower initial dosages, particularly for children, are used to avoid unwanted effects. Fewer studies have examined side effects in children. To avoid side effects and improve treatment adherence, clinicians should start the medication at a low dosage and increase the dosage slowly as indicated and tolerated. During the acute phase of treatment, patients should be treated with adequate and tolerable dosages for at least 4–6 weeks. Clinical response should be assessed at 4- to 6-week intervals, and the dosage can be increased if a complete response has not been obtained. If only a partial response has been achieved at the point of assessment, the physician may consider strategies described in the subsection "Treatment-Resistant Depression" later in this chapter. At each step, adequate time should be allowed for clinical response, and frequent, early dosage adjustments should be avoided.

Given the small but significant association between antidepressants and worsening or emergent spontaneous SREs, all patients receiving these medications for suicidal and other symptoms should be carefully monitored, particularly during the first weeks of treatment. The FDA recommends that patients be seen every week for the first 4 weeks and biweekly thereafter. If weekly face-to-face appointments cannot be scheduled, evaluations should be carried out briefly by phone. However, there are currently no data available to suggest that the face-to-face monitoring schedule proposed by the FDA or telephone calls have any impact on the risk of suicide. Although monitoring is important for all patients, it should be more carefully done for patients who have a history of suicidal ideation or suicide attempts or who show behavior associated with an increased risk for suicide (e.g., prior suicidality, impulsivity, substance abuse, history of sexual abuse, psychosis, mixed manic/hypomanic episodes) (Gould et al. 1996; Shaffer and Craft 1999); patients who have become agitated, disinhibited, or irritable while taking an antidepressant; and those with family history of bipolar disorder or suicide.

Treatment of Major Depressive Disorder Subtypes and Bipolar Depression

Bipolar Depression

Many children and adolescents seeking treatment for depression are usually experiencing their first depressive episode. Because the symptoms of unipolar and bipolar depression are similar, it is difficult to decide whether a patient needs only an antidepressant or treatment with other medications or psychotherapies. Some symptoms, such as psychosis, greater mood lability, pharmacologically induced mania/hypomania, and family history of bipolar disorder, may alert the clinician to the risk that the child could develop a manic or hypomanic episode (Diler et al. 2017). Also, the presence of subthreshold manic or hypomanic episodes (currently called "major depressive disorder, with mixed features" in DSM-5 [American Psychiatric Association 2022] if there are at least three manic symptoms but not enough for mania/hypomania) may indicate the existence of bipolar disorder.

Lurasidone and the olanzapine-fluoxetine combination were more efficacious than placebo for youth with bipolar depression in RCTs, whereas studies suggest potential benefits with quetiapine, risperidone, and ziprasidone (cited by DelBello et al. 2017; Rengasamy and Birmaher 2019). In adults, RCTs have found positive effects with lithium carbonate, valproate, and some of the second-generation antipsychotics, such as quetiapine and lurasidone, either alone or in combination with mood stabilizers for treatment of bipolar depression. Similarly, for MDD with mixed features, adult studies have found that second-generation antipsychotics (e.g. lurasidone or ziprasidone) may be efficacious (Kennedy et al. 2016). Lamotrigine as monotherapy or as an adjunctive treatment appears to be efficacious in preventing relapses or recurrences of depression, and a meta-analysis showed modest effects for the acute treatment of bipolar depression in adults (Geddes et al. 2009). SSRIs and bupropion combined with mood stabilizers may be beneficial for the treatment of bipolar depression in adults (American Psychiatric Association 2002; Gijsman et al. 2004; Hirschfeld 2007). Moreover, one RCT found that monotherapy with fluoxetine was better than placebo for the management of depressed adult patients with bipolar II disorder and did not induce significant increases in manic switches (Amsterdam et al. 1998). However, antidepressants must be used cautiously because they may induce a switch to mania/hypomania.

Children and adolescents do not always respond to medications in the same way as adults, and they may be more prone to switch to mania with antidepressant treatment. In particular, youth who have subthreshold manic symptoms or a family history of bipolar disorder may be at the greatest risk for conversion to mania with antidepressant use (Baumer et al. 2006; Goldsmith et al. 2011). Therefore, these recommendations must be followed with caution until results from controlled studies of children and adolescents are made available.

Psychotic Depression

No controlled studies of psychotic depression in children and adolescents have been done. Because only 20%–40% of adults respond to antidepressant monotherapy (American Psychiatric Association 2010), recommended treatment often consists of antidepressants combined with an antipsychotic. In clinical practice, the antipsychotic is usually tapered after remission of the depression. However, at least in adults, the second-generation antipsychotic medications are beneficial as monotherapy for depression, raising a question about the need to discontinue them unless they are inducing significant side effects (e.g., metabolic or neurological side effects). Electroconvulsive therapy (ECT) is particularly effective for the psychotic subtype of depression in adults (American Psychiatric Association 2010) and may be useful for depressed adolescents as well (Ghaziuddin et al. 2004). Treatment with antidepressants in psychotic depressed children should be conducted with caution because the presence of psychosis is a marker for possible development of bipolar disorder (Geller et al. 1994; Strober and Carlson 1982).

Seasonal Affective Disorder

Studies in adults have shown that SSRIs and bright-light therapy are beneficial for the treatment of subjects with recurrent seasonal affective disorder. One small RCT ($n=28$) suggested that bright-light therapy is efficacious for the treatment of children and adolescents with seasonal affective disorder (Swedo et al. 1997), but no studies with antidepressants have been conducted in this younger population.

Treatment-Resistant Depression

As in adults (American Psychiatric Association 2010), up to 60% of youth with MDD experience a partial treatment response (moderate response on the CGI-I; presence of significant symptoms of MDD but not the full syndrome), and 20%–30% may have no response at all (Birmaher et al. 2000; Brent et al. 2009; Emslie et al. 2008; March et al. 2004). Patients with a partial response have a significantly higher rate of relapse during the first 6 months following therapy and have significantly more psychosocial, occupational, and medical problems (American Psychiatric Association 2010). Moreover, among children, chronic depression does not usually remit spontaneously and is not responsive to placebo (American Academy of Child and Adolescent Psychiatry 1998; American Psychiatric Association 2010), indicating the need for more aggressive treatments for patients with these conditions.

The first step in treatment for patients with treatment-resistant depression is to establish the nonresponse. Several definitions of *nonresponse* have been used, including the presence of a significant number of depressive symptoms, symptom improvement of less than 50% as measured by rating scales (e.g., the CDRS-R), and no change or worsening per CGI scores. After establishing that the patient's symptoms have not responded, the clinician must learn why. The most common reasons for treatment failure are inappropriate diagnoses, inappropriate or inadequate drug/psychosocial therapy dosage or length of trial, treatment noncompliance, pharmacokinetic/pharmacodynamic factors, comorbidity with other psychiatric disorders (e.g., persistent depressive disorder, anxiety, ADHD, covert substance abuse, personality disorders) or medical illnesses (e.g., hypothyroidism), presence of subthreshold manic/hypomanic symptoms, psychosocial issues and stressors (e.g., abuse, conflicts), and persistent or intolerable side effects (American Psychiatric Association 2010; Brent et al. 1998, 2009; Hughes et al. 1999). Other factors associated with nonresponse include severe depression, long depression, suicidality, lack of response or mild response after 2–4 weeks of treatment, hopelessness, and inadequate treatment by the therapist (e.g., poor-quality CBT) or a poor "fit" between patient/family and therapist. Carefully evaluating for subtle symptoms of hypomania is important to determine whether bipolar disorder may be the reason that the patient's symptoms are not responding to treatment or are even worsening with antidepressant treatment.

The Treatment of SSRI-Resistant Depression in Adolescents (TORDIA) study (Brent et al. 2008) is the only RCT of youth with treatment-refractory depression. This study of a large sample of adolescents with MDD indicated that the combination of CBT and an antidepressant was more efficacious than the antidepressant alone (54.8% vs. 40.5%). No differences were found among the antidepressants used in the study (fluoxetine, citalopram, venlafaxine). The expected variables were associated with poor response (e.g., more severe depression, comorbid disorder, abuse). Follow-up assessments showed continuous remission, with approximately 60% of patients achieving remission by 72 weeks. About 25% of those who had achieved remission later experienced relapse (Emslie et al. 2010; Vitiello et al. 2011).

Once treatment noncompliance has been ruled out, the following strategies, based on the TORDIA study and the adult research literature, have been recommended:

1. *Optimize initial treatments.* Although few studies have evaluated the efficacy of this strategy, initial treatment can be maximized by increasing the length of the trial or the dosage.
   a. *Extend the initial medication trial.* For patients who experience at least a partial response after receiving a therapeutic dose of an antidepressant for 6 weeks, the first and simplest strategy is to extend the treatment for another 2–4 weeks if the patient's clinical and functional status allows (American Psychiatric Association 2010; Thase and Rush 1997).
   b. *Increase the dosage.* This strategy can be utilized for partial responders. Dosages can be increased to the maximum dosages unless the patient develops side effects (American Psychiatric Association 2010; Heiligenstein et al. 2006).
2. *Switch strategies.* For patients whose symptoms do not respond to a specific antidepressant medication or who cannot tolerate its side effects, another antidepressant of the same class or a different class (e.g., venlafaxine for a patient who did not respond to a SSRI) can be tried. The few adult studies published to date suggest that, because of the probable heterogeneity in depression mechanisms, the more efficacious approach is to switch antidepressant classes rather than stay within the same class. Also, severe depression appears to respond better to antidepressants with both serotonergic and adrenergic properties (e.g., venlafaxine) (Poirier and Boyer 1999). MAOIs have been found beneficial for patients whose symptoms have not responded to other medications (American Psychiatric Association 2010; Thase and Rush 1997), but their use in children and adolescents is complicated because of the dietary restrictions. An open study suggested that symptoms of depression in adolescents that had not responded to TCAs did respond to MAOIs (Ryan et al. 1988b). However, the adolescents' symptoms may not have responded to TCAs because this group of medications is not efficacious for the treatment of pediatric MDD (Birmaher et al. 1996a).
3. *Augment or combine strategies.* The TORDIA study (Brent et al. 2009) provided evidence that the combination of an antidepressant and CBT is

efficacious for adolescents with treatment-resistant MDD. However, pharmacological augmentation has not been well studied in youth. In adults, the most common augmentation or combination strategies include adding atypical antipsychotics (aripiprazole, quetiapine, or lurasidone), atypical antidepressants (bupropion or mirtazapine), lithium carbonate at therapeutic levels for a period of 4 weeks, or L-triiodothyronine (25–50 μg/day). Esketamine (intranasal form) and brexpiprazole were recently FDA approved for augmentation of MDD in adults. Less common augmentation strategies include adding a stimulant or omega-3 fatty acids or combining an SSRI with a TCA (American Psychiatric Association 2010; Bauer et al. 2000). In adults, the combination of lithium and antidepressants has yielded response rates of 50%–65% in studies that administered lithium at therapeutic levels for at least 4 weeks (e.g., American Psychiatric Association 2010; Thase and Rush 1997). The interval before response to lithium augmentation has been reported to be from several days to 3 weeks. After this period, the chance to observe improvement with lithium decreases.

In adolescents with MDD, an open-label study showed significant improvement of refractory depressive symptoms after augmentation of TCA treatment with lithium (Ryan et al. 1988a). Another open-label study, however, did not replicate this finding (Strober et al. 1992). Observational studies suggest that augmentation using quetiapine and aripiprazole may be beneficial for overall functioning or for reducing self-injury (Bildik et al. 2012; Pathak et al. 2005).

Case reports have suggested that adding stimulant medications or combining an SSRI with a TCA may also be effective (American Psychiatric Association 2010), but these combinations must be used with caution because of the possibility of interactions (as with, e.g., SSRIs and TCAs). In adolescents and adults, the combination of antidepressants and psychotherapy (CBT, interpersonal psychotherapy) for patients with severe or treatment-resistant depression has also been found useful (Keller et al. 2000; March et al. 2004).

4. *Consider ECT.* ECT is one of the most efficacious treatments for adults with nonresistant MDD (70% response) and resistant MDD (50% response) (American Psychiatric Association 2010; Ghaziuddin et al. 2004). However, because of its invasiveness, ECT remains the treatment of choice only for the most severe, incapacitating forms of resistant depres-

sion. No controlled studies have been conducted in adolescents, although retrospective chart reviews suggest similar response rates (e.g., 58%) and that ECT is safe in adolescents (cited in Cullen et al. 2019). Approximately 60% of adult patients who are treated successfully with ECT tend to experience relapse after 6 months (American Psychiatric Association 2010). Therefore, they require maintenance treatment with antidepressants and sometimes maintenance ECT. However, maintenance ECT has never been reported in adolescents.

5. *Try other biological treatments.* Other innovative treatments, such as intravenous ketamine, intravenous clomipramine, transcranial magnetic stimulation (TMS), transcranial direct current stimulation (tDCS), and vagal nerve stimulation (VNS), have been used for the treatment of adults with depression that has not responded to standard treatment (American Psychiatric Association 2010). Promisingly, intravenous ketamine/esketamine has demonstrated significantly greater reduction in depressive symptoms compared with placebo in several adult RCTs, with effects lasting from several hours up to 1 week after ketamine administration (Marcantoni et al. 2020). Ketamine, although generally well tolerated, requires postinfusion medical monitoring for 2–4 hours. Several ongoing RCTs are investigating ketamine for the treatment of MDD in youth, with one open-label trial ($n = 13$) suggesting efficacy and tolerability (cited in Kim et al. 2021). In adolescents, intravenous clomipramine has been shown to be efficacious for patients whose symptoms have failed to respond to other antidepressant treatment (Sallee et al. 1997). In addition, preliminary open-label/naturalistic studies suggest that TMS may be safe and effective, although no studies exist examining tDCS or VNS in depressed youth (cited by Cullen et al. 2019). Activity-based interventions (e.g., aerobic exercise or yoga) may also be beneficial for some depressed youth (James-Palmer et al. 2020; Wegner et al. 2020). Although some supplements (e.g., vitamin D and *N*-acetylcysteine) may be safe and have some preliminary evidence suggesting potential benefit as an augmentation treatment for MDD in youth, caution should be taken in using over-the-counter herbs or supplements because the quality of such compounds may vary, and some supplements may have adverse effects (e.g., psychosis with kratom) or may interact with antidepressant treatments (e.g., St. John's wort).

All of the strategies described require implementation in a systematic fashion (for reviews, see American Academy of Child and Adolescent Psychiatry 1998; American Psychiatric Association 2010; Thase and Rush 1997). Comparing these strategies with other treatments of medical disorders can be useful to help patients and their families understand the medication plan and to improve compliance with and tolerance of treatment. The example of hypertension is appropriate: diuretics may be used alone or combined with other antihypertensives in different trials, according to response. Psychoeducation for the patient and family is also required to avoid the development of hopelessness in the patient and family as well as in the clinician.

Treatment of Comorbid Conditions and Suicidality

Comorbid disorders may influence the onset, maintenance, and recurrence of depression (Birmaher et al. 1996a, 1996b; Emslie et al. 2010). Thus, in addition to treating the depressive symptoms, clinicians should treat the comorbid conditions that often accompany depressive disorders (Hughes et al. 1999).

For example, depressed adolescents with comorbid ADHD respond less well to treatment than do those with depression alone (Hamilton and Bridge 1999). For patients with depression and ADHD—especially those for whom the ADHD seems to be the primary problem—and because the stimulants exert their effect quickly, it is recommended that the ADHD be treated first. Thereafter, if the depressive symptoms continue after the ADHD is stabilized, an SSRI should be added (Hughes et al. 1999; Pliszka 2000). This strategy, however, has not been validated. An open study using bupropion suggested that this medication can be efficacious in treating both MDD and ADHD (Daviss et al. 2001), although the effect of bupropion on ADHD is not as impressive as that obtained by treatment with stimulants (Conners et al. 1996). It has been suggested that atomoxetine may help both ADHD and depression, but this medication is a weak antidepressant and has notably weaker effects compared with stimulants in the treatment of ADHD.

The treatment of comorbid anxiety, which more often precedes depression than vice versa, is essential both because it contributes to improvement and because the anxiety, if left untreated, may predispose the individual to future depressive episodes (Hayward et al. 2000; Kovacs et al. 1989). Fortunately, similar pharmacotherapy and psychotherapy treatments found useful for the treatment of MDD have also been found beneficial for the treatment of youth with anxiety disorders (e.g., CBT, SSRIs) (Birmaher et al. 2003; Kendall 1994; Research Unit on Pediatric Psychopharmacology Anxiety Study Group 2001).

Other comorbid conditions, such as OCD, conduct disorder, eating disorders, and PTSD, have also been found to affect treatment response. These comorbid conditions must be addressed in order for the treatment of depressed youth to be successful (Birmaher et al. 1996b; Brent et al. 1998; Goodyer et al. 1997).

Suicidal ideation and behavior are common symptoms accompanying major depression and are more likely to occur in the face of comorbid disruptive disorders, mixed manic/hypomanic symptoms, substance abuse, physical or sexual abuse, impulsive behaviors, prior suicide attempts, and family history of suicidal behavior (e.g., Gould et al. 1996). Assessing suicidality, securing any lethal agents (e.g., medications, firearms), and developing safety plans with the patient and family are essential components of the management of the suicidal depressed patient. Patients who cannot formulate a safety plan (or have low confidence in their ability to use such a plan) and those at higher future risk of acting on suicidal thoughts (e.g., those with ongoing suicidal ideation with intent, a plan, or a recent suicide attempt) may require inpatient hospitalization. Treatment of the underlying depression may be necessary but not sufficient to prevent recurrent attempts. Other contributors to suicidality, such as sexual abuse, drug and alcohol use, ADHD, conduct problems, impulsivity and aggression, personality disorders, and family discord, must be assessed and targeted (Brent et al. 1999).

An important consideration is that in the TADS, the combination of CBT and fluoxetine was associated with lower risk for suicidality (March et al. 2004). However, not all studies have found the protective effect of CBT (e.g., TORDIA; Goodyer et al. 2007; Spirito et al. 2011).

Continuation Therapy

Naturalistic longitudinal studies and open follow-up studies following acute RCTs have shown that the rate of MDD relapse is very high (e.g., 25%–48% within 1 year) (Birmaher et al. 2002; Kennard et al. 2009a, 2009b, 2014; Vitiello et al. 2011). An RCT of fluoxetine discontinuation showed that, compared with a switch to placebo, continuing fluoxetine was associated with a much lower rate of relapse (22% vs. 48%) (Emslie et al. 2008). Similar results have been reported in adults with MDD (American Psychiatric Association 2010). Therefore, until further research results are available, clinicians should offer all patients continuation treatment for 6–12 months after complete symptom remission to consolidate the response and prevent relapse of symptoms. During this phase, patients should be seen biweekly or monthly depending on the their clinical status, functioning, support systems, environmental stressors, motivation for treatment, and other psychiatric or medical disorders. Patients and their families should be taught to recognize early signs of relapse.

One study openly administered fluoxetine for 6 weeks to a large sample of children and adolescents with MDD (Kennard et al. 2014). Responders were offered to continue fluoxetine alone or fluoxetine + relapse-prevention CBT for an additional 6 months. Relapse-prevention CBT was effective in reducing the risk of relapse compared with fluoxetine alone (9% vs. 27%) but not in accelerating time to remission.

During the continuation phase, antidepressants must be maintained at the same dosage used to attain remission of acute symptoms, provided that the medication causes no significant side effects or dosage-related negative effects on the patient's compliance (American Psychiatric Association 2010). At the end of the continuation phase, if a decision is made to discontinue the antidepressant, the medication should be tapered gradually (e.g., over a period of 6 weeks) to avoid withdrawal effects (e.g., sleep disturbance, irritability, gastrointestinal symptoms) that may lead the clinician to misinterpret the need for continued medication treatment. In addition, clinical practice has suggested that rapid discontinuation of antidepressants may precipitate a relapse or recurrence of depression. Ideally, treatment discontinuation should occur while children and adolescents are on extended vacation, rather than during the school year.

If relapse occurs, the clinician should first determine whether the patient has been compliant with treatment. If the patient has not been compliant, the antidepressant medication should be resumed. If the patient has been compliant and their symptoms had been previously responding to the medication (without significant side effects), the clinician should consider the presence of ongoing stressors (e.g., conflict, abuse), comorbid psychiatric disorders (e.g., anxiety disorder; ADHD, predominantly inattentive or combined presentation; substance abuse; persistent depressive disorder; subthreshold manic/hypomanic symptoms or undetected bipolar II disorder; or eating disorder), and medical illnesses. Depending on the circumstances, an increase in the medication dosage, a change to another medication, augmentation strategies, or psychotherapy may be indicated. For patients receiving only psychotherapy, the clinician should consider adding medications or using new psychotherapeutic strategies.

Maintenance Therapy

After the patient has been asymptomatic for approximately 6–12 months (continuation phase), the clinician must decide whether the patient should receive maintenance therapy, which therapy to use, and for how long. The main goal of the maintenance phase is to prevent recurrences. This phase may last from 1 year to much longer and is typically conducted with a visit frequency of every 1–3 months depending on the patient's clinical status, functioning, support systems, environmental stressors, motivation for treatment, and other psychiatric or medical disorders.

Determining Who Should Receive Maintenance Therapy

The recommendation for maintenance therapy depends on several factors, such as severity of the initial depressive episode (e.g., suicidality, psychosis, functional impairment), number and severity of prior depressive episodes, chronicity, comorbid disorders, family psychopathology, presence of support, patient and family willingness to adhere to the treatment program, and contraindications to treatment.

Factors associated with increased risk for recurrence in naturalistic studies and open follow-ups after acute RCTs of depressed children and adolescents may serve as a guide for the clinician in deciding who needs maintenance treatment. These factors include a history of prior depressive episodes, female sex, late onset, suicidality, "double" depression, subsyndromal depressive symptoms, poor functioning, comorbid disorders, personality disorders, exposure to negative events (e.g., abuse, conflicts), and family history of recurrence (two or more family members with a history of MDD recurrence) (Birmaher et al. 1996a,

1996b; Goodyer et al. 1998; Kennard et al. 2009a, 2009b; Klein et al. 2001; Vitiello et al. 2011; Wagner et al. 2004).

No maintenance RCTs in depressed children and adolescents have been reported to date. Among depressed adults, those who have had only a single uncomplicated episode of depression, mild episodes, or lengthy intervals between episodes (e.g., 5 years) probably should not start maintenance treatment (American Psychiatric Association 2010), whereas those who have had three or more depressive episodes (especially if they occur in a short period of time and have deleterious consequences), chronic depressions, and severe depressions should receive maintenance treatment.

Controversy exists about using maintenance treatment to treat patients who have had two previous episodes. Overall, maintenance treatment has been recommended for adult depressed patients who have had two depressive episodes and who meet one or more of the following criteria (American Psychiatric Association 2002; Depression Guideline Panel 1993): 1) the family has a history of bipolar disorder or recurrent depression, 2) the first depressive episode occurred before age 20 years, and 3) both episodes were severe or life-threatening and occurred during the previous 3 years. Given that depression in youth has a similar clinical presentation, sequelae, and natural course as in adults, these guidelines should probably also be applied for children and adolescents who have experienced two previous major depressive episodes.

Deciding Which Treatment to Use

For practical reasons, unless there is any contraindication (e.g., medication side effects), the treatment that was efficacious in the induction of remission of the acute episode should be continued for maintenance therapy. However, patients whose symptoms are being maintained with medications should also be offered psychotherapy to help them cope with the psychosocial scars induced by the depression. Furthermore, many depressed youth live in environments charged with stressful situations, and their parents usually have psychiatric disorders; therefore, multimodal treatments are ideal.

When selecting a medication for maintenance therapy, the clinician should consider the side effect profile and the way the side effects may affect the patient's compliance. For example, dry mouth, weight gain, increased sweating, sexual dysfunction, and polyuria (if the patient is taking lithium) may be very troublesome and may induce discontinuation of treatment. In addition, in children and adolescents, the long-term consequences of using antidepressant medications (e.g., chronic inhibition of serotonin reuptake by an SSRI) are unknown.

Other factors—such as a patient's embarrassment with friends, uneasiness about the idea of having their mind "controlled by a medication," view of treatment with medications as a sign of "weakness," and uncertainty about the risk of relapse in spite of doing well while taking medications—should all be addressed with both the patient and parents.

Determining How Long the Maintenance Phase Should Last

Adult patients with second episodes who fulfill the criteria for maintenance therapy noted earlier in this section should be maintained for several years (up to 5 years in adult studies) with the same antidepressant dosage used to achieve clinical remission during the acute treatment phase. However, patients with three or more episodes and patients with second episodes associated with psychosis, severe impairment, and severe suicidality that proved very difficult to treat should be considered for longer periods of treatment or even lifelong treatment.

TCAs, SSRIs, and lithium have been found to be efficacious for the prevention of depressive recurrences in adult patients (American Psychiatric Association 2010). However, given the apparent lack of efficacy of TCAs in youth, as well as the advantages of SSRIs and their efficacy in the acute treatment of MDD, the SSRIs are considered first-line medications in maintenance therapy in this population. Antidepressant medication, unless it is not tolerated, should be continued at the full dosage used to exert the initial therapeutic effect.

For most children and adolescents, multimodal therapies are recommended. In addition to antidepressant medications, psychosocial maintenance strategies should be implemented to help the patient's inner and interpersonal conflicts, improve their coping and social skills, help them deal with the psychosocial and personal scars left by the depression, and improve their academic and social functioning. The reduction of family stress, promotion of a supportive environment, and effective treatment of parents and siblings with psychiatric disorders may also help diminish the risk for recurrence.

Disruptive Mood Dysregulation Disorder

DSM-5 (American Psychiatric Association 2013) added a new disorder to the mood disorders category, *disruptive mood dysregulation disorder* (DMDD). This disorder is characterized by frequent, severe, recurrent temper outbursts and chronically irritable and/or angry mood, both of which must have been present for at least 1 year and must not be accounted for by other mood disorders. DMDD was mainly included in DSM-5 to reduce the misdiagnosis of bipolar disorder in children with chronic irritability and temper outbursts without the episodicity that characterizes bipolar disorder (Axelson 2013). However, the high degree of overlap with symptoms of depression and oppositional defiant disorder (ODD) and similar course and outcome of youth with ODD has raised questions as to whether DMDD represents a distinct disorder or is simply a more severe form of ODD or bipolar disorder (Axelson et al. 2012; Copeland et al. 2014; Leibenluft 2011; Rowe et al. 2010; Stringaris et al. 2009). It could also be asked whether it was premature to include DMDD in DSM-5 because of the scarce literature available, the fact that irritable mood and temper outbursts are ubiquitous across psychiatric disorders, its high comorbidity with other disorders, and the low reliability of the diagnosis.

Few pharmacological studies have examined treatments for DMDD or severe mood dysregulation (SMD) (Leibenluft 2011), a syndrome from which DMDD was derived. However, in contrast to DMDD, SMD also includes some symptoms of ADHD, mania, and depression. A recent RCT of youth with SMD/DMDD ($n=53$) found greater response (defined by improvement in irritability) to treatment with a combination of citalopram and methylphenidate compared with placebo and methylphenidate (Towbin et al. 2020). Other smaller studies (Ns<35) of youth with SMD/DMDD suggest reductions in irritability with risperidone and methylphenidate but not with lithium (cited by Benarous et al. 2017). Until the diagnosis of DMDD is clear, clinicians should be careful when assessing children with chronic irritability and temper tantrums and should search for the presence of underlying disorders for which there are known treatments, rather rush to DMDD.

Clinical Pearls

- Inform patients and families that the treatment of major depressive disorder (MDD) includes three phases: acute, continuation, and maintenance.
- Remember that the goal of treatment is not only to achieve response but also to achieve remission and good psychosocial functioning.
- Offer education and support to depressed youth and their families during all phases of treatment. Some mildly depressed youth may respond well to short-term management with education and support.
- Depending on the severity and chronicity of the youth's depression and other factors, use antidepressants (selective serotonin reuptake inhibitors [SSRIs] as first line) and/or psychotherapy (cognitive-behavioral therapy [CBT] and interpersonal psychotherapy) during the acute phase.
- Question youth and families about side effects because children and adolescents treated with SSRIs may uncommonly exhibit onset or worsening of suicidal ideation and, more rarely, suicide attempts.
- After successful acute treatment, offer all youth continuation treatment with the same dosage of antidepressants and psychotherapy (e.g., CBT) for 6–12 months to prevent relapses.
- After the continuation phase, provide maintenance treatment with antidepressants and/or psychotherapy for 1 year or longer to prevent recurrences, especially for depressed youth with severe depressions or frequent recurrences. For some, treatment may last years. In these cases, intermittent trials without medications are warranted to observe whether the patient needs further treatment.

- Manage comorbid disorders (with evidence-based treatments for each of these conditions), ongoing conflicts, and family psychopathology to help patients achieve remission.
- In managing resistant depressions, consider factors associated with poor response to treatment, such as severe depression, long depressions, poor treatment adherence, misdiagnoses, ongoing negative life events (e.g., abuse), presence of comorbid disorders (e.g., subthreshold manic/hypomanic symptoms, anxiety, ADHD, eating disorders), and poor adherence to treatment.
- Until the disruptive mood dysregulation disorder (DMDD) diagnosis is clarified, look for and treat the underlying disorders in children with DMDD.

References

Alderman J, Wolkow R, Chung M, Johnston HF: Sertraline treatment of children and adolescents with obsessive-compulsive disorder or depression: pharmacokinetics, tolerability, and efficacy. J Am Acad Child Adolesc Psychiatry 37(4):386–394, 1998 9549959

American Academy of Child and Adolescent Psychiatry: Practice parameters for the assessment and treatment of children and adolescents with depressive disorders. J Am Acad Child Adolesc Psychiatry 37(10 Suppl):63S–83S, 1998 9785729

American Psychiatric Association: Diagnostic and Statistical Manual of Mental Disorders, 4th Edition. Washington, DC, American Psychiatric Association, 1994

American Psychiatric Association: Practice guideline for the treatment of patients with bipolar disorder (revision). Am J Psychiatry 159(4 Suppl):1–50, 2002 11958165

American Psychiatric Association: Practice Guideline for the Treatment of Patients With Major Depressive Disorder, 3rd Edition. Arlington, VA, American Psychiatric Association, 2010

American Psychiatric Association: Diagnostic and Statistical Manual of Mental Disorders, 5th Edition. Arlington, VA, American Psychiatric Association, 2013

American Psychiatric Association: Diagnostic and Statistical Manual of Mental Disorders, 5th Edition, Text Revision. Washington, DC, American Psychiatric Association, 2022

Amsterdam JD, Garcia-España F, Fawcett J, et al: Efficacy and safety of fluoxetine in treating bipolar II major depressive episode. J Clin Psychopharmacol 18(6):435–440, 1998 9864074

Apter A, Lipschitz A, Fong R, et al: Evaluation of suicidal thoughts and behaviors in children and adolescents taking paroxetine. J Child Adolesc Psychopharmacol 16(1–2):77–90, 2006 16553530

Arango C, Buitelaar JK, Fegert JM, et al: Safety and efficacy of agomelatine in combination with psychosocial counselling in children and adolescents with major depressive disorder: a double-blind, randomised, controlled, phase 3 trial in nine countries. Lancet Psychiatry 9(2):113–124, 2021 34919834

Atkinson SD, Prakash A, Zhang Q, et al: A double-blind efficacy and safety study of duloxetine flexible dosing in children and adolescents with major depressive disorder. J Child Adolesc Psychopharmacol 24(4):180–189, 2014 24813026

Atkinson S, Lubaczewski S, Ramaker S, et al: Desvenlafaxine versus placebo in the treatment of children and adolescents with major depressive disorder. J Child Adolesc Psychopharmacol 28(1):55–65, 2018 29185786

Axelson D: Taking disruptive mood dysregulation disorder out for a test drive. Am J Psychiatry 170(2):136–139, 2013 23377631

Axelson D, Perel J, Rudolph G, et al: Sertraline pediatric/adolescent PK-PD parameters: dose/plasma level ranging for depression. Clin Pharmacol Ther 67:169, 2000a

Axelson D, Perel J, Rudolph G, et al: Significant differences in pharmacokinetics/dynamics of citalopram between adolescents and adults: implications for clinical dosing, in Proceedings of the 39th Annual Meeting of the American College of Neuropsychopharmacology, San Juan, Puerto Rico, December 2000b, p 122

Axelson D, Findling RL, Fristad MA, et al: Examining the proposed disruptive mood dysregulation disorder diagnosis in children in the Longitudinal Assessment of Manic Symptoms study. J Clin Psychiatry 73(10):1342–1350, 2012 23140653

Bauer M, Bschor T, Kunz D, et al: Double-blind, placebo-controlled trial of the use of lithium to augment antidepressant medication in continuation treatment of unipolar major depression. Am J Psychiatry 157(9):1429–1435, 2000 10964859

Baumer FM, Howe M, Gallelli K, et al: A pilot study of antidepressant-induced mania in pediatric bipolar disorder: characteristics, risk factors, and the serotonin transporter gene. Biol Psychiatry 60(9):1005–1012, 2006 16945343

Beck AT: Depression: Clinical, Experimental and Theoretical Aspects. New York, Harper and Row, 1967

Benarous X, Consoli A, Guilé JM, et al: Evidence-based treatments for youths with severely dysregulated mood: a qualitative systematic review of trials for SMD and DMDD. Eur Child Adolesc Psychiatry 26(1):5–23, 2017 27662894

Berard R, Fong R, Carpenter DJ, et al: An international, multicenter, placebo-controlled trial of paroxetine in adolescents with major depressive disorder. J Child Adolesc Psychopharmacol 16(1–2):59–75, 2006 16553529

Bildik T, et al: Effectiveness and tolerability of aripiprazole in a real-world outpatient population of youth. Klinik Psikofarmakol Bulteni 22(3):225–234, 2012

Birmaher B: Remission of a mother's depression is associated with her child's mental health. Am J Psychiatry 168(6):563–565, 2011 21642476

Birmaher B, Ryan ND, Williamson DE, et al: Childhood and adolescent depression: a review of the past 10 years part I. J Am Acad Child Adolesc Psychiatry 35(11):1427–1439, 1996a 8936909

Birmaher B, Ryan ND, Williamson DE, et al: Childhood and adolescent depression: a review of the past 10 years part II. J Am Acad Child Adolesc Psychiatry 35(12):1575–1583, 1996b 8973063

Birmaher B, Brent DA, Kolko D, et al: Clinical outcome after short-term psychotherapy for adolescents with major depressive disorder. Arch Gen Psychiatry 57(1):29–36, 2000 10632230

Birmaher B, Arbelaez C, Brent D: Course and outcome of child and adolescent major depressive disorder. Child Adolesc Psychiatr Clin N Am 11(3):619–637, 2002 12222086

Birmaher B, Axelson DA, Monk K, et al: Fluoxetine for the treatment of childhood anxiety disorders. J Am Acad Child Adolesc Psychiatry 42(4):415–423, 2003 12649628

Birmaher B, Brent D, Bernet W, et al: Practice parameter for the assessment and treatment of children and adolescents with depressive disorders. J Am Acad Child Adolesc Psychiatry 46(11):1503–1526, 2007 18049300

Boyer EW, Shannon M: The serotonin syndrome. N Engl J Med 352(11):1112–1120, 2005 15784664

Brent DA: Antidepressants and pediatric depression: the risk of doing nothing. N Engl J Med 351(16):1598–1601, 2004 15483276

Brent DA, Poling K, McKain B, Baugher M: A psychoeducational program for families of affectively ill children and adolescents. J Am Acad Child Adolesc Psychiatry 32(4):770–774, 1993 8340297

Brent DA, Holder D, Kolko D, et al: A clinical psychotherapy trial for adolescent depression comparing cognitive, family, and supportive therapy. Arch Gen Psychiatry 54(9):877–885, 1997 9294380

Brent DA, Kolko DJ, Birmaher B, et al: Predictors of treatment efficacy in a clinical trial of three psychosocial treatments for adolescent depression. J Am Acad Child Adolesc Psychiatry 37(9):906–914, 1998 9735610

Brent DA, Kolko DJ, Birmaher B, et al: A clinical trial for adolescent depression: predictors of additional treatment in the acute and follow-up phases of the trial. J Am Acad Child Adolesc Psychiatry 38(3):263–270, discussion 270–271, 1999 10087687

Brent D, Emslie G, Clarke G, et al: Switching to another SSRI or to venlafaxine with or without cognitive behavioral therapy for adolescents with SSRI-resistant depression: the TORDIA randomized controlled trial. JAMA 299(8):901–913, 2008 18314433

Brent DA, Emslie GJ, Clarke GN, et al: Predictors of spontaneous and systematically assessed suicidal adverse events in the treatment of SSRI-resistant depression in adolescents (TORDIA) study. Am J Psychiatry 166(4):418–426, 2009 19223438

Bridge JA, Iyengar S, Salary CB, et al: Clinical response and risk for reported suicidal ideation and suicide attempts in pediatric antidepressant treatment: a meta-analysis of randomized controlled trials. JAMA 297(15):1683–1696, 2007 17440145

Bridge JA, Birmaher B, Iyengar S, et al: Placebo response in randomized controlled trials of antidepressants for pediatric major depressive disorder. Am J Psychiatry 166(1):42–49, 2009 19047322

Cheung AH, Emslie GJ, Mayes TL: Review of the efficacy and safety of antidepressants in youth depression. J Child Psychol Psychiatry 46(7):735–754, 2005 15972068

Clarke G, Debar L, Lynch F, et al: A randomized effectiveness trial of brief cognitive-behavioral therapy for depressed adolescents receiving antidepressant medication. J Am Acad Child Adolesc Psychiatry 44(9):888–898, 2005 16113617

Clein PD, Riddle MA: Pharmacokinetics in children and adolescents. Child Adolesc Psychiatr Clin N Am 4:59–75, 1995

Conners CK, Casat CD, Gualtieri CT, et al: Bupropion hydrochloride in attention deficit disorder with hyperactivity. J Am Acad Child Adolesc Psychiatry 35(10):1314–1321, 1996 8885585

Copeland WE, Shanahan L, Egger H, et al: Adult diagnostic and functional outcomes of DSM-5 disruptive mood dysregulation disorder. Am J Psychiatry 171(6):668–674, 2014 24781389

Cullen KR, Padilla LE, Papke VN, Klimes-Dougan B: New somatic treatments for child and adolescent depression. Curr Treat Options Psychiatry 6(4):380–400, 2019 33312841

Daviss WB, Bentivoglio P, Racusin R, et al: Bupropion sustained release in adolescents with comorbid attention-deficit/hyperactivity disorder and depression. J Am Acad Child Adolesc Psychiatry 40(3):307–314, 2001 11288772

Daviss WB, Perel JM, Rudolph GR, et al: Steady-state pharmacokinetics of bupropion SR in juvenile patients. J Am Acad Child Adolesc Psychiatry 44(4):349–357, 2005 15782082

DelBello MP, Hochadel TJ, Portland KB, et al: A double-blind, placebo-controlled study of selegiline transdermal system in depressed adolescents. J Child Adolesc Psychopharmacol 24(6):311–317, 2014 24955812

DelBello MP, Goldman R, Phillips D, et al: Efficacy and safety of lurasidone in children and adolescents with bipolar I depression: a double-blind, placebo-controlled study. J Am Acad Child Adolesc Psychiatry 56(12):1015–1025, 2017 29173735

Depression Guideline Panel: Depression in Primary Care, Vol 2: Treatment of Major Depression (Clinical Practice Guideline No 5). AHCPR Publication No 93-0551. Rockville, MD, Agency for Health Care Policy and Research, Public Health Service, U.S. Department of Health and Human Services, April 1993

Diler RS, Goldstein TR, Hafeman D, et al: Distinguishing bipolar depression from unipolar depression in youth: preliminary findings. J Child Adolesc Psychopharmacol 27(4):310–319, 2017 28398819

Donnelly CL, Wagner KD, Rynn M, et al: Sertraline in children and adolescents with major depressive disorder. J Am Acad Child Adolesc Psychiatry 45(10):1162–1170, 2006 17003661

Dugas M, Mouren MC, Halfon O, Moron P: Treatment of childhood and adolescent depression with mianserin. Acta Psychiatr Scand Suppl 320:48–53, 1985 3863468

Durgam S, Chen C, Migliore R, et al: A phase 3, double-blind, randomized, placebo-controlled study of vilazodone in adolescents with major depressive disorder. Paediatr Drugs 20(4):353–363, 2018 29633166

Emslie GJ, Rush AJ, Weinberg WA, et al: A double-blind, randomized, placebo-controlled trial of fluoxetine in children and adolescents with depression. Arch Gen Psychiatry 54(11):1031–1037, 1997 9366660

Emslie GJ, Walkup JT, Pliszka SR, Ernst M: Nontricyclic antidepressants: current trends in children and adolescents. J Am Acad Child Adolesc Psychiatry 38(5):517–528, 1999 10230183

Emslie GJ, Heiligenstein JH, Wagner KD, et al: Fluoxetine for acute treatment of depression in children and adolescents: a placebo-controlled, randomized clinical trial. J Am Acad Child Adolesc Psychiatry 41(10):1205–1215, 2002 12364842

Emslie GJ, Wagner KD, Kutcher S, et al: Paroxetine treatment in children and adolescents with major depressive disorder: a randomized, multicenter, double-blind, placebo-controlled trial. J Am Acad Child Adolesc Psychiatry 45(6):709–719, 2006 16721321

Emslie GJ, Findling RL, Yeung PP, et al: Venlafaxine ER for the treatment of pediatric subjects with depression: results of two placebo-controlled trials. J Am Acad Child Adolesc Psychiatry 46(4):479–488, 2007 17420682

Emslie GJ, Kennard BD, Mayes TL, et al: Fluoxetine versus placebo in preventing relapse of major depression in children and adolescents. Am J Psychiatry 165(4):459–467, 2008 18281410

Emslie GJ, Ventura D, Korotzer A, Tourkodimitris S: Escitalopram in the treatment of adolescent depression: a randomized placebo-controlled multisite trial. J Am Acad Child Adolesc Psychiatry 48(7):721–729, 2009 19465881

Emslie GJ, Mayes T, Porta G, et al: Treatment of Resistant Depression in Adolescents (TORDIA): week 24 outcomes. Am J Psychiatry 167(7):782–791, 2010 20478877

Emslie GJ, Prakash A, Zhang Q, et al: A double-blind efficacy and safety study of duloxetine fixed doses in children and adolescents with major depressive disorder. J Child Adolesc Psychopharmacol 24(4):170–179, 2014 24815533

Findling RL, Reed MD, Myers C, et al: Paroxetine pharmacokinetics in depressed children and adolescents. J Am Acad Child Adolesc Psychiatry 38(8):952–959, 1999 10434486

Findling RL, Preskorn SH, Marcus RN, et al: Nefazodone pharmacokinetics in depressed children and adolescents. J Am Acad Child Adolesc Psychiatry 39(8):1008–1016, 2000 10939229

Findling RL, McNamara NK, Stansbrey RJ, et al: The relevance of pharmacokinetic studies in designing efficacy trials in juvenile major depression. J Child Adolesc Psychopharmacol 16(1–2):131–145, 2006 16553534

Findling RL, Groark J, Chiles D, et al: Safety and tolerability of desvenlafaxine in children and adolescents with major depressive disorder. J Child Adolesc Psychopharmacol 24(4):201–209, 2014 24611442

Findling RL, DelBello MP, Zuddas A, et al: Vortioxetine for major depressive disorder in adolescents: 12-week randomized, placebo-controlled, fluoxetine-referenced, fixed-dose study. J Am Acad Child Adolesc Psychiatry 61(9):1106–1118, 2022 35033635

Geddes JR, Calabrese JR, Goodwin GM: Lamotrigine for treatment of bipolar depression: independent meta-analysis and meta-regression of individual patient data from five randomised trials. Br J Psychiatry 194(1):4–9, 2009 19118318

Geller B, Fox LW, Clark KA: Rate and predictors of prepubertal bipolarity during follow-up of 6- to 12-year-old depressed children. J Am Acad Child Adolesc Psychiatry 33(4):461–468, 1994 8005898

Ghaziuddin N, Kutcher SP, Knapp P, et al: Practice parameter for use of electroconvulsive therapy with adolescents. J Am Acad Child Adolesc Psychiatry 43(12):1521–1539, 2004 15564821

Gibbons RD, Hur K, Bhaumik DK, Mann JJ: The relationship between antidepressant medication use and rate of suicide. Arch Gen Psychiatry 62(2):165–172, 2005 15699293

Gijsman HJ, Geddes JR, Rendell JM, et al: Antidepressants for bipolar depression: a systematic review of randomized, controlled trials. Am J Psychiatry 161(9):1537–1547, 2004 15337640

Goldsmith M, Singh M, Chang K: Antidepressants and psychostimulants in pediatric populations: is there an association with mania? Paediatr Drugs 13(4):225–243, 2011 21692547

Goodyer IM, Herbert J, Secher SM, Pearson J: Short-term outcome of major depression I: comorbidity and severity at presentation as predictors of persistent disorder. J Am Acad Child Adolesc Psychiatry 36(2):179–187, 1997 9031570

Goodyer IM, Herbert J, Altham PM: Adrenal steroid secretion and major depression in 8- to 16-year-olds, III: influence of cortisol/DHEA ratio at presentation on subsequent rates of disappointing life events and persistent major depression. Psychol Med 28(2):265–273, 1998 9572084

Goodyer I, Dubicka B, Wilkinson P, et al: Selective serotonin reuptake inhibitors (SSRIs) and routine specialist care with and without cognitive behaviour therapy in adolescents with major depression: randomised controlled trial. BMJ 335(7611):142, 2007 17556431

Gould MS, Fisher P, Parides M, et al: Psychosocial risk factors of child and adolescent completed suicide. Arch Gen Psychiatry 53(12):1155–1162, 1996 8956682

Graovac M: The therapeutic effects of tianeptine on adolescents. Eur Psychiatry 24(Suppl 1):1, 2009

Guy W: Clinical global impressions, in ECDEU Assessment Manual for Psychopharmacology, Revised (NIMH Publ No 76-338). Rockville, MD, National Institute of Mental Health, 1976, pp 218–222

Hamilton JD, Bridge J: Outcome at 6 months for 50 adolescents with major depression treated in a health maintenance organization. J Am Acad Child Adolesc Psychiatry 38(11):1340–1346, 1999 10560219

Hamilton M: A rating scale for depression. J Neurol Neurosurg Psychiatry 23:56–62, 1960 14399272

Hammad TA, Laughren T, Racoosin J: Suicidality in pediatric patients treated with antidepressant drugs. Arch Gen Psychiatry 63(3):332–339, 2006 16520440

Hayward C, Killen JD, Kraemer HC, Taylor CB: Predictors of panic attacks in adolescents. J Am Acad Child Adolesc Psychiatry 39(2):207–214, 2000 10673832

Hazell P, O'Connell D, Heathcote D, Henry D: Tricyclic drugs for depression in children and adolescents. Cochrane Database Syst Rev (2):CD002317, 2002 12076448

Heiligenstein JH, Hoog SL, Wagner KD, et al: Fluoxetine 40–60 mg versus fluoxetine 20 mg in the treatment of children and adolescents with a less-than-complete response to nine-week treatment with fluoxetine 10–20 mg: a pilot study. J Child Adolesc Psychopharmacol 16(1–2):207–217, 2006 16553541

Hirschfeld RMA: Guideline watch (November 2005): Practice Guideline for the Treatment of Patients With Bipolar Disorder, 2nd Edition. Focus 5(1):34–39, 2007

Hughes CW, Emslie GJ, Crismon ML, et al: The Texas Children's Medication Algorithm Project: report of the Texas Consensus Conference Panel on Medication Treatment of Childhood Major Depressive Disorder. J Am Acad Child Adolesc Psychiatry 38(11):1442–1454, 1999 10560232

James-Palmer A, Anderson EZ, Zucker L, et al: Yoga as an intervention for the reduction of symptoms of anxiety and depression in children and adolescents: a systematic review. Front Pediatr 8:78, 2020 32232017

Katz LY, Kozyrskyj AL, Prior HJ, et al: Effect of regulatory warnings on antidepressant prescription rates, use of health services and outcomes among children, adolescents and young adults. CMAJ 178(8):1005–1011, 2008 18390943

Keller MB, McCullough JP, Klein DN, et al: A comparison of nefazodone, the cognitive behavioral-analysis system of psychotherapy, and their combination for the treatment of chronic depression. N Engl J Med 342(20):1462–1470, 2000 10816183

Keller MB, Ryan ND, Strober M, et al: Efficacy of paroxetine in the treatment of adolescent major depression: a randomized, controlled trial. J Am Acad Child Adolesc Psychiatry 40(7):762–772, 2001 11437014

Kendall PC: Treating anxiety disorders in children: results of a randomized clinical trial. J Consult Clin Psychol 62(1):100–110, 1994 8034812

Kennard BD, Silva SG, Mayes TL, et al; TADS: Assessment of safety and long-term outcomes of initial treatment with placebo in TADS. Am J Psychiatry 166(3):337–344, 2009a 19147693

Kennard BD, Silva SG, Tonev S, et al: Remission and recovery in the Treatment for Adolescents with Depression Study (TADS): acute and long-term outcomes. J Am Acad Child Adolesc Psychiatry 48(2):186–195, 2009b 19127172

Kennard BD, Emslie GJ, Mayes TL, et al: Sequential treatment with fluoxetine and relapse: prevention CBT to improve outcomes in pediatric depression. Am J Psychiatry 171(10):1083–1090, 2014 24935082

Kennedy SH, Lam RW, McIntyre RS, et al: Canadian Network for Mood and Anxiety Treatments (CANMAT) 2016 clinical guidelines for the management of adults with major depressive disorder: section 3. Pharmacological treatments. Can J Psychiatry 61(9):540–560, 2016

Kim SM, Han DH, Lee YS, Renshaw PF: Combined cognitive behavioral therapy and bupropion for the treatment of problematic on-line game play in adolescents with major depressive disorder. Comput Human Behav 28(5):1954–1959, 2012

Kim S, Rush BS, Rice TR: A systematic review of therapeutic ketamine use in children and adolescents with treatment-resistant mood disorders. Eur Child Adolesc Psychiatry 30(10):1485–1501, 2021 32385697

Klein DN, Lewinsohn PM, Seeley JR, Rohde P: A family study of major depressive disorder in a community sample of adolescents. Arch Gen Psychiatry 58(1):13–20, 2001 11146753

Kovacs M, Goldston D: Cognitive and social cognitive development of depressed children and adolescents. J Am Acad Child Adolesc Psychiatry 30(3):388–392, 1991 1711524

Kovacs M, Gatsonis C, Paulauskas SL, Richards C: Depressive disorders in childhood IV: a longitudinal study of comorbidity with and risk for anxiety disorders. Arch Gen Psychiatry 46(9):776–782, 1989 2774847

Lake MB, Birmaher B, Wassick S, et al: Bleeding and selective serotonin reuptake inhibitors in childhood and adolescence. J Child Adolesc Psychopharmacol 10(1):35–38, 2000 10755580

Leibenluft E: Severe mood dysregulation, irritability, and the diagnostic boundaries of bipolar disorder in youths. Am J Psychiatry 168(2):129–142, 2011 21123313

Leonard HL, March J, Rickler KC, Allen AJ: Pharmacology of the selective serotonin reuptake inhibitors in children and adolescents. J Am Acad Child Adolesc Psychiatry 36(6):725–736, 1997 9183126

Lewinsohn PM, Allen NB, Seeley JR, Gotlib IH: First onset versus recurrence of depression: differential processes of psychosocial risk. J Abnorm Psychol 108(3):483–489, 1999 10466272

Libby AM, Orton HD, Valuck RJ: Persisting decline in depression treatment after FDA warnings. Arch Gen Psychiatry 66(6):633–639, 2009 19487628

Mandoki MW, Tapia MR, Tapia MA, et al: Venlafaxine in the treatment of children and adolescents with major depression. Psychopharmacol Bull 33(1):149–154, 1997 9133767

Mann JJ, Emslie G, Baldessarini RJ, et al: ACNP Task Force report on SSRIs and suicidal behavior in youth. Neuropsychopharmacology 31(3):473–492, 2006 16319919

Marcantoni WS, Akoumba BS, Wassef M, et al: A systematic review and meta-analysis of the efficacy of intravenous ketamine infusion for treatment resistant depression: January 2009–January 2019. J Affect Disord 277:831–841, 2020 33065824

March J, Silva S, Petrycki S, et al: Fluoxetine, cognitive-behavioral therapy, and their combination for adolescents with depression: Treatment for Adolescents With Depression Study (TADS) randomized controlled trial. JAMA 292(7):807–820, 2004 15315995

Martin A, Young C, Leckman JF, et al: Age effects on antidepressant-induced manic conversion. Arch Pediatr Adolesc Med 158(8):773–780, 2004 15289250

Mufson L, Dorta KP, Wickramaratne P, et al: A randomized effectiveness trial of interpersonal psychotherapy for depressed adolescents. Arch Gen Psychiatry 61(6):577–584, 2004 15184237

Olfson M, Shaffer D, Marcus SC, Greenberg T: Relationship between antidepressant medication treatment and suicide in adolescents. Arch Gen Psychiatry 60(10):978–982, 2003 14557142

Pathak S, Johns ES, Kowatch RA: Adjunctive quetiapine for treatment-resistant adolescent major depressive disorder: a case series. J Child Adolesc Psychopharmacol 15(4):696–702, 2005 16190801

Pilowsky DJ, Wickramaratne P, Poh E, et al: Psychopathology and functioning among children of treated depressed fathers and mothers. J Affect Disord 164:107–111, 2014 24856562

Pine DS, Cohen P, Gurley D, et al: The risk for early adulthood anxiety and depressive disorders in adolescents with anxiety and depressive disorders. Arch Gen Psychiatry 55(1):56–64, 1998 9435761

Pliszka SR: Patterns of psychiatric comorbidity with attention-deficit/hyperactivity disorder. Child Adolesc Psychiatr Clin N Am 9(3):525–540, vii, 2000

Poirier MF, Boyer P: Venlafaxine and paroxetine in treatment-resistant depression: double-blind, randomised comparison. Br J Psychiatry 175:12–16, 1999 10621762

Poznanski EO, Freeman LN, Mokros HB: Children's Depression Rating Scale–Revised. Psychopharmacol Bull 21:979–989, 1985

Puig-Antich J, Lukens E, Davies M, et al: Psychosocial functioning in prepubertal major depressive disorders. II. Interpersonal relationships after sustained recovery from affective episode. Arch Gen Psychiatry 42(5):511–517, 1985 3985761

Rao U, Ryan ND, Birmaher B, et al: Unipolar depression in adolescents: clinical outcome in adulthood. J Am Acad Child Adolesc Psychiatry 34(5):566–578, 1995 7775352

Renaud J, Brent DA, Baugher M, et al: Rapid response to psychosocial treatment for adolescent depression: a two-year follow-up. J Am Acad Child Adolesc Psychiatry 37(11):1184–1190, 1998 9808930

Rengasamy M, Birmaher B: Bipolar II disorder in childhood and adolescence, in Bipolar II Disorder: Recognition, Understanding, and Treatment. Edited by Swartz HA, Suppes T. Washington, DC, American Psychiatric Association Publishing, 2019, pp 241–262

Research Unit on Pediatric Psychopharmacology Anxiety Study Group: Fluvoxamine for the treatment of anxiety disorders in children and adolescents. N Engl J Med 344(17):1279–1285, 2001 11323729

Rowe R, Costello EJ, Angold A, et al: Developmental pathways in oppositional defiant disorder and conduct disorder. J Abnorm Psychol 119(4):726–738, 2010 21090876

Ryan ND, Meyer V, Dachille S, et al: Lithium antidepressant augmentation in TCA-refractory depression in adolescents. J Am Acad Child Adolesc Psychiatry 27(3):371–376, 1988a 3379022

Ryan ND, Puig-Antich J, Rabinovich H, et al: MAOIs in adolescent major depression unresponsive to tricyclic antidepressants. J Am Acad Child Adolesc Psychiatry 27(6):755–758, 1988b 3198564

Safer DJ, Zito JM: Treatment-emergent adverse events from selective serotonin reuptake inhibitors by age group: children versus adolescents. J Child Adolesc Psychopharmacol 16(1–2):159–169, 2006 16553536

Sallee FR, Vrindavanam NS, Deas-Nesmith D, et al: Pulse intravenous clomipramine for depressed adolescents: double-blind, controlled trial. Am J Psychiatry 154(5):668–673, 1997 9137123

Shaffer D, Craft L: Methods of adolescent suicide prevention. J Clin Psychiatry 60(Suppl):70–74, discussion 75–76, 113–116, 1999

Shaffer D, Gould MS, Brasic J, et al: A Children's Global Assessment Scale (CGAS). Arch Gen Psychiatry 40(11):1228–1231, 1983 6639293

Simeon JG, Dinicola VF, Ferguson HB, Copping W: Adolescent depression: a placebo-controlled fluoxetine treatment study and follow-up. Prog Neuropsychopharmacol Biol Psychiatry 14(5):791–795, 1990 2293257

Simon GE, Savarino J, Operskalski B, Wang PS: Suicide risk during antidepressant treatment. Am J Psychiatry 163(1):41–47, 2006 16390887

Spirito A, Esposito-Smythers C, Wolff J, Uhl K: Cognitive-behavioral therapy for adolescent depression and suicidality. Child Adolesc Psychiatr Clin N Am 20(2):191–204, 2011 21440850

Stein D, Williamson DE, Birmaher B, et al: Parent-child bonding and family functioning in depressed children and children at high risk and low risk for future depression. J Am Acad Child Adolesc Psychiatry 39(11):1387–1395, 2000 11068894

Stringaris A, Cohen P, Pine DS, Leibenluft E: Adult outcomes of youth irritability: a 20-year prospective community-based study. Am J Psychiatry 166(9):1048–1054, 2009 19570932

Strober M, Carlson G: Bipolar illness in adolescents with major depression: clinical, genetic, and psychopharmacologic predictors in a three- to four-year prospective follow-up investigation. Arch Gen Psychiatry 39(5):549–555, 1982 7092488

Strober M, Freeman R, Rigali J, et al: The pharmacotherapy of depressive illness in adolescence II: effects of lithium augmentation in nonresponders to imipramine. J Am Acad Child Adolesc Psychiatry 31(1):16–20, 1992 1537769

Strober M, Lampert C, Schmidt S, Morrell W: The course of major depressive disorder in adolescents I: recovery and risk of manic switching in a follow-up of psychotic and nonpsychotic subtypes. J Am Acad Child Adolesc Psychiatry 32(1):34–42, 1993 8428882

Swedo SE, Allen AJ, Glod CA, et al: A controlled trial of light therapy for the treatment of pediatric seasonal affective disorder. J Am Acad Child Adolesc Psychiatry 36(6):816–821, 1997 9183137

Thase ME, Rush AJ: When at first you don't succeed: sequential strategies for antidepressant nonresponders. J Clin Psychiatry 58(Suppl 13):23–29, 1997 9402916

Toren P, Goldstein G, Ben-Amitay G, et al: Reboxetine: a randomized controlled open-label study in children and adolescents with major depression. Isr J Psychiatry Relat Sci 56(1):26–33, 2019

Towbin K, Vidal-Ribas P, Brotman MA, et al: A double-blind randomized placebo-controlled trial of citalopram adjunctive to stimulant medication in youth with chronic severe irritability. J Am Acad Child Adolesc Psychiatry 59(3):350–361, 2020 31128268

Valuck RJ, Libby AM, Sills MR, et al: Antidepressant treatment and risk of suicide attempt by adolescents with major depressive disorder: a propensity-adjusted retrospective cohort study. CNS Drugs 18(15):1119–1132, 2004 15581382

Vieta E, Locklear J, Günther O, et al: Treatment options for bipolar depression: a systematic review of randomized, controlled trials. J Clin Psychopharmacol 30(5):579–590, 2010 20814319

Vitiello B, Emslie G, Clarke G, et al: Long-term outcome of adolescent depression initially resistant to selective serotonin reuptake inhibitor treatment: a follow-up study of the TORDIA sample. J Clin Psychiatry 72(3):388–396, 2011 21208583

von Knorring AL, Olsson GI, Thomsen PH, et al: A randomized, double-blind, placebo-controlled study of citalopram in adolescents with major depressive disorder. J Clin Psychopharmacol 26(3):311–315, 2006 16702897

Wagner KD, Ambrosini P, Rynn M, et al: Efficacy of sertraline in the treatment of children and adolescents with major depressive disorder: two randomized controlled trials. JAMA 290(8):1033–1041, 2003 12941675

Wagner KD, Robb AS, Findling RL, et al: A randomized, placebo-controlled trial of citalopram for the treatment of major depression in children and adolescents. Am J Psychiatry 161(6):1079–1083, 2004 15169696

Wagner KD, Jonas J, Findling RL, et al: A double-blind, randomized, placebo-controlled trial of escitalopram in the treatment of pediatric depression. J Am Acad Child Adolesc Psychiatry 45(3):280–288, 2006 16540812

Wegner M, Amatriain-Fernández S, Kaulitzky A, et al: Systematic review of meta-analyses: exercise effects on depression in children and adolescents. Front Psychiatry 11:81, 2020 32210847

Weihs KL, Murphy W, Abbas R, et al: Desvenlafaxine versus placebo in a fluoxetine-referenced study of children and adolescents with major depressive disorder. J Child Adolesc Psychopharmacol 28(1):36–46, 2018 29189044

Wilens TE, Wyatt D, Spencer TJ: Disentangling disinhibition. J Am Acad Child Adolesc Psychiatry 37(11):1225–1227, 1998 9808935

Zheng W, Cai DB, Xiang YQ, et al: Adjunctive intranasal esketamine for major depressive disorder: a systematic review of randomized double-blind controlled-placebo studies. J Affect Disord 265:63–70, 2020 31957693

6

Bipolar Disorders

Tiffany Thomas-Lakia, M.D.
Baris Olten, M.D.
Robert L. Findling, M.D., M.B.A.

Research over the past 20 years has helped better define the phenomenology and course of bipolar disorder in children and adolescents. Pediatric bipolar disorder (PBD) has been shown to have a chronic course with high rates of subsyndromal and syndromal episodes, as well as little interepisode recovery, and therefore can lead to substantive psychosocial dysfunction (Biederman et al. 2004; Birmaher et al. 2009; Findling et al. 2001; Geller et al. 2004). For these reasons, effective treatments are needed for youth with PBD. The purpose of this chapter is to present a rational, practical, and common-sense approach to the pharmacotherapeutic management of bipolar disorder in children and adolescents.

Pharmacotherapy guidelines and practice parameters for treating PBD have been published (Kowatch et al. 2005; McClellan et al. 2007), with more recent studies in children and adolescents providing clinicians with additional valuable information on the treatment of PBD. Briefly, the use of lithium or one of several atypical antipsychotics as monotherapy is suggested in the initial treatment of manic or mixed bipolar presentations in outpatients without psychosis. Partial response to monotherapy with a given agent should be addressed by adding another drug from a different class of compounds to the preexisting pharmacological regimen. A rational approach to patients whose symptoms do not respond at all to a given agent might be to treat the youth with a medication from a different drug class.

In this chapter, we review medications that have been studied in the treatment of pediatric bipolar illness and summarize the extant evidence for the treatment of acute manic or mixed states, maintenance therapy, bipolar depression, and combination pharmacotherapy.

Treatment of Acute Manic or Mixed States

Lithium

Our focus in this section is on lithium monotherapy for the treatment of manic/mixed states. The use of lithium in bipolar depression and as part of combination therapy is described further in the sections "Treatment of Pediatric Bipolar Depression" and "Combination Pharmacotherapy."

Lithium was the first medication approved by the FDA for use in treating bipolar disorder in children and adolescents ages 12 years or older. In 2006, the Collaborative Lithium Trials (CoLT) group began definitive testing of lithium in juvenile mania under the auspices of a National Institute of Child Health and Human Development contract. These innovative studies provided data to inform the labeling of lithium for children and adolescents with bipolar disorder. The CoLT trials provided definitive data on 1) evidence-based dosing strategies for lithium, 2) pharmacokinetic and biodisposition of lithium in pediatric patients, 3) acute efficacy of lithium in pediatric bipolar illness, 4) long-term effectiveness of lithium treatment, and 5) short- and long-term safety of lithium (Findling et al. 2008, 2013c). Based on this extensive work, lithium is now an FDA-approved treatment for acute manic and mixed episodes and a maintenance treatment for patients age 7 years or older with bipolar I disorder.

Supporting Studies in Youth

The published literature on lithium provides evidence to suggest that lithium is both effective and reasonably well tolerated in the treatment of PBD. Under the auspices of CoLT, Findling et al. (2015c) performed an 8-week randomized, double-blind, placebo-controlled study of youth ages 7–17 years and found lithium to be superior to placebo in reducing manic symptoms. Other trials have found lithium combined with divalproex or antipsychotics to be useful as well (Findling et al. 2003; Kafantaris et al. 2003). However, in head-to-head studies comparing lithium with divalproex or risperidone in youth, both divalproex and risperidone demonstrated superiority over lithium for acute mania (Geller et al. 2012; Kowatch et al. 2007).

In summary, although lithium can be a complicated medication to use, and perhaps has a more modest acute response than antipsychotics in the treatment of mania, compelling evidence supports its effectiveness.

Formulations

Lithium is available in tablet, liquid, and long-acting formulations. Lithium carbonate is perhaps the most widely used formulation and comes in generic tablets at strengths of 150 mg, 300 mg, and 600 mg. Lithobid, a sustained-release preparation in film-coated dissolving tablets, is available in 300-mg strength. A generic version of extended-release lithium carbonate is also available in 300- and 450-mg strengths. Lithium citrate is an oral solution of lithium with a concentration of 300 mg/tsp (8 mEq/5 mL).

Preliminary Evaluation

Prior to initiating any medication regimen, clinicians should give thoughtful consideration to the target symptoms and their severity, anticipated barriers to medication adherence, and their patient's ability to swallow pills. Before lithium treatment is initiated, a careful medical history should be obtained. Particular attention should be paid to reviewing organ systems known to be affected by lithium administration, including the renal, endocrine, neurological, and cardiovascular systems. Given that lithium is known to be a teratogen, increasing the likelihood of Ebstein's anomaly, especially during the first trimester of pregnancy, a pregnancy test should be completed for females of childbearing potential prior to initiating treatment.

Table 6–1. FDA-recommended lithium dosing for bipolar I disorder

Patient group	Adult and pediatric patients weighing >30 kg	Pediatric patients weighing 20–30 kg
Formulation	Tablets	Tablets
Starting dosage, *mg*	300 tid	300 bid
Dosage titration, *mg*	300 every 3 days	300 weekly
Acute goal		
Serum level, *mEq/L*	0.8–1.2	0.8–1.2
Usual dosage, *mg*	600 bid to tid	600–1,500 in divided doses daily
Maintenance goal		
Serum level, *mEq/L*	0.8–1.0	0.8–1.0
Usual dosage, *mg*	300–600 bid to tid	600–1,200 in divided doses daily

Discussion with females of childbearing potential should also be considered both before and throughout treatment to assess whether these patients are sexually active or intend to become pregnant. Baseline laboratory work, including blood urea nitrogen (BUN)/creatinine, electrolytes, and thyrotropin (thyroid-stimulating hormone [TSH]), should be obtained to evaluate for the possibility of any preexisting renal impairment, electrolyte imbalances, or hypothyroidism that may lead the clinician to eschew prescribing lithium to the patient. We also recommend obtaining a pretreatment electrocardiogram (ECG) for each patient to rule out any cardiac conduction abnormalities.

Medication Dosing

We advise that the FDA-recommended dosing guidelines be followed for the administration of immediate-release lithium in children and adolescents with bipolar I disorder (Table 6–1).

Findling et al. (2010) investigated the first-dose pharmacokinetics of oral lithium carbonate in children and adolescents ages 7–17 years after administration of immediate-release capsules of 600 mg or 900 mg. Lithium plasma concentrations were followed over 48–72 hours in 39 subjects. Lithium clearances did not vary systematically with age, dose, sex, or creatinine clearances. Allometrically scaled clearance and volume of distribution from the population analysis were within the range reported in adults. Single-dose profiles of lithium in these young patients did show marked variability. This finding indicates that ongoing serum monitoring is needed during continued lithium therapy. Serum levels at the higher end of this therapeutic range appear to be associated with better symptom amelioration but also with greater side effects.

The FDA recommends obtaining serum lithium concentration assays 3 days after medication initiation. For immediate-release formulations, the level should be drawn 12 hours after the last dose and regularly until the patient is stabilized. For sustained-release formulations, a trough level should be obtained prior to the next dose. When the lithium dosage is stable, we recommend that screening laboratory work be repeated. Subsequently, lithium levels, calcium levels, TSH, and renal function (BUN/creatinine or creatinine clearance) should be evaluated every 2–3 months or more frequently if necessary.

In addition to regular monitoring of serum lithium levels, the FDA recommends that levels be reassessed any time there is a change in dosage, an addition or change in dosage of a concurrent medication, or a marked change in strenuous physical activity or in the event of a concomitant disease or illness.

Side Effects

Adverse effects from lithium are common and involve the CNS and the renal, dermatological, endocrine, and gastrointestinal systems (Table 6–2). While side effects during lithium treatment are common, they generally do not lead to lithium discontinuation. It appears that gastrointestinal symptoms (e.g., stomachache, nausea, vomiting, and diarrhea) are the most common side effects noted. Often, gastrointestinal side effects can be addressed by recommending that the patient take lithium with food, dividing the doses more frequently throughout the course of the day, or administering lithium in the liquid citrate formulation. Persistent nausea, vomiting, and diarrhea (as well as other side effects noted later) may all signal the presence of lithium toxicity; for this reason, careful inquiry and reassessment of serum lithium levels should be considered for patients presenting with these concerns. If the lithium level is indeed high, lithium doses may be stopped for 24 hours while the level is rechecked and reinitiation at a lower dosage is considered.

Table 6–2. Management of common lithium side effects

System	Side effect	Suggested intervention
Gastrointestinal	Nausea, emesis, diarrhea	Reduce dosage or split dose.
		Take with food.
		Change to citrate formulation.
CNS	Tremor, ataxia, slowed mentation	Reduce dosage or split dose.
Renal	Polyuria, changes in renal function	Allow for bathroom breaks.
		Monitor kidney function every 3 months.
Dermatological	Acne, rash	Educate patient/family about side effects.
Endocrine	Weight gain, thyroid abnormalities.	Educate patient/family about appropriate diet and exercise.
		Monitor thyroid function every 3–6 months.

Other side effects appear to be less common. CNS side effects reported include tremor, ataxia, and slowed mentation. Tremor is usually mild and can be aided by dosage reduction. Although propranolol has been described as a treatment for lithium-related tremor in adults, this management strategy is not one we generally recommend for youth. Renal side effects include polyuria, polydipsia, and possible morphological changes to the kidney after long-term use. Unfortunately, insufficient data are available regarding the long-term renal effects of lithium in young patients. Dermatologically, an acne-like rash can be a troubling side effect for adolescents, and patients should be educated concerning this possibility. Rash and hair loss have been infrequently described in relation to lithium therapy. Last, endocrine side effects can include weight gain and hypothyroidism.

Drug Interactions and Cautions

Lithium is excreted by the kidney. Thus, medication interactions may occur as a result of modification of renal excretion by other agents. Concomitant use of other medications or substances may either increase or decrease lithium levels.

For example, nonsteroidal anti-inflammatory drugs (NSAIDs) can increase lithium levels by reducing renal excretion. Although the use of NSAIDs is not necessarily contraindicated for patients prescribed lithium, care should be given if NSAIDs are taken during lithium therapy, with particular attention to symptoms of lithium toxicity. Thiazide diuretics, although not commonly used in young people, may substantively increase lithium levels; theophylline and caffeine may decrease lithium levels by enhancing renal excretion. Because sodium chloride can also affect the renal excretion of lithium, excessive intake of salty snack foods or salt-repleting sports drinks can lower the lithium level. These medication interactions, dietary considerations, and adequate hydration, especially during summer months and during vigorous physical activities, should be discussed with the patient.

In summary, lithium use in PBD is supported by the literature and at present is one of the FDA-approved treatments for PBD. Although the use of lithium has substantive burdens in terms of monitoring and its side effect profile, its potential for significant benefit allows it to remain a potential agent in the treatment of PBD.

Anticonvulsants

Although anticonvulsants appear to be widely used in the treatment of PBD, no anticonvulsants have been FDA-approved for treating acute mania or as a maintenance therapy for bipolar disorder in children and adolescents. In adults, divalproex sodium, lamotrigine, and extended-release carbamazepine are approved for bipolar disorder. Carbamazepine, oxcarbazepine, divalproex sodium, lamotrigine, and topiramate have all been investigated in youth with bipolar illness. Other, newer agents such as zonisamide, levetiracetam, and tiagabine have not yet received rigorous testing in youth with bipolar disorder.

Carbamazepine

Carbamazepine was the first anticonvulsant extensively studied as a potential treatment for bipolar disorder in adults. However, carbamazepine is not commonly used in the treatment of bipolar disorder in children and adolescents. This is most likely attributable to a paucity of clinical trial data for carbamazepine use in youth, compared with lithium or divalproex sodium. Another possible contributing factor is that challenges associated with the administration of carbamazepine might complicate its use, including the possibility of medication interactions, concerns regarding aplastic anemia and agranulocytosis, and metabolic autoinduction.

Supporting studies in youth. The limited data that exist on the use of carbamazepine in PBD suggest that it may be useful in the treatment of children and adolescents. In an open-label trial comparing carbamazepine, lithium, and divalproex sodium, 5 of 13 participants (ages 6–18 years) with bipolar I or bipolar II disorder achieved a 50% reduction in manic symptoms within 6 weeks of initiating carbamazepine therapy (Kowatch et al. 2003). One prospective, 8-week, open-label trial investigated the use of extended-release carbamazepine monotherapy in 27 youth (ages 6–12 years) with bipolar disorder. Extended-release carbamazepine was initiated at 200 mg/day, and the dosage was increased by 100 mg in the first 2 weeks and by 200 mg weekly thereafter per clinician judgment based on tolerability and response. The maximum dosage used in the study was 1,200 mg/day (not to exceed 35 mg/kg body weight or serum concentrations >12 μg/mL). In this trial, extended-release carbamazepine was found to have modest antimanic effects and a somewhat better antidepressive and antipsychotic response. Although the medication was well tolerated in this trial, high dropout rates occurred, predominantly due to lack of response (Joshi et al. 2010). Another open-label trial of extended-release carbamazepine studied a total of 60 children (ages 10–12) and 97 adolescents (ages 13–17) with bipolar I disorder who were experiencing acute or manic episodes (Findling et al. 2014). The investigators concluded that extended-release carbamazepine may be an effective treatment but that more definitive studies are needed (Findling and Ginsberg 2014).

Formulations. Carbamazepine is available in several forms. Generic carbamazepine is available as 100-mg tablets and chewable tablets, 200-mg tablets, and an 100-mg/5-mL oral solution. These formulations are generally dosed three or four times daily. An extended-release form of carbamazepine (Carbatrol) is also available in capsule form in strengths of 100 mg, 200 mg, and 300 mg, which allows twice-daily dosing. The contents of a Carbatrol capsule may be sprinkled over food, such as applesauce. This form is similar to the extended-release formulation (Equetro), which is available in sprinkle capsules in strengths of 100 mg, 200 mg, and 300 mg. The tablet version of extended-release carbamazepine, Tegretol-XR, is available in strengths of 100 mg, 200 mg, and 400 mg.

Preliminary evaluation. A thorough medical history should be obtained before carbamazepine is prescribed. Particular attention should be paid to any history of hepatic dysfunction, hematological abnormalities, cardiac conduction problems, or immunological concerns. Laboratory work should include a complete blood count (CBC) with differential and platelets, electrolytes, BUN/creatinine, transaminases, and a urine pregnancy test, if applicable. Careful discussion about the teratogenic potential of carbamazepine should occur with all patients of childbearing potential, both before initiating treatment and throughout maintenance therapy. In addition, carbamazepine-induced Stevens-Johnson syndrome/toxic epidermal necrolysis is strongly associated with the *HLA-B*1502* allele, which is highly prevalent in populations with ancestry across broad areas of Asia. Patients with ancestry in genetically at-risk populations should be screened for the presence of the *HLA-B*1502* allele prior to beginning treatment with carbamazepine, and the drug should be avoided in those testing positive. Because carbamazepine can autoinduce its metabolism, blood levels should be monitored carefully and dosage adjustments made accordingly (Kudriakova et al. 1992). In addition, carbamazepine can significantly affect the metabolism of numerous other medications, so a use of concomitant medications should be fully assessed.

Medication dosing. Carbamazepine use in the child and adolescent population has been extensively studied in the pediatric neurology literature, and the following recommendations are based on those studies. In children younger than 6 years, carbamazepine should be initiated at 10–20 mg/kg/day bid or tid, and the dosage should be titrated at weekly intervals until symptom resolution or until dosage-limiting side effects develop. The maximum daily dosage in this age group is 35 mg/kg/day. As noted in the earlier section "Formulations," the carbamazepine oral solution should be administered in a three- or four-times-daily dosing regimen to minimize any side effects from the higher peak serum levels seen with this formulation. In children ages 6–12 years, carbamazepine may be initiated at a dosage of 100 mg bid and the dosage increased weekly by 100 mg, with the total daily dose not to exceed 1 g. For those older than 12 years, carbamazepine can be initiated at a dosage of 200 mg bid and the total daily dose titrated by 200 mg weekly. Adequate serum levels in individuals older than 12 years are generally achieved at dosages similar to those used in adults (800–1,200 mg/day). Of note, in the open-label study to compare carbamazepine, lithium, and divalproex sodium in children and adolescents with bipolar disorder, all of the subjects in the carbamazepine arm had the drug initiated at a dosage of 15 mg/kg/day (Kowatch et al. 2000). Joshi et al. (2010) studied extended-release carbamazepine in an open-label trial mentioned previously (see the earlier subsection "Supporting Studies in Youth"). In this study, extended-release carbamazepine was initiated at 200 mg/day, and the dosage was increased by 100 mg in the first 2 weeks and 200 mg weekly thereafter. The maximum dosage used in the study was 1,200 mg/day (not to exceed 35 mg/kg body weight or serum concentrations >12 µg/mL).

We have generally found that initiating carbamazepine at a dosage of approximately 15 mg/kg/day is reasonably well tolerated. The therapeutic serum level range is 4–12 µg/mL, with 7–10 µg/mL being a common maintenance drug level. Because autoinduction may occur during carbamazepine therapy, dosages initially found to be therapeutic may subsequently be inadequate. For this reason, careful laboratory and symptom monitoring is indicated. We recommend that drug levels, CBC with differential and platelets, and liver enzyme measurements be completed at least every other week during the first 2 months of treatment, then at least every 3 months thereafter.

Side effects. Common side effects of carbamazepine affect both the gastrointestinal system and the CNS. Nausea and sedation are commonly experienced and can often be minimized with gradual titration of treatment and divided dosing. Blurred vision and ataxia also may be noted.

Hematological, dermatological, and hepatic side effects seem to be less common. Mild leukopenia and thrombocytopenia may occur in some individuals. Rarely, some patients develop aplastic anemia or agranulocytosis. Transient skin rashes may occur. Stevens-Johnson syndrome may occur very rarely with carbamazepine use; this risk increases in individuals with the *HLA-B*1502* allele, and at-risk populations should be tested before initiating treatment, as described earlier (see "Preliminary Evaluation"). Transaminase levels may become mildly elevated with carbamazepine administration. Hyponatremia has been reported in some patients in addition to abnormal renal function. Weight gain does not appear to be a substantive problem with this medication.

Drug interactions and cautions. Carbamazepine is metabolized through the cytochrome P450 (CYP) 3A3 and CYP3A4 systems and therefore has the potential to interact with many commonly used medications. A partial listing of drugs that can *increase* carbamazepine levels includes fluoxetine, fluvoxamine, valproate, tricyclic antidepressants, prednisolone, and macrolide antibiotics (erythromycin). Use of carbamazepine may *decrease* blood levels of oral contraceptives (and possibly cause contraceptive failure), benzodiazepines, theophylline, sertraline, and neuroleptics, among other medications. Carbamazepine has been associated with fetal abnormalities when used by pregnant females during the first trimester.

In summary, data on carbamazepine's effectiveness in treating pediatric mania are limited. No randomized, double-blind trials currently exist to support its routine use. In addition, the numerous risks related to carbamazepine use and its extensive interactions with other concomitant medications suggest that it should be considered a second-line or adjunctive agent in treating PBD until further studies are performed. At this time, we do not recommend carbamazepine as a first-line agent for the treatment of PBD.

Divalproex Sodium

Divalproex sodium received FDA approval for treatment of mania in adults in 1994. It appears that valproate, unlike carbamazepine, is commonly prescribed to children and adolescents with bipolar disorder.

Supporting studies in youth. Acute treatment of manic, hypomanic, and mixed mania symptoms in youth has been evaluated in open-label trials of up to 8 weeks in duration (Papatheodorou et al. 1995; Scheffer et al. 2005; Wagner et al. 2002). These studies suggest that divalproex may be effective in the treatment of bipolar disorder in young patients. Headache, gastrointestinal complaints, and sedation were commonly observed side effects in these reports.

Findling et al. (2005) evaluated the longer-term use of divalproex sodium in PBD. Their study reported on an 18-month, double-blind, maintenance comparison of lithium and divalproex sodium in youth ages 5–18 years with bipolar disorder. Divalproex was initiated in divided doses, and the dosage was gradually increased to a target of 20 mg/kg/day. In this trial, lithium and divalproex treatment appeared to have similar effectiveness as maintenance treatments. Gastrointestinal complaints, tremor, and headache were commonly reported side effects.

The National Institute of Mental Health (NIMH) funded a double-blind comparison study of lithium, divalproex, and placebo over an 8-week period.

In that trial, divalproex was found to be superior to placebo (Kowatch et al. 2007). However, in a randomized, double-blind, industry-sponsored study of extended-release divalproex use in youth with bipolar disorder (*N*=150), no statistically significant improvement in acute manic symptoms was found for those given divalproex versus those given placebo (Wagner et al. 2009). An explanation for the discrepant results between these two studies may be related to between-site variability. The NIMH-supported study was conducted at substantially fewer sites than the industry-sponsored trial; therefore, intersite variability may have contributed to the results of the industry-supported trial. Furthermore, combination pharmacotherapy studies have suggested that divalproex may be beneficial when coadministered with lithium, quetiapine, or risperidone (Findling et al. 2003; Kowatch et al. 2003).

Formulations. Standard valproic acid without enteric coating is available as Depakene in 250-mg capsules and as a 250-mg/5-mL elixir. Enteric-coated valproic acid (divalproex sodium) is available as Depakote in 125-mg, 250-mg, and 500-mg tablets. Depakote Sprinkle Capsules are available in 125-mg strength. The beaded contents of the capsules can be sprinkled over applesauce for children who have difficulty swallowing pills. Extended-release Depakote is available in 250- and 500-mg tablets, and once-daily dosing may be possible with this form.

Preliminary evaluation. A detailed medical history is recommended prior to beginning treatment with valproate. Particular attention should be paid to any history of hepatic or hematological dysfunction. Concomitant medications that are hepatically metabolized should also be reviewed. The teratogenic potential for neural tube defects has been well established with valproate therapy, and urine pregnancy testing and documentation of education regarding this possibility is suggested for patients of childbearing potential. Concerns regarding polycystic ovary syndrome (PCOS) have prompted some clinicians to document patients' pretreatment menstrual patterns in order to facilitate the identification of any changes in menses that might occur during valproate therapy. Baseline laboratory work should include a CBC with differential and platelets as well as an assessment of liver function (e.g., transaminases, bilirubin). Because treatment with divalproex may lead to weight gain, monitoring of weight and height prior to and during treatment is also recommended.

Medication dosing. Enteric-coated preparations are generally preferred over generic valproic acid for the treatment of pediatric patients with bipolar illness, given that enteric-coated formulations are associated with a reduced risk for gastrointestinal side effects such as dyspepsia and abdominal pain. For outpatients, we generally recommend initiating divalproex sodium at a dosage of approximately 10–15 mg/kg/day in divided doses. Then, based on the results of serum levels and on clinical response, dosage increases in 250-mg to 500-mg increments may be considered. Serum levels of valproic acid should be obtained shortly after treatment initiation, during dosage titration periods, or as clinically indicated. Valproic acid levels should be drawn 12 hours after the last dose (trough level), and in clinical practice it is generally collected before the first morning dose. Adequate serum levels have been reported in the 50- to 125-μg/mL range, and the total daily dose should not exceed 60 mg/kg. After dosage stabilization, liver function tests, CBC with differential and platelets, and serum levels should be obtained at least every 6 months or whenever clinical symptoms change.

Side effects. Side effects that have been associated with divalproex pharmacotherapy in the pediatric bipolar population have included weight gain as well as gastrointestinal, CNS, hematological, and hepatic events (Table 6–3). CNS effects that have been reported include cognitive dulling, headache, tremor, and somnolence. Although the enteric-coated preparations can minimize gastrointestinal symptoms, patients taking these formulations have reported nausea, stomach pain, diarrhea, and emesis. Rare cases of hepatic failure and potentially fatal pancreatitis have also been observed. Specifically, cases of fatal valproate-induced acute liver failure have been reported in patients with mitochondrial disease caused by mutations of the mitochondrial DNA polymerase gamma gene *POLG*. Hence, valproate is contraindicated in patients with mitochondrial disorders caused by *POLG* mutations and in children younger than 2 years who are suspected of having a mitochondrial disorder, as stated in the boxed warning for the drug. We routinely advise patients to notify their physician about new-onset symptoms of nausea, lethargy, jaundice, or anorexia. Thrombocytopenia also may occur, so patients should be monitored for bleeding or easy bruising.

The issue surrounding PCOS has received substantive interest. PCOS is a syndrome of hyperandrogenism (menstrual irregularities, hirsutism, acne, and

Table 6–3. Management of divalproex sodium–related side effects

System	Side effect	Suggested intervention
Gastrointestinal	Nausea, emesis, stomach pain, diarrhea	Take with food. Switch to Depakote formulation. Consider checking serum level for toxicity.
CNS	Tremor, headache, sedation, cognitive dulling	Reduce dosage or split dose.
Hematological	Leukopenia, thrombocytopenia	Consider hematology consultation. Consider medication discontinuation.
Hepatic	Elevated transaminases/pancreatic enzymes	Consider rechecking laboratory values. Consider medication discontinuation.
Endocrine	Menstrual irregularities, hyperandrogenism	Consider referral to an endocrinologist. Consider switching mood-stabilizing agents.
General	Weight gain	Educate patient/family about appropriate diet and exercise. Consider nutrition consultation.

alopecia). Small studies have failed to consistently show a relationship between PCOS and valproate use among patients without seizure disorders (H. Joffe et al. 2003; R.T. Joffe et al. 2003). However, Qin et al. (2006) identified a functional single nucleotide polymorphism, –71G, that may contribute to the creation of excessive testosterone production. Furthermore, valproate has been shown to potentiate this gene's expression in ovarian cells (Nelson-DeGrave et al. 2004; Wood et al. 2005). In sum, valproate treatment may play a role in the potentiation of PCOS in certain patients, so careful monitoring may be indicated until a clearer picture of the association between valproate administration and PCOS is available.

Drug interactions and cautions. Like many other psychotropic agents, valproate is metabolized in the liver. Because of the possibility of medication interactions, care should be used when valproate is prescribed with concomitant agents. Commonly used drugs that can *increase* valproate levels include erythromycin, fluoxetine, aspirin, and ibuprofen. Similarly, carbamazepine may *decrease* valproate levels during concomitant use.

Valproate can lead to substantive increases in lamotrigine levels when both agents are used together, which may result in serious dermatological reactions. Therefore, dosing of lamotrigine should be modified when prescribed concomitantly with valproate.

Other Anticonvulsants

Evidence for the use of other, newer anticonvulsants in the acute treatment of PBD is sparse. For this reason, we generally do not prescribe these compounds to patients unless other agents with more extensive empirical support fail to provide adequate therapeutic benefit.

Lamotrigine is indicated for the maintenance treatment of adults with bipolar disorder, although its acute management of mood episodes in adults is not well established. Findling et al. (2015a) aimed to compare the efficacy of adjunctive lamotrigine versus placebo in children ages 10–17 years with bipolar I disorder who were receiving conventional bipolar disorder treatment. In this randomized withdrawal trial, patients with bipolar I disorder of at least moderate severity received lamotrigine during an open-label phase (up to 18 weeks). Patients who maintained a stable lamotrigine dosage for 2 weeks or longer and met specific clinical improvement criteria were randomly assigned to double-blind lamotrigine or to placebo for up to 36 weeks. Data from the open-label phase indicated that most patients experienced benefit in mood symptoms with lamotrigine treatment. However, data analysis of the randomized double-blind phase failed to detect a benefit of adjunctive lamotrigine. Data analysis also indicated that lamotrigine may be effective in a subset of older adolescents.

One methodologically stringent, double-blind, placebo-controlled clinical trial by Delbello et al. (2005) examined the use of topiramate in children ages 6–17 years with bipolar I disorder. Topiramate appeared to trend toward having some therapeutic efficacy, but the trial was ended before the entire planned sample was ascertained because results of concurrent adult mania studies failed to demonstrate efficacy for the compound. Definitive conclusions about the short-term efficacy of topiramate cannot be made on the basis of this pediatric trial because of its limited sample size and therefore reduced statistical power to detect a difference between medication and placebo.

Similar to what had been suggested previously in adults (Benedetti et al. 2004; Hummel et al. 2002), oxcarbazepine was described in two separate case reports as possibly being beneficial in the treatment of PBD (Davanzo et al. 2004; Teitelbaum 2001). However, in a large, multisite, randomized, double-blind, placebo-controlled study in children and adolescents, treatment with oxcarbazepine was found not to be superior to treatment with placebo (Wagner et al. 2006).

Although some published reports have considered zonisamide, levetiracetam, and tiagabine in the adult literature, these studies were not placebo-controlled and generally lacked methodological rigor. At present, we do not prescribe these three agents to youth for management of PBD given the lack of data to support their use.

Atypical Antipsychotics

At present, the atypical antipsychotic agents that are available to clinicians in the United States include aripiprazole, asenapine, clozapine, lurasidone, olanzapine, paliperidone (the active metabolite of risperidone), quetiapine, risperidone, and ziprasidone. In addition, brexpiprazole, cariprazine, iloperidone, and lumateperone have been marketed in the United States but remain unstudied in children and adolescents currently experiencing manic or mixed episodes. We do not yet have a head-to-head randomized trial comparing the efficacy of different atypical antipsychotics in children and adolescents, but efficacy appears to be comparable across separate trials (Correll et al. 2010). Researchers in pediatric bipolar illness continue to explore the usefulness of atypical antipsychotics as a monotherapy and as an adjunctive therapy in this often difficult-to-treat population.

General Evaluation and Monitoring

Before any atypical antipsychotic medication is prescribed, care must be taken to obtain an accurate psychiatric, medical, and family history. Particular attention should be paid to the patient's medical and family history and a physical examination that considers weight/obesity, endocrine, and cardiovascular system issues as well as neurological status and movement disorders. When prescribing any psychotropic medication to children and adolescents, clinicians should review its potential for short- and long-term side effects with both the patient and their guardian. In addition to considerations pertaining to this entire class of medications, some issues are specific to individual agents; these are reviewed in the respective discussions of each agent later in the chapter.

One of the key aspects that confers *atypicality* to this drug class is its reduced propensity to cause extrapyramidal side effects (EPS) compared with the older, *typical* antipsychotics. However, neurological side effects such as dystonia, parkinsonism, and tardive dyskinesia have been reported with these agents. The potential for these risks should be reviewed with patients and their guardians. We also recommend paying extra attention to the assessment of EPS prior to and during the course of treatment with this group of drugs. Tardive dyskinesia is a possibly irreversible side effect of atypical antipsychotics, and we recommend carefully evaluating and monitoring patients for this possibility. A commonly used instrument to facilitate this process is the Abnormal Involuntary Movement Scale (National Institute of Mental Health 1985).

The potential for metabolic/endocrine and cardiovascular complications in patients taking atypical antipsychotics has been greatly discussed. The American Academy of Child and Adolescent Psychiatry has developed practice parameters to assist clinicians with suggested monitoring strategies when using atypical antipsychotic medications in children and adolescents (Findling et al. 2011). Preliminary data suggest that metformin might decrease the weight gain associated with atypical antipsychotics in this population; however, additional high-quality evidence is needed (Ellul et al. 2018).

Avoiding medication interactions with atypical antipsychotics generally involves avoiding specific concomitant therapies. Because atypical antipsychotic medications can be sedating, caution should be used when combining them with other CNS depressants. Medications that affect cardiac conduction by lengthening the QT interval should be used cautiously and with regular cardiac monitoring. Concomitant use of medications affecting hepatic metabolism can reduce (e.g., carbamazepine) or increase (e.g., fluvoxamine, atomoxetine) blood levels of certain atypical antipsychotics.

Aripiprazole (Abilify)

Aripiprazole is currently FDA approved for the acute and maintenance treatment of manic and mixed episodes associated with bipolar I disorder in patients ages 10–17 years. Of the atypical antipsychotics, aripiprazole is distinct because it acts as a partial dopamine agonist.

Supporting studies. One randomized, double-blind, placebo-controlled study of 296 patients ages 10–17 years with bipolar I disorder showed that aripiprazole, at dosages of 10 mg/day and 30 mg/day, was superior to placebo in the acute treatment of manic and mixed episodes (Findling et al. 2009). A meta-analysis of the efficacy and safety of aripiprazole across pediatric bipolar disorder trials and observational studies revealed that this agent was effective, and its safety profile was comparable with that of other medications, with significantly lower risk of hyperprolactinemia (Meduri et al. 2016).

Formulations. Aripiprazole is available in both tablet and liquid formulations. Tablets are available in strengths of 2 mg, 5 mg, 10 mg, 15 mg, 20 mg, and 30 mg. The liquid preparation is available as a 1-mg/mL elixir. An orally disintegrating tablet formulation is available in strengths of 10 mg, 15 mg, 20 mg, and 30 mg. Aripiprazole is also available in an injectable form that has not yet been studied in children.

Medication dosing. Given its long half-life, aripiprazole is routinely prescribed in once-daily dosing. The FDA recommends a starting dosage of 2 mg/day in pediatric patients (ages 10–17), with titration to 5 mg/day after 2 days and a target dosage of 10 mg/day after 2 additional days. We do not recommend exceeding the FDA-approved maximum dosage of 30 mg/day.

Side effects. Common side effects reported with aripiprazole in youth include sedation, motoric activation, nausea, and emesis (Table 6–4). Studies in adults suggest that aripiprazole may have a reduced propensity for inducing weight gain compared with some of the other atypical agents; however, it does appear to be associated with weight gain in youth. Clinically significant ECG changes do not appear to be common with aripiprazole. In addition, because of aripiprazole's distinct partial dopamine agonism, prolactin levels seem to decrease during therapy with this medication.

Asenapine (Saphris)

Asenapine has been approved by the FDA for the acute treatment of manic or mixed episodes associated with bipolar disorder in children and adolescents ages 10–17 years. This approval was based on a 3-week randomized controlled

Table 6–4. Management of aripiprazole side effects

System	Side effect	Suggested intervention
Gastrointestinal	Nausea, emesis	Take with food.
		Titrate more slowly.
		Reduce dosage.
CNS	Headache, sedation, activation, akathisia	Reduce or split dosage.
		Change time of daily administration.
General	Weight gain	Educate patient and family about appropriate diet and exercise.
		Consider nutrition consultation.
		Switch to another treatment.

trial (RCT) involving 403 children and adolescents who were assigned to either placebo or to one of three fixed doses of asenapine (2.5 mg, 5 mg, or 10 mg) twice daily. The patients assigned asenapine all showed statistically significant improvement in symptoms. The most common side effect reported was sedation (>30% with asenapine vs. 6% with placebo). Other, more common side effects in this study included dizziness, nausea, increased appetite, weight gain, strange taste sensation, and numbing of the mouth. The latter two side effects are likely related to the sublingual formulation of asenapine. Overall, asenapine was generally well tolerated in this study population (Findling et al. 2015b).

Clozapine (Clozaril)

Whereas the other atypical antipsychotics are considered first-line agents, clozapine is generally reserved for patients whose symptoms fail to respond to other forms of therapy, and it appears to be used only rarely in pediatric patients with bipolar illness because of its associated risk for potentially fatal agranulocytosis. Also, clozapine can lower the seizure threshold and lead to both electroencephalographic changes and overt seizures in youth who take this medication.

Some evidence suggests that clozapine may be of benefit to adolescents with treatment-resistant bipolar illness (Masi et al. 2002). Unfortunately, no prospective RCTs of clozapine have been reported in this population.

Olanzapine (Zyprexa, Zydis)

Olanzapine is FDA approved for the acute treatment of manic or mixed episodes associated with bipolar I disorder in youth ages 13–17 years. Weight gain and endocrine abnormalities (e.g., diabetes, dyslipidemias) associated with olanzapine therapy have received attention in adults and are of important clinical concern for children and adolescents, who may be at greater risk for antipsychotic-related weight gain.

Supporting studies. In a 3-week double-blind, placebo-controlled, randomized trial (Tohen et al. 2007), adolescent patients (ages 13–17 years) with mania were randomly assigned to olanzapine ($n=107$) at dosages ranging from 2.5 mg/day to 20 mg/day or to placebo ($n=54$). The investigators found that, compared with placebo, treatment with olanzapine was associated with greater reduction in manic symptoms. Patients given olanzapine gained more weight (3.7 kg) than those given placebo (0.3 kg). Furthermore, the olanzapine-treated group showed significantly greater changes in levels of prolactin, fasting glucose, fasting total cholesterol, uric acid, and the hepatic enzymes aspartate transaminase and alanine transaminase. Post hoc analysis of this study revealed that early response to olanzapine at week 1 in acute pediatric manic or mixed episodes was strongly associated with ultimate response and remission at week 3 (Xiao et al. 2017). These results suggest that the benefits of olanzapine for the treatment of PBD should be considered within the context of its safety profile. This may lead clinicians to consider this medication only after other atypical antipsychotics have been tried first.

Formulations. Olanzapine is available in tablets, in an intramuscular preparation (short- and long-acting), and in the dissolving formulation Zydis. Tablets are available in strengths of 2.5 mg, 5 mg, 7.5 mg, 10 mg, 15 mg, and 20 mg. Zydis orally disintegrating tablets, available in strengths of 5 mg, 10 mg, 15 mg, and 20 mg, may be useful for children who are unable to swallow tablets. The short-acting injectable form of olanzapine is generally reserved for management of emergencies and potentially dangerous situations, whereas the long-acting intramuscular injection (Zyprexa Relprevv) is available for maintenance therapy.

Preliminary evaluation. Given that olanzapine therapy may be associated with weight gain and endocrine dysfunction, care should be exercised to establish any history of endocrine dysfunction or obesity in both the child or ad-

Table 6–5. Management of olanzapine side effects

System	Side effect	Suggested intervention
Endocrine	Glucose intolerance	Monitor fasting glucose and hemoglobin A1C at least annually.
		Consider nutrition consultation.
	Prolactin elevation	Monitor for changes in menses, galactorrhea, or gynecomastia.
CNS	Headache, sedation	Reduce dosage or split dose.
		Administer dose at bedtime.
General	Weight gain	Educate patient/family about appropriate diet and exercise.
		Consider nutrition consultation.
		Switch to another atypical antipsychotic.
		Consider adding metformin or topiramate.

olescent and their biological family prior to therapy. Discussions with patients and their families should include both short- and long-term risks noted in pediatric trials. We also suggest that the patient and family actively participate in monitoring of side effects.

Medication dosing. The FDA-approved dosing guidelines recommend that oral olanzapine be initiated at dosages of 2.5 mg/day or 5 mg/day, with a target dosage of 10 mg/day. Dosing adjustments in increments of 2.5 mg or 5 mg are recommended. Dosages greater than 20 mg/day have not been clinically evaluated in the pediatric population.

Side effects. Side effects associated with olanzapine include glucose intolerance, prolactin elevation, headache, sedation, and weight gain (Table 6–5). Weight gain has been noted in published pediatric bipolar trials. Although sedation is commonly reported with olanzapine use, gastrointestinal problems appear to be relatively uncommon. Unfortunately, methodologically stringent long-term studies of olanzapine in this patient population are lacking. Therefore, the magnitude of weight gain associated with long-term olanzapine therapy in the pediatric population has yet to be adequately characterized.

Quetiapine (Seroquel)

Quetiapine is FDA approved for the acute treatment of manic episodes in pediatric patients ages 10–17 years with bipolar I disorder.

Supporting studies. In one prospective study, 50 patients ages 12–18 years with mania were randomly assigned to treatment with either quetiapine (at dosages ranging from 400 mg/day to 600 mg/day) or divalproex (at dosages necessary to achieve serum levels of 80–120 μg/mL) for up to 4 weeks (Delbello et al. 2006). The authors found both medications to be equally effective in ameliorating manic symptoms, and both were reasonably well tolerated. Another randomized, placebo-controlled trial of 277 patients ages 10–17 years found that quetiapine at dosages of 400 mg/day and 600 mg/day was more effective than placebo in treating acute manic symptoms in PBD (Pathak et al. 2013).

Other studies have evaluated the usefulness of quetiapine as an adjunctive treatment in PBD. These clinical trials are discussed in the "Combination Pharmacotherapy" section later in this chapter.

Formulations. Quetiapine is available in 25-, 50-, 100-, 200-, 300-, and 400-mg strengths. A long-acting formulation of quetiapine (Seroquel XR) is available in 50-, 150-, 200-, 300-, and 400-mg strengths.

Medication dosing. For adolescents, the FDA recommends that the total daily dose for the initial 5 days of therapy be 50 mg (day 1), 100 mg (day 2), 200 mg (day 3), 300 mg (day 4), and 400 mg (day 5). After day 5, the dosage should be adjusted within the recommended range of 400–600 mg/day on the basis of response and tolerability. Dosage adjustments should be in increments no greater than 100 mg/day. No additional benefit has been shown in prescribing more than 600 mg/day for adolescents. The dosing schedule for immediate-release formulations should be divided twice or three times daily as necessary.

Side effects/preliminary evaluation. The management of the common side effects of quetiapine is described in Table 6–6. The adult research literature notes blood pressure elevation, sedation, and orthostatic hypotension as common adverse effects with quetiapine treatment. Although we have observed weight gain with quetiapine in our clinical practice, it appears to be less than that noted with olanzapine and clozapine treatment. The risk of EPS may be relatively modest with quetiapine compared with the other atypical agents.

Table 6–6. Management of quetiapine side effects

System	Side effect	Suggested intervention
Cardiovascular	Elevated blood pressure (both systolic and diastolic)	Monitor blood pressure closely; adjust dosage as necessary to minimize blood pressure changes.
CNS	Sedation, orthostasis	Reduce or split dosage to three times daily, with the larger dose at night.
		Caution patient to be careful when getting out of bed and standing up.
Visual	Cataracts	Educate patient about possible changes in eyesight.
		Recommend regular ophthalmological evaluation.
General	Weight gain	Educate patient about appropriate diet and exercise.
		Consider nutrition consultation.
		Consider switching to another agent.

Cataract formation has been noted in laboratory animals administered quetiapine. Although a relationship between quetiapine use and cataract formation has not been established in humans, clinicians may want to consider recommending ophthalmological examinations for patients prescribed this medication, in addition to the other evaluations that should be considered before beginning atypical antipsychotic therapy (see "General Evaluation and Monitoring" earlier in this chapter).

Risperidone (Risperdal)

Risperidone was the first atypical antipsychotic to receive FDA approval for the treatment of acute mania or mixed episodes associated with bipolar I disorder in youth ages 10–17 years.

Supporting studies. Haas et al. (2009) conducted a randomized study of risperidone versus placebo in the acute treatment of manic or mixed episodes in 169 patients ages 10–17 years. Risperidone was found to be superior to placebo and was relatively well tolerated at dosages as low as 0.5–2.5 mg/day. Geller et al. (2012) compared risperidone with valproic acid or lithium in an 8-week RCT assessing their comparative efficacy in pediatric bipolar manic or mixed episodes. The study demonstrated that risperidone was more efficacious than valproic acid and lithium for the initial treatment of a manic episode but had potentially serious metabolic side effects.

Formulations. Risperidone is available in tablet, liquid, disintegrating tablet, and long-acting injectable forms. The tablets and oral disintegrating tablets are available in 0.25-, 0.5-, 1-, 2-, 3-, and 4-mg strengths. The concentration of the liquid formulation is 1 mg/mL. Data are limited on the use of injectable Risperdal Consta and long-acting oral paliperidone (Invega) in youth.

Preliminary evaluation. As recommended before any atypical antipsychotic initiation, clinicians should obtain an accurate psychiatric, medical, and family history (see "General Evaluation and Monitoring" earlier in this chapter). Risperidone, compared with other atypical antipsychotics, appears to have a greater propensity to increase prolactin concentrations. In our experience, prolactin-related side effects are not often problematic. Therefore, we generally do not monitor prolactin concentrations over time. However, we do recommend that a pretreatment prolactin level be obtained for youth prior to initiating risperidone. Then, if side effects that might be attributable to prolactin (e.g., irregular menses/amenorrhea, galactorrhea, breast enlargement) develop de novo and a prolactin measurement is subsequently obtained, the clinician has a baseline level for comparison.

Medication dosing. The FDA-recommended starting dosage of risperidone in youth with bipolar disorder is 0.5 mg/day, administered as a single daily dose in either the morning or evening. Dose adjustments, if indicated, should occur at intervals of not less than 24 hours, in increments of 0.5 mg/day or 1 mg/day (administered daily or divided twice daily), as tolerated, to a recommended dosage of 2.5 mg/day. Although efficacy at dosages between 0.5 mg/day and 6 mg/day has been demonstrated in studies of pediatric patients with bipolar mania, no additional benefit was seen for dosages higher than 2.5 mg/day, and these higher dosages were associated with more adverse events. Dosages greater than 6 mg/day have not been studied. In our experience, dosage-limiting side effects during risperidone titration are sedation and EPS.

Table 6–7. Management of risperidone side effects

System	Side effect	Suggested intervention
CNS	Sedation, headache	Reduce the total dosage.
		Administer more of the daily dose at night.
Endocrine	Glucose intolerance, prolactin elevation	Monitor fasting glucose.
		Monitor for changes in menses, galactorrhea, or gynecomastia.
General	Weight gain	Educate patient/family about appropriate diet and exercise.
		Consider switching to another agent.

For younger children, we generally suggest starting at 0.25 mg/day, with titration every 2–3 days, to a total dosage that does not exceed 2 mg/day. This total daily dosage is typically administered in two relatively equal doses. For older children and adolescents (typically weighing >40 kg), we generally consider a similar dosing strategy that employs 0.5-mg dosing increments and a total dosage that does not exceed 4 mg/day.

Side effects. The most commonly reported side effects during risperidone treatment include weight gain, headache, and sedation (Table 6–7). A more rapid rate of dosage titration, as well as higher final total daily dosages, seems to increase the risk of EPS during pediatric risperidone therapy. As noted (see earlier subsection "Preliminary Evaluation"), rates of hyperprolactinemia seem higher with risperidone than with other atypical antipsychotics.

Ziprasidone (Geodon)

Ziprasidone is FDA approved as monotherapy for schizophrenia and for acute treatment of manic or mixed episodes associated with bipolar I disorder in adults. The European Medicines Agency (EMA) has approved ziprasidone as an acute treatment for pediatric mania in patients ages 10–17 years. To date, the FDA has not yet approved ziprasidone for any pediatric indication.

Supporting studies. One randomized, placebo-controlled trial of 237 patients ages 10–17 years with a manic or mixed episode associated with bipolar I disorder found that ziprasidone at dosages of 40–160 mg/day was effective for the treatment of bipolar disorder and was generally well tolerated, with a neutral metabolic profile (Findling et al. 2013a).

More recently, Findling et al. (2022) investigated the acute efficacy, safety, and tolerability of flexibly dosed ziprasidone in youth with bipolar I disorder. In a 4-week double-blind study, participants ages 10–17 years were randomly assigned to ziprasidone (20–80 mg bid) or placebo. Some were then enrolled in a 26-week open-label extension study. Based on the results of the double-blind phase, the authors concluded that ziprasidone was effective for youth with bipolar I disorder in a manic episode. Overall, ziprasidone was safe and well tolerated, with no meaningful effects on weight or metabolic parameters.

Formulations. Ziprasidone is available in capsules and as an intramuscular injection. The capsule form is available in 20-mg, 40-mg, 60-mg, and 80-mg strengths. The injectable form is reserved for acute agitation; although its use has been described in case reports (Hazaray et al. 2004; Staller 2004), this formulation has not been examined in methodologically stringent research in the pediatric population.

Preliminary evaluation. The evaluation prior to initiating ziprasidone therapy is similar to that mentioned earlier for the other atypical antipsychotics (see "General Evaluation and Monitoring"). Particular attention should be paid to any individual or family history of cardiac conduction problems or symptoms associated with cardiac disease (e.g., syncope, arrhythmias, or family history of sudden cardiac death). The EMA reports that ziprasidone was associated with a mild to moderate dose-related prolongation of the QT interval in pediatric bipolar clinical trials, similar to that seen in the adult population. Ziprasidone should not be given together with medicinal products known to prolong the QT interval, and caution is advised regarding its use in patients with significant bradycardia. Electrolyte disturbances such as hypokalemia and hypomagnesemia increase the risk for malignant arrhythmias and should be corrected before treatment with ziprasidone is started. If patients with stable cardiac disease are treated, an ECG should be considered before treatment is started. In clinical practice, we recommend that ECGs be obtained prior to and during the course of ziprasidone therapy (see subsection "Side Effects").

Medication dosing. The EMA's recommended dosage of ziprasidone in the acute treatment of pediatric (ages 10–17 years) bipolar mania is a single 20-mg dose on day 1. The drug should subsequently be administered in two divided doses daily and titrated over 1–2 weeks to a target range of 120–160 mg/day for patients weighing 45 kg or more or 60–80 mg/day for those weighing less than 45 kg. Subsequent dosing should be adjusted based on clinical status, within the weight-based ranges of 80–160 mg/day or 40–80 mg/day, respectively. The EMA warns against exceeding the weight-based maximum dose (160 mg/day or 80 mg/day) because ziprasidone's safety profile at these dosages has not been confirmed, and it is associated with dose-related QT interval prolongation.

In addition, because taking ziprasidone with food increases its bioavailability, we generally recommend that patients take ziprasidone with food consistently in order to achieve predictable drug exposure.

Side effects. Sedation, akathisia, and elevated heart rates have been noted when ziprasidone is prescribed to youth (Barnett 2004) (Table 6–8). Unlike with many other atypical agents, substantive weight increases and dyslipidemias do not appear to be associated with ziprasidone therapy in adults. Ziprasidone does have a generally modest effect on intracardiac conduction in adults, but the risks associated with this effect appear to be modest (Daniel 2003). Although concerns have been raised (Blair et al. 2005), the effects of ziprasidone on cardiac electrophysiology have not yet been fully characterized in children or adolescents. In the absence of definitive information regarding the magnitude of QTc prolongation that may occur in youth, no definitive recommendations about ECG monitoring in those treated with ziprasidone can be made. However, in our practice, in addition to a baseline ECG, we generally suggest that an ECG be repeated after every 40- to 60-mg/day increase in dosage.

Ziprasidone-associated mania has also been described (Keating et al. 2005). The mechanism for this action and frequency of this occurrence in young people remain empirical questions for which further research is needed.

Lurasidone (Latuda)

Lurasidone is not currently approved by the FDA for the treatment of mixed or manic states in PBD but is approved for the treatment of pediatric patients (ages 10–17) with bipolar I disorder experiencing an acute depressive episode.

Lurasidone is available in 20-, 40-, 60-, and 80-mg tablets. The FDA recommends initiating lurasidone at a dosage of 20 mg given once daily as mono-

Table 6–8. Management of ziprasidone side effects

System	Side effect	Suggested intervention
CNS	Sedation, akathisia, extrapyramidal side effects	Reduce the daily dosage.
		Administer the total daily dosage three times daily rather than in twice-daily divided doses.
		Administer a larger proportion of the total daily dose at bedtime.
Cardiovascular	QTc prolongation, elevated heart rates	Monitor for any syncopal events or dizziness.
		Consider medication dosage decrease or discontinuation.
		Consider electrocardiographic monitoring at baseline and during upward dosage titration.
		Consider electrocardiographic monitoring when optimal dosage is achieved, then periodically or if symptoms change.

therapy. Initial dosage titration is not required. The dosage may be increased after 1 week based on clinical response. Lurasidone has been shown to be effective in a dosage range of 20–80 mg/day as monotherapy.

In a 6-week randomized, double-blind, placebo-controlled trial, lurasidone showed significant efficacy in the treatment of pediatric bipolar depression in patients ages 10–17 within the dosage range of 20–80 mg/day (DelBello et al. 2017). It was well tolerated, with no significant metabolic side effects. Patients who completed the acute phase were enrolled in a 2-year, open-label extension phase. The study results demonstrated that lurasidone was generally well tolerated and effective for up to 2 years, with low rates of discontinuation due to adverse events (DelBello et al. 2021).

Further information on lurasidone can be found in Chapter 5 ("Major Depressive Disorder").

Maintenance Therapy

Bipolar illness is a chronic, long-term condition. However, many pharmacotherapy studies in the pediatric bipolar literature have lasted no longer than 8 weeks. Limited studies are available to provide physicians with long-term efficacy and safety information. Although the pediatric neurology literature provides some insights into the long-term safety of several of the anticonvulsants, data are limited regarding the long-term effectiveness and use of these medications in children and adolescents with bipolar illness.

Maintenance therapy with lithium has been investigated. The CoLT group studied the long-term effect of lithium following acute treatment of mania. The average length of treatment after stabilization was 14.9 weeks. Investigators found that lithium is safe and effective at maintaining remission for patients whose symptoms initially responded to lithium for the treatment of mania. However, patients who only partially responded to lithium during acute treatment did not demonstrate substantial improvement during the long-term phase, despite the ability to receive adjunctive medications (Findling et al. 2013c). The CoLT trials provided further evidence in support of lithium for the maintenance treatment of pediatric bipolar I disorder. In this double-blind, placebo-controlled discontinuation study, participants ages 7–17 experiencing a manic or mixed episode received 24 weeks of lithium treatment in one of the prior CoLT trials (CoLT 1 or CoLT 2). Those who responded clinically to lithium were randomly assigned to continue lithium or cross-titrated to placebo for up to 28 weeks. The results of this study indicated that lithium maintenance treatment was generally safe and well tolerated (Findling et al. 2019).

One 18-month study evaluating the effectiveness of lithium monotherapy versus divalproex monotherapy in PBD found lithium to be as useful as divalproex monotherapy, and both drugs were generally well tolerated (Findling et al. 2005). Evidence indicated that lithium was superior to placebo in maintenance treatment of PBD, and lithium and divalproex seemed to perform similarly, which implies that divalproex might also be superior to placebo for maintenance treatment. Further research is necessary to answer this question.

The superiority of aripiprazole in maintenance therapy has also been demonstrated. Findling et al. (2013b) conducted a 30-week randomized, double-blind, placebo-controlled study involving youth ages 10–17 with bipolar I disorder with manic or mixed episodes, with or without psychosis. By study completion, the participants randomly assigned to either aripiprazole 10 mg/day or 30 mg/day showed statistically significant improvement in manic symptoms versus placebo. The medication was generally well tolerated, although a high attrition rate was noted in all treatment arms.

In another study, following mood stability with up to 16 weeks of open-label aripiprazole treatment, patients ages 4–9 years with bipolar disorder were randomly assigned in a double-blind manner to either continue aripiprazole or switch to a placebo for up to 72 weeks. The study results indicated that patients given aripiprazole had lower rates of symptom relapse compared with those given placebo (Findling et al. 2012).

Maintenance therapy with quetiapine was investigated in an open-label study (Duffy et al. 2009). Following mood stabilization and discontinuation of other psychotropic medications, 13 of 18 youth maintained mood stability for 40 weeks on quetiapine monotherapy. No patients in the study withdrew because of lack of tolerability.

Nearly all maintenance studies in youth have focused on manic symptoms. Findling et al. (2015a) studied the efficacy of adjunctive lamotrigine for manic, depressed, and mixed states. In a randomized, double-blind, placebo-controlled withdrawal study, youth ages 10–17 assigned to lamotrigine experienced delayed time to onset of bipolar events compared with those assigned to placebo, although the results were not statistically significant. In subgroup analysis, however, results were statistically significant for adolescents ages 13–17.

Although more evidence is emerging, additional studies are needed to address the long-term effectiveness and safety of maintenance medication options in the pediatric bipolar population.

Treatment of Pediatric Bipolar Depression

Treatment of pediatric bipolar depression is covered in Chapter 5. Please refer to the section in that chapter titled "Treatment of Major Depressive Disorder Subtypes and Bipolar Depression."

Combination Pharmacotherapy

Much of the recent treatment research into PBD suggests that lithium, mood stabilizers, or atypical antipsychotics may be effective as drug monotherapy in treating this illness. Increasing evidence suggests that combination pharmacotherapy, consisting of more than one agent, also might be appropriate for some patients, including inpatients, youth with psychosis, and patients who experience only a partial symptom response to one class of medications.

The combination of lithium with divalproex sodium has demonstrated effectiveness in treating pediatric mania (Findling et al. 2003). Other data suggest that lithium in combination with other antipsychotics may also be a rational therapeutic strategy (Kafantaris et al. 2001). Similarly, adjunctive administration of quetiapine with divalproex has been found to be an effective approach in adolescent mania (Delbello et al. 2002).

One of the goals of the CoLT studies was to investigate monotherapy with lithium versus combination therapy. Most patients (25 of 41) were prescribed multiple psychotropics; 13 patients were concomitantly prescribed divalproex and/or an antipsychotic for refractory mania. Researchers found that for patients with refractory mania, the addition of other psychotropics provided little to no improvement in symptoms (Findling et al. 2013c).

Clinicians may infer from these data that many, but not all, patients will require more than one psychotropic agent. Unfortunately, at present, it is not possible to identify prior to treatment initiation which patients will or will not experience a response to drug monotherapy. Traditionally, monotherapy with a mood stabilizer was the preferred initial treatment for patients with less severe mania and mania without psychosis. However, a recent meta-analysis found that second-generation antipsychotics were more efficacious in the treatment of mania, albeit more likely to cause side effects (Correll et al. 2010). Clearly, more research is needed in this area.

Because psychiatric comorbidity is the rule (not the exception) in PBD, clinicians should pay careful attention to discerning whether other psychiatric conditions are present when they are faced with a young patient with bipolarity. Unfortunately, very few data are available about how to treat psychiatric comorbidities in PBD.

The best evidence available regarding psychiatric comorbidities in PBD pertains to the treatment of comorbid ADHD. Scheffer et al. (2005) demonstrated that the addition of mixed amphetamine salts was effective in treating ADHD symptoms following mood stabilization with divalproex monotherapy. Similarly, in youth who had achieved a stable mood with lithium and/or divalproex sodium, those treated with stimulants did not have an increased risk of relapse compared with those who were not treated with a psychostimulant (Findling et al. 2005).

Another study investigated the short-term efficacy of methylphenidate in 16 youth with bipolar disorder and ADHD who were euthymic when taking at least one mood stabilizer but continued to experience clinically significant ADHD symptoms. Participants received 1 week each of placebo, methylphenidate 5 mg bid, methylphenidate 10 mg bid, and methylphenidate 15 mg bid in a crossover design. Findings demonstrated that treatment with methylphenidate was superior to placebo in treating ADHD symptoms, and its administration was not associated with mood destabilization (Findling et al. 2007).

In patients who have not achieved mood stability, Vitiello et al. (2012) found that patients with comorbid ADHD were more likely to respond to risperidone versus lithium compared with peers without ADHD. The authors suggested this difference may be due to risperidone improving hyperactivity/impulsivity, although caution should be used in interpreting these findings.

Conclusion

Quite a bit of progress has occurred since the start of this century in the pharmacological treatment of PBD. Clinicians are now better able to recognize and more effectively treat this condition. Continued research into the phenomenology, longitudinal course, genetics, and therapeutics of this spectrum of illnesses will eventually provide insights into the pathophysiology of PBD. Those insights, in turn, should contribute to the development of a broader, evidence-based foundation for the identification and management of PBD. As research into those domains continues and as a better appreciation and understanding of the development and course of the illness develops, it is possible that these avenues of research may eventually lead to useful preventive strategies for this chronic, debilitating illness.

Clinical Pearls

- Be sure the diagnosis is correct. Because pediatric bipolar disorder can be difficult to diagnose, it is important to be sure the right patients are receiving the correct interventions.

- Select a medication regimen that is based on scientific data from pediatric populations.
- Use the right dosage of medication. Some medicines require therapeutic drug concentration monitoring. In addition, many agents will be less effective if underdosed or may be less safe if prescribed at too high a dosage.
- Continue the medication trial for an adequate period of time. Some drugs do not provide noteworthy salutary effects until after several weeks of treatment at an appropriate dosage.
- Be aware of any psychiatric comorbidities that might contribute to what seemingly is "treatment nonresponse."
- Carefully assess for side effects because the medications used in the treatment of pediatric bipolarity may be associated with substantive risks.
- Remove agents that might be exacerbating the illness. Some medications can worsen the course of illness in some patients.

References

Barnett MS: Ziprasidone monotherapy in pediatric bipolar disorder. J Child Adolesc Psychopharmacol 14(3):471–477, 2004 15650505

Benedetti A, Lattanzi L, Pini S, et al: Oxcarbazepine as add-on treatment in patients with bipolar manic, mixed or depressive episode. J Affect Disord 79(1–3):273–277, 2004 15023507

Biederman J, Mick E, Faraone SV, et al: A prospective follow-up study of pediatric bipolar disorder in boys with attention-deficit/hyperactivity disorder. J Affect Disord 82(Suppl 1):S17–S23, 2004 15571786

Birmaher B, Axelson D, Goldstein B, et al: Four-year longitudinal course of children and adolescents with bipolar spectrum disorders: the Course and Outcome of Bipolar Youth (COBY) study. Am J Psychiatry 166(7):795–804, 2009 19448190

Blair J, Scahill L, State M, Martin A: Electrocardiographic changes in children and adolescents treated with ziprasidone: a prospective study. J Am Acad Child Adolesc Psychiatry 44(1):73–79, 2005 15608546

Correll CU, Sheridan EM, DelBello MP: Antipsychotic and mood stabilizer efficacy and tolerability in pediatric and adult patients with bipolar I mania: a comparative analysis of acute, randomized, placebo-controlled trials. Bipolar Disord 12(2):116–141, 2010 20402706

Daniel DG: Tolerability of ziprasidone: an expanding perspective. J Clin Psychiatry 64(Suppl 19):40–49, 2003 14728089

Davanzo P, Nikore V, Yehya N, Stevenson L: Oxcarbazepine treatment of juvenile-onset bipolar disorder. J Child Adolesc Psychopharmacol 14(3):344–345, 2004 15650489

Delbello MP, Schwiers ML, Rosenberg HL, Strakowski SM: A double-blind, randomized, placebo-controlled study of quetiapine as adjunctive treatment for adolescent mania. J Am Acad Child Adolesc Psychiatry 41(10):1216–1223, 2002 12364843

Delbello MP, Findling RL, Kushner S, et al: A pilot controlled trial of topiramate for mania in children and adolescents with bipolar disorder. J Am Acad Child Adolesc Psychiatry 44(6):539–547, 2005 15908836

Delbello MP, Kowatch RA, Adler CM, et al: A double-blind randomized pilot study comparing quetiapine and divalproex for adolescent mania. J Am Acad Child Adolesc Psychiatry 45(3):305–313, 2006 16540815

DelBello MP, Goldman R, Phillips D, et al: Efficacy and safety of lurasidone in children and adolescents with bipolar I depression: a double-blind, placebo-controlled study. J Am Acad Child Adolesc Psychiatry 56(12):1015–1025, 2017 29173735

DelBello MP, Tocco M, Pikalov A, et al: Tolerability, safety, and effectiveness of two years of treatment with lurasidone in children and adolescents with bipolar depression. J Child Adolesc Psychopharmacol 31(7):494–503, 2021 34324397

Duffy A, Milin R, Grof P: Maintenance treatment of adolescent bipolar disorder: open study of the effectiveness and tolerability of quetiapine. BMC Psychiatry 9:4, 2009 19200370

Ellul P, Delorme R, Cortese S: Metformin for weight gain associated with second-generation antipsychotics in children and adolescents: a systematic review and meta-analysis. CNS Drugs 32(12):1103–1112. 2018 30238318

Findling RL, Ginsberg LD: The safety and effectiveness of open-label extended-release carbamazepine in the treatment of children and adolescents with bipolar I disorder suffering from a manic or mixed episode. Neuropsychiatr Dis Treat 10:1589–1597, 2014 25210452

Findling RL, Gracious BL, McNamara NK, et al: Rapid, continuous cycling and psychiatric co-morbidity in pediatric bipolar I disorder. Bipolar Disord 3(4):202–210, 2001 11552959

Findling RL, McNamara NK, Gracious BL, et al: Combination lithium and divalproex sodium in pediatric bipolarity. J Am Acad Child Adolesc Psychiatry 42(8):895–901, 2003 12874490

Findling RL, McNamara NK, Youngstrom EA, et al: Double-blind 18-month trial of lithium versus divalproex maintenance treatment in pediatric bipolar disorder. J Am Acad Child Adolesc Psychiatry 44(5):409–417, 2005 15843762

Findling RL, Short EJ, McNamara NK, et al: Methylphenidate in the treatment of children and adolescents with bipolar disorder and attention-deficit/hyperactivity disorder. J Am Acad Child Adolesc Psychiatry 46(11):1445–1453, 2007 18049294

Findling RL, Frazier JA, Kafantaris V, et al: The Collaborative Lithium Trials (CoLT): specific aims, methods, and implementation. Child Adolesc Psychiatry Ment Health 2(1):21, 2008 18700004

Findling RL, Nyilas M, Forbes RA, et al: Acute treatment of pediatric bipolar I disorder, manic or mixed episode, with aripiprazole: a randomized, double-blind, placebo-controlled study. J Clin Psychiatry 70(10):1441–1451, 2009 19906348

Findling RL, Landersdorfer CB, Kafantaris V, et al: First-dose pharmacokinetics of lithium carbonate in children and adolescents. J Clin Psychopharmacol 30(4):404–410, 2010 20531219

Findling RL, Drury SS, Jensen PS, et al: Practice Parameter for the Use of Atypical Antipsychotic Medications in Children and Adolescents. Washington, DC, American Academy of Child and Adolescent Psychiatry, 2011. Available at: https://www.aacap.org/App_Themes/AACAP/docs/practice_parameters/Atypical_Antipsychotic_Medications_Web.pdf. Accessed October 2015.

Findling RL, Youngstrom EA, McNamara NK, et al: Double-blind, randomized, placebo-controlled long-term maintenance study of aripiprazole in children with bipolar disorder. J Clin Psychiatry 73(1):57–63, 2012 22152402

Findling RL, Cavuş I, Pappadopulos E, et al: Efficacy, long-term safety, and tolerability of ziprasidone in children and adolescents with bipolar disorder. J Child Adolesc Psychopharmacol 23(8):545–557, 2013a 24111980

Findling RL, Correll CU, Nyilas M, et al: Aripiprazole for the treatment of pediatric bipolar I disorder: a 30-week, randomized, placebo-controlled study. Bipolar Disord 15(2):138–149, 2013b 23437959

Findling RL, Kafantaris V, Pavuluri M, et al: Post-acute effectiveness of lithium in pediatric bipolar I disorder. J Child Adolesc Psychopharmacol 23(2):80–90, 2013c 23510444

Findling RL, Pathak S, Earley WR, et al: Efficacy and safety of extended-release quetiapine fumarate in youth with bipolar depression: an 8 week, double-blind, placebo-controlled trial. J Child Adolesc Psychopharmacol 24(6):325–335, 2014 24956042

Findling RL, Chang K, Robb A, et al: Adjunctive maintenance lamotrigine for pediatric bipolar I disorder: a placebo-controlled, randomized withdrawal study. J Am Acad Child Adolesc Psychiatry 54(12):1020–1031.e3, 2015a 26598477

Findling RL, Landbloom RL, Szegedi A, et al: Asenapine for the acute treatment of pediatric manic or mixed episode of bipolar I disorder. J Am Acad Child Adolesc Psychiatry 54(12):1032–1041, 2015b 26598478

Findling RL, Robb A, McNamara NK, et al: Lithium in the acute treatment of bipolar I disorder: a double-blind, placebo-controlled study. Pediatrics 136(5):885–894, 2015c 26459650

Findling RL, McNamara NK, Pavuluri M, et al: Lithium for the maintenance treatment of bipolar I disorder: a double-blind, placebo-controlled discontinuation study. J Am Acad Child Adolesc Psychiatry 58(2):287–296, 2019 30738555

Findling RL, Atkinson S, Bachinsky M, et al: Efficacy, safety, and tolerability of flexibly dosed ziprasidone in children and adolescents with mania in bipolar I disorder: a randomized placebo-controlled replication study. J Child Adolesc Psychopharmacol 32(3):143–152, 2022 35394365

Geller B, Tillman R, Craney JL, Bolhofner K: Four-year prospective outcome and natural history of mania in children with a prepubertal and early adolescent bipolar disorder phenotype. Arch Gen Psychiatry 61(5):459–467, 2004 15123490

Geller B, Luby JL, Joshi P, et al: A randomized controlled trial of risperidone, lithium, or divalproex sodium for initial treatment of bipolar I disorder, manic or mixed phase, in children and adolescents. Arch Gen Psychiatry 69(5):515–528, 2012 22213771

Haas M, Delbello MP, Pandina G, et al: Risperidone for the treatment of acute mania in children and adolescents with bipolar disorder: a randomized, double-blind, placebo-controlled study. Bipolar Disord 11(7):687–700, 2009 19839994

Hazaray E, Ehret J, Posey DJ, et al: Intramuscular ziprasidone for acute agitation in adolescents. J Child Adolesc Psychopharmacol 14(3):464–470, 2004 15650504

Hummel B, Walden J, Stampfer R, et al: Acute antimanic efficacy and safety of oxcarbazepine in an open trial with an on-off-on design. Bipolar Disord 4(6):412–417, 2002 12519102

Joffe H, Hall JE, Cohen LS, et al: A putative relationship between valproic acid and polycystic ovarian syndrome: implications for treatment of women with seizure and bipolar disorders. Harv Rev Psychiatry 11(2):99–108, 2003 12868510

Joffe RT, Brasch JS, MacQueen GM: Psychiatric aspects of endocrine disorders in women. Psychiatr Clin North Am 26(3):683–691, 2003 14563103

Joshi G, Wozniak J, Mick E, et al: A prospective open-label trial of extended-release carbamazepine monotherapy in children with bipolar disorder. J Child Adolesc Psychopharmacol 20(1):7–14, 2010 20166791

Kafantaris V, Coletti DJ, Dicker R, et al: Adjunctive antipsychotic treatment of adolescents with bipolar psychosis. J Am Acad Child Adolesc Psychiatry 40(12):1448–1456, 2001 11765291

Kafantaris V, Coletti D, Dicker R, et al: Lithium treatment of acute mania in adolescents: a large open trial. J Am Acad Child Adolesc Psychiatry 42(9):1038–1045, 2003 12960703

Keating AM, Aoun SL, Dean CE: Ziprasidone-associated mania: a review and report of 2 additional cases. Clin Neuropharmacol 28(2):83–86, 2005 15795551

Kowatch RA, Suppes T, Carmody TJ, et al: Effect size of lithium, divalproex sodium, and carbamazepine in children and adolescents with bipolar disorder. J Am Acad Child Adolesc Psychiatry 39(6):713–720, 2000 10846305

Kowatch RA, Sethuraman G, Hume JH, et al: Combination pharmacotherapy in children and adolescents with bipolar disorder. Biol Psychiatry 53(11):978–984, 2003 12788243

Kowatch RA, Fristad M, Birmaher B, et al: Treatment guidelines for children and adolescents with bipolar disorder. J Am Acad Child Adolesc Psychiatry 44(3):213–235, 2005 15725966

Kowatch RA, Findling RL, Scheffer RE, et al: Pediatric bipolar collaborative mood stabilizer trial. Poster presented at the annual meeting of the American Academy of Child and Adolescent Psychiatry. Boston, MA, October 23–28, 2007

Kudriakova TB, Sirota LA, Rozova GI, Gorkov VA: Autoinduction and steady-state pharmacokinetics of carbamazepine and its major metabolites. Br J Clin Pharmacol 33(6):611–615, 1992 1389933

Masi G, Mucci M, Millepiedi S: Clozapine in adolescent inpatients with acute mania. J Child Adolesc Psychopharmacol 12(2):93–99, 2002 12188978

McClellan J, Kowatch R, Findling RL: Practice parameter for the assessment and treatment of children and adolescents with bipolar disorder. J Am Acad Child Adolesc Psychiatry 46(1):107–125, 2007 17195735

Meduri M, Gregoraci G, Baglivo V, et al: A meta-analysis of efficacy and safety of aripiprazole in adult and pediatric bipolar disorder in randomized controlled trials and observational studies. J Affect Disord 191:187–208, 2016 26674213

National Institute of Mental Health: Abnormal Involuntary Movement Scale (AIMS). Psychopharmacol Bull 21:1077–1080, 1985

Nelson-DeGrave VL, Wickenheisser JK, Cockrell JE, et al: Valproate potentiates androgen biosynthesis in human ovarian theca cells. Endocrinology 145(2):799–808, 2004 14576182

Papatheodorou G, Kutcher SP, Katic M, Szalai JP: The efficacy and safety of divalproex sodium in the treatment of acute mania in adolescents and young adults: an open clinical trial. J Clin Psychopharmacol 15(2):110–116, 1995 7782483

Pathak S, Findling RL, Earley WR, et al: Efficacy and safety of quetiapine in children and adolescents with mania associated with bipolar I disorder: a 3-week, double-blind, placebo-controlled trial. J Clin Psychiatry 74(1):e100–e109, 2013 23419231

Qin K, Ehrmann DA, Cox N, et al: Identification of a functional polymorphism of the human type 5 17beta-hydroxysteroid dehydrogenase gene associated with polycystic ovary syndrome. J Clin Endocrinol Metab 91(1):270–276, 2006 16263811

Scheffer RE, Kowatch RA, Carmody T, Rush AJ: Randomized, placebo-controlled trial of mixed amphetamine salts for symptoms of comorbid ADHD in pediatric bipolar disorder after mood stabilization with divalproex sodium. Am J Psychiatry 162(1):58–64, 2005 15625202

Staller JA: Intramuscular ziprasidone in youth: a retrospective chart review. J Child Adolesc Psychopharmacol 14(4):590–592, 2004 15662151

Teitelbaum M: Oxcarbazepine in bipolar disorder. J Am Acad Child Adolesc Psychiatry 40(9):993–994, 2001 11556642

Tohen M, Kryzhanovskaya L, Carlson G, et al: Olanzapine versus placebo in the treatment of adolescents with bipolar mania. Am J Psychiatry 164(10):1547–1556, 2007 17898346

Vitiello B, Riddle MA, Yenokyan G, et al: Treatment moderators and predictors of outcome in the Treatment of Early Age Mania (TEAM) study. J Am Acad Child Adolesc Psychiatry 51(9):867–878, 2012 22917200

Wagner KD, Weller EB, Carlson GA, et al: An open-label trial of divalproex in children and adolescents with bipolar disorder. J Am Acad Child Adolesc Psychiatry 41(10):1224–1230, 2002 12364844

Wagner KD, Kowatch RA, Emslie GJ, et al: A double-blind, randomized, placebo-controlled trial of oxcarbazepine in the treatment of bipolar disorder in children and adolescents. Am J Psychiatry 163(7):1179–1186, 2006 16816222

Wagner KD, Redden L, Kowatch RA, et al: A double-blind, randomized, placebo-controlled trial of divalproex extended-release in the treatment of bipolar disorder in children and adolescents. J Am Acad Child Adolesc Psychiatry 48(5):519–532, 2009 19325497

Wood JR, Nelson-Degrave VL, Jansen E, et al: Valproate-induced alterations in human theca cell gene expression: clues to the association between valproate use and metabolic side effects. Physiol Genomics 20(3):233–243, 2005 15598877

Xiao L, Ganocy SJ, Findling RL, et al: Baseline characteristics and early response at week 1 predict treatment outcome in adolescents with bipolar manic or mixed episode treated with olanzapine: results from a 3-week, randomized, placebo-controlled trial. J Clin Psychiatry 78(9):e1158–e1166, 2017 28922591

7

Autism Spectrum Disorder

Michelle L. Palumbo, M.D.

Christopher J. Keary, M.D.

Christopher J. McDougle, M.D.

In 1943, Leo Kanner presented 11 case histories illustrating a syndrome in which the "pathognomonic, fundamental disorder is the children's inability to relate themselves in the ordinary way to people and situations from the beginning of life" (Kanner 1943, p. 242). He described several common characteristics, such as an autistic aloneness, impaired language development, stereotypies, literalness, and a need for sameness. In this compelling article, Kanner illustrated the clinical entity known today as autism spectrum disorder (ASD).

We want to thank the Nancy Lurie Marks Family Foundation for their support of this work. We also thank Drs. Kimberly A. Stigler and Craig A. Erickson for their contributions to a previous version of this chapter.

Thirty-seven years later, the publication of DSM-III (American Psychiatric Association 1980) heralded the inclusion of infantile autism among its formal diagnoses. Many of Kanner's initial findings were reflected in the criteria in DSM-III as well as in subsequent revisions. DSM-IV (American Psychiatric Association 1994) recharacterized the disorder under the larger umbrella term of pervasive developmental disorders (PDDs), including autistic disorder (autism), Asperger's disorder, Rett's disorder, childhood disintegrative disorder, and pervasive developmental disorder not otherwise specified (PDD-NOS). Similar to Kanner's observations, these criteria emphasized severe impairments in social interaction and communication as well as restricted interests and activities as being core features. More recently, DSM-5 (American Psychiatric Association 2013) collapsed autistic disorder, Asperger's disorder, and PDD-NOS into one term, *autism spectrum disorder*, in an attempt to simplify diagnosis while still capturing the heterogeneity of the disorder. In this vein, designations of mild, moderate, and severe can be assigned and impairments in verbal communication are no longer a requirement for diagnosis.

Recent estimates have calculated the prevalence of intellectual developmental disorder (intellectual disability) in children with ASD at 31% and 40%, respectively (Van Naarden Braun et al. 2015; Wingate et al. 2014). These estimates, which are lower than rates of co-occurring intellectual disability seen in the mid-1990s, may reflect the increasing prevalence of ASD among children with average, above-average, or borderline intellectual ability compared with that of children with intellectual disability (Van Naarden Braun et al. 2015).

In this chapter, we focus on the pharmacotherapy of ASD. The therapeutic approach to the management of ASD is multimodal. Treatments must take into account the global cognitive functioning of the individual, highlighting the importance of educational interventions. In addition, many people with ASD have delays in language development, thus making speech therapy essential to improving outcomes. Occupational therapy, social skills training, and physical therapy are also frequently necessary. Educating caregivers in behavioral management techniques can be very useful and may decrease the use of pharmacotherapy in this population.

In addition to nonpharmacological approaches, medication is often required to treat co-occurring psychiatric diagnoses or behavioral concerns.

Such treatments can significantly improve the patient's ability to benefit from behavioral and educational interventions. Yet no medication carries expert consensus as a treatment for the core symptoms of ASD. To date, risperidone and aripiprazole are the only drugs with an FDA approval specifically for use in populations with ASD in the treatment of irritability. Although no other medications have obtained FDA approval for specific use in patients with ASD, various drugs are used to treat interfering associated target symptoms in this population. In this chapter, we present current evidence regarding the pharmacotherapy of ASD (Table 7–1), review the adverse effects of the medications used, and outline practical management strategies.

Atypical Antipsychotics

Research into the pharmacotherapy of ASD began in the 1960s with the typical antipsychotics. Because of significant adverse effects associated with the low-potency antipsychotics (e.g., chlorpromazine, thioridazine), the high-potency antipsychotic haloperidol was systematically investigated in numerous well-designed studies (Anderson et al. 1989; Campbell et al. 1978; Cohen et al. 1980). However, haloperidol's potent dopamine D_2 receptor antagonism frequently led to acute dystonic reactions as well as drug-induced and withdrawal-related dyskinesias (Campbell et al. 1997). Currently, the typical antipsychotics as a whole are reserved for patients with severe treatment-resistant symptoms.

Concerns regarding the typical antipsychotics directed researchers toward the development of the atypical antipsychotics. These drugs, with their profile of potent antagonism at serotonin and dopamine receptors, have a purported decreased risk of acute extrapyramidal symptoms (EPS) and tardive dyskinesia.

Clozapine

Clozapine is an antagonist at the serotonin 5-HT_{2A}, 5-HT_{2C}, and 5-HT_3 receptors and the dopamine D_1, D_2, D_3, and D_4 receptors (Baldessarini and Frankenburg 1991). Four case reports and one small retrospective study have been published on the use of clozapine for irritability in ASD (defined as severe tantrums, aggression, and self-injury) (Beherec et al. 2011; Chen et al. 2001; Gobbi and Pulvirenti 2001; Lambrey et al. 2010; Zuddas et al. 1996). Overall, the lack of research on clozapine in patients with ASD is largely due to the

Table 7–1. Selected published double-blind, placebo-controlled trials in ASD

Drug	Study	Subjects		Design	Results	Target symptom
		N	Age, *years*			
Antipsychotics						
Aripiprazole	Marcus et al. 2009	218	6–17	8 weeks, parallel groups	Aripiprazole > placebo (29/52 responders [56%])	Irritability
	Owen et al. 2009	98	6–17	8 weeks, parallel groups	Aripiprazole > placebo (24/46 responders [52%])	Irritability
	Findling et al. 2014	85	6–17	16 weeks, parallel groups (extension study)	Aripiprazole = placebo (measuring rate of relapse)	Irritability
Haloperidol	Anderson et al. 1989	45	2–7	12 weeks, crossover	Haloperidol > placebo	Hyperactivity, irritability
Lurasidone	Loebel et al. 2016	150	6–17	6 weeks parallel groups	Lurasidone 20 mg/day = lurasidone 60 mg/day = placebo	Irritability
Risperidone	McDougle et al. 1998b	31	18–43	12 weeks, parallel groups	Risperidone > placebo (8/14 responders [57%])	Repetitive and aggressive behavior
	McCracken et al. 2002	101	5–17	8 weeks, parallel groups	Risperidone > placebo (34/49 responders [69%])	Irritability
	Shea et al. 2004	79	5–12	8 weeks, parallel groups	Risperidone > placebo (35/40 responders [87%])	Irritability

Table 7–1. Selected published double-blind, placebo-controlled trials in ASD *(continued)*

		Subjects				
Drug	**Study**	***N***	**Age, *years***	**Design**	**Results**	**Target symptom**
Risperidone *(continued)*	Kent et al. 2013	96	5–17	6 weeks, parallel groups	High-dose risperidone > placebo; low-dose risperidone = placebo	Irritability
Serotonin reuptake inhibitors						
Citalopram	King et al. 2009	149	5–17	12 weeks, parallel groups	Citalopram = placebo	Repetitive behavior
Clomipramine	Gordon et al. 1993	24	6–23	10 weeks, crossover	Clomipramine > placebo; clomipramine > desipramine (19/28 responders [68%])	Anger and obsessive-compulsive behavior
	Remington et al. 2001	36	10–36	7 weeks, crossover	Clomipramine > placebo	Irritability, stereotypy
Fluoxetine	Hollander et al. 2005	39	5–16	20 weeks, crossover	Fluoxetine > placebo	Repetitive behaviors
	Hollander et al. 2012	37	18–60	12 weeks, parallel groups	Fluoxetine > placebo	Compulsive behavior
	Reddihough et al. 2019	109	7.5–18	16 weeks, parallel groups	Fluoxetine = placebo	Repetitive behavior
	Herscu et al. 2020	158	5–17	14 weeks, parallel groups	Fluoxetine = placebo	Repetitive behavior

Table 7–1. Selected published double-blind, placebo-controlled trials in ASD *(continued)*

Drug	Study	Subjects		Design	Results	Target symptom
		N	Age, *years*			
Fluvoxamine	McDougle et al. 1996a	30	18–53	12 weeks, parallel groups	Fluvoxamine > placebo (8/15 responders [53%])	Repetitive behavior
	McDougle et al. 2000	34	5–18	12 weeks, parallel groups	Fluvoxamine = placebo	Repetitive behavior
	Sugie et al. 2005	18	3–8	12 weeks, parallel groups	Fluvoxamine > placebo	Global improvement
α_2-Adrenergic agonists						
Clonidine	Jaselskis et al. 1992	8	5–13	14 weeks, crossover	Clonidine > placebo by teacher and parent ratings but not clinician ratings (6/8 responders [75%]	Inattention, impulsivity, hyperactivity
Clonidine (transdermal)	Fankhauser et al. 1992	9	5–33	10 weeks, crossover	Clonidine > placebo (6/9 responders) [67%])	Social relationships, affectual and sensory responses
Guanfacine ER	Scahill et al. 2015	62	5–14	8 weeks, parallel groups	Guanfacine ER > placebo (15/30 responders [50%])	Hyperactivity

Table 7–1. Selected published double-blind, placebo-controlled trials in ASD *(continued)*

		Subjects				
Drug	**Study**	***N***	**Age, *years***	**Design**	**Results**	**Target symptom**
Psychostimulants						
Methylphenidate	Quintana et al. 1995	10	7–11	4 weeks, crossover	Methylphenidate > placebo	Hyperactivity
	Handen et al. 2000	13	5–11	3 weeks, crossover	Methylphenidate > placebo (8/13 responders [62%])	Hyperactivity
	Research Units on Pediatric Psychopharmacology Autism Network 2005a	72	5–14	4 weeks, crossover	Methylphenidate > placebo (35/72 responders [49%])	Hyperactivity
Selective norepinephrine reuptake inhibitors						
Atomoxetine	Harfterkamp et al. 2012	97	6–17	8 weeks, parallel groups	Atomoxetine > placebo (9/43 responders [20.9%])	ADHD symptoms
Atomoxetine ± parent training	Handen et al. 2015	128	5–14	10 weeks, parallel groups	Atomoxetine = atomoxetine + parent training > placebo	ADHD symptoms

Note. ASD = autism spectrum disorder; ER = extended release.

drug's adverse effect profile. Its propensity to lower the seizure threshold is troubling, particularly in a patient population that is predisposed to develop seizures. In addition, individuals with cognitive limitations and an impaired ability to communicate would have difficulty conveying information regarding symptoms associated with agranulocytosis and tolerating frequent venipuncture.

Risperidone

Risperidone is FDA approved for the treatment of irritability in children and adolescents ages 5–16 years with ASD. Risperidone has negligible affinities for muscarinic receptors and high affinities for serotonin 5-HT_{1D}, 5-HT_{2A}, and 5-HT_{2C} receptors; dopamine D_2, D_3, and D_4 receptors; α_1-adrenergic receptors; and H_1-histaminic receptors (Leysen et al. 1988). Several open-label studies have demonstrated that risperidone effectively targets core and related symptoms of ASD (Findling et al. 1997; Masi et al. 2001a; McDougle et al. 1997; Nicolson et al. 1998). The efficacy of risperidone was considered in a 12-week, double-blind, placebo-controlled study of irritability and repetitive behaviors in adults with autism (n=17) or PDD-NOS (n=14) (McDougle et al. 1998b). Of 14 subjects randomly assigned to risperidone (mean dosage 2.9 mg/day), 8 (57%) were deemed responders as measured by the Clinical Global Impression–Improvement (CGI-I) subscale versus none in the placebo group. The most common adverse effect was transient somnolence. Weight gain was reported in only two of the subjects in the risperidone group.

The first double-blind, placebo-controlled study of risperidone in youth with autism was conducted by the Research Units on Pediatric Psychopharmacology (RUPP) Autism Network (McCracken et al. 2002). In this 8-week study, 101 children and adolescents (mean age, 8.8 years) with target symptoms of tantrums, aggression, or self-injurious behavior were treated with risperidone or placebo. Risperidone treatment at a mean dosage of 1.8 mg/day (range, 0.5–3.5 mg/day) was found to reduce Aberrant Behavior Checklist (ABC) Irritability subscale scores by 56.9% compared with a 14.1% reduction with placebo. Overall, 69% of risperidone-treated subjects were judged responders compared with only 12% of those given placebo. Adverse effects of risperidone compared with placebo included weight gain (mean, 2.7 kg vs. 0.8 kg), increased appetite, sedation, dizziness, and sialorrhea. Further analyses revealed the medication to be significantly more effective than placebo for reducing interfering stereotypic and repetitive behaviors (McDougle et al. 2005).

The RUPP Autism Network subsequently published the results of a risperidone open-label extension study. This 16-week study involved 63 of the subjects whose symptoms responded to risperidone in the 8-week trial. The mean risperidone dosage remained stable. Subjects in this study continued to gain weight (mean, 5.1 kg over 24 weeks). Overall, only 8% discontinued the drug because of loss of efficacy; one subject discontinued the drug because of adverse effects (constipation). At the end of this phase, 32 subjects considered responders were then randomly assigned either to continued risperidone or to gradual substitution with placebo over a duration of 4 weeks. A statistically significant difference in relapse rate was reported, with 10 of the 16 subjects (62.5%) switched to placebo experiencing relapse versus 2 of the 16 (12.5%) who continued risperidone (Research Units on Pediatric Psychopharmacology Autism Network 2005b). A follow-up trial an average of 21 months later reported that 84 of these subjects continued taking risperidone with ongoing therapeutic benefit but also with persistent elevated appetite, weight gain, and enuresis (Aman et al. 2015).

In a second double-blind, placebo-controlled study of risperidone for the treatment of irritability in children and adolescents with PDDs, Shea et al. (2004) randomly assigned 79 youth ages 5–12 years to risperidone at a mean dosage of 1.2 mg/day or placebo over a duration of 8 weeks. Overall, 87% of risperidone-treated subjects had improved CGI-I scores compared with 40% of those given placebo. In addition, there was a 64% reduction in ABC Irritability subscale scores for children given risperidone versus a 31% reduction for those given placebo. Regarding adverse effects, weight gain was more common in the risperidone group than in the placebo group (2.7 kg vs. 1.0 kg), as were increased sedation, heart rate, and systolic blood pressure.

A 6-week, double-blind, placebo-controlled study of risperidone in children and adolescents ages 5–17 years with ASD examined the efficacy and side effect profile of risperidone dosages less than 0.25 mg/day (Kent et al. 2013). The findings replicated the efficacy of higher dosages (1.25 mg/day and 1.75 mg/day) in the treatment of irritability; however, the investigators did not find efficacy at dosages below 0.25 mg/day.

Olanzapine

Olanzapine has high affinity for the dopamine D_1, D_2, and D_4 receptors; serotonin 5-HT_{2A}, 5-HT_{2C}, and 5-HT_3 receptors; α_1-adrenergic receptors; H_1-histaminic receptors; and muscarinic receptors (Bymaster et al. 1996). Olanzapine is reported to be beneficial in the treatment of irritability in ASD according to case reports, open-label trials, and a small double-blind, placebo-controlled trial (Hollander et al. 2006b; Malone et al. 2001; Potenza et al. 1999). However, significant weight gain and its possible associated metabolic sequelae have restricted its use in this population. A small 8-week, double-blind, placebo-controlled trial evaluated olanzapine in 11 youth ages 6–14 years with PDD (Hollander et al. 2006b). At a mean dosage of 10 mg/day (range, 7.5–12.5 mg/day), 3 of 6 subjects (50%) in the olanzapine group were considered responders based on the CGI-I scale measure of global functioning compared with 1 of 5 subjects (20%) in the placebo group. Olanzapine was associated with sedation and increased appetite as well as considerable weight gain compared with placebo (3.4 kg±2.2 kg vs. 0.68 kg±0.68 kg).

Quetiapine

Quetiapine has affinity for the dopamine D_1 and D_2 receptors, the serotonin 5-HT_{2A} and 5-HT_{1A} receptors, and the histaminic H_1 receptors (Arnt and Skarsfeldt 1998). It has been studied in an uncontrolled fashion, with mixed findings. A retrospective review of quetiapine was conducted with data for patients in an outpatient autism clinic (Corson et al. 2004). Twenty patients ages 5–28 years (mean, 12.1 years) were included in the study and received quetiapine (mean dosage, 248.7 mg/day; range, 25–600 mg/day) over a mean duration of 59.8 weeks (range, 4–180 weeks). Of the 20 patients, 8 (40%) were considered responders to quetiapine based on results on the CGI-I scale anchored to irritability and hyperactivity. Adverse effects were reported in 50% of the patients, and 15% subsequently discontinued quetiapine.

Three notable open-label trials have been conducted with varying results. The first, a 16-week trial, involved six subjects (mean age, 10.9 years) (Martin et al. 1999). Two participants who completed the trial were considered responders. Three withdrew because of sedation and lack of effectiveness, and one dropped out after a possible seizure. Overall, no statistically significant improvement was reported. Findling et al. (2004) conducted a 12-week open-label study of quetiapine (mean dosage, 292 mg/day; range, 100–400 mg/day) in nine youth ages 12–17 years (mean, 14.6±2.3 years) with autism. Two patients (22%) experienced a response to treatment, as assessed with the CGI-I anchored to global functioning. The most common adverse effects included sedation, weight gain, and increased agitation. Golubchik et al. (2011) conducted an 8-week open-label trial of low-dosage quetiapine (mean, 122 mg/day) in 11 high-functioning adolescents ages 13–17 with ASD. Although only a trend toward improvement in the CGI Severity subscale score was found, significant reductions in aggression and sleep disturbances were reported. Moreover, tolerability was favorable compared with previous studies, with improved rates of study completion and no significant change in body weight.

Ziprasidone

Ziprasidone is a potent antagonist at the dopamine D_1 and D_2 receptors and the serotonin 5-HT_{2A} and 5-HT_{2C} receptors (Tandon et al. 1997). It is also a 5-HT_{1A} receptor agonist that inhibits serotonin and norepinephrine reuptake. In a case series of ziprasidone that included 12 youth ages 8–20 years (mean, 11.6 ±4.4 years) with autism (n=9) or PDD-NOS (n=3), 6 patients (50%) experienced a response to ziprasidone at a mean dosage of 59.2 mg/day (range, 20–120 mg/day) over a duration of at least 6 weeks (McDougle et al. 2002). Treatment resulted in improvement, as assessed with the CGI-I, in symptoms of aggression, agitation, and irritability. The most common adverse effect was transient sedation. The mean weight change was −2.6 kg (range, −16.1 kg to +2.7 kg). No cardiovascular adverse effects were reported. Malone et al. (2007) conducted a 6-week open-label study of ziprasidone for irritability in 12 youth (mean age, 14.5 years; range, 12–18 years) with autism. Nine subjects (75%) were judged treatment responders as assessed with the CGI-I. Ziprasidone was associated with mild to moderate sedation, and dystonic reactions occurred in two subjects. The authors reported that the medication was weight neutral. Although the mean QTc interval seen on electrocardiograms (ECGs) increased by 14.7 msec, the clinical significance of this finding was unclear.

Aripiprazole

Aripiprazole is FDA approved for the treatment of irritability in youth ages 6–17 years with ASD. The drug is a partial dopamine D_2 and serotonin 5-HT_{1A}

agonist and a serotonin 5-HT_{2A} antagonist (Burris et al. 2002). A 14-week, prospective, open-label study of aripiprazole for irritability was conducted in 25 children and adolescents with PDD-NOS and Asperger's disorder (mean age, 8.6 years; range, 5–17 years) (Stigler et al. 2009). Of the 25 study participants, 22 (88%) were considered responders to aripiprazole at a mean dosage of 7.8 mg/day (range, 2.5–15 mg/day), as assessed with the CGI-I and the ABC Irritability subscale. Aripiprazole was well tolerated, with tiredness and weight gain among the more commonly recorded adverse effects.

Two larger-scale controlled studies of aripiprazole were subsequently conducted in children and adolescents with autism and associated irritability. Marcus et al. (2009) conducted an 8-week double-blind, placebo-controlled, fixed-dose study in 218 youth ages 6–17 years. Subjects were randomly assigned to placebo or to aripiprazole (5 mg/day, 10 mg/day, or 15 mg/day). Improvement in irritability was seen on the ABC Irritability subscale at all dosages. Adverse effects included sedation, weight gain, and EPS, among others. Owen et al. (2009) conducted an 8-week, double-blind, placebo-controlled trial of flexibly dosed aripiprazole (2–15 mg/day) in 98 youth ages 6–17 years with autism. They reported significant improvement in irritability, as demonstrated with the CGI-I and the ABC Irritability subscale. Weight gain, drooling, tremor, vomiting, and sedation were among the adverse effects recorded, with post hoc analysis revealing higher mean increases in weight and rates of somnolence, sedation, and fatigue in antipsychotic-naive subjects (Mankoski et al. 2013).

The long-term safety and tolerability of aripiprazole (range, 2–15 mg/day) for irritability in children and adolescents ages 6–17 years with autism was examined in a 52-week open-label, flexibly dosed study (Marcus et al. 2011b). In addition to de novo subjects, patients from the aforementioned studies by Marcus et al. (2009) and Owen et al. (2009) were eligible to enroll. Of the 300 participants, 199 (66%) completed 52 weeks of treatment. Common adverse effects included weight gain, vomiting, and increased appetite, among others. Efficacy, a secondary objective after safety and tolerability, was evaluated using the CGI-I and the ABC Irritability subscale (Marcus et al. 2011a). Concomitant psychotropic agents were permitted during the study (except α_2-adrenergic agonists, carbamazepine, oxcarbazepine, and other antipsychotics). At end point, most subjects had a CGI-I score of "much improved" or "very much improved." The authors concluded that aripiprazole reduced symptoms of irritability associated with autism in youth ages 6–17 years.

A separate blind, placebo-controlled study examined the efficacy of long-term aripiprazole usage compared with placebo among children and adolescents with autism whose symptoms had responded to short-term aripiprazole treatment (Findling et al. 2014). An initial 157 subjects completed 13–26 weeks of single-blinded aripiprazole treatment. Eighty-five subjects whose symptoms responded to treatment, as defined by a change in ABC Irritability subscale and CGI-I scores, were randomly assigned to blinded allocation to placebo or to ongoing aripiprazole treatment for 16 additional weeks (mean dosage at study completion, 9.7 mg/day). No statistically significant differences in Kaplan-Meier relapse rates were found between aripiprazole and placebo; however, a post hoc analysis demonstrated a number needed to treat of 6 to prevent one additional relapse, which the authors concluded signified that some patients could benefit from maintenance treatment. The most significant common long-term adverse events were upper respiratory tract infection (10.3%), constipation (5.1%), and movement disorder (5.1%).

A more recent double-blind, placebo-controlled trial sought to compare the efficacy and tolerability of risperidone and aripiprazole in children and adolescents ages 6–17 years with ASD and significant irritability (DeVane et al. 2019). By the end of a 10-week, double-blind treatment phase, there was a nonsignificant trend toward superiority for risperidone as measured using the ABC Irritability subscale, and there were no differences in CGI-I scores. Efficacy results between the two treatment arms were similar after an additional 12-week open-label extension. Both groups demonstrated significant reductions in ABC Irritability subscale and CGI-I scores compared with baseline. Mean weight gain in the aripiprazole treatment arm was significantly less than that in the risperidone group at 10 weeks (1.38 kg vs. 3.31 kg), but the difference between groups became nonsignificant for the 31 participants who completed the 12-week extension.

Paliperidone

Paliperidone (9-hydroxy-risperidone) is FDA approved for the treatment of schizophrenia in adolescents ages 12–17 years. Stigler et al. (2012) evaluated the effectiveness and tolerability of paliperidone for irritability in autism. In this 8-week, prospective, open-label study, 21 of 25 subjects (84%) with autism (mean age, 15.3 years; range, 12–21 years) were considered responders to paliperidone (mean dosage, 7.1 mg/day; range, 3–12 mg/day), based on CGI-I and ABC Irritability subscale scores. Mean serum prolactin increased from 5.3 ng/mL (baseline) to 41.4 ng/mL (end point); however, no signs or symptoms associated with hyperprolactinemia were observed or reported. Weight gain, sedation, and EPS were among the adverse effects reported.

Lurasidone

Lurasidone antagonizes dopamine D_2 and serotonin 5-HT_{2A} receptor systems with high affinity and is FDA approved for the treatment of schizophrenia and bipolar I depression in adults. Loebel et al. (2016) evaluated the effectiveness and tolerability of lurasidone for irritability in ASD in a 6-week, double-blind, placebo-controlled study of outpatients ages 6–17 years with ASD. The study had three treatment arms: placebo (n=51), lurasidone 20 mg/day (n=50), and lurasidone 60 mg/day (n=49). By 6 weeks, there were no differences between either the 20-mg/day or 60-mg/day groups versus placebo on the primary outcome measures of ABC Irritability subscale or CGI-I scores. Vomiting and somnolence were the most common side effects. Subjects in the 60-mg/day treatment arm showed greater rates of weight gain compared with placebo, but those in the 20-mg/day arm did not.

Metformin

Metformin hydrochloride is a biguanide medication that increases insulin sensitivity and decreases intestinal glucose absorption and hepatic glucose production. It is approved for the treatment of type 2 diabetes and has been found to stop or reverse weight gain associated with antipsychotic medications (Zheng et al. 2015). Anagnostou et al. (2016) published a 16-week, double-blind, placebo-controlled study to evaluate the tolerability and efficacy of metformin for weight gain rate reduction in 60 subjects ages 6–17 years with ASD. Metformin was titrated up to 500 mg bid for children ages 6–9 years and 850 mg bid for those ages 10–17 years. For subjects with weight gain associated with starting an atypical antipsychotic, metformin reduced rates of BMI increase (*z* score) and weight gain compared with placebo. A small percentage of subjects (11%) taking metformin experienced a decrease in BMI of 8%–9%. A difference between treatment and placebo arms was not apparent until after 8 weeks of treatment. Gastrointestinal adverse events were the most common, and five subjects in the treatment arm discontinued due to adverse events (agitation, $n=4$; sedation, $n=1$). A 16-week, open-label follow-up study of the same participants found that improvements in the rate of weight gain seen in the treatment arm were maintained but without additional decreases in BMI or weight (Handen et al. 2017).

Serotonin Reuptake Inhibitors

Research into the pathophysiology of ASD identified some abnormalities in serotonergic system function. Schain and Freedman (1961) first reported on elevated whole-blood levels of serotonin in children with autism compared with control children. Additional reports have pointed to the possibility of abnormal maturational processes of the serotonergic system in youth with autism, as exhibited by a lack of age-related decline in blood levels of serotonin as seen in typically developing subjects (Anderson et al. 1987; Leboyer et al. 1999).

Research into the genetic basis of a potential serotonergic abnormality in autism has yielded mixed results. Some studies have noted nominally significant excess transmission of alleles of the serotonin transporter gene, whereas other studies have reported no excess transmission (Conroy et al. 2004).

Other evidence suggesting the potential utility of medications affecting serotonin in patients with ASD comes from findings of an exacerbation of behavioral symptoms in medication-free adults with autism experiencing acute dietary depletion of the serotonin precursor tryptophan (McDougle et al. 1996b).

Clomipramine

Clomipramine is a tricyclic antidepressant that potently inhibits serotonin reuptake and affects norepinephrine and dopamine reuptake (Greist et al. 1995). Clomipramine is FDA approved for the treatment of OCD in youth ages 10–17 years.

One open-label and two controlled studies have evaluated clomipramine in patients with ASD. In a 12-week open-label trial of clomipramine (mean dosage, 139.4 ± 50.4 mg/day) in 35 adults with PDDs, 18 of the 33 participants (55%) who completed the trial were judged, based on their CGI-I scores, to have a treatment response (Brodkin et al. 1997). Improvement in aggression, self-injurious behavior, repetitive phenomena, and social relatedness was recorded. Thirteen patients (39%) experienced significant adverse effects, including seizures ($n=3$), weight gain, constipation, sedation, and agitation.

In another study, clomipramine (mean dosage, 152±56 mg/day) was shown to be superior to the relatively selective norepinephrine reuptake inhibitor desipramine (mean dosage, 127±52 mg/day) and to placebo in a 10-week, randomized crossover study of 24 children with autism (mean age, 9.6 years) (Gordon et al. 1993). Improvement with clomipramine was associated with decreased anger and obsessive-compulsive symptoms. Adverse effects included tachycardia, QTc interval prolongation, and a grand mal seizure in one subject. Similar tolerability issues were noted by Remington et al. (2001) in their report on a 7-week, double-blind, placebo-controlled trial of clomipramine (mean dosage, 128 mg/day), haloperidol (mean dosage, 1.3 mg/day), and placebo in 36 patients ages 10–36 years with autism. Among patients who completed this trial, clomipramine and haloperidol were similarly effective in reducing irritability and stereotypy. However, significantly fewer individuals receiving clomipramine versus haloperidol were able to complete the trial (37.5% vs. 69.7%). Reasons for leaving the trial that were associated with clomipramine included lack of efficacy and the emergence of adverse effects, among which sedation and tremor were most prevalent. Because of tolerability issues, the use of clomipramine in patients with ASD remains limited.

Fluvoxamine

Fluvoxamine is a selective serotonin reuptake inhibitor (SSRI) FDA-approved for use in children and adolescents ages 8–17 years with OCD. In a double-blind, placebo-controlled study, fluvoxamine (mean dosage, 276.7 mg/day) reduced repetitive and maladaptive behavior in 8 of 15 adults with autism (53%) randomly assigned to the active drug (McDougle et al. 1996a). In these adults, fluvoxamine was generally well tolerated, with adverse effects including sedation and nausea. A double-blind, placebo-controlled study did not find fluvoxamine (mean dosage, 107 mg/day) effective for repetitive behavior in 34 children and adolescents with PDDs (McDougle et al. 2000). In these younger patients, fluvoxamine was poorly tolerated, with 14 patients experiencing adverse effects, including hyperactivity, insomnia, aggression, and agitation. In an open-label report of 18 youth (mean age, 11.3 ±3.6 years) with PDDs treated with low-dosage fluvoxamine (1.5 mg/kg/day) for 10 weeks, the drug was similarly not associated with a significant treatment response (Martin et al. 2003). In a 12-week, double-blind, placebo-controlled crossover study of fluvoxamine in 18 children with autism, Sugie et al. (2005) noted that 10 patients (55%) had at least a *mild* treatment response, with 5 (28%) showing an *excellent* drug response in terms of global improvement on the CGI-I scale. In this report, fluvoxamine was generally well tolerated. Three children (17%) had to exit the study due to behavioral activation. Overall, although findings are mixed, fluvoxamine appears to be better tolerated in adults than in youth with ASD.

Fluoxetine

Fluoxetine is an SSRI that is FDA-approved in children and adolescents for the treatment of OCD (ages 7–17 years) and major depressive disorder (ages 8–17 years). Two open-label trials and three small, placebo-controlled crossover trials suggested fluoxetine may be effective for repetitive symptoms in patients with autism (Buchsbaum et al. 2001; DeLong et al. 2002; Fatemi et al. 1998; Hollander et al. 2005, 2012). Hollander et al. (2005) performed a 20-week, placebo-controlled, crossover study of fluoxetine (mean dosage, 9.9 mg/day; range 2.4–20 mg/day) in 39 children (mean age, 8.2 years) with PDDs. They found that the medication performed significantly better than placebo in reducing repetitive behaviors. No improvement in measures of speech or social interaction was noted, and adverse effects were not significantly different between fluoxetine and placebo. Moreover, Hollander et al. (2012) performed a trial of fluoxetine among mostly higher-functioning adults with ASD (mean age, 34.3 years) in a 12-week, placebo-controlled study design. Similarly, subjects receiving the active drug (mean dosage, 64.76 mg/day) showed statistically significant reductions in compulsive behavior as measured by the Yale-Brown Obsessive Compulsive Scale (Y-BOCS) and general improvement in repetitive symptoms as measured with the CGI.

In contrast, the Study of Fluoxetine in Autism (SOFIA) study—a large-scale, 14-week, double-blind, placebo-controlled study in 158 children and adolescents ages 5–17 years with autism—determined that fluoxetine (dosage, 2–18 mg/day) was no more effective than placebo for repetitive behavior (Herscu et al. 2020). Subjects with ASD in this larger study had, on average, lower intellectual and adaptive functioning than those in the earlier Hollander et al. (2012) trial. A 16-week, double-blind, placebo-controlled study (Reddihough et al. 2019) included 146 youth ages 7.5–18 years with ASD and examined fluoxetine for the treatment of repetitive behavior. Although the study used higher dosages (20–30 mg) and included higher-functioning subjects (only 30% with intellectual disability), the results were equivocal. At study end point, the difference in change in Children's Yale-Brown Obsessive Compulsive Scale (CY-BOCS) PDD scores (3.72-point decrease in the fluoxetine group vs. 2.53-point decrease in placebo group) became nonsignificant after controlling for group differences. Moreover, there was no difference in CGI-I scores between the treatment and placebo groups. In summary, results with fluoxetine bear similarities to those with fluvoxamine, supporting a stronger research basis for the use of SSRIs in adults with ASD than for youth with the disorder.

Sertraline

To date, only open-label trials have described the use of the SSRI sertraline in the treatment of ASD. Sertraline is approved for the treatment of OCD in children ages 6–17 years. In a 12-week open-label study of 42 adults with PDDs, McDougle et al. (1998a) found that sertraline (mean dosage, 122 mg/day) was effective for reducing aggression and repetitive behavior. Participants with autism and PDD-NOS showed significantly more improvement than did those with Asperger's disorder. The authors attributed this response to the possibility that subjects with Asperger's disorder had been less symptomatic at baseline. Three patients (7%) dropped out of the study because of worsening agitation and anxiety. An open-label trial of sertraline (25–50 mg/day for 2–8 weeks) was conducted in nine children ages 6–12 years with autism (Steingard et al. 1997). Eight children (88%) showed improvement during the trial, manifesting reduced irritability, anxiety, and need for sameness.

Paroxetine

The SSRI paroxetine has been the subject of a few uncontrolled reports in ASD. Case reports have noted decreased irritable behavior associated with paroxetine use in a 15-year-old boy with autism (Snead et al. 1994) and a 7-year-old boy with autism (Posey et al. 1999). In a heterogeneous sample, 15 adults with intellectual disability with or without a concomitant diagnosis of PDD received 16 weeks of open-label treatment with paroxetine (20–50 mg/day) (Davanzo et al. 1998). The drug was associated with reduced aggression after 1 month but not at the 4-month follow-up.

Citalopram

A 12-week, double-blind, placebo-controlled study of citalopram (mean dosage, 16.5±6.5 mg/day) for repetitive behavior was conducted in 149 children and adolescents (mean age, 9.4 years; range, 5–17 years) with PDDs (King et al. 2009). In contrast to the positive preliminary findings of the retrospective studies, this large-scale controlled study found citalopram to be ineffective for repetitive behaviors. In addition, citalopram was more likely to be associated with adverse effects, including increased energy level, impulsiveness, hyperactivity, decreased concentration, stereotypy, and insomnia, among others.

Escitalopram

Escitalopram, the *S*-enantiomer of citalopram, is approved for the treatment of major depressive disorder in adolescents ages 12–17 years. A 10-week open-label study of escitalopram (mean dosage, 11.1 mg/day) in 28 youth (mean age, 10.4 years) with PDDs found that 17 (61%) were treatment responders, with response defined as a 50% reduction in parent-rated ABC Irritability subscale scores (Owley et al. 2005). A wide variety of dose response was noted, with some participants unable to tolerate the medication at 10 mg/day and others showing positive response at the lowest dosage of 2.5 mg/day.

Other Medications With Serotonergic Effects

Mirtazapine

Mirtazapine, a drug with both serotonergic and noradrenergic properties, was evaluated in an open-label trial in patients with ASD (Posey et al. 2001). Twenty-six subjects with ASD were given mirtazapine (range, 7.5–45 mg/day) over a mean duration of 150 days. Nine patients (35%) were considered treatment responders, as measured with the CGI-I, with reduced aggression, self-injury, irritability, hyperactivity, anxiety, insomnia, and depression. No effect on social relatedness or communication impairment was noted. Adverse effects were considered mild and included increased appetite, irritability, and sedation. A retrospective study investigated the effectiveness of mirtazapine (mean dosage, 21.6 mg/day; range, 15–30 mg/day) for inappropriate sexual behavior (e.g., excessive masturbation) in 10 youth ages 5–16 years with autistic disorder (Coskun et al. 2009). Eight of the 10 patients were deemed by their CGI-I scores as having "much improved" or "very much improved" in the symptom of excessive masturbation. Increased appetite, weight gain, and sedation were among the most frequently reported adverse effects.

A recent 10-week, double-blind, placebo-controlled pilot trial examined mirtazapine for the treatment of anxiety in youth ages 5–17 years with ASD (McDougle et al. 2022). Thirty subjects were randomly assigned to mirtazapine (mean dosage, 41.8 ± 5.2 mg) or placebo in a 2:1 ratio, with the CGI-I measuring anxiety and the Pediatric Anxiety Rating Scale (PARS) as primary outcome measures. A nonsignificant trend toward superiority of mirtazapine compared with placebo was observed with the PARS (effect size, 0.63). For 47% of participants assigned to mirtazapine, symptoms were considered much improved (CGI-I = 2) or very much improved (CGI-I = 1) compared with 20% of those assigned to placebo. No subjects withdrew due to adverse effects. Although the most common side effects with mirtazapine were sedation/drowsiness, appetite increase, and irritability, no statistically significant difference was found in the frequency of adverse effects between the placebo and the active drug. Although the results were not statistically significant, the authors concluded that mirtazapine showed favorable tolerability and efficacy, which warrant conducting a controlled trial of mirtazapine for anxiety in a larger population of subjects with ASD.

Venlafaxine

Venlafaxine is a dual serotonin and norepinephrine reuptake inhibitor. Low-dose venlafaxine (18.75 mg/day) was associated with decreased hyperactivity and irritability in two adolescents and one young adult with autistic disorder over 6 months of treatment (Carminati et al. 2006). A retrospective review of 10 children, adolescents, and young adults with ASD treated with venlafaxine (6.25–50 mg/day) found that 6 (60%) were responders, as defined by the CGI-I (Hollander et al. 2000). The medication was reportedly well tolerated, and improvement in repetitive behaviors, socialization, communication, and inattention was noted. One case report noted increased aggressive behavior when venlafaxine (37.5 mg increased to 75 mg/day) was added to the treatment regimen of an adolescent female with autistic disorder who was also taking a stable dosage of olanzapine (10 mg/day) (Marshall et al. 2003).

Buspirone

Buspirone is a serotonin 5-HT_{1A} receptor partial agonist with FDA approval for the treatment of generalized anxiety disorder in adults. Several case reports and small open-label studies have reported on the effectiveness of buspirone in patients with ASD. Larger open-label studies have generated conflicting results. An open-label study of buspirone (30–60 mg/day for 28–413 days) found it to be ineffective in treating target symptoms, including aggression and self-injury, in a sample of 26 adults with intellectual disability, which included 9 patients with ASD (King and Davanzo 1996). In another open-label study, however, 22 children and adolescents with ASD were treated with buspirone (15–45 mg/day) for 6–8 weeks (Buitelaar et al. 1998). Nine patients (41%) showed significant improvement as measured with the CGI-I, addressing target symptoms of anxiety and irritability. During a continuation phase for treatment responders, one child developed an orofacial-lingual dyskinesia after 10 months of treatment that remitted following drug discontinuation.

In an 8-week, randomized, double-blind, placebo-controlled trial of buspirone in combination with risperidone in children and adolescents ages 4–17 years with autistic disorder, investigators found that buspirone added to risperidone was more effective than risperidone alone in the treatment of ASD-related irritability (Ghanizadeh and Ayoobzadehshirazi 2015). Concomitant medications were allowed as long as they were stable for the study duration. A total of 40 subjects participated in the study, and the target dosages of risperidone were 2 mg/day for subjects weighing less than 40 kg and 3 mg/day for those weighing more than 40 kg. The target dosages of buspirone were 10 mg/day for subjects weighing less than 40 kg and 20 mg/day for those weighing more than 40 kg. Both medications reached the target dosage by week 2 and could be modified afterward based on efficacy and side effects; dosages could not exceed the targets set. A positive response was defined as a 25% or greater decrease in ABC Irritability subscale score. The results showed that 81.2% of subjects in the buspirone group were classified as responders compared with 44.4% in the placebo group. The mean risperidone dosage between groups was not statistically different. Side effects were most common in the buspirone group and included increased appetite, drowsiness, and fatigue. Both appetite increase and decrease and dry mouth were reported in the placebo group (Ghanizadeh and Ayoobzadehshirazi 2015).

A larger double-blind, placebo-controlled study of low-dose buspirone in young children with ASD examined the drug's effect in reducing core symptoms of autism (Chugani et al. 2016). The 166-subject trial was conducted in children ages 2–6 years with ASD over 48 weeks of treatment, with the Autism Diagnostic Observation Schedule (ADOS) as the primary outcome measure. No significant differences were seen in total ADOS score between the placebo and treatment arms, and there were no significant differences in adverse events between the placebo group and the 2.5-mg-bid and 5-mg-bid groups. A decrease in the ADOS restricted repetitive behaviors subcategory was seen in the 2.5-mg-bid group compared with the placebo and the 5-mg-bid groups. However, the authors acknowledged limitations in the use of the ADOS as an outcome measure for autism severity. Further trials exploring the use of buspirone for repetitive behaviors in ASD are required.

Psychostimulants

Psychostimulants are considered first-line agents for the treatment of hyperactivity and inattention in patients diagnosed with ADHD (Greenhill et al. 2002b). Whereas some preliminary research concluded that stimulants were generally ineffective and associated with adverse effects in patients with autistic disorder (Aman 1982; Campbell 1975; Stigler et al. 2004a), other trials have suggested that they may be effective in this population. Methylphenidate is FDA-approved for the treatment of ADHD in children and adolescents ages 6–17 years. A double-blind, crossover study (2-week treatment phases) of methylphenidate (10 mg or 20 mg bid) was conducted in 10 children ages 7–11 years with autistic disorder (Quintana et al. 1995). Overall, a modest benefit of methylphenidate treatment over placebo was found. Adverse effects included insomnia, irritability, and decreased appetite. Another double-blind, placebo-controlled crossover study of methylphenidate (0.3 mg/kg/day and 0.6 mg/kg/day) found a 50% reduction in the Conners' Hyperactivity Index scores in 8 of 13 children (62%) ages 5–11 years with autistic disorder (Handen et al. 2000). Adverse effects, which were more common with the 0.6-mg/kg/day dosage, included social withdrawal and irritability.

The RUPP Autism Network completed the largest controlled trial of a psychostimulant in patients with ASD to date. This study involved 72 youth ages 5–14 years with target symptoms of moderate to severe hyperactivity. Subjects entered a 1-week test-dosage phase in which placebo and three doses (low, medium, and high) of methylphenidate were administered. The 66 subjects who tolerated the test-dosage phase received 1 week each of placebo and methylphenidate at three different dosages in random order during a 4-week, double-blind, crossover phase. Those whose symptoms responded to methylphenidate then entered an 8-week open-label phase. Overall, 35 of 72 enrolled subjects (49%) experienced a response to methylphenidate. Discontinuation of study medication due to adverse effects occurred in 13 of 72 subjects (18%) (Research Units on Pediatric Psychopharmacology Autism Network 2005a). These results are consistent with the findings of a smaller study of methylphenidate in 13 youth with ASD (Di Martino et al. 2004) in which five participants developed increased hyperactivity, stereotypy, dysphoria, or tics within 1 hour of a single test dose (0.4 mg/kg) and were unable to tolerate the medication. Symptoms in six of the remaining eight subjects responded to the methylphenidate, resulting in an overall response rate of 46%.

In contrast with these findings, data from the National Institute of Mental Health Multimodal Treatment of ADHD (MTA) study showed that 69% of typically developing youth with ADHD experienced a response to methylphenidate treatment, with only 1.4% discontinuing due to adverse effects (Greenhill et al. 2002a). Methylphenidate is less effective and is associated with more frequent adverse effects in youth with ASD and ADHD than in typically developing youth with ADHD. A within-subjects crossover, double-blind, placebo-controlled study of three different dosages (low, 0.21 mg/kg; medium, 0.35 mg/kg; and high, 0.48 mg/kg) of extended-release methylphenidate was published in 2013 (Pearson et al. 2013). The specific extended-release formulation used mimicked twice-daily dosing, with a morning dose of extended-release methylphenidate that was combined with a dose of immediate-release methylphenidate in the afternoon. This study included 24 school-age children (mean age, 8.8±1.7 years; mean IQ, 85±16.8) with ASD. In the double-blind phase, subjects were given 1 week at each dosage level, including placebo. Decreases in hyperactivity and impulsivity based on parent and teacher measures were found at both the high and medium dosage levels. Teachers were able to detect a small difference with the lower dosage. Reduction in oppositional behavior and improvement in social skills were also found on parent measures. The side effect profile of the long-acting stimulant preparation was similar to the immediate-release formulation, with trouble sleeping and appetite changes being the predominant side effects. Of note, no significant increase in irritability, repetitive behavior, or repetitive language was observed in this study. In a follow-up study completed with the same cohort, extended-release methylphenidate demonstrated improvements in cognitive performance, specifically in the areas of sustained attention, impulsivity/inhibition, and selective attention (Pearson et al. 2020).

Kim et al. (2017) completed a 6-week pilot study with 27 children ages 5–15 years with ASD and ADHD to examine the dose-effect response to long-acting liquid methylphenidate. Initially, participants were randomly assigned to one of three dosage groups: very low (5–10 mg/day), low (5–20 mg/day), and moderate (5–40 mg/day). Because the maximum tolerated dosage was 20 mg/day in all but two participants in the moderate-dosage group, that and the low-dosage group were combined and renamed the medium-dosage group. The ADHD Rating Scale was administered by a blinded clinician, and the scores showed a significant linear downward trend in both dosage groups. By the end of week 6, the CGI-I score was "much improved" or "very much improved" in 83% of the medium-dosage group compared with 33% of the low-dosage group. The medium-dosage group also displayed improvement in all five subscales of the ABC, a secondary measure. No serious adverse events were reported in this study. In the medium-dosage group, aggression, irritability, and end-of-the-day rebound decreased from baseline.

Other Drug Treatments for ADHD

Clonidine

Clonidine is an α_2-adrenergic agonist, and its extended-release formulation (clonidine ER) has been FDA approved for the treatment of ADHD in children and adolescents ages 6–17 years. Clonidine has been evaluated in two small controlled trials involving youth with autism/autistic disorder. A double-blind, placebo-controlled, crossover trial (6-week treatment periods) of clonidine (4–10 µg/kg/day) was conducted in eight young males with autism (mean age, 8.1 years) with symptoms of inattention, impulsivity, and hyperactivity (Jaselskis et al. 1992). The drug was associated with decreased hyperactivity and irritability on teacher and parent ratings, but no treatment-associated differences on clinician ratings were found. Adverse effects of clonidine included hypotension, sedation, and irritability. Transdermal clonidine (5 μg/kg/day) was evaluated in a double-blind, placebo-controlled, crossover study (4-week treatment phases) involving nine males ages 5–33 years with autistic disorder (Fankhauser et al. 1992). Significant improvement in hyperactivity and anxiety was recorded. The most commonly reported adverse effects were sedation and fatigue. To date, no studies of effectiveness of clonidine ER specifically in individuals with ASD have been published.

Guanfacine

Guanfacine is an α_2-adrenergic agonist, and its extended-release formulation (guanfacine ER) is FDA-approved for the treatment of ADHD in youth ages 6–17 years. Preliminary research suggested that guanfacine may be well tolerated and beneficial for hyperactivity symptoms in children and adolescents with ASD (Posey et al. 2004b). A prospective, open-label trial was conducted in 25 youth (mean age, 9 years; range, 5–14 years) with autism and hyperactivity whose symptoms had previously not responded to methylphenidate (Scahill et al. 2006). In this study, 48% of patients showed improvement in hyperactivity at total daily doses of 1–3 mg. Decreased frustration tolerance and tearfulness led three patients to discontinue the study. A small double-blind, placebo-controlled trial of guanfacine was completed in 11 children with hyperactivity and intellectual disability and/or autism (Handen et al. 2008). Forty-five percent of participants had a significant reduction in hyperactivity. The most common adverse effects included increased irritability and drowsiness. To date, one case report of guanfacine ER in patients with autism/ASD has been published (Blankenship et al. 2011). The authors found improvement in inattention, hyperactivity, and impulsivity in two patients (ages 4 and 9 years) at total daily dosages of 2–3 mg. Adverse effects included sedation and reduced blood pressure. An 8-week, randomized, double-blind, placebo-controlled trial of guanfacine ER was conducted in 62 youth (mean age, 8.5 ± 2.5 years) with ASD (Scahill et al. 2015). Subjects were classified as positive responders if their CGI-I score was "much improved" or "very much improved." Fifty percent of participants in the guanfacine ER group were classified as responders compared with 9.4% of the placebo group. The guanfacine ER group also exhibited significant improvement compared with the placebo group on the ABC Hyperactivity subscale. The maximum dosage of guanfacine ER was 3 mg/day for participants weighing less than 25 kg and 4 mg/day for those weighing more than 25 kg. The dosage schedule was not fixed, and dosages could be adjusted to manage side effects. With the exception of stable doses of antiepileptic medications, no other medications were allowed in this study. Sedation, fatigue, and decreased appetite were the most common side effects. Blood pressure was lower than baseline in the guanfacine ER group for approximately 4 weeks and returned to nearly baseline values by week 8. No clinically significant ECG changes were observed in this study.

Atomoxetine

The selective norepinephrine reuptake inhibitor atomoxetine is approved for the treatment of youth ages 6–17 years with ADHD. Results of two open-label studies suggested that the drug may decrease symptoms of motor hyperactivity and inattention in less severely affected children and adolescents with ASD (Posey et al. 2006; Troost et al. 2006). In the study by Posey et al. (2006), 16 youth ages 6–14 years with autism received atomoxetine at a mean dosage of 1.2 mg/kg/day. Of these 16 subjects, 12 (75%) were deemed responders. The medication was well tolerated, aside from two patients who discontinued due to irritability. A 10-week open-label study of atomoxetine (mean dosage, 1.2 mg/kg/day) was conducted in 12 youth with ASD (Troost et al. 2006). Although treatment led to a 44% reduction in ADHD symptoms, five subjects (42%) discontinued the study due to adverse effects such as irritability, nausea, and anxiety. A placebo-controlled, crossover pilot study of atomoxetine was completed in 16 youth ages 5–15 years with autism and hyperactivity (Arnold et al. 2006). Of the 16 participants, 9 (56%) demonstrated a significant reduction in symptoms of hyperactivity. One patient was rehospitalized for recurrent irritability on the drug. Upper gastrointestinal symptoms and fatigue were the most frequently reported adverse effects. A randomized 8-week, double-blind, placebo-controlled study of atomoxetine for ADHD symptoms in children with ASD demonstrated a moderate improvement in ADHD symptoms. There were a total of 97 subjects in the study, with an age range of 6–17 years. All had an IQ of at least 60. Dosages were titrated up over a 3-week period to atomoxetine 1.2 mg/kg/day or placebo. After 8 weeks of treatment, ADHD Rating Scale total and subscale scores improved significantly in the atomoxetine group, and the mean Conners' Teacher Rating Scale hyperactivity score decreased significantly. No serious adverse events were reported, and nausea, decreased appetite, headache, and fatigue were the most common side effects. One subject in the atomoxetine group discontinued the trial secondary to fatigue.

As has been seen with other medication trials for ADHD symptoms in subjects with ASD, lower rates of response to treatment were observed compared with similar trials in more typically developing subjects with ADHD alone. The studies of typically developing children with ADHD found no difference between improvement in hyperactivity and improvement in inattention with atomoxetine, whereas the study of children with ASD and ADHD found greater improvement in hyperactivity over inattention (Harfterkamp et al. 2012). No beneficial effect was observed in social interaction. There were, however, some signs of beneficial effects of atomoxetine in regard to inappropriate speech, fear of change, and stereotypies. Eighty-eight subjects (42 in the atomoxetine group and 46 who initially received placebo) were followed for an additional 20 weeks in an open-label extension phase (Harfterkamp et al. 2014). No drug-related serious adverse events occurred during this phase. Subjects in this phase demonstrated continued improvement in ADHD symptoms as well as subsiding adverse effects (Harfterkamp et al. 2014).

Combining non-drug interventions with psychopharmacology is a common question of interest in many psychiatric disorders, including ADHD. In a 10-week, randomized, double-blind placebo-controlled study, adding parent training to atomoxetine did not result in a statistically significant improvement in response rate versus drug alone. The study had 128 subjects ages 5–14 years; 99 completed the study. Responders were characterized by a CGI-I score of 2 or less and a decrease in Swanson, Nolan, and Pelham (SNAP) Teacher and Parent Rating Scale score of 30 or more. The results showed that 45.2% of subjects in the atomoxetine group were classified as responders compared with 46.9% in the combined treatment group. This difference was not statistically significant. Although adding parent training to atomoxetine did not result in a significant difference compared with atomoxetine alone, parent training alone was significantly better than placebo. Atomoxetine was well tolerated; however, complaints of abdominal pain and decreased appetite were significantly higher in the atomoxetine group (Handen et al. 2015). At the end of a 24-week open-label extension of this study, 68% of responders originally in the atomoxetine group continued to meet response criteria. Subjects who participated in the open-label trial were more likely to be considered responders with a combination of parent therapy and atomoxetine (Smith et al. 2016). At 1.5 years, most of the subjects retained their 34-week improvement; only 34% were still taking atomoxetine, 27% were taking stimulants, and 25% were taking no medication (Arnold et al. 2018).

Mood Stabilizers

Valproic Acid

The mood stabilizer and antiepileptic drug valproic acid (divalproex sodium) has been investigated in open-label and double-blind, placebo-controlled studies in individuals with autism (Hellings et al. 2005; Hollander et al. 2001, 2006a, 2010).

An 8-week, double-blind, placebo-controlled study of valproic acid (mean blood level, 77.8 μg/mL at 8 weeks) was conducted in 30 youth ages 6–20 years with autism and significant aggressive behavior (Hellings et al. 2005). In this trial, treatment was not associated with significant improvement in irritability as measured by the ABC Irritability subscale or in global symptoms as measured with the CGI-I. One participant developed a rash, which remitted following drug discontinuation, and two others developed elevated serum ammonia. In an 8-week, double-blind, placebo-controlled trial of valproic acid in 13 youth with autism and interfering repetitive behaviors, treatment was associated with a significant reduction in repetitive phenomena as measured with the CY-BOCS (Hollander et al. 2006a). Overall, the medication was well tolerated. A 12-week, double-blind, placebo-controlled study of valproic acid was completed in 27 youth ages 5–15 years with ASD and irritability (Hollander et al. 2010). The authors reported that 62.5% of the valproic acid group experienced a response to treatment versus 9% of the placebo group (mean blood level, 89.8 μg/mL for responders vs. 64.3 μg/mL for nonresponders). Irritability, insomnia, headache, and weight gain were among the adverse effects reported.

Lithium

Lithium is a mood stabilizer that is FDA-approved for the treatment of bipolar disorder in youth ages 12–17 years. Three case reports have described the use of lithium in patients with ASD. Two reports have noted reduced manic-like symptoms in individuals with ASD and a family history of bipolar disorder

(Kerbeshian et al. 1987; Steingard and Biederman 1987). A single report of lithium augmentation of fluvoxamine in an adult with autistic disorder noted improvement in symptoms of aggression and irritability after 2 weeks of treatment, as measured with the CGI-I (Epperson et al. 1994). A retrospective chart review was conducted in 30 psychiatrically hospitalized subjects with ASD who were prescribed lithium for mood disorder and/or irritability (Siegel et al. 2014). The mean age of this sample was 13.6 years, and 53.3% of the subjects had a full-scale IQ of less than 70. Overall, 43% of participants demonstrated improvement based on a CGI-I score of 1 or 2. A greater effect was noted when at least two pretreatment mood symptoms were present, especially mania and euphoria/elevated mood. The mean lithium blood level was 0.70 mEq/L. Improved status on the CGI-I did not correlate with lithium blood levels. Most study participants were also taking other psychotropic medications, and all had a history of exposure to atypical antipsychotics. The average length of treatment was 29.7 days. A high rate of side effects (47%) was reported, with the most common being vomiting (13%), tremor (10%), fatigue (10%), irritability (7%), and enuresis (7%) (Siegel et al. 2014).

Lamotrigine

Lamotrigine is an anticonvulsant and mood stabilizer that attenuates some forms of glutamate release via inhibition of sodium, calcium, and potassium channels. The use of lamotrigine (mean dosage, 4.5 mg/kg/day) over a mean duration of 14 months was described in 13 children ages 3–13 years with autism and intractable epilepsy (Uvebrant and Bauzienè 1994). Eight subjects (62%) showed a decrease in autism symptoms. Adverse effects included sleep disturbance and rash. In a 4-week, double-blind, placebo-controlled trial of lamotrigine (5 mg/kg/day) in 14 children ages 3–11 years with autistic disorder, Belsito et al. (2001) reported no treatment-associated benefit as measured by the ABC, Childhood Autism Rating Scale, and Pre-Linguistic Autism Diagnostic Observation Scale. Insomnia and hyperactivity were the most common side effects reported.

Levetiracetam

Levetiracetam is an anticonvulsant with inhibitory and neuroprotective properties. A 10-week, double-blind, placebo-controlled trial of the drug (mean dosage, 862.5 mg/day; range, 500–1,250 mg/day) was conducted in 20 youth ages 5–17 years with ASD (Wasserman et al. 2006). No significant difference was found between levetiracetam and placebo on global measures of autism or on measures of irritability, affective instability, and repetitive behavior. Overall, the drug was well tolerated, with mild agitation, aggression, and hyperactivity among the adverse effects reported.

Cholinesterase Inhibitors

Donepezil

The cholinesterase inhibitor donepezil has been evaluated in two open-label reports in patients with ASD. Improved speech was noted in 25 young males (mean age, 6.6 years) given donepezil (2.5 mg/day or 5 mg/day) over 12 weeks of open-label treatment (Chez et al. 2000). No improvement in social relatedness was noted. Adverse effects included aggression, irritability, sedation, and sleep disturbance. In a retrospective review of open-label donepezil add-on treatment (mean dosage, 9.4±1.8 mg/day), Hardan and Handen (2002) reported that four of eight patients (50%) ages 7–19 years with autistic disorder who were taking other psychotropic medications experienced a positive response to treatment as measured with the CGI-I. In addition, scores decreased on the Hyperactivity and Irritability subscales of the ABC. In this study, donepezil was generally well tolerated, with one patient developing nausea and vomiting and one patient reporting mild irritability. Handen et al. (2011) investigated the efficacy and tolerability of donepezil on executive functioning in 34 patients ages 8–17 years with autism. The study involved a 10-week, double-blind, placebo-controlled trial of donepezil (5 mg/day and 10 mg/day), followed by a 10-week open-label trial for placebo nonresponders. No significant differences were found between donepezil and placebo on measures of executive functioning. Mild adverse effects associated with the drug included diarrhea, headache, and fatigue.

Rivastigmine

The cholinesterase inhibitor rivastigmine was evaluated in a 12-week open-label trial in 32 participants with autistic disorder (Chez et al. 2004). Improvement with treatment was noted in expressive speech and overall autistic behavior using standardized measures.

Galantamine

Galantamine is a cholinesterase inhibitor and nicotinic receptor modulator. A 12-week open-label trial (mean dosage, 18.4 mg/day; range, 12–24 mg/day) was conducted in 13 youth ages 4–17 years with autistic disorder (Nicolson et al. 2006). The medication was well tolerated and considered beneficial for reducing symptoms of aggression, behavioral dyscontrol, and inattention. A 10-week, randomized, double-blind, placebo-controlled, parallel-groups study of galantamine in combination with risperidone in 40 children ages 4–12 years with ASD was published in 2014 (Ghaleiha et al. 2014). Compared with placebo, the group that received galantamine demonstrated improvement in the ABC Irritability and Lethargy/Social Withdrawal subscale scores. No significant differences in side effects between groups were reported (Ghaleiha et al. 2014).

Glutamatergic Agents

Amantadine

Amantadine, a compound used to treat influenza, herpes zoster, and Parkinson's disease, has known noncompetitive *N*-methyl-D-aspartate (NMDA) antagonist activity (Kornhuber et al. 1994). In one 4-week, double-blind, placebo-controlled trial in 39 youth ages 5–19 years with autistic disorder, amantadine (final dosage, 5 mg/kg/day) was associated with improved clinician ratings in the domains of hyperactivity and inappropriate speech on the ABC (King et al. 2001). No significant treatment-associated improvements were noted on parent ratings. The medication was reportedly well tolerated. A double-blind, placebo-controlled study using amantadine in conjunction with risperidone in 40 children ages 4–12 years with ASD demonstrated a beneficial effect in terms of hyperactivity and irritability as well as overall general improvement with amantadine (100–150 mg bid) compared with placebo. No significant differences in adverse effects between groups were seen (Mohammadi et al. 2013).

Memantine

Memantine is an uncompetitive NMDA antagonist used in the treatment of Alzheimer's disease. Initial open-label studies suggested improvement in social behavior and other core symptoms of autism (Chez et al. 2007) as well as in irritability, hyperactivity, and memory (Owley et al. 2006). Despite these promising findings, larger double-blind, placebo-controlled trials examining the extended-release formulation (memantine ER) for social impairment in ASD have failed to show differences from placebo (Aman et al. 2017; Hardan et al. 2019). These trials have used the Social Responsiveness Scale (SRS) as a primary outcome measure and employed multiple trial designs, including a 12-week randomized, placebo-controlled, open-label extension and a randomized treatment withdrawal. More than 1,000 youth ages 6–12 years with ASD participated in the trials. Secondary measures including the ABC for children and the CGI-I also failed to show significant differences between the placebo and treatment groups. High placebo responses on the SRS were noted. Within the 12-week trial and the 48-week open-label extension, irritability was the most common treatment-emergent adverse effect (6.7% in the treatment group vs. 3.3% in the placebo group).

D-Cycloserine

D-Cycloserine is an antibiotic traditionally used to treat tuberculosis. It is also an NMDA partial agonist shown to reduce the negative symptoms associated with schizophrenia (Goff et al. 1999). Ten medication-free patients with autistic disorder (mean age, 10±7.7 years) participated in an 8-week trial that began with a 2-week placebo lead-in phase followed by 2 weeks at each of three dosages: 0.7 mg/kg/day, 1.4 mg/kg/day, and 2.8 mg/kg/day (Posey et al. 2004a). D-Cycloserine was associated with improvement on the CGI-I and the Social Withdrawal subscale of the ABC. Four participants (40%) were considered responders based on CGI-I ratings of "much improved." Two patients (20%) had to drop out of the study due to development of a transient motor tic and increased echolalia, respectively. In a 10-week randomized, double-blind trial conducted by Urbano et al. (2014, 2015), 20 adolescents with ASD were randomly assigned to D-cycloserine, either 50 mg/day or 50 mg/week. Mean ages of participants were 17.9 years (SD 2.51) and 17.3 years (SD 2.83) for the daily-dose and weekly-dose groups, respectively. The groups received D-cycloserine for 8 weeks and were followed up for 2 weeks afterward for a total of 10 weeks. Participants were not required to stop all other psychiatric medications; however, those medications had to be maintained at their current dosage for the duration of the trial. A 37% decrease in the ABC Stereotypy subscale score was found (Urbano et al. 2014). Significant improvement was also seen on both the SRS and the ABC Social Withdrawal/Lethargy subscale (Urbano et al. 2015). There was no significant difference related to whether the dose was given on a daily or weekly basis.

N-Acetylcysteine

N-Acetylcysteine (NAC) is a prodrug of cysteine used as a treatment for acetaminophen overdose–induced liver injury. It acts to inhibit the vesicular release of glutamate through a complex mechanism mediated via the cellular uptake of cystine, a byproduct of oxidized cysteine. This mechanism reduces glutamatergic neurotransmission, which is proposed to address the excitatory-inhibitory imbalances in glutamate, as well as oxidative stress, that are hypothesized to underlie some forms of ASD. A randomized, double-blind, controlled pilot trial of oral NAC was conducted by Hardan et al. (2012) to examine its effect in reducing irritability in children ages 3.2–10.7 years with autism. Thirty-three participants were randomly assigned 1:1 to 12 weeks of NAC and uptitrated to 900 mg tid or to placebo, with the ABC Irritability subscale as the primary outcome measure. NAC treatment significantly improved irritability compared with placebo (F=6.80; P<0.001; d=0.96), whereas secondary measures of core symptoms of ASD showed no differences. In contrast, a more recent randomized, double-blind, placebo-controlled trial of 31 youth ages 4–12 years with ASD failed to find a difference between placebo and NAC over 12 weeks on measures of irritability using the ABC Irritability subscale (Wink et al. 2016). This more recent study used the CGI-I anchored to core social impairment as the primary outcome, with the SRS, ABC, and Vineland Adaptive Behavioral Scales, Second Edition, as secondary outcome measures. No significant differences between the placebo and NAC groups were observed on any of the outcome measures. The average daily dose of NAC at the conclusion of the trial was 56.2±9.7 mg/kg. Although efficacy results of NAC use in ASD have been mixed, both trials suggested good tolerability. Gastrointestinal side effects (nausea, vomiting, and diarrhea) were most common in the 2012 trial, whereas upper respiratory symptoms, headache, and stomachache were most common in the 2016 trial.

Other Compounds

β-Adrenergic Antagonists

β-Adrenergic blockers block norepinephrine receptors, thus limiting norepinephrine neurotransmission. Eight hospitalized adults with autistic disorder were described as having improved speech and socialization following open-label treatment with propranolol or nadolol (mean dosage, 225 mg/day over 14.2 months) (Ratey et al. 1987). All patients showed a marked decrease in aggression. Six patients (75%) demonstrated improvement in social skills, and four (50%) developed improved speech during treatment. Seven patients were taking concomitant antipsychotics, with five able to decrease and one able to discontinue the antipsychotic during the trial. The investigators thought the improvement noted was due to decreased hyperarousal. A 13-year-old male patient with severe ASD and impairing hypersexual behaviors that occurred across settings and were unresponsive to behavioral interventions was given propranolol 10 mg bid (0.3 mg/kg/day) to target the hypersexual behaviors (Deepmala and Agrawal 2014). Improvement was noticed as early as 2 weeks after starting treatment. His hypersexual behaviors subsequently increased when the medication was discontinued due to an unfilled prescription, and they improved when it was resumed. Of note, this patient was taking risperidone (1.5 mg bid) concomitantly. At the time of the case report, he had been taking propranolol for 1 year at the same dosage with no adverse effects.

Naltrexone

The opiate receptor antagonist naltrexone has been evaluated in four controlled studies in patients with autism. This research was stimulated by findings of elevated endorphin levels in the blood (Weizman et al. 1984) and cerebrospinal fluid (Gillberg et al. 1985; Ross et al. 1987) of individuals with autism. Although the initial reports were promising, subsequent larger, double-blind, placebo-controlled studies did not demonstrate significant efficacy regarding core or associated symptoms of autism (Campbell et al. 1993; Feldman et al. 1999; Leboyer et al. 1992; Willemsen-Swinkels et al. 1995). Overall, most of the evidence points toward naltrexone as ineffective in improving ASD symptoms or self-injurious behavior and as potentially having a modest effect in the treatment of hyperactivity.

Secretin

The gastrointestinal peptide secretin stimulates secretion of water and bicarbonate from the pancreas and supports the activity of cholecystokinin, which, in turn, further activates pancreatic secretion. Extensive study of this compound in autism occurred following an initial report of successful open-label treatment in three patients who experienced improvement in maladaptive behavior and core ASD symptoms (Horvath et al. 1998). After initial reports of secretin's success were described in the mainstream media, its use spread to the point that more than 500,000 doses had been administered to patients with autism by 1999 (Kamińska et al. 2002). Fifteen double-blind, placebo-controlled trials have now evaluated the use of secretin in patients with ASD, and none of the reports concluded that the drug was effective (Sturmey 2005). These reports included single-dose and multiple-dose trials of human or porcine secretin. Although secretin represents one of the most studied compounds in patients with ASD, no evidence yet supports its use in this diagnostic group.

Oxytocin

Oxytocin is a neuropeptide synthesized in the hypothalamus that acts peripherally in the body in the induction of milk letdown and the facilitation of uterine contractions. Treatment roles for oxytocin in humans include the management of postpartum hemorrhage and the induction of labor. It is also involved in social behavior and is thought to play a role in mother-child and adult-adult interpersonal bonds as well as in social memory and recognition (for review, see Preti et al. 2014). Many initial studies among primarily high-functioning subjects with autism that assessed emotional recognition found improvement attributable to oxytocin administration (Anagnostou et al. 2012; Domes et al. 2014; Guastella et al. 2010; Hollander et al. 2007; Watanabe et al. 2014), but this was not the case in all studies (Dadds et al. 2014). Some studies using functional MRI measures found changes in activation in response to oxytocin in areas of the brain hypothesized to mediate social behavior (Domes et al. 2014; Watanabe et al. 2014). Results have been more mixed for oxytocin's effect on restricted repetitive behaviors or eye gaze, and two studies (Anagnostou et al. 2012; Dadds et al. 2014) failed to find differences in global measures of clinical improvement in response to oxytocin.

Two more recent, large, placebo-controlled, double-blind trials in youth with ASD have, unfortunately, failed to find benefit with oxytocin for social behavior compared with placebo. The first study (Sikich et al. 2021) was conducted in 290 children and adolescents ages 3–17 years with ASD and included subjects with and without intellectual disability. The trial was 24 weeks long and failed to find a difference between intranasal oxytocin and placebo groups using the ABC modified Social Withdrawal subscale as the primary outcome measure. The second study (Yamasue et al. 2020) was conducted in 106 adults ages 18–48 years with ASD without intellectual disability. The study failed to find improvement on the primary outcome measure, the social reciprocity score on ADOS module 4. In the pediatric study by Sikich et al. (2021), adverse events included increased appetite, increased energy, restlessness, weight loss, increased thirst, inattention, and myalgia. Three subjects withdrew due to irritability. One participant in the adult trial by Yamasue et al. (2020) experienced temporary gynecomastia.

Folinic Acid

Folate (vitamin B_9) is a water-soluble vitamin essential for neurodevelopment. Deficiencies in folate and metabolism may be linked to ASD (Frye et al. 2020). Past evidence for folic acid and its related derivatives has been limited to case series and case reports. More recently, three randomized, double-blind placebo-controlled trials have been published.

Frye et al. (2018) published a 12-week randomized, double-blind, placebo-controlled trial of high-dose folinic acid (2 mg/kg/day; maximum, 50 mg/day) in 48 children and adolescents ages 3–14 years with nonsyndromic ASD with language impairment (preverbal, fewer than 25 functional words). They reported a medium to large effect size (Cohen's d=0.70) on verbal communication in participants receiving folinic acid compared with those receiving placebo. The investigators also studied biomarkers for altered folate metabolism, including the folate receptor autoantibody and a glutathione redox ratio. The presence of folate receptor autoantibody was associated with an even larger effect size (Cohen's d=0.91). No serious adverse events were reported in the folinic acid group. The difference in adverse events between groups was not significant.

Renard et al. (2020) published findings of a 12-week randomized, placebo-controlled study of folinic acid in 19 children ages 3–12 years with ASD. Participants receiving folinic acid did not demonstrate a statistically significant improvement in ADOS scores, the primary outcome measure. However, there was a significant difference in scores on the ADOS Communication and Social Interaction subscales compared with placebo. No serious adverse events were reported in this study.

Looking at folinic acid as an adjunct treatment to risperidone, Batebi et al. (2021) completed a 10-week randomized, double-blind, placebo-controlled study in 55 youth ages 4–12 years with ASD. Both groups received risperidone concurrently. In this trial, no other concomitant medications were allowed. There was a significant effect in time×treatment on the Inappropriate Speech subscale of the ABC, the primary outcome measure ($P = 0.044$). Appetite stimulation and diarrhea were the most common side effects reported in the treatment group. The difference in side effects was not statistically significant between groups.

Cannabinoids

The cannabis plant contains more than 100 cannabinoids, the most common being Δ-9-tetrahydrocannabinol (THC) and cannabidiol (CBD). THC is considered the psychoactive part of the cannabis plant. CBD has become a compound of interest for various psychiatric disorders, including psychotic disorders, anxiety disorders, substance use disorders, insomnia, PTSD, ADHD, mood disorders, and ASD. Despite its popularity, evidence for its use is limited. A few small, nonrandomized studies of CBD have suggested positive behavioral effects in individuals with ASD (Aran et al. 2019; Bar-Lev Schleider et al. 2019; Bilge and Ekici 2021; Fleury-Teixeira et al. 2019), but only one randomized, double-blind placebo-controlled trial of CBD in ASD has been published (Aran et al. 2021). In this study, 150 participants ages 5–21 years with ASD received either a 20:1 CBD/THC compound, pure cannabinoids, or placebo for 12 weeks, followed by a 4-week washout and crossover for an additional 12 weeks. The primary outcome measures for this study included the Home Situations Questionnaire–Autism Spectrum Disorder (HSQ-ASD) and the CGI-I based on disruptive behavior. The difference in the HSQ-ASD between groups was not statistically significant. A CGI-I rating of much improved or very much improved was found in 49% of patients treated with whole-plant CBD compared with 21% of those given placebo. Subjects treated with whole-plant CBD demonstrated an improvement of 14.9 points on the SRS-2, a secondary outcome measure, which was statistically significant compared with the control group (P=0.009). The most common adverse events during the study were sleepiness and decreased appetite. No serious adverse events occurred during the trial (Aran et al. 2021).

Safety Issues

In this portion of the chapter, we focus on adverse effects reported for selected classes of medications that are used in the pharmacotherapy of ASD. This is not meant to be an extensive review of all adverse effects for all drugs previously discussed but, rather, to highlight major adverse effects of several commonly used classes of drugs that should be brought to the reader's attention. When selecting a medication, the clinician must educate the patient and caregivers about its potential adverse effects.

Atypical Antipsychotics

Atypical antipsychotics are associated with a risk of several adverse events that warrant monitoring. Although they purportedly have a decreased risk of EPS and tardive dyskinesia in comparison with the typical antipsychotics, these events have been reported in individuals with ASD taking atypical agents (Correll et al. 2011; Kidd 2018; Malone et al. 2002; Zuddas et al. 2000). Hyperprolactinemia is another adverse effect that may occur during treatment with an atypical antipsychotic. With the exception of aripiprazole, which can decrease prolactin, all other atypical antipsychotics can cause elevations in prolactin levels. Studies of risperidone and paliperidone found significant elevation in prolactin levels in patients with ASD, despite the fact that no participants showed clinical signs of hyperprolactinemia (Gagliano et al. 2004; Masi et al. 2001b, 2003; Stigler et al. 2012). Chronic hyperprolactinemia can lead to disordered growth, sexual dysfunction, and osteoporosis (Saito et al. 2004).

In children and adolescents, olanzapine is associated with a considerable risk of weight gain, whereas quetiapine, risperidone, aripiprazole, and paliperidone are associated with a moderate risk (De Hert et al. 2011; Stigler et al. 2012). In contrast, published data in youth suggest that ziprasidone may be associated with a *decreased* risk of weight gain. The association between weight gain and atypical antipsychotic use in patients with ASD is of significant concern. Evidence has implicated this class of drugs in the onset or exacerbation of diabetes and hyperlipidemia (De Hert et al. 2011; Stigler et al. 2004b). Regular monitoring of patient weight, as well as fasting glucose, hemoglobin A1C, and lipids, is highly recommended. In addition, selection of a particular antipsychotic may warrant monitoring of liver functions, blood count, and ECG depending on the choice of agent and additional clinical history.

Selective Serotonin Reuptake Inhibitors

In 2004, the FDA required SSRI manufacturers to include a black box warning describing the potential for increased suicidality in children and adolescents taking these medications, especially in the first few months of treatment. With this in mind, regular assessment for suicidality must be part of the treatment plan for patients with ASD taking any of these agents. Prepubertal patients with ASD who are taking SSRIs also may be at increased risk of behavioral activation and irritability during treatment compared with postpubertal patients (McDougle et al. 2000). Given these concerns, clinicians should consider initially prescribing low dosages of SSRIs for patients and slowly titrating toward an effective dosage.

Psychostimulants

Psychostimulants may be less well tolerated in youth with ASD than in typically developing children with ADHD (Research Units on Pediatric Psychopharmacology Autism Network 2005a). Adverse effects that warrant close monitoring include increased irritability, agitation, hyperactivity, decreased appetite, weight loss, insomnia, exacerbation/development of tics, and psychosis (rarely). In addition, this drug class rarely may be associated with cardiovascular adverse events, which places individuals with preexisting heart conditions at higher risk. A baseline medical history and physical examination are recommended to identify at-risk individuals with structural cardiac abnormalities or other cardiovascular symptoms (Correll et al. 2011).

α_2-Adrenergic Agonists

α_2-Adrenergic agonists are typically well tolerated, aside from possible adverse effects of sedation and hypotension. Depressive symptoms may worsen or be induced as well. A baseline ECG prior to beginning this class of drugs should be considered, particularly in patients with a significant history of cardiovascular problems. Constipation can also occur with this particular class of medications.

Atomoxetine

In 2005, the FDA required manufacturers of atomoxetine to include a black box warning regarding potential increased suicidal ideation in children and adolescents treated with this drug. Because of this risk, regular assessment for suicidality in patients prescribed atomoxetine is warranted. In addition, rare cases of hepatic dysfunction associated with atomoxetine use warrant ongoing assessment for signs and symptoms of liver failure in ASD patients taking this medication (Bangs et al. 2008; Erdogan et al. 2011).

Mood Stabilizers

Among the mood stabilizers, the anticonvulsant valproic acid is frequently used to treat persons with ASD. Drug levels should be monitored on a regular basis to ensure that they remain in the therapeutic range. Patients should be regularly assessed for symptoms of valproic acid toxicity, including nausea, vomiting, ataxia, tremor, dizziness, headache, confusion, and somnolence. Hepatotoxicity is a possible serious adverse effect associated with the drug, warranting periodic liver function tests (Dreifuss et al. 1987). Pancreatitis is another rare but potentially life-threatening complication. In addition, due to the risk of thrombocytopenia, a blood count including platelets should be obtained for all patients receiving this medication.

Risks from taking another mood stabilizer, lithium, include impaired renal and thyroid function, thus warranting regular monitoring (Scahill et al. 2001). In addition, baseline ECGs are recommended. Lithium levels must be monitored on a regular basis during treatment. Toxic levels of lithium are often close to the therapeutic range (0.6–1.2 μg/mL), thus making it essential to monitor for signs and symptoms of lithium toxicity during treatment. Signs of toxicity include lethargy, nausea, vomiting, diarrhea, tremor, weakness, and seizures.

Practical Management Strategies

A multimodal approach to the management of ASD is essential. This often incorporates speech therapy, occupational therapy, physical therapy, educational interventions, and social skills training. Ongoing collaboration with the patient's educational team at school can ease transitions, decrease maladaptive behaviors, and optimize learning in the classroom setting. In addition, behavior therapy may be of particular importance because it may decrease the need for pharmacotherapy in patients with ASD. Even with the use of such interventions, however, medication is often required to decrease the serious behavioral problems commonly observed in youth with ASD.

The pharmacotherapy of ASD is currently based on a target symptom approach. As described in this chapter, a variety of medications may impact specific target symptom domains in this population. The algorithm shown in Figure 7–1 provides an overview of drug treatment strategies for three symptom domains commonly encountered in ASD: irritability (tantrums, aggression, self-injury), motor hyperactivity and inattention, and interfering repetitive phenomena.

Clinical Pearls

- Use a multimodal therapeutic approach to the management of autism spectrum disorder (ASD).
- Prescribe medication to reduce maladaptive behaviors, allowing youth with ASD to maximize benefit from therapy and educational services.
- Base pharmacotherapy of ASD on a target symptom approach. Three major target symptom domains in ASD are irritability (tantrums, aggression, self-injury), hyperactivity/inattention, and interfering repetitive interests/activities.

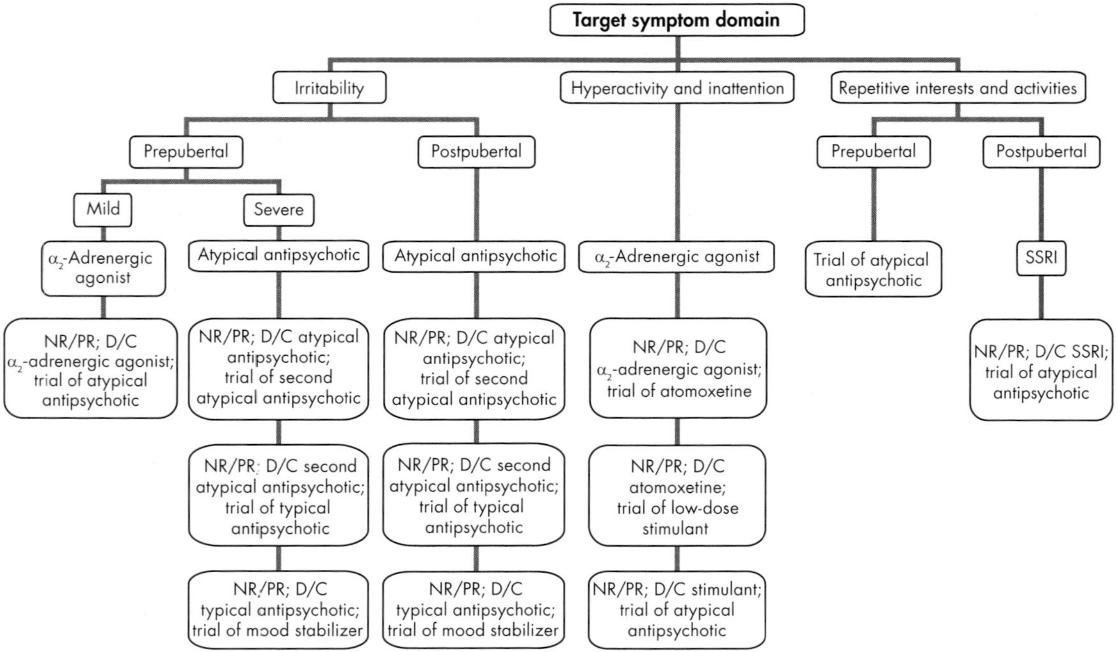

Figure 7–1. A target symptom approach to the pharmacotherapy of autism spectrum disorder (ASD).

This algorithm provides an overview of drug treatment strategies for three symptom domains commonly encountered in ASD: irritability (tantrums, aggression, self-injury), motor hyperactivity and inattention, and interfering repetitive phenomena. For repetitive behaviors, behavioral therapy is recommended as the first-line treatment. There is better evidence to support a trial of an SSRI prior to an atypical antipsychotic for postpubertal patients than for prepubertal patients.

D/C=discontinue; NR/PR=nonresponse/partial response; SSRI=selective serotonin reuptake inhibitor.

- Try prescribing an α_2-adrenergic agonist for youth with mild aggression or self-injury or an atypical antipsychotic for individuals with more severe symptoms.
- Consider risperidone and aripiprazole for the treatment of irritability in youth with ASD because these medications are FDA approved.
- Keep in mind that prepubertal versus postpubertal patients with ASD may be at increased risk of behavioral activation and irritability during selective serotonin reuptake inhibitor (SSRI) treatment for interfering repetitive phenomena.
- Remember that stimulants appear less well tolerated and less effective in youth with ASD compared with typically developing children with ADHD.
- Consider a trial of guanfacine prior to atomoxetine or a stimulant for symptoms of hyperactivity and inattention in ASD.
- Given the increased challenges with the safety and tolerability of SSRIs in prepubertal children with ASD, consider a trial of buspirone before using an SSRI or serotonin-norepinephrine reuptake inhibitor.

References

Aman MG: Stimulant drug effects in developmental disorders and hyperactivity: toward a resolution of disparate findings. J Autism Dev Disord 12(4):385–398, 1982 6131061

Aman M, Rettiganti M, Nagaraja HN, et al: Tolerability, safety, and benefits of risperidone in children and adolescents with autism: 21-month follow-up after 8-week placebo-controlled trial. J Child Adolesc Psychopharmacol 25(6):482–493, 2015 26262903

Aman MG, Findling RL, Hardan AY, et al: Safety and efficacy of memantine in children with autism: randomized placebo-controlled study and open-label extension. J Child Adolesc Psychopharmacol 27(5):403–412, 2017 26978327

American Psychiatric Association: Diagnostic and Statistical Manual of Mental Disorders, 3rd Edition. Washington, DC, American Psychiatric Association, 1980

American Psychiatric Association: Diagnostic and Statistical Manual of Mental Disorders, 4th Edition. Washington, DC, American Psychiatric Association, 1994

American Psychiatric Association: Diagnostic and Statistical Manual of Mental Disorders, 5th Edition, Arlington, VA, American Psychiatric Association, 2013

Anagnostou E, Soorya L, Chaplin W, et al: Intranasal oxytocin versus placebo in the treatment of adults with autism spectrum disorders: a randomized controlled trial. Mol Autism 3(1):16, 2012 23216716

Anagnostou E, Aman MG, Handen BL, et al: Metformin for treatment of overweight induced by atypical antipsychotic medication in young people with autism spectrum disorder: a randomized clinical trial. JAMA Psychiatry 73(9):928–937, 2016 27556593

Anderson GM, Freedman DX, Cohen DJ, et al: Whole blood serotonin in autistic and normal subjects. J Child Psychol Psychiatry 28(6):885–900, 1987 3436995

Anderson LT, Campbell M, Adams P, et al: The effects of haloperidol on discrimination learning and behavioral symptoms in autistic children. J Autism Dev Disord 19(2):227–239, 1989 2663834

Aran A, Cassuto H, Lubotzky A, et al: Brief report: cannabidiol-rich cannabis in children with autism spectrum disorder and severe behavioral problems-a retrospective feasibility study. J Autism Dev Disord 49(3):1284–1288, 2019 30382443

Aran A, Harel M, Cassuto H, et al: Cannabinoid treatment for autism: a proof-of-concept randomized trial. Mol Autism 12(1):6, 2021 33536055

Arnold LE, Aman MG, Cook AM, et al: Atomoxetine for hyperactivity in autism spectrum disorders: placebo-controlled crossover pilot trial. J Am Acad Child Adolesc Psychiatry 45(10):1196–1205, 2006 17003665

Arnold LE, Ober N, Aman MG, et al: A 1.5-year follow-up of parent training and atomoxetine for attention-deficit/hyperactivity disorder symptoms and noncompliant/disruptive behavior in autism. J Child Adolesc Psychopharmacol 28(5):322–330, 2018 29694241

Arnt J, Skarsfeldt T: Do novel antipsychotics have similar pharmacological characteristics? A review of the evidence. Neuropsychopharmacology 18(2):63–101, 1998 9430133

Baldessarini RJ, Frankenburg FR: Clozapine: a novel antipsychotic agent. N Engl J Med 324(11):746–754, 1991 1671793

Bangs ME, Jin L, Zhang S, et al: Hepatic events associated with atomoxetine treatment for attention-deficit hyperactivity disorder. Drug Saf 31(4):345–354, 2008 18366245

Bar-Lev Schleider L, Mechoulam R, Saban N, et al: Real life experience of medical cannabis treatment in autism: analysis of safety and efficacy. Sci Rep 9(1):200, 2019 30655581

Batebi N, Moghaddam HS, Hasanzadeh A, et al: Folinic acid as adjunctive therapy in treatment of inappropriate speech in children with autism: a double-blind and placebo-controlled randomized trial. Child Psychiatry Hum Dev 52(5):928–938, 2021 33029705

Beherec L, Lambrey S, Quilici G, et al: Retrospective review of clozapine in the treatment of patients with autism spectrum disorder and severe disruptive behaviors. J Clin Psychopharmacol 31(3):341–344, 2011 21508854

Belsito KM, Law PA, Kirk KS, et al: Lamotrigine therapy for autistic disorder: a randomized, double-blind, placebo-controlled trial. J Autism Dev Disord 31(2):175–181, 2001 11450816

Bilge S, Ekici B: CBD-enriched cannabis for autism spectrum disorder: an experience of a single center in Turkey and reviews of the literature. J Cannabis Res 3(1):53, 2021 34911567

Blankenship K, Erickson CA, Stigler KA, et al: Guanfacine extended release in two patients with pervasive developmental disorders. J Child Adolesc Psychopharmacol 21(3):287–290, 2011 21663433

Brodkin ES, McDougle CJ, Naylor ST, et al: Clomipramine in adults with pervasive developmental disorders: a prospective open-label investigation. J Child Adolesc Psychopharmacol 7(2):109–121, 1997 9334896

Buchsbaum MS, Hollander E, Haznedar MM, et al: Effect of fluoxetine on regional cerebral metabolism in autistic spectrum disorders: a pilot study. Int J Neuropsychopharmacol 4(2):119–125, 2001 11466160

Buitelaar JK, van der Gaag RJ, van der Hoeven J: Buspirone in the management of anxiety and irritability in children with pervasive developmental disorders: results of an open-label study. J Clin Psychiatry 59(2):56–59, 1998 9501886

Burris KD, Molski TF, Xu C, et al: Aripiprazole, a novel antipsychotic, is a high-affinity partial agonist at human dopamine D2 receptors. J Pharmacol Exp Ther 302(1):381–389, 2002 12065741

Bymaster FP, Hemrick-Luecke SK, Perry KW, Fuller RW: Neurochemical evidence for antagonism by olanzapine of dopamine, serotonin, alpha 1-adrenergic and muscarinic receptors in vivo in rats. Psychopharmacology (Berl) 124(1–2):87–94, 1996 8935803

Campbell M: Pharmacotherapy in early infantile autism. Biol Psychiatry 10(4):399–423, 1975 240449

Campbell M, Anderson LT, Meier M, et al: A comparison of haloperidol and behavior therapy and their interaction in autistic children. J Am Acad Child Psychiatry 17(4):640–655, 1978 370186

Campbell M, Anderson LT, Small AM, et al: Naltrexone in autistic children: behavioral symptoms and attentional learning. J Am Acad Child Adolesc Psychiatry 32(6):1283–1291, 1993 8282676

Campbell M, Armenteros JL, Malone RP, et al: Neuroleptic-related dyskinesias in autistic children: a prospective, longitudinal study. J Am Acad Child Adolesc Psychiatry 36(6):835–843, 1997 9183140

Carminati GG, Deriaz N, Bertschy G: Low-dose venlafaxine in three adolescents and young adults with autistic disorder improves self-injurious behavior and attention deficit/hyperactivity disorders (ADHD)-like symptoms. Prog Neuropsychopharmacol Biol Psychiatry 30(2):312–315, 2006 16307837

Chen NC, Bedair HS, McKay B, et al: Clozapine in the treatment of aggression in an adolescent with autistic disorder. J Clin Psychiatry 62(6):479–480, 2001 11465533

Chez MG, Nowinski CV, Buchanan CP, et al: Donepezil (Aricept) use in children with autistic spectrum disorders. Ann Neurol 48:541, 2000

Chez MG, Aimonovitch M, Buchanan T, et al: Treating autistic spectrum disorders in children: utility of the cholinesterase inhibitor rivastigmine tartrate. J Child Neurol 19(3):165–169, 2004 15119476

Chez MG, Burton Q, Dowling T, et al: Memantine as adjunctive therapy in children diagnosed with autistic spectrum disorders: an observation of initial clinical response and maintenance tolerability. J Child Neurol 22(5):574–579, 2007 17690064

Chugani DC, Chugani HT, Wiznitzer M, et al: Efficacy of low-dose buspirone for restricted repetitive behavior in young children with autism spectrum disorder: a randomized trial. J Pediatr 170:45–53, 2016 26746121

Cohen IL, Campbell M, Posner D, et al: Behavioral effects of haloperidol in young autistic children: an objective analysis using a within-subjects reversal design. J Am Acad Child Psychiatry 19(4):665–677, 1980 7204797

Conroy J, Meally E, Kearney G, et al: Serotonin transporter gene and autism: a haplotype analysis in an Irish autistic population. Mol Psychiatry 9(6):587–593, 2004 14708029

Correll CU, Kratochvil CJ, March JS: Developments in pediatric psychopharmacology: focus on stimulants, antidepressants, and antipsychotics. J Clin Psychiatry 72(5):655–670, 2011 21658348

Corson AH, Barkenbus JE, Posey DJ, et al: A retrospective analysis of quetiapine in the treatment of pervasive developmental disorders. J Clin Psychiatry 65(11):1531–1536, 2004 15554768

Coskun M, Karakoc S, Kircelli F, Mukaddes NM: Effectiveness of mirtazapine in the treatment of inappropriate sexual behaviors in individuals with autistic disorder. J Child Adolesc Psychopharmacol 19(2):203–206, 2009 19364298

Dadds MR, MacDonald E, Cauchi A, et al: Nasal oxytocin for social deficits in childhood autism: a randomized controlled trial. J Autism Dev Disord 44(3):521–531, 2014 23888359

Davanzo PA, Belin TR, Widawski MH, King BH: Paroxetine treatment of aggression and self-injury in persons with mental retardation. Am J Ment Retard 102(5):427–437, 1998 9544340

Deepmala D, Agrawal M: Use of propranolol for hypersexual behavior in an adolescent with autism. Ann Pharmacother 48(10):1385–1388, 2014 24965689

De Hert M, Dobbelaere M, Sheridan EM, et al: Metabolic and endocrine adverse effects of second-generation antipsychotics in children and adolescents: a systematic review of randomized, placebo controlled trials and guidelines for clinical practice. Eur Psychiatry 26(3):144–158, 2011 21295450

DeLong GR, Ritch CR, Burch S: Fluoxetine response in children with autistic spectrum disorders: correlation with familial major affective disorder and intellectual achievement. Dev Med Child Neurol 44(10):652–659, 2002 12418789

DeVane CL, Charles JM, Abramson RK, et al: Pharmacotherapy of autism spectrum disorder: results from the randomized BAART clinical trial. Pharmacotherapy 39(6):626–635, 2019 31063671

Di Martino A, Melis G, Cianchetti C, Zuddas A: Methylphenidate for pervasive developmental disorders: safety and efficacy of acute single dose test and ongoing therapy: an open-pilot study. J Child Adolesc Psychopharmacol 14(2):207–218, 2004 15319018

Domes G, Kumbier E, Heinrichs M, Herpertz SC: Oxytocin promotes facial emotion recognition and amygdala reactivity in adults with Asperger syndrome. Neuropsychopharmacology 39(3):698–706, 2014 24067301

Dreifuss FE, Santilli N, Langer DH, et al: Valproic acid hepatic fatalities: a retrospective review. Neurology 37(3):379–385, 1987 3102998

Epperson CN, McDougle CJ, Anand A: Lithium augmentation of fluvoxamine in autistic disorder: a case report. J Child Adolesc Psychopharmacol 4:201–207, 1994

Erdogan A, Ozcay F, Piskin E, et al: Idiosyncratic liver failure probably associated with atomoxetine: a case report. J Child Adolesc Psychopharmacol 21(3):295–297, 2011 21663435

Fankhauser MP, Karumanchi VC, German ML, et al: A double-blind, placebo-controlled study of the efficacy of transdermal clonidine in autism. J Clin Psychiatry 53(3):77–82, 1992 1548248

Fatemi SH, Realmuto GM, Khan L, Thuras P: Fluoxetine in treatment of adolescent patients with autism: a longitudinal open trial. J Autism Dev Disord 28(4):303–307, 1998 9711486

Feldman HM, Kolmen BK, Gonzaga AM: Naltrexone and communication skills in young children with autism. J Am Acad Child Adolesc Psychiatry 38(5):587–593, 1999 10230191

Findling RL, Maxwell K, Wiznitzer M: An open clinical trial of risperidone monotherapy in young children with autistic disorder. Psychopharmacol Bull 33(1):155–159, 1997 9133768

Findling RL, McNamara NK, Gracious BL, et al: Quetiapine in nine youths with autistic disorder. J Child Adolesc Psychopharmacol 14(2):287–294, 2004 15319025

Findling RL, Mankoski R, Timko K, et al: A randomized controlled trial investigating the safety and efficacy of aripiprazole in the long-term maintenance treatment of pediatric patients with irritability associated with autistic disorder. J Clin Psychiatry 75(1):22–30, 2014 24502859

Fleury-Teixeira P, Caixeta FV, Ramires da Silva LC, et al: Effects of CBD-enriched cannabis sativa extract on autism spectrum disorder symptoms: an observational study of 18 participants undergoing compassionate use. Front Neurol 10:1145, 2019 31736860

Frye RE, Slattery J, Delhey L, et al: Folinic acid improves verbal communication in children with autism and language impairment: a randomized double-blind placebo-controlled trial. Mol Psychiatry 23(2):247–256, 2018 27752075

Frye RE, Rossingol DA, Scahill L, et al: Treatment of folate metabolism abnormalities in autism spectrum disorder. Semin Pediatr Neurol 10:35, 2020

Gagliano A, Germanò E, Pustorino G, et al: Risperidone treatment of children with autistic disorder: effectiveness, tolerability, and pharmacokinetic implications. J Child Adolesc Psychopharmacol 14(1):39–47, 2004 15142390

Ghaleiha A, Ghyasvand M, Mohammadi MR, et al: Galantamine efficacy and tolerability as an augmentative therapy in autistic children: a randomized, double-blind, placebo-controlled trial. J Psychopharmacol 28(7):677–685, 2014 24132248

Ghanizadeh A, Ayoobzadehshirazi A: A randomized double-blind placebo-controlled clinical trial of adjuvant buspirone for irritability in autism. Pediatr Neurol 52(1):77–81, 2015 25451017

Gillberg C, Terenius L, Lönnerholm G: Endorphin activity in childhood psychosis: spinal fluid levels in 24 cases. Arch Gen Psychiatry 42(8):780–783, 1985 4015322

Gobbi G, Pulvirenti L: Long-term treatment with clozapine in an adult with autistic disorder accompanied by aggressive behaviour. J Psychiatry Neurosci 26(4):340–341, 2001 11590976

Goff DC, Tsai G, Levitt J, et al: A placebo-controlled trial of d-cycloserine added to conventional neuroleptics in patients with schizophrenia. Arch Gen Psychiatry 56(1):21–27, 1999 9892252

Golubchik P, Sever J, Weizman A: Low-dose quetiapine for adolescents with autistic spectrum disorder and aggressive behavior: open-label trial. Clin Neuropharmacol 34(6):216–219, 2011 21996644

Gordon CT, State RC, Nelson JE, et al: A double-blind comparison of clomipramine, desipramine, and placebo in the treatment of autistic disorder. Arch Gen Psychiatry 50(6):441–447, 1993 8498878

Greenhill LL, Findling RL, Swanson JM, et al: A double-blind, placebo-controlled study of modified-release methylphenidate in children with attention-deficit/hyperactivity disorder. Pediatrics 109(3):E39, 2002a 11875167

Greenhill LL, Pliszka S, Dulcan MK, et al: Practice parameter for the use of stimulant medications in the treatment of children, adolescents, and adults. J Am Acad Child Adolesc Psychiatry 41(2 Suppl):26S–49S, 2002b 11833633

Greist JH, Jefferson JW, Kobak KA, et al: Efficacy and tolerability of serotonin transport inhibitors in obsessive-compulsive disorder: a meta-analysis. Arch Gen Psychiatry 52(1):53–60, 1995 7811162

Guastella AJ, Einfeld SL, Gray KM, et al: Intranasal oxytocin improves emotion recognition for youth with autism spectrum disorders. Biol Psychiatry 67(7):692–694, 2010 19897177

Handen BL, Johnson CR, Lubetsky M: Efficacy of methylphenidate among children with autism and symptoms of attention-deficit hyperactivity disorder. J Autism Dev Disord 30(3):245–255, 2000 11055460

Handen BL, Sahl R, Hardan AY: Guanfacine in children with autism and/or intellectual disabilities. J Dev Behav Pediatr 29(4):303–308, 2008 18552703

Handen BL, Johnson CR, McAuliffe-Bellin S, et al: Safety and efficacy of donepezil in children and adolescents with autism: neuropsychological measures. J Child Adolesc Psychopharmacol 21(1):43–50, 2011 21309696

Handen BL, Aman MG, Arnold LE, et al: Atomoxetine, parent training, and their combination in children with autism spectrum disorder and attention-deficit/hyperactivity disorder. J Am Acad Child Adolesc Psychiatry 54(11):905–915, 2015 26506581

Handen BL, Anagnostou E, Aman MG, et al: A randomized, placebo-controlled trial of metformin for the treatment of overweight induced by antipsychotic medication in young people with autism spectrum disorder: open-label extension. J Am Acad Child Adolesc Psychiatry 56(10):849–856, 2017 28942807

Hardan AY, Handen BL: A retrospective open trial of adjunctive donepezil in children and adolescents with autistic disorder. J Child Adolesc Psychopharmacol 12(3):237–241, 2002 12427297

Hardan AY, Fung LK, Libove RA, et al: A randomized controlled pilot trial of oral N-acetylcysteine in children with autism. Biol Psychiatry 71(11):956–961, 2012 22342106

Hardan AY, Hendren RL, Aman MG, et al: Efficacy and safety of memantine in children with autism spectrum disorder: results from three phase 2 multicenter studies. Autism 23(8):2096–2111, 2019 31027422

Harfterkamp M, van de Loo-Neus G, Minderaa RB, et al: A randomized double-blind study of atomoxetine versus placebo for attention-deficit/hyperactivity disorder symptoms in children with autism spectrum disorder. J Am Acad Child Adolesc Psychiatry 51(7):733–741, 2012 22721596

Harfterkamp M, Buitelaar JK, Minderaa RB, et al: Atomoxetine in autism spectrum disorder: no effects on social functioning; some beneficial effects on stereotyped behaviors, inappropriate speech, and fear of change. J Child Adolesc Psychopharmacol 24(9):481–485, 2014 25369243

Hellings JA, Weckbaugh M, Nickel EJ, et al: A double-blind, placebo-controlled study of valproate for aggression in youth with pervasive developmental disorders. J Child Adolesc Psychopharmacol 15(4):682–692, 2005 16190799

Herscu P, Handen BL, Arnold LE, et al: The SOFIA study: negative multicenter study of low dose fluoxetine on repetitive behaviors in children adolescents with autistic disorder. J Autism Dev Disord 50(9):3233–3244, 2020 31267292

Hollander E, Kaplan A, Cartwright C, Reichman D: Venlafaxine in children, adolescents, and young adults with autism spectrum disorders: an open retrospective clinical report. J Child Neurol 15(2):132–135, 2000 10695900

Hollander E, Dolgoff-Kaspar R, Cartwright C, et al: An open trial of divalproex sodium in autism spectrum disorders. J Clin Psychiatry 62(7):530–534, 2001 11488363

Hollander E, Phillips A, Chaplin W, et al: A placebo controlled crossover trial of liquid fluoxetine on repetitive behaviors in childhood and adolescent autism. Neuropsychopharmacology 30(3):582–589, 2005 15602505

Hollander E, Soorya L, Wasserman S, et al: Divalproex sodium vs. placebo in the treatment of repetitive behaviours in autism spectrum disorder. Int J Neuropsychopharmacol 9(2):209–213, 2006a 16316486

Hollander E, Wasserman S, Swanson EN, et al: A double-blind placebo-controlled pilot study of olanzapine in childhood/adolescent pervasive developmental disorder. J Child Adolesc Psychopharmacol 16(5):541–548, 2006b 17069543

Hollander E, Bartz J, Chaplin W, et al: Oxytocin increases retention of social cognition in autism. Biol Psychiatry 61(4):498–503, 2007 16904652

Hollander E, Chaplin W, Soorya L, et al: Divalproex sodium vs placebo for the treatment of irritability in children and adolescents with autism spectrum disorders. Neuropsychopharmacology 35(4):990–998, 2010 20010551

Hollander E, Soorya L, Chaplin W, et al: A double-blind placebo-controlled trial of fluoxetine for repetitive behaviors and global severity in adult autism spectrum disorders. Am J Psychiatry 169(3):292–299, 2012 22193531

Horvath K, Stefanatos G, Sokolski KN, et al: Improved social and language skills after secretin administration in patients with autistic spectrum disorders. J Assoc Acad Minor Phys 9(1):9–15, 1998 9585670

Jaselskis CA, Cook EH Jr, Fletcher KE, Leventhal BL: Clonidine treatment of hyperactive and impulsive children with autistic disorder. J Clin Psychopharmacol 12(5):322–327, 1992 1479049

Kamińska B, Czaja M, Kozielska E, et al: Use of secretin in the treatment of childhood autism. Med Sci Monit 8(1):RA22–RA26, 2002 11782669

Kanner L: Autistic disturbances of affective contact. Nerv Child 2:217–250, 1943

Kent JM, Kushner S, Ning X, et al: Risperidone dosing in children and adolescents with autistic disorder: a double-blind, placebo-controlled study. J Autism Dev Disord 43(8):1773–1783, 2013 23212807

Kerbeshian J, Burd L, Fisher W: Lithium carbonate in the treatment of two patients with infantile autism and atypical bipolar symptomatology. J Clin Psychopharmacol 7(6):401–405, 1987 3429701

Kidd V: Risperidone-induced tardive dyskinesia in an autistic child. Prim Care Companion CNS Disord 20(6):18l02283, 2018 30549485

Kim SJ, Shonka S, French WP, et al: Dose-response effects of long-acting liquid methylphenidate in children with attention deficit/hyperactivity disorder (ADHD) and autism spectrum disorder (ASD): a pilot study. J Autism Dev Disord 47(8):2307–2313, 2017 28474229

King BH, Davanzo P: Buspirone treatment of aggression and self-injury in autistic and nonautistic persons with severe mental retardation. Dev Brain Dysfunct 9:22–31, 1996

King BH, Wright DM, Handen BL, et al: Double-blind, placebo-controlled study of amantadine hydrochloride in the treatment of children with autistic disorder. J Am Acad Child Adolesc Psychiatry 40(6):658–665, 2001 11392343

King BH, Hollander E, Sikich L, et al: Lack of efficacy of citalopram in children with autism spectrum disorders and high levels of repetitive behavior: citalopram ineffective in children with autism. Arch Gen Psychiatry 66(6):583–590, 2009 19487623

Kornhuber J, Weller M, Schoppmeyer K, Riederer P: Amantadine and memantine are NMDA receptor antagonists with neuroprotective properties. J Neural Transm Suppl 43(Suppl 43):91–104, 1994 7884411

Lambrey S, Falissard B, Martin-Barrero M, et al: Effectiveness of clozapine for the treatment of aggression in an adolescent with autistic disorder. J Child Adolesc Psychopharmacol 20(1):79–80, 2010 20166802

Leboyer M, Bouvard MP, Launay JM, et al: Brief report: a double-blind study of naltrexone in infantile autism. J Autism Dev Disord 22(2):309–319, 1992 1345670

Leboyer M, Philippe A, Bouvard M, et al: Whole blood serotonin and plasma beta-endorphin in autistic probands and their first-degree relatives. Biol Psychiatry 45(2):158–163, 1999 9951562

Leysen JE, Gommeren W, Eens A, et al: Biochemical profile of risperidone, a new antipsychotic. J Pharmacol Exp Ther 247(2):661–670, 1988 2460616

Loebel A, Brams M, Goldman RS, et al: Lurasidone for the treatment of irritability associated with autistic disorder. J Autism Dev Disord 46(4):1153–1163, 2016 26659550

Malone RP, Cater J, Sheikh RM, et al: Olanzapine versus haloperidol in children with autistic disorder: an open pilot study. J Am Acad Child Adolesc Psychiatry 40(8):887–894, 2001 11501687

Malone RP, Maislin G, Choudhury MS, et al: Risperidone treatment in children and adolescents with autism: short- and long-term safety and effectiveness. J Am Acad Child Adolesc Psychiatry 41(2):140–147, 2002 11837403

Malone RP, Delaney MA, Hyman SB, Cater JR: Ziprasidone in adolescents with autism: an open-label pilot study. J Child Adolesc Psychopharmacol 17(6):779–790, 2007 18315450

Mankoski R, Stockton G, Manos G, et al: Aripiprazole treatment of irritability associated with autistic disorder and the relationship between prior antipsychotic exposure, adverse events, and weight change. J Child Adolesc Psychopharmacol 23(8):572–576, 2013 24138011

Marcus RN, Owen R, Kamen L, et al: A placebo-controlled, fixed-dose study of aripiprazole in children and adolescents with irritability associated with autistic disorder. J Am Acad Child Adolesc Psychiatry 48(11):1110–1119, 2009 19797985

Marcus RN, Owen R, Manos G, et al: Aripiprazole in the treatment of irritability in pediatric patients (aged 6–17 years) with autistic disorder: results from a 52-week, open-label study. J Child Adolesc Psychopharmacol 21(3):229–236, 2011a 21663425

Marcus RN, Owen R, Manos G, et al: Safety and tolerability of aripiprazole for irritability in pediatric patients with autistic disorder: a 52-week, open-label, multicenter study. J Clin Psychiatry 72(9):1270–1276, 2011b 21813076

Marshall BL, Napolitano DA, McAdam DB, et al: Venlafaxine and increased aggression in a female with autism. J Am Acad Child Adolesc Psychiatry 42(4):383–384, 2003 12649624

Martin A, Koenig K, Scahill L, Bregman J: Open-label quetiapine in the treatment of children and adolescents with autistic disorder. J Child Adolesc Psychopharmacol 9(2):99–107, 1999 10461820

Martin A, Koenig K, Anderson GM, Scahill L: Low-dose fluvoxamine treatment of children and adolescents with pervasive developmental disorders: a prospective, open-label study. J Autism Dev Disord 33(1):77–85, 2003 12708582

Masi G, Cosenza A, Mucci M, Brovedani P: Open trial of risperidone in 24 young children with pervasive developmental disorders. J Am Acad Child Adolesc Psychiatry 40(10):1206–1214, 2001a 11589534

Masi G, Cosenza A, Mucci M: Prolactin levels in young children with pervasive developmental disorders during risperidone treatment. J Child Adolesc Psychopharmacol 11(4):389–394, 2001b 11838821

Masi G, Cosenza A, Mucci M, Brovedani P: A 3-year naturalistic study of 53 preschool children with pervasive developmental disorders treated with risperidone. J Clin Psychiatry 64(9):1039–1047, 2003 14628979

McCracken JT, McGough J, Shah B, et al: Risperidone in children with autism and serious behavioral problems. N Engl J Med 347(5):314–321, 2002 12151468

McDougle CJ, Naylor ST, Cohen DJ, et al: A double-blind, placebo-controlled study of fluvoxamine in adults with autistic disorder. Arch Gen Psychiatry 53(11):1001–1008, 1996a 8911223

McDougle CJ, Naylor ST, Cohen DJ, et al: Effects of tryptophan depletion in drug-free adults with autistic disorder. Arch Gen Psychiatry 53(11):993–1000, 1996b 8911222

McDougle CJ, Holmes JP, Bronson MR, et al: Risperidone treatment of children and adolescents with pervasive developmental disorders: a prospective open-label study. J Am Acad Child Adolesc Psychiatry 36(5):685–693, 1997 9136504

McDougle CJ, Brodkin ES, Naylor ST, et al: Sertraline in adults with pervasive developmental disorders: a prospective open-label investigation. J Clin Psychopharmacol 18(1):62–66, 1998a 9472844

McDougle CJ, Holmes JP, Carlson DC, et al: A double-blind, placebo-controlled study of risperidone in adults with autistic disorder and other pervasive developmental disorders. Arch Gen Psychiatry 55(7):633–641, 1998b 9672054

McDougle CJ, Kresch LE, Posey DJ: Repetitive thoughts and behavior in pervasive developmental disorders: treatment with serotonin reuptake inhibitors. J Autism Dev Disord 30(5):427–435, 2000 11098879

McDougle CJ, Kem DL, Posey DJ: Case series: use of ziprasidone for maladaptive symptoms in youths with autism. J Am Acad Child Adolesc Psychiatry 41(8):921–927, 2002 12164181

McDougle CJ, Scahill L, Aman MG, et al: Risperidone for the core symptom domains of autism: results from the study by the Autism Network of the Research Units on Pediatric Psychopharmacology. Am J Psychiatry 162:1142–1148, 2005 15930063

McDougle CJ, Thom RP, Ravichandran CT, et al: A randomized double-blind, placebo-controlled pilot trial of mirtazapine for anxiety in children and adolescents with autism spectrum disorder. Neuropsychopharmacol 47(6): 1263–1270, 2022 35241779

Mohammadi MR, Yadegari N, Hassanzadeh E, et al: Double-blind, placebo-controlled trial of risperidone plus amantadine in children with autism: a 10-week randomized study. Clin Neuropharmacol 36(6):179–184, 2013 24201232

Nicolson R, Awad G, Sloman L: An open trial of risperidone in young autistic children. J Am Acad Child Adolesc Psychiatry 37(4):372–376, 1998 9549957

Nicolson R, Craven-Thuss B, Smith J: A prospective, open-label trial of galantamine in autistic disorder. J Child Adolesc Psychopharmacol 16(5):621–629, 2006 17069550

Owen R, Sikich L, Marcus RN, et al: Aripiprazole in the treatment of irritability in children and adolescents with autistic disorder. Pediatrics 124(6):1533–1540, 2009 19948625

Owley T, Walton L, Salt J, et al: An open-label trial of escitalopram in pervasive developmental disorders. J Am Acad Child Adolesc Psychiatry 44(4):343–348, 2005 15782081

Owley T, Salt J, Guter S, et al: A prospective, open-label trial of memantine in the treatment of cognitive, behavioral, and memory dysfunction in pervasive developmental disorders. J Child Adolesc Psychopharmacol 16(5):517–524, 2006 17069541

Pearson DA, Santos CW, Aman MG, et al: Effects of extended release methylphenidate treatment on ratings of attention-deficit/hyperactivity disorder (ADHD) and associated behavior in children with autism spectrum disorders and ADHD symptoms. J Child Adolesc Psychopharmacol 23(5):337–351, 2013 23782128

Pearson DA, Santos CW, Aman MG, et al: Effects of extended-release methylphenidate treatment on cognitive task performance in children with autism spectrum disorder and attention-deficit/hyperactivity disorder. J Child Adolesc Psychopharmacol 30(7):414–426, 2020 32644833

Posey DI, Litwiller M, Koburn A, McDougle CJ: Paroxetine in autism. J Am Acad Child Adolesc Psychiatry 38(2):111–112, 1999 9951204

Posey DJ, Guenin KD, Kohn AE, et al: A naturalistic open-label study of mirtazapine in autistic and other pervasive developmental disorders. J Child Adolesc Psychopharmacol 11(3):267–277, 2001 11642476

Posey DJ, Kem DL, Swiezy NB, et al: A pilot study of d-cycloserine in subjects with autistic disorder. Am J Psychiatry 161(11):2115–2117, 2004a 15514414

Posey DJ, Puntney JI, Sasher TM, et al: Guanfacine treatment of hyperactivity and inattention in pervasive developmental disorders: a retrospective analysis of 80 cases. J Child Adolesc Psychopharmacol 14(2):233–241, 2004b 15319020

Posey DJ, Wiegand RE, Wilkerson J, et al: Open-label atomoxetine for attention-deficit/hyperactivity disorder symptoms associated with high-functioning pervasive developmental disorders. J Child Adolesc Psychopharmacol 16(5):599–610, 2006 17069548

Potenza MN, Holmes JP, Kanes SJ, McDougle CJ: Olanzapine treatment of children, adolescents, and adults with pervasive developmental disorders: an open-label pilot study. J Clin Psychopharmacol 19(1):37–44, 1999 9934941

Preti A, Melis M, Siddi S, et al: Oxytocin and autism: a systematic review of randomized controlled trials. J Child Adolesc Psychopharmacol 24(2):54–68, 2014 24679173

Quintana H, Birmaher B, Stedge D, et al: Use of methylphenidate in the treatment of children with autistic disorder. J Autism Dev Disord 25(3):283–294, 1995 7559293

Ratey JJ, Bemporad J, Sorgi P, et al: Open trial effects of beta-blockers on speech and social behaviors in 8 autistic adults. J Autism Dev Disord 17(3):439–446, 1987 3654495

Reddihough DS, Marraffa C, Mouti A, et al: Effect of fluoxetine on obsessive-compulsive in children and adolescents with autism spectrum disorders: a randomized clinical trial. JAMA 322(16):1561–1569, 2019 31638682

Remington G, Sloman L, Konstantareas M, et al: Clomipramine versus haloperidol in the treatment of autistic disorder: a double-blind, placebo-controlled, crossover study. J Clin Psychopharmacol 21(4):440–444, 2001 11476129

Renard E, Leheup B, Guéant-Rodriguez RM, et al: Folinic acid improves the score of autism in the EFFET placebo-controlled randomized trial. Biochimie 173:57–61, 2020 32387472

Research Units on Pediatric Psychopharmacology (RUPP) Autism Network: Randomized, controlled, crossover trial of methylphenidate in pervasive developmental disorders with hyperactivity. Arch Gen Psychiatry 62(11):1266–1274, 2005a 16275814

Research Units on Pediatric Psychopharmacology (RUPP) Autism Network: Risperidone treatment of autistic disorder: longer-term benefits and blinded discontinuation after 6 months. Am J Psychiatry 162(7):1361–1369, 2005b 15994720

Ross DL, Klykylo WM, Hitzemann R: Reduction of elevated CSF beta-endorphin by fenfluramine in infantile autism. Pediatr Neurol 3(2):83–86, 1987 2977280

Saito E, Correll CU, Gallelli K, et al: A prospective study of hyperprolactinemia in children and adolescents treated with atypical antipsychotic agents. J Child Adolesc Psychopharmacol 14(3):350–358, 2004 15650492

Scahill L, Farkas L, Hamrin V: Lithium in children and adolescents. J Child Adolesc Psychiatr Nurs 14(2):89–93, 2001 11883628

Scahill L, Aman MG, McDougle CJ, et al: A prospective open trial of guanfacine in children with pervasive developmental disorders. J Child Adolesc Psychopharmacol 16(5):589–598, 2006 17069547

Scahill L, McCracken JT, King BH, et al: Extended-release guanfacine for hyperactivity in children with autism spectrum disorder. Am J Psychiatry 172(12):1197–1206 2015 26315981

Schain RJ, Freedman DX: Studies on 5-hydroxyindole metabolism in autistic and other mentally retarded children. J Pediatr 58:315–320, 1961 13747230

Shea S, Turgay A, Carroll A, et al: Risperidone in the treatment of disruptive behavioral symptoms in children with autistic and other pervasive developmental disorders. Pediatrics 114(5):e634–e641, 2004 15492353

Siegel M, Beresford CA, Bunker M, et al: Preliminary investigation of lithium for mood disorder symptoms in children and adolescents with autism spectrum disorder. J Child Adolesc Psychopharmacol 24(7):399–402, 2014 25093602

Sikich L, Kolevzon A, King BH, et al: Intranasal oxytocin in children and adolescents with autism spectrum disorder. N Engl J Med 385(16):1462–1473, 2021 34644471

Smith T, Aman MG, Arnold LE, et al: Atomoxetine and parent training for children with autism and attention-deficit/hyperactivity disorder: a 24-week extension study. J Am Acad Child Adolesc Psychiatry 55(10):868–876, 2016 27663942

Snead RW, Boon F, Presberg J: Paroxetine for self-injurious behavior. J Am Acad Child Adolesc Psychiatry 33(6):909–910, 1994 8083152

Steingard R, Biederman J: Lithium responsive manic-like symptoms in two individuals with autism and mental retardation. J Am Acad Child Adolesc Psychiatry 26(6):932–935, 1987 2892825

Steingard RJ, Zimnitzky B, DeMaso DR, et al: Sertraline treatment of transition-associated anxiety and agitation in children with autistic disorder. J Child Adolesc Psychopharmacol 7(1):9–15, 1997 9192538

Stigler KA, Desmond LA, Posey DJ, et al: A naturalistic retrospective analysis of psychostimulants in pervasive developmental disorders. J Child Adolesc Psychopharmacol 14(1):49–56, 2004a 15142391

Stigler KA, Potenza MN, Posey DJ, McDougle CJ: Weight gain associated with atypical antipsychotic use in children and adolescents: prevalence, clinical relevance, and management. Paediatr Drugs 6(1):33–44, 2004b 14969568

Stigler KA, Diener JT, Kohn AE, et al: Aripiprazole in pervasive developmental disorder not otherwise specified and Asperger's disorder: a 14-week, prospective, open-label study. J Child Adolesc Psychopharmacol 19(3):265–274, 2009 19519261

Stigler KA, Mullett JE, Erickson CA, et al: Paliperidone for irritability in adolescents and young adults with autistic disorder. Psychopharmacology (Berl) 223(2):237–245, 2012 22549762

Sturmey P: Secretin is an ineffective treatment for pervasive developmental disabilities: a review of 15 double-blind randomized controlled trials. Res Dev Disabil 26(1):87–97, 2005 15590241

Sugie Y, Sugie H, Fukuda T, et al: Clinical efficacy of fluvoxamine and functional polymorphism in a serotonin transporter gene on childhood autism. J Autism Dev Disord 35(3):377–385, 2005 16119478

Tandon R, Harrigan E, Zorn SH: Ziprasidone: a novel antipsychotic with unique pharmacology and therapeutic potential. J Serotonin Res 4:159–177, 1997

Troost PW, Steenhuis MP, Tuynman-Qua HG, et al: Atomoxetine for attention-deficit/hyperactivity disorder symptoms in children with pervasive developmental disorders: a pilot study. J Child Adolesc Psychopharmacol 16(5):611–619, 2006 17069549

Urbano M, Okwara L, Manser P, et al: A trial of d-cycloserine to treat stereotypies in older adolescents and young adults with autism spectrum disorder. Clin Neuropharmacol 37(3):69–72, 2014 24824660

Urbano M, Okwara L, Manser P, et al: A trial of cycloserine to treat the social deficit in older adolescents and young adults with autism spectrum disorders. J Neuropsychiatry Clin Neurosci 27(2):133–138, 2015 25923852

Uvebrant P, Bauzienè R: Intractable epilepsy in children: the efficacy of lamotrigine treatment, including non-seizure-related benefits. Neuropediatrics 25(6):284–289, 1994 7770124

Van Naarden Braun K, Christensen D, Doernberg N, et al: Trends in the prevalence of autism spectrum disorder, cerebral palsy, hearing loss, intellectual disability, and vision impairment, metropolitan Atlanta, 1991–2010. PLoS One 10(4):e0124120, 2015 25923140

Wasserman S, Iyengar R, Chaplin WF, et al: Levetiracetam versus placebo in childhood and adolescent autism: a double-blind placebo-controlled study. Int Clin Psychopharmacol 21(6):363–367, 2006 17012983

Watanabe T, Abe O, Kuwabara H, et al: Mitigation of sociocommunicational deficits of autism through oxytocin-induced recovery of medial prefrontal activity: a randomized trial. JAMA Psychiatry 71(2):166–175, 2014 24352377

Weizman R, Weizman A, Tyano S, et al: Humoral-endorphin blood levels in autistic, schizophrenic and healthy subjects. Psychopharmacology (Berl) 82(4):368–370, 1984 6427830

Willemsen-Swinkels SHN, Buitelaar JK, Nijhof GJ, van England H: Failure of naltrexone hydrochloride to reduce self-injurious and autistic behavior in mentally retarded adults: double-blind placebo-controlled studies. Arch Gen Psychiatry 52(9):766–773, 1995 7654128

Wingate M, Kriby RS, Pettygrove S, et al. Prevalence of autism spectrum disorder among children aged 8 years—Autism and Developmental Disabilities Monitoring Network, 11 sites, United States, 2010. MMWR Surveill Summ 63(2):1–21, 2014 24670961

Wink LK, Adams R, Wang Z, et al: A randomized placebo-controlled pilot study of N-acetylcysteine in youth with autism spectrum disorder. Mol Autism 7:26, 2016 27103982

Yamasue H, Okada T, Munesue T, et al: Effect of intranasal oxytocin on the core social symptoms of autism spectrum disorder: a randomized clinical trial. Mol Psychiatry 25(8):1849–1858, 2020 29955161

Zheng W, Li XB, Tang YL, et al: Metformin for weight gain and metabolic abnormalities associated with antipsychotic treatment: meta-analysis of randomized placebo-controlled trials. J Clin Psychopharmacol 35(5):499–509, 2015 26280837

Zuddas A, Ledda MG, Fratta A, et al: Clinical effects of clozapine on autistic disorder. Am J Psychiatry 153(5):738, 1996 8615435

Zuddas A, Di Martino A, Muglia P, Cianchetti C: Long-term risperidone for pervasive developmental disorder: efficacy, tolerability, and discontinuation. J Child Adolesc Psychopharmacol 10(2):79–90, 2000 10933118

8

Tic Disorders

Lawrence Scahill, M.S.N., Ph.D.
Sarah Lytle, M.D.
Stephanie Pope, M.D.
Basim Mikhail, M.D.

Tic disorders, including Tourette's disorder, are movement disorders that begin in childhood and are defined by the presence of enduring motor tics, phonic tics, or both. The tics of Tourette's disorder show an extraordinary range from mild to severe across patients and a fluctuating course within patients (Lin et al. 2002; Roessner et al. 2011). In addition to the association with tics, Tourette's disorder is frequently connected with hyperactivity, impulsiveness, distractibility, obsessive-compulsive symptoms, and anxiety (Jankovic 2009). Therefore, the assessment and treatment of children and adolescents with Tourette's disorder correctly includes consideration of these multiple sources of impairment. Indeed, although the referral question may be about tics, the presence of ADHD, OCD, or an anxiety disorder may be more pressing than the tic symptoms. In assessment and treatment planning, clinicians must take into account, in addition to the sources of impairment, the domains of functioning that may be adversely affected.

We begin with a brief review of the epidemiology of tic disorders to underscore their public health importance, followed by a review of the diagnosis and treatment of children with tic disorders. Our major focus in this chapter is the pharmacological treatment of children with tic disorders. Because of the common co-occurrence of OCD and ADHD in individuals with tic disorders, we also examine the treatment of these disorders in the pediatric population. Behavioral treatments for Tourette's disorder, which are beyond the scope of this chapter, can also play an key role in treatment, as reported in a meta-analysis by McGuire et al. (2014). Although there is growing interest in deep brain stimulation and repetitive transcranial magnetic stimulation, these approaches are not discussed (for a review of surgical approaches to the treatment of refractory Tourette's disorder, see Deeb and Malaty 2020 and Schrock et al. 2015).

Epidemiology

Transient tics are relatively common, affecting up to 20% of school-age children (Scahill et al. 2014). Tic disorders are defined in DSM-5 (American Psychiatric Association 2022) by the duration and types of tics present. DSM-5 also stipulates that the tics must begin before the child reaches 18 years of age. In practice, tics usually begin in early school age, between the ages of 5 and 7.

Historically, Tourette's disorder has been considered a rare and uniformly severe condition. However, prior estimates of its prevalence were frequently based on counts of clinically ascertained cases. This method resulted in a systematic undercount because it failed to include cases that had not come to clinical attention—perhaps milder cases or cases with poor access to care. To correct this problem, later studies surveyed community samples, which has resulted in higher estimates of prevalence.

In a previous study, the CDC conducted a national telephone survey of nearly 64,000 households with children ages 6–17 years (Centers for Disease Control and Prevention 2009). A lifetime diagnosis of Tourette's disorder was reported in 3 per 1,000 children, for an estimated total count of 148,000 cases nationwide, with a male-to-female ratio of 3:1. Because most cases were described as mild according to the parents, missing mild cases are not likely to provide a complete explanation. The survey also reported a rate of 3.9 per 1,000 in non-Hispanic white children compared with 1.6 per 1,000 for Hispanic children and 1.5 per 1,000 for Black children, suggesting that race and ethnicity may affect rates of identified cases. With regard to comorbidities, 64% of the children with Tourette's disorder also had a diagnosis of ADHD, 43% had a history of disruptive behavior, and 40% had a history of anxiety problems.

Another challenge to determining the prevalence of tics over time has been the changing criteria with evolving DSM editions. This can be seen in comparing the determined prevalence rates between the Isle of Wight study (Rutter et al. 1970) and a study from Costello et al. (1996). In the time between these two studies, the introduction of DSM-III (American Psychiatric Association 1980) specified and broadened the diagnostic criteria. Specifically, in the Isle of Wight study, Rutter et al. (1970) evaluated a sample of 3,000 children ages 10–12 years. In that sample, 4.4% of the children were identified as having tics, but no cases of Tourette's disorder were identified. In contrast, using DSM-III-R criteria (American Psychiatric Association 1987), Costello et al. (1996) reported a prevalence of 4.2% for all tic disorders combined (transient tic disorder, chronic tic disorder, and Tourette's disorder) in a similar age group of children who were participants in the Great Smoky Mountains Study. The differences in diagnostic classification across these two studies appear to be attributable to differences in definitions rather than true differences in the prevalence of tic disorders.

Several reviews have also examined prevalence rates. Knight et al. (2012) completed a systematic review and meta-analysis looking at this question. They reported a prevalence of Tourette's disorder in children of 0.77% overall. When comparing the prevalence of Tourette's disorder between boys and girls, the researchers found a rate of 1.06% versus 0.25%, respectively. Transient tic disorder prevalence for children was much higher at 2.99%.

In a critical review of the literature including 11 published surveys, Scahill et al. (2014) found that transient tics are relatively common, affecting up to 20% of school-age children, with a male-to-female ratio between 2:1 and 3.5:1. Meanwhile, the prevalence of Tourette's disorder has been estimated from a lower bound of 2.6 per 1,000 to an upper bound of 38 per 1,000. This level of imprecision is not ideal for judging public health importance and service need, and this same review proposed a narrower range of 3–8 cases per 1,000. Indeed, five studies reviewed reported 4–6 cases per 1,000.

Other literature assessing this question includes a review of prevalence studies that also considered participant location, race, comorbid illness, and study methodology. The authors concluded that prevalence is within the range of 0.3%–5.7% (Robertson 2015). Another review in that same year reported a prevalence of 0.3%–0.9% (Scharf et al. 2015) but suggested that study limitations likely led to lower estimates than what is most likely true.

Diagnosis and Assessment

Any assessment of a child suspected of having a tic disorder begins with a review of tic symptoms and exploration of associated problems, such as inattention, hyperactivity, and obsessive-compulsive symptoms. Pertinent information about tic symptoms includes the age at onset and course of symptoms, current severity of motor and phonic tics, presence of premonitory sensations and capacity for tic suppression, overall burden caused by the tics, and treatment approaches implemented to date.

Tics tend to be rapid movements or brief vocalizations that are performed in a stereotyped manner. Tics also tend to occur in brief or extended clusters, followed by a period of relative quiescence. In mild cases, the bouts of tics are brief, with relatively long tic-free periods (an hour to several hours), and may go unnoticed by casual observers. By contrast, individuals with moderate or marked severity may have bouts of forceful tics consisting of multiple movements and vocalizations with only brief tic-free periods. Frequent and forceful movements or vocalizations may be easily noticeable across settings and may interfere with everyday activities.

Many patients with Tourette's disorder describe a warning or urge prior to the performance of a tic. This may be described as a vague feeling of tension or a physical feeling occurring in a specific body region. In fact, the body region involved may be the same muscle group inherent in tic expression (Leckman et al. 1993; Woods et al. 2005). Patients with Tourette's disorder also describe an ability to suppress their tics—at least momentarily. The relationship between premonitory sensations and tic suppression is intriguing but not completely understood.

Young children, usually between ages 7 and 10 years, may not spontaneously report either of these phenomena. However, by age 10 years, most children with Tourette's disorder describe both the warning before some of their tics and at least a fleeting capacity to suppress them. Children and adults often report that the act of suppressing a tic intensifies the urge to perform it. This accentuation pushes the urge to a crescendo and ultimately makes the tic irresistible (Leckman et al. 1993). Although many patients describe the capacity to suppress tics, at least momentarily, few can explain how this is accomplished. The effort to suppress tics may reflect the individual's gradual awareness that the tics can have social consequences. In other words, as children with Tourette's disorder begin to understand the social consequences of tics, they increase their vigilance about the tics and recruit conscious effort to suppress them. This increased vigilance may promote the evolution of premonitory sensations as the child becomes more aware of the earliest signs of tic behavior. This conceptualization has not been specifically tested and remains speculative.

The differential diagnosis of Tourette's disorder and tic disorders is based on the type of tics present (motor or vocal) and the duration of symptoms (American Psychiatric Association 2022). Provisional tic disorder is defined by the presence of motor and/or vocal tics for less than a year. The diagnosis of persistent (chronic) motor or vocal tic disorder is made when the child has motor or vocal tics (but not both) for longer than a year. Tourette's disorder is defined by the presence of both motor and phonic tics for more than a year. Diagnosis of Tourette's disorder does not require that both motor and phonic tics be present at the same time but does require that both be present during the course of illness (and may wax and wane). Other key elements in these diagnoses include onset before age 18 years and exclusion of other causes for the tics, such as medication or other medical conditions. For example, a child who only showed tics while being treated with a psychostimulant would not be diagnosed with Tourette's disorder.

Another important aspect to consider when assessing for tics is the phenomenon of a seemingly abrupt upsurge, such as was seen with a possible association to "Tik Tok tics" in 2020 and 2021 (Olvera et al. 2021). This sudden increase in tics was also noted by the CDC, which examined data from the National Syndromic Surveillance Program and found that visits to emergency departments for a variety of mental health issues increased following the National Emergency Declaration for COVID-19 in March 2020. Among the increased mental health concerns was an increase in tics and tic-like behavior, particularly among females ages 12–17 years. This was atypical, given the known prevalence of tics presenting at a younger age and usually in males

(Radhakrishnan et al. 2022). Thus, when evaluating patients with new-onset tics, clinicians should ask about online and social media activities, assess timelines in terms of onset of symptoms, and evaluate thoroughly for other causes of tic-like symptoms.

Several tic symptom checklists and clinician interviews are available for the assessment of tic severity. Two commonly used instruments are the Tic Symptom Self-Report (Allen et al. 2005; Scahill et al. 1997) and the Yale Global Tic Severity Scale (YGTSS; Leckman et al. 1989). In addition, a thorough developmental, family, and social history can help distinguish Tourette's disorder from other medical or psychiatric conditions and guide treatment decisions.

Treatment of Tics in Children With Tourette's Disorder

The first-line treatment for tics in children with Tourette's disorder is *education*, particularly the following points:

1. Tourette's disorder is not a progressive condition.
2. In most cases, tics are mild to moderate in severity.
3. Treating tics may not improve symptoms of ADHD or other disruptive behavior.
4. Tics have a fluctuating course, even when the individual is taking a tic-suppressing medication.
5. Most children with Tourette's disorder will show a decline in tics by early adulthood (Bloch et al. 2006b).

Understandably, parents and children may overfocus on the child's tics. The clinician's role is to help refocus them on the child's most pressing problems and to keep the parents mindful of the child's overall development. This discussion may extend to teachers and other school personnel as well. For example, children may attempt to suppress tics, which can affect their focus. Children with tics may also be subject to bullying. When tics interfere with a child's functioning, including social sequelae or self-esteem, pharmacotherapy may be considered.

Antipsychotics

The FDA-approved medications for Tourette's disorder are haloperidol for children ages 3–12 years, pimozide for adolescents ages 12 years or older, and aripiprazole for individuals ages 7–17 years. Other antipsychotics have been studied and are discussed here as well.

Early randomized trials demonstrated that the potent dopamine D_2 receptor antagonists haloperidol and pimozide were superior to placebo for suppressing tics in adults with Tourette's disorder (Ross and Moldofsky 1978; Shapiro and Shapiro 1984). Two randomized controlled trials (RCTs) compared pimozide with haloperidol; one study found better results with haloperidol in adults (Shapiro et al. 1989), whereas the other study, which involved youth, found no difference (Sallee et al. 1997). However, the latter trial indicated that haloperidol had more severe side effects than pimozide at equivalent dosages (Sallee et al. 1997). Compared with current practice, earlier studies used high dosages of these medications (up to 20 mg/day for haloperidol and up to 48 mg/day for pimozide). In contemporary clinical practice, the trend is clearly toward the use of lower dosages, such as 1–4 mg/day for haloperidol and 2–6 mg/day for pimozide (Roessner et al. 2011; Scahill et al. 2006).

Fluphenazine has also been studied. In an open-label trial with subjects that included children and adults, fluphenazine was effective for 17 of 21 patients at dosages ranging from 2 mg/day to 15 mg/day given in two divided doses. Most of the subjects who had previous experience with haloperidol preferred fluphenazine (Goetz et al. 1984). Another study reviewed charts of children and adults treated with fluphenazine (dosage range, 0.5–1.2 mg/day) for Tourette's disorder over a 26-year period, with many of the participants taking fluphenazine for months. Of the 268 participants, 211 showed marked improvement (Wijemanne et al. 2014).

The atypical antipsychotic medications currently available in the United States include aripiprazole, asenapine, brexpiprazole, cariprazine, clozapine, iloperidone, lumateperone, lurasidone, olanzapine, paliperidone, quetiapine, risperidone, and ziprasidone, which have serotonin-blocking effects and variable D_2-blocking properties (Table 8–1).

As mentioned earlier, aripiprazole is FDA-approved for the treatment of Tourette's disorder. A number of open-label studies provided preliminary evidence for its safety and efficacy. (Cui et al. 2010; Lyon et al. 2009; Wang et al.

Table 8–1. Dosing guidelines for antipsychotic drugs used in the treatment of tics of moderate or greater severity

Medication[a]	Starting dosage, *mg/day*	Usual dosage range, *mg/day*	Placebo-controlled trial?
Aripiprazole	2–5	5–10	Yes[b]
Asenapine	NR		No
Brexpiprazole	NR		No
Cariprazine	NR		No
Fluphenazine	0.5–1.0	1.5–10	No
Haloperidol	0.25–0.5	1–4	Yes[b]
Iloperidone	NR		No
Lumateperone	NR		No
Lurasidone	NR		No
Olanzapine	2.5–5.0	2.5–12.5	No
Paliperidone	3	3–6	No
Pimozide	0.5–1.0	2–6	Yes[b]
Quetiapine	25–50	75–150	No
Risperidone	0.25–0.5	1–3	Yes[b]
Ziprasidone	5–10	10–40	Yes[c]

Note. NR=no reports in Tourette's disorder.
[a]Clozapine is not listed because of its complexity of use and failure to show efficacy.
[b]Superior to placebo in more than one study.
[c]Superior to placebo in one study.

2016). A 10-week multicenter, double-blind, randomized, placebo-controlled trial of 61 youth ages 6–18 years with Tourette's disorder reported a significant reduction in tics on the YGTSS (P=0.0196) in participants given aripiprazole compared with those who given placebo, and the drug was well tolerated (Yoo et al. 2013). A multicenter, randomized, double-blind, placebo-controlled trial of aripiprazole in 133 children and adolescents ages 7–17 years with Tourette's disorder reported that aripiprazole was a safe and efficacious treatment for the disorder in this age group (Sallee et al. 2017). Dosing guidelines suggest a starting dosage of 2 mg/day, with recommended and maximum dosages of 5 mg/day and 10 mg/day, respectively, for patients who weigh less than 50 kg, and recommended and maximum dosages of 10 mg/day and 20 mg/day, respectively, for those who weigh 50 kg or more.

Aripiprazole was also studied in head-to-head trials with other medications. In an open-label study comparing aripiprazole and haloperidol, 48 youth ages 6–15 years with tics were treated with either aripiprazole 5–20 mg/day or haloperidol 0.75–4.5 mg/day for 8 weeks. Both medications were similarly efficacious in reducing tic symptoms. Improvement was noted in the first follow-up visit at week 2 and was sustained during the rest of the 8-week trial (Yoo et al. 2011). A double-blind trial compared risperidone and aripiprazole for children with tics. This study included 60 children, with a duration of 8 weeks. Participants in both groups were found to have at least 35% reduction in their Total Tic Severity Scale score. There was no significant difference between the groups (Ghanizadeh and Haghighi 2014).

A number of meta-analyses also have concluded that aripiprazole is a generally tolerable and effective treatment for children with tics (Cox et al. 2016; Wang et al. 2017; Yang et al. 2015, 2019; W. Zheng et al. 2016).

Risperidone has also been well studied. It was found to be superior to placebo for tic reduction in two trials (Dion et al. 2002; Scahill et al. 2003b) and in other studies was found to be equally as effective as pimozide (Bruggeman et al. 2001; Gilbert et al. 2004), clonidine (Gaffney et al. 2002), and aripiprazole (Ghanizadeh and Haghighi 2014). Ziprasidone was well tolerated and found to be superior to placebo in a randomized trial of 28 children with Tourette's disorder (Sallee et al. 2000). Two open-label trials of olanzapine in a total of 30 adult patients offer some encouraging results for the treatment of tics (Budman et al. 2001; Stamenkovic et al. 2000). One small study of 10 children ages 7–13 years with Tourette's disorder and aggression had statistically significantly lowered YGTSS scores (Stephens et al. 2004). To date, only two small case series are available for quetiapine (Mukaddes and Abali 2003). Clozapine was no better than placebo for the treatment of tics (Caine et al. 1979). When considered in light of the effectiveness of haloperidol and pimozide, the failure of clozapine suggests that dopamine D_2 blockade is an important mechanism in tic suppression. One small case series is available for extended-release paliperidone (Yamamuro et al. 2014). No studies for individuals with tic disorders have been completed for the other antipsychotic medications.

The appeal of the atypical antipsychotics is their demonstrated lower probability for neurological side effects such as dystonia, dyskinesia, tremor, and parkinsonism. Atypical antipsychotics are less likely to cause tardive dyskinesia in the long term and have a lower likelihood of neurological side effects in the short term (Findling and McNamara 2004). One study examined motor side effects in 80 children treated with antipsychotics (mostly atypical) versus treatment without antipsychotics for 6 months or longer. Nine percent of the subjects who were given antipsychotics exhibited hyperkinesia compared with none of those who were not given antipsychotics. Of note, a higher percentage of African American youth (15%) exhibited hyperkinesia compared with European American youth (4%) (Wonodi et al. 2007). A systematic review of the literature including 10 studies with a total of 783 children and adolescents given mainly risperidone (n=737; mean dosage, 1.58 mg/day), quetiapine (n=27), and olanzapine (n=19) reported an annualized tardive dyskinesia rate of 0.38% (Correll and Kane 2007). A meta-analysis of 41 studies including 2,114 youth reported a mean extrapyramidal symptom rate of 17.1% for aripiprazole (Bernagie et al. 2016).

Other adverse effects of clozapine include increased appetite, weight gain, and the potential for metabolic abnormalities (Meyer and Koro 2004). Based on reports from non–Tourette's disorder clinical populations, clozapine appears to be associated with the highest risk of weight gain, followed (in order) by olanzapine, quetiapine, risperidone, and ziprasidone (Allison and Casey 2001). A systematic review and pooled analysis of youth treated for pediatric bipolar disorder also found an association between atypical antipsychotics and weight gain. A large retrospective study of 3.7 million patients taking an antipsychotic (of whom 82,754 were prescribed an atypical antipsychotic) between 1998 and 2004 found a higher association with diabetes, which was higher still in younger patients (Hammerman et al. 2008). Other adverse events reported in children and adolescents include social phobia, constipation, drooling, sedation, and cognitive blunting (Aman et al. 2005; Scahill et al. 2003b).

Clinical concerns have also been raised about alterations in cardiac conduction times, such as QTc prolongation. This issue is not new, given that similar concerns have been expressed about pimozide. Although the occurrence of QTc prolongation is presumed to be rare in the dosage ranges used in the treatment of tics, clinicians should obtain electrocardiograms (ECGs) for patients before starting treatment with pimozide, during the dosage-adjustment phase, and annually during ongoing treatment (Scahill et al. 2006). Pimozide also appears to interact with medications that inhibit CYP3A4, such as clarithromycin (Desta et al. 1999). In a study comparing aripiprazole and pimozide, the group given pimozide showed decreases in blood pressure and increases in QTc, whereas those given aripiprazole showed increases in blood pressure but no significant change in QTc (Gulisano et al. 2011). Of the atypical antipsychotics, ziprasidone appears to increase QTc to a mild degree. In a series of 20 children with various psychiatric conditions, a modest increase in QTc occurred during treatment with ziprasidone (Blair et al. 2005). Unlike pimozide, however, ziprasidone does not seem to be vulnerable to drug interactions because it does not rely on a single hepatic pathway. The package insert for ziprasidone mentions that it is contraindicated in patients with a known history of QTc prolongation. Until more data are available to inform practice, guidelines similar to those used for pimozide have been recommended (Scahill et al. 2006). Medications for tic disorders studied in RCTs are listed in Table 8–2.

Non-Antipsychotic Medications

Over the past decade, various non-antipsychotic medications have been tried for the treatment of tics, including baclofen, botulinum toxin, clonidine, D-serine, ecopipam, guanfacine, intravenous immunoglobulin, levetiracetam, mecamylamine, metoclopramide, *N*-acetylcysteine, nicotine, omega-3 fatty acids, ondansetron, pergolide, pramipexole, riluzole, tetrabenazine, topiramate, valproic acid, and 5-Ling granule (an herbal medicine). Most have not been well studied; the medications that have been studied in RCTs with more than 20 subjects with tics are listed in Table 8–2.

Following encouraging results in three open studies (Jankovic 1994; Kwak et al. 2000; Marras et al. 2001), Porta et al. (2004) conducted a placebo-controlled trial of botulinum toxin in Tourette's disorder. The authors reported about a 40% difference between active drug and placebo. Treatment with botulinum toxin involves direct injection into the selected muscle of the motor tic, or the laryngeal folds in the case of a vocal tic (Porta et al. 2004). In open-label studies, the botulinum toxin injections appeared to reduce both the premonitory sensations at the injection site and the actual tic. Adverse effects included transient soreness at the injection site, weakness of the injected muscle, and

Table 8–2. Randomized placebo-controlled trials ($N>20$) focused on tic reduction using YGTSS Total Tic score[a]

Study	Drug	*N*	Duration, *weeks*	Treatment effect[b]	Active > placebo?	Dropouts, *N*
Sallee et al. 2000	Ziprasidone	28	8	6.9	Yes	2
Cummings et al. 2002	Guanfacine	24	4	5.6	No	NR
Scahill et al. 2003b[b]	Risperidone	34	8	6.0	Yes	2
Nicolson et al. 2005[c]	Metoclopramide	28	8	5.9	Yes	4
Toren et al. 2005	Ondansetron	30	3	2.0	No	3
Jankovic et al. 2010	Topiramate	29	10	8.5	Yes	16
Yoo et al. 2013	Aripiprazole	61	10	5.4	Yes	1
Sallee et al. 2017	Aripiprazole	13	8	6.26	Yes	14

Note. Trials with mecamylamine, botulinum toxin, and tetrahydrocannabinol were not included in the table. Trials did not use YGTSS Total Tic score. Levetiracetam was not included because report did not include results for the first arm of the crossover trial.

NR=not reported; YGTSS=Yale Global Tic Severity Scale.

[a]Several other trials (e.g., atomoxetine, guanfacine, selegiline) evaluated tic outcomes on the YGTSS but were primarily focused on ADHD.

[b]Change in active drug vs. change in placebo.

[c]Four subjects dropped out; three additional subjects were excluded for protocol violations.

loss of voice volume if the vocal cords were the target of treatment. Because benefit is generally confined to the injected muscle group, botulinum toxin should only be considered in cases with a prominent tic or interfering tics. The dosage and frequency of repeat injections have not been standardized. More study is needed to answer these critical issues, particularly in youth.

Levetiracetam has been examined in open trials and three RCTs. An open-label trial included 60 youth ages 6–18 years with tics or Tourette's disorder. All 60 patients had improvement in tics (YGTSS score, –17.2, P=0.05; mean total tic score, –5.0, P=0.03) over the course of 1 year (Awaad et al. 2005). Four years later, the same authors published a randomized, placebo-controlled trial of levetiracetam for pediatric tics that included 24 children ages 6–18 years with Tourette's disorder. Of the 12 patients in the levetiracetam group, 10 noted improvements in Clinical Global Impression (CGI) scores compared with 1 of 12 patients in the placebo group. (Awaad et al. 2009).

Another RCT compared active levetiracetam with placebo (N=22) (Smith-Hicks et al. 2007), whereas yet another (N=22) compared it with clonidine and included adults up to age 27 years (Hedderick et al. 2009). Both trials used a crossover design and did not provide interpretable information on the first arm of the trial, thereby making it difficult to compare these results with those of other trials. Nonetheless, the results of these trials do not support the use of levetiracetam in children with Tourette's disorder.

Ondansetron is a selective serotonin 5-HT_3 receptor antagonist that was developed as an antiemetic. A placebo-controlled trial provided encouraging although inconclusive results (Toren et al. 2005). In this study, 30 subjects ages 14–46 years were randomly assigned to ondansetron 24 mg/day (8 mg tid) or placebo for the 3-week trial. On one measure of tic severity, a significant difference was found between the active drug and placebo, but no difference was found between groups in the more frequently used YGTSS Total Tic score. Ondansetron was well tolerated, but the study had significant limitations. This drug is not currently recommended for the treatment of tics in youth.

Topiramate is an anticonvulsant that is also used to treat migraine. Its mechanism of action is not completely understood, but it appears to enhance GABA-mediated inhibition at $GABA_A$ receptors. It may also have glutamate-blocking properties. Jankovic et al. (2010) enrolled 29 children and adults in a 10-week, placebo-controlled trial. Topiramate was started at 25 mg/day and increased slowly in 25-mg increments to an average dosage of 118 mg/day. The medication is typically administered on a twice-daily schedule. As shown in Table 8–2, the treatment effect on the YGTSS Total Tic score was the largest over any other listed medication, including risperidone (the only studied medication showing superiority to placebo in more than one trial [Dion et al. 2002; Scahill et al. 2003b]). However, the attrition rate in the topiramate trial was considerably larger than in the other trials presented in the table. The statistical analysis followed the intent-to-treat convention with last observation carried forward. Attrition was greater in the placebo group, suggesting that higher YGTSS scores were carried forward to end point in the placebo group. Thus, although these results are encouraging, the relatively large treatment effect of topiramate may be misleading.

A recent meta-analysis of articles compared topiramate with other medications for children with Tourette's disorder, using risk ratios to report efficacy and safety. In the 15 studies, which included 1,070 individuals ages 2–17 years, topiramate was found to be more effective than the control medication (Yu et al. 2020). However, current evidence is insufficient to support the use of topiramate because high-quality, placebo-controlled trials are needed. Reports on the risk of birth defects following fetal exposure to topiramate and the risk, albeit apparently low, of metabolic acidosis warrant discussion of the risk-benefit ratio of this drug in the treatment of Tourette's disorder. A survey of some 800,000 live births in Denmark over a 12-year period identified 1,532 infants exposed to newer anticonvulsants, including topiramate (Mølgaard-Nielsen and Hviid 2011). The authors reported a slight but not significant increase in the risk of birth defects in infants exposed to topiramate (4.6%) compared with unexposed infants (2.4%). In a large study of insurance claims between 2002 and 2019, the frequency of oral clefts in children exposed in utero was 0.23% for topiramate and 0.17% for other antiepileptic medications (RR 1.39) (Green et al. 2012).

An 8-week study of 603 youth ages 5–18 years investigated 5-Ling granule versus tiapride versus placebo (Y. Zheng et al. 2016). The investigators found that both the 5-Ling granule and tiapride significantly reduced YGTSS scores. Participants treated with 5-Ling granule also showed less fatigue, sleep disturbance, and dizziness compared with the tiapride group.

In an open study of 10 children treated with metoclopramide, many of whom had comorbid conditions such as ADHD, all experienced improvement in tics based on YGTSS scores. On average, these participants saw an improvement of 55% in YGTSS scores (Acosta and Castellanos 2004). In an 8-week RCT, 27 children ages 7–18 years were given metoclopramide or placebo for tics. The medication group (average dosage,32.9 ± 5.1 mg/day) was found to have a nearly 39% reduction in YGTSS scores versus 13% in the placebo group ($P = 0.001$) (Nicolson et al. 2005). Side effects did not significantly differ between groups. Future studies are needed to confirm the efficacy and safety of metoclopramide in treating Tourette's disorder.

Summary of Pharmacotherapy for Tics

For children and adolescents with mild tics, medications aimed at reducing their tics may not be necessary. For children who have tics that are frequent and forceful and that interfere with activities of daily living, medication is likely indicated. Effective pharmacological treatment typically reduces the frequency and intensity of tics, but it does not eliminate them. The antipsychotic medications haloperidol, pimozide, and aripiprazole appear to be the most effective. Risperidone, ziprasidone, and fluphenazine have also demonstrated some benefit. Although it is considered effective, haloperidol has fallen out of use due to concerns about its short- and long-term adverse effects. Pimozide is effective and generally well tolerated at low dosages but requires cardiac monitoring and is vulnerable to medication interactions. Aripiprazole and risperidone are the best studied of the newer atypical antipsychotics and are superior to placebo. Despite a lower risk of neurological side effects with these agents, weight gain remains an important clinical concern. Ziprasidone also appears to be effective, but supportive data are limited to one RCT. Botulinum toxin may be considered for patients with a single interfering tic. However, treatment guidelines on the dosage and frequency of injection remain somewhat uncertain.

Comorbid Illnesses With Tics or Tourette's Disorder

Epidemiology of Comorbid Illnesses

Tourette's disorder has a high association with comorbid OCD and ADHD, and they are thought to be of closely related and interconnected pathophysiology (Bloch et al. 2006b; Coffey et al. 1998; Denckla 2006; Lewin et al. 2010; Peterson et al. 2001; Sukhodolsky et al. 2003). In DSM-5 (American

Psychiatric Association 2022), OCD includes a specifier for "tic-related" if a patient "has a current or past history of a tic disorder." One study examined OCD, ADHD, and other comorbidities with a larger sample size. In this multisite trial, 1,374 participants ages 6 years or older with Tourette's disorder were assessed. Of all the participants, 85.7% had at least one comorbidity diagnosis and 57.7% had two or more comorbid diagnoses. The most common comorbidities were ADHD (54.3%) and OCD (50.0%), with 72.1% of patients having either ADHD or OCD. Most interestingly, of these participants, 29.5% had Tourette's disorder with OCD and ADHD, 22.4% had Tourette's disorder with ADHD, 20.2% had Tourette's disorder with OCD, and only 27.9% had Tourette's disorder without ADHD or OCD. Other comorbidities included mood disorders (29.8%), anxiety disorders (36.1%), disruptive behavior disorders (28.7%), elimination disorders (16.2%), and low rates of psychotic and substance use disorders (most likely related to the young age of the participants) (Hirschtritt et al. 2015).

The evaluation and treatment of comorbid psychiatric illnesses is an important component of the successful management of a tic disorder. The management of OCD and ADHD comorbid with tic disorders is covered in further detail in the discussion that follows.

Pharmacotherapy of OCD With Tics or Tourette's Disorder

Diagnosis and Assessment of OCD With Tics or Tourette's Disorder

OCD is characterized in DSM-5 by recurrent and persistent thoughts, urges, or images (obsessions) that are difficult to dislodge and/or repetitive behaviors or mental acts that the person feels driven to perform (compulsions). Many patients report that attempts to resist the performance of compulsions increases anxiety as well as the urge to perform the compulsion. According to DSM-5, the obsessions or compulsions must be time-consuming (taking up at least 1 hour per day) or cause clinically significant distress or impairment. Adolescents and adults with OCD acknowledge that their obsessions or compulsions are excessive. This realization may not be present in younger children.

In the assessment of children with tic disorders and OCD, it may be difficult to distinguish between tics and compulsive behaviors. For example, some children may describe a recurring concern that "something bad will happen" if a specific touching ritual is not completed. Another child may perform a similar-appearing ritual but will describe a need or an urge to carry out the behavior in response to an urge that is not related to a fear. This description often sounds similar to satisfying the premonitory sensations preceding a tic. Children with these behaviors who are driven by a sensation or urge will often describe a need to "get it right" or achieve a sense of completion. In a series of 80 children and adolescents, investigators observed differences in the OCD symptom picture according to the presence or absence of chronic tics (Scahill et al. 2003a). Children with OCD without tics tended to perform rituals to prevent harm. By contrast, children with chronic tics and OCD appeared to carry out repetitive behaviors to achieve a sense of completion rather than for harm reduction. These findings suggest that assessment should consider the events and situations associated with the ritualized behaviors and what seems to drive them—harm reduction or a need to achieve completion.

Pharmacotherapy

Selective serotonin reuptake inhibitors (SSRIs) are often effective in treating OCD, but unfortunately most RCTs of SSRIs in children and adolescents with OCD have excluded subjects with Tourette's disorder, making it unclear how these results translate to naturalistic clinical samples (Geller et al. 2003b). In addition, some evidence in children and adults suggests that tic-related OCD may be a distinct subtype of OCD (Leckman et al. 1994; Scahill et al. 2003a). OCD with comorbidities responds differently to medications. In a post hoc study of a previously reported 32-week multisite, efficacy study of paroxetine in 335 youth with OCD that included those with comorbidities, comorbid disorders included generalized anxiety disorder (20%), ADHD (19%), specific phobia (16%), tic disorder (15%), separation anxiety disorder (10%), dysthymia (8%), oppositional defiant disorder (8%), and major depressive disorder (6%). The response rate to paroxetine for all participants was 71% and was significantly lower in those with comorbid ADHD (56%), tic disorder (53%), and oppositional defiant disorder (39%) (Geller et al. 2003a).

Another study used the data sample from the Pediatric OCD Treatment Study (POTS) published in 2004. Of the 112 participants, 17 had comorbid tics. When this group of 17 patients was analyzed separately, their treatment response was higher for cognitive-behavioral therapy (CBT) + sertraline combination treatment than for CBT alone. Sertraline was not found to be more effective than placebo in the comorbid group. These results differed from the original POTS, which reported that OCD without tics responded better to the CBT + sertraline combination than to either CBT or sertraline alone (Pediatric OCD Treatment Study Team 2004).

These results suggest that SSRIs may not be as effective in the treatment of children and adolescents with OCD and comorbid tics compared with those with OCD who do not have comorbid tics. Others have suggested using augmentation strategies. One study that looked at augmenting an SSRI included youth ages 7–18 years with OCD who had not responded to SSRI monotherapy. The 69 nonresponders were randomly assigned to continue treatment with adjunctive risperidone or aripiprazole for 12 weeks, and 68.1% saw an improvement in their tics with the addition of the antipsychotic (Masi et al. 2013).

The adult research literature includes studies examining OCD in adult patients with or without tics. For example, one retrospective study showed that patients with comorbid tic disorder responded to the addition of haloperidol, whereas none of those with and without comorbid tics in the placebo group had improvement in OCD symptoms (McDougle et al. 1994). A systematic review examined augmentation strategies for treating adults with OCD with or without tics. The results indicated that antipsychotics, specifically risperidone and haloperidol, are appropriate augmentation for SSRI nonresponders because one-third of those whose symptoms did not respond to SSRI monotherapy improved with an adjunctive antipsychotic medication. This was particularly true for those with comorbid tic disorder (Bloch et al. 2006a). In addition, an open-label study of aripiprazole in 16 youth ages 8–17 years with Tourette's disorder or chronic tic disorder, in which 12 had comorbid OCD, demonstrated statistically significant improvements in Child's Yale-Brown Obsessive Compulsive Scale obsessions ($P<0.002$), compulsions ($P<0.003$), and total ($P<0.0003$) scores (Murphy et al. 2009).

Pharmacotherapy of ADHD With Tics or Tourette's Disorder

Stimulants

Stimulants are the first-line agents for the treatment of ADHD (MTA Cooperative Group 1999; see also Chapter 2, "Attention-Deficit/Hyperactivity Disorder"). Because of the lack of efficacy or adverse effects, trials of stimulants fail in 10%–20% of children with ADHD (Elia et al. 1991; MTA Cooperative Group 1999). Case reports over the past three decades suggest that stimulants may induce the emergence of tics or an increase in preexisting tics in children with ADHD (Erenberg et al. 1985; Golden 1974; Lipkin et al. 1994; Lowe et al. 1982; Riddle et al. 1995; Varley et al. 2001). Two placebo-controlled trials that excluded children with tic disorders (Barkley et al. 1990; Borcherding et al. 1990) also reported the emergence of tics in a small percentage of children treated with stimulants.

However, meta-analyses have examined this purported association. One study examined the risk of developing de novo tics or of exacerbating existing tics with psychostimulant treatment of ADHD in children (Cohen et al. 2015). This meta-analysis included 22 double-blind, randomized, placebo-controlled trials. The authors found that de novo tics and exacerbation of tics were reported in both the psychostimulant and the placebo groups (5.7% vs. 6.5%). The risk of de novo tics or exacerbation of tics between psychostimulant and placebo was similar, with a relative risk of 0.99. Dosage, length of treatment, and type of psychostimulant did not alter the risk of de novo tics or tic exacerbation (Cohen et al. 2015). These and other analyses have concluded that evidence from RCTs does not support an association between the use of psychostimulants and worsening preexisting tics (Bloch et al. 2009; Pringsheim and Steeves 2011), as discussed later in this chapter.

Two naturalistic studies also provide information on the longer-term effects of stimulants in youth with Tourette's disorder (Gadow et al. 1999; Law and Schachar 1999). Although most children in these longer-term studies did not show an increase in tics, acute exacerbations did occur in a few participants, resulting in either discontinuation of the stimulant or the addition of a tic-suppressing medication. Taken together, these findings suggest that stimulants should be considered in the treatment of children with ADHD and tics (Bloch et al. 2009).

Nonstimulants

Various nonstimulant medications have been used in the treatment of children with ADHD, including the selective norepinephrine reuptake inhibitors atomoxetine and desipramine, the antidepressant bupropion, modafinil, and selegiline as well as the α_2-adrenergic agonists clonidine and guanfacine. Table 8–3 shows the starting dosages and usual maintenance dosages of nonstimulant

Table 8–3. Dosing guidelines for nonstimulant medications used in the treatment of children with tics and ADHD

			Placebo-controlled trial?	
Medication[a]	**Starting dosage, *mg***	**Usual dosage range, *mg/day***	**ADHD**[b]	**ADHD + tics**[c]
Atomoxetine	18–25	36–100	Yes	Yes
Bupropion	25–50	75–150	Yes	No
Clonidine	0.025–0.05	0.2–0.3	Yes	Yes
Clonidine ER	0.1	0.2–0.3	Yes	No
Guanfacine	0.25–0.5	2–3	No	Yes
Guanfacine ER	1	2–4	Yes	No
Modafinil	50–100	200–400	Yes	No
Pindolol	5–10	15–40	Yes	No
Selegiline	5	5–10	No	Yes

Note. ER=extended release.
[a]Desipramine is not listed, having fallen out of use due to concerns about QTc prolongation.
[b]Children with ADHD without a tic disorder.
[c]Children with ADHD plus a chronic tic disorder.

medications that have been evaluated in the treatment of ADHD (see Chapter 2 for descriptions of other nonstimulants used in the treatment of ADHD).

Four nonstimulant drugs are now FDA-approved for the treatment of children with ADHD: guanfacine ER (extended release), clonidine ER, atomoxetine, and viloxazine ER. Viloxazine ER was FDA-approved for the treatment of ADHD in children and adolescents in 2021, but there are currently no studies of this medication in individuals with tic disorders.

Three RCTs comparing atomoxetine with placebo in children with ADHD showed greater efficacy for atomoxetine (Kelsey et al. 2004; Michelson et al. 2001, 2002). An 18-week, placebo-controlled study conducted by Allen et al. (2005) evaluated the efficacy and safety of atomoxetine in 148 children (mean age, 11.2 years) with ADHD and a chronic tic disorder. Atomoxetine resulted in a 28% improvement on a clinician-rated measure of ADHD symptoms compared with 14% for placebo. This level of improvement in ADHD symptoms is similar to but slightly lower than that seen with guanfacine, clonidine, and desipramine in this population. Treatment with atomoxetine also showed a reduction in tic severity compared with placebo, although this association was not statistically significant. Atomoxetine treatment was associated with a greater reduction in tic severity at end point relative to placebo, approaching significance (YGTSS total score, -5.5 ± 6.9 vs. -3.0 ± 8.7; $P=0.063$). The adverse effects in this study were also similar to those in other reports for atomoxetine in children with ADHD. Nausea, vomiting, decreased appetite, and weight loss were significantly more frequent in the atomoxetine group than the placebo group. Insomnia, which has been reported in other pediatric ADHD studies, was no different from placebo in this study.

The α_2-adrenergic agonists clonidine and guanfacine are also used to treat children with ADHD and co-occurring tic disorders, and further information can be found Chapter 2. Indeed, this class of medications is perhaps the most commonly used for the treatment of tics and ADHD in tic disorder clinics (Freeman et al. 2000). The use of clonidine in children with tic disorders has been evaluated mainly in small studies (e.g., Hunt et al. 1985). The randomized, placebo-controlled trial of desipramine by Singer et al. (1995) involving 34 children also included a clonidine arm in the crossover design. In that study, clonidine was deemed to be no better than placebo.

In a randomized, placebo-controlled trial, Scahill et al. (2001) evaluated 34 children ages 7–14 years with ADHD and a chronic tic disorder treated with guanfacine. After 8 weeks of treatment with dosages ranging from 1.5 mg/day to 3.0 mg/day given in three divided doses, the guanfacine group showed 37% improvement on the teacher-rated ADHD Rating Scale, compared with 8% for the placebo group. Sedation led to discontinuation by only one subject. Other adverse effects included a slight drop in mean blood pressure and pulse and mid-sleep awakening in a few subjects. The three-times-daily dosing may have been protective against hypotensive effects by minimizing the fluctuation of the medication level across the day. For example, in a case series of 200 children from a Tourette's disorder clinic who were treated with guanfacine, four participants had syncopal episodes (King et al. 2006). In this case series, guanfacine was administered in a single bedtime dose. A review by Scahill et al. (2006) indicated that cardiac monitoring with routine ECGs is not necessary when treating children with clonidine or guanfacine. Clearly, the patient's blood pressure and pulse should be monitored during dosage adjustment and during the maintenance phase.

An extended-release formulation of guanfacine was approved for the treatment of ADHD in 2009. This approval was supported by two large-scale trials that compared multiple fixed doses of guanfacine ER with placebo and established its short-term efficacy and safety in children with ADHD (Biederman et al. 2008; Sallee et al. 2009). However, a multisite, 8-week, randomized, double-blind, placebo-controlled trial found that guanfacine ER did not have a large effect on tic severity in youth with chronic tic disorders (Murphy et al. 2017).

The tricyclic antidepressant desipramine has also been used in the treatment of ADHD. Placebo-controlled trials in the 1980s and 1990s showed that it was effective for the treatment of ADHD in children without co-occurring tic disorders (Biederman et al. 1989) and in children with ADHD and tic disorders (Singer et al. 1995). Spencer et al. (2002) conducted a 6-week placebo-controlled study in 41 children with ADHD and a chronic tic disorder. At total dosages averaging 3.4 mg/kg/day given in two divided doses, desipramine was superior to placebo on an ADHD symptom rating scale, improving by 42%, compared with little change in the placebo group. Tics improved by 30% on average in the desipramine group, compared with no change in the placebo group. Adverse effects included decreased appetite, insomnia, and dry mouth. The investigators detected a significant increase in pulse and blood pressure in the desipramine group but no abnormalities on ECG. Despite these overall positive results, desipramine is falling out of use due to concerns about prolonged cardiac conduction times and reports of sudden death.

Selegiline is a selective monoamine oxidase inhibitor that directly enhances dopamine function in the brain. In addition, it is metabolized to an amphetamine compound in the brain, which may further enhance central catecholamine function. To date, there have been two controlled studies of selegiline in children with ADHD. In the first study, Mohammadi et al. (2004) compared selegiline with methylphenidate in a double-blind, randomized trial involving 40 children ages 6–15 years with ADHD without co-occurring tics. Following 60 days of treatment at a maximum total dosage of methylphenidate 40 mg/day or selegiline 10 mg/day (both dispensed in two divided doses), there was a 54% decrease in the teacher rating for children receiving methylphenidate and a 50% improvement for those receiving selegiline. Results on parent ratings were slightly more favorable for both medications.

Headache and decreased appetite were more frequent in the methylphenidate group; otherwise, both medications were well tolerated.

In the second study, Feigin et al. (1996) studied selegiline in 24 children with Tourette's disorder and ADHD using a double-blind, crossover design. Subjects were randomly assigned either to selegiline followed by placebo or to placebo followed by selegiline. Despite the 6-week washout between phases, the study design poses serious problems to the interpretation of the results. First, more than one-third of the sample dropped out of the study. Second, there was a clear order effect, in that the participants who received selegiline first showed benefit compared with those assigned to placebo. By contrast, the participants who received selegiline second actually showed a mean worsening of ADHD symptoms. Overall, selegiline was no better than placebo. However, a secondary analysis showed a significant effect for selegiline in the first phase, although the medication had no apparent impact on tics. Selegiline appears to be well tolerated. At low dosages, it requires no dietary restrictions, and medication interaction is not a major concern. However, given the inconsistent results to date, more study is needed to demonstrate its efficacy for ADHD symptoms.

Comparison Studies of Stimulants and Nonstimulants

In the 16-week Treatment of ADHD in Children with Tic disorders (TACT) trial conducted by the Tourette's Syndrome Study Group (2002), 136 children with ADHD and a tic disorder were randomly assigned to placebo, clonidine alone, methylphenidate alone, or clonidine plus methylphenidate. Although the effects were modest, tics declined in all active treatment groups. Approximately one-quarter of the participants in the methylphenidate-only group showed an increase in tics, which was only slightly higher than the rate seen in the placebo group. Monotherapy with either clonidine or methylphenidate was effective in reducing teacher-rated ADHD symptoms, but the magnitude was small (38% and 36%, respectively, with no correction for placebo) compared with the level of improvement documented for methylphenidate in the multisite Multimodal Treatment of ADHD (MTA) study (56% for the medication-only group) (MTA Cooperative Group 1999). In contrast, participants who were randomly assigned to clonidine plus methylphenidate showed a 57% improvement on ADHD outcomes. The dosage of methylphenidate in the TACT study was relatively low compared with that given in the MTA study (25.7 mg/day in two divided doses vs. 31–38 mg/day in three divided doses). The more conservative approach used in the TACT study may explain the lower level of improvement observed in the methylphenidate group. The level of improvement for monotherapy with clonidine in this study is consistent with the results of another study that employed the same design in children with ADHD uncomplicated by tic disorders (Palumbo et al. 2008). Taken together, the results of the TACT trial indicate that methylphenidate can be used safely in youth with Tourette's disorder. Given the conservative dosing for methylphenidate used in that study, clinicians may decide against taking the more aggressive approach described in the MTA study; although the more conservative approach may be associated with a lower magnitude of effect, it may also be associated with a lower likelihood of adverse effects, including tics.

In more support of the safety of stimulants in treating ADHD with tics, a meta-analysis by Bloch et al. (2009) included nine RCTs that examined the use of stimulants and nonstimulants for children with ADHD and comorbid tics. The study medications in these studies included dextroamphetamine, methylphenidate, clonidine, guanfacine, desipramine, atomoxetine, and deprenyl. The authors concluded that methylphenidate was the most effective medication for treating ADHD and did not worsen tics, whereas clonidine and guanfacine were the most effective in treating both tics and ADHD.

In another meta-analysis, Pringsheim and Steeves (2011) included eight RCTs of stimulants and nonstimulants for children with tics and ADHD. They found that tics improved in children treated with guanfacine, desipramine, methylphenidate, clonidine, and the combination of methylphenidate and clonidine.

One small 12-week, open-label study of aripiprazole in 28 children and adolescents ages 8–16 years with Tourette's disorder and comorbid ADHD demonstrated a significant improvement in tics based on YGTSS scores and DSM-IV ADHD Rating Scale scores (Masi et al. 2012).

Summary of Pharmacotherapy of ADHD With Tics or Tourette's Disorder

Stimulants are an appropriate option for the treatment of ADHD in individuals with comorbid tics. The exacerbation of tics or appearance of de novo tics should be considered a potential side effect, although evidence has not shown that stimulants worsen tics. Meanwhile, atomoxetine and the α_2-adrenergic agonists are also rational choices for the treatment of ADHD in children with chronic tic disorders, especially if an adequate stimulant trial has been unsuccessful. Further data on viloxazine are needed. The α_2-adrenergic agonists may also be used in combination with stimulants. For families who decline treatment with a stimulant, the α_2-adrenergic agonists may be a rational alternative.

Conclusion

The proper diagnosis and assessment of children and adolescents with tic disorders is important to ensure accurate treatment recommendations. Although the first-line treatment for tic disorders is education, medications may be warranted for individuals with frequent, forceful, and interfering tics. Habit reversal training can also be effective in the treatment of tic disorders. Atypical antipsychotics, including aripiprazole and risperidone, have demonstrated effectiveness in reducing tics and have a better safety profile than older typical antipsychotics. Tics are also often comorbid with OCD and ADHD. SSRIs typically do not lead to improvement in tics; therefore, children and adolescents with comorbid OCD and tic disorders may require treatment with both an SSRI and an augmenting agent for the tic disorder. Youth with comorbid ADHD and tic disorder may be treated with stimulant medications because newer evidence suggests that stimulants do not worsen tics. Atomoxetine and the α_2-adrenergic agonists may also be used to treat ADHD in youth with tic disorders.

Clinical Pearls

- Advise patients and their families that Tourette's disorder is frequently associated with ADHD, obsessive-compulsive symptoms, and anxiety.
- Consider education to be the first-line treatment for tics in children with Tourette's disorder.
- Remember that pharmacotherapy specifically targeted at reducing tics may not be needed for children and adolescents with mild tics.
- Consider psychostimulants, particularly methylphenidate, as a treatment option for children with ADHD and tics.

References

Acosta MT, Castellanos FX: Use of the "inverse neuroleptic" metoclopramide in Tourette syndrome: an open case series. J Child Adolesc Psychopharmacol 14(1):123–128, 2004 15142399

Allen AJ, Kurlan RM, Gilbert DL, et al: Atomoxetine treatment in children and adolescents with ADHD and comorbid tic disorders. Neurology 65(12):1941–1949, 2005 16380617

Allison DB, Casey DE: Antipsychotic-induced weight gain: a review of the literature. J Clin Psychiatry 62(Suppl 7):22–31, 2001 11346192

Aman MG, Arnold LE, McDougle CJ, et al: Acute and long-term safety and tolerability of risperidone in children with autism. J Child Adolesc Psychopharmacol 15(6):869–884, 2005 16379507

American Psychiatric Association: Diagnostic and Statistical Manual of Mental Disorders, 3rd Edition. Washington, DC, American Psychiatric Association, 1980

American Psychiatric Association: Diagnostic and Statistical Manual of Mental Disorders, 3rd Edition, Revised. Washington, DC, American Psychiatric Association, 1987

American Psychiatric Association: Diagnostic and Statistical Manual of Mental Disorders, 5th Edition, Text Revision. Washington, DC, American Psychiatric Association, 2022

Awaad Y, Michon AM, Minarik S: Use of levetiracetam to treat tics in children and adolescents with Tourette syndrome. Mov Disord 20(6):714–718, 2005 15704204

Awaad Y, Michon AM, Minarik S, Rink T: Levetiracetam in Tourette syndrome: a randomized double blind, placebo controlled study. J Pediatr Neurol 7(3):257–263, 2009

Barkley RA, McMurray MB, Edelbrock CS, Robbins K: Side effects of methylphenidate in children with attention deficit hyperactivity disorder: a systemic, placebo-controlled evaluation. Pediatrics 86(2):184–192, 1990 2196520

Bernagie C, Danckaerts M, Wampers M, De Hert M: Aripiprazole and acute extrapyramidal symptoms in children and adolescents: a meta-analysis. CNS Drugs 30(9):807–818, 2016 27395403

Biederman J, Baldessarini RJ, Wright V, et al: A double-blind placebo controlled study of desipramine in the treatment of ADD, I: efficacy. J Am Acad Child Adolesc Psychiatry 28(5):777–784, 1989 2676967

Biederman J, Melmed RD, Patel A, et al: A randomized, double-blind, placebo-controlled study of guanfacine extended release in children and adolescents with attention-deficit/hyperactivity disorder. Pediatrics 121(1):e73–e84, 2008 18166547

Blair J, Scahill L, State M, Martin A: Electrocardiographic changes in children and adolescents treated with ziprasidone: a prospective study. J Am Acad Child Adolesc Psychiatry 44(1):73–79, 2005 15608546

Bloch MH, Landeros-Weisenberger A, Kelmendi B, et al: A systematic review: antipsychotic augmentation with treatment refractory obsessive-compulsive disorder. Mol Psychiatry 11(7):622–632, 2006a 16585942

Bloch MH, Peterson BS, Scahill L, et al: Adulthood outcome of tic and obsessive-compulsive symptom severity in children with Tourette syndrome. Arch Pediatr Adolesc Med 160(1):65–69, 2006b 16389213

Bloch MH, Panza KE, Landeros-Weisenberger A, Leckman JF: Meta-analysis: treatment of attention-deficit/hyperactivity disorder in children with comorbid tic disorders. J Am Acad Child Adolesc Psychiatry 48(9):884–893, 2009 19625978

Borcherding BG, Keysor CS, Rapoport JL, et al: Motor/vocal tics and compulsive behaviors on stimulant drugs: is there a common vulnerability? Psychiatry Res 33(1):83–94, 1990 2217661

Bruggeman R, van der Linden C, Buitelaar JK, et al: Risperidone versus pimozide in Tourette's disorder: a comparative double-blind parallel-group study. J Clin Psychiatry 62(1):50–56, 2001 11235929

Budman CL, Gayer A, Lesser M, et al: An open-label study of the treatment efficacy of olanzapine for Tourette's disorder. J Clin Psychiatry 62(4):290–294, 2001 11379844

Caine ED, Polinsky RJ, Kartzinel R, Ebert MH: The trial use of clozapine for abnormal involuntary movement disorders. Am J Psychiatry 136(3): 317–320, 1979 154301

Centers for Disease Control and Prevention: Prevalence of diagnosed Tourette syndrome in persons aged 6–17 years—United States, 2007. MMWR Morb Mortal Wkly Rep 58(21):581–585, 2009 19498335

Coffey BJ, Miguel EC, Biederman J, et al: Tourette's disorder with and without obsessive-compulsive disorder in adults: are they different? J Nerv Ment Dis 186(4):201–206, 1998 9569887

Cohen SC, Mulqueen JM, Ferracioli-Oda E, et al: Meta-analysis: risk of tics associated with psychostimulant use in randomized, placebo-controlled trials. J Am Acad Child Adolesc Psychiatry 54(9):728–736, 2015 26299294

Correll CU, Kane JM: One-year incidence rates of tardive dyskinesia in children and adolescents treated with second-generation antipsychotics: a systematic review. J Child Adolesc Psychopharmacol 17(5):647–656, 2007 17979584

Costello EJ, Angold A, Burns BJ, et al: The Great Smoky Mountains Study of Youth: goals, design, methods, and the prevalence of DSM-III-R disorders. Arch Gen Psychiatry 53(12):1129–1136, 1996 8956679

Cox JH, Seri S, Cavanna AE: Safety and efficacy of aripiprazole for the treatment of pediatric Tourette syndrome and other chronic tic disorders. Pediatric Health Med Ther 7:57–64, 2016 29388585

Cui YH, Zheng Y, Yang YP, et al: Effectiveness and tolerability of aripiprazole in children and adolescents with Tourette's disorder: a pilot study in China. J Child Adolesc Psychopharmacol 20(4):291–298, 2010 20807067

Cummings DD, Singer HS, Krieger M, et al: Neuropsychiatric effects of guanfacine in children with mild Tourette syndrome: a pilot study. Clin Neuropharmacol 25(6):325–332, 2002 12469007

Deeb W, Malaty I: Deep brain stimulation for Tourette syndrome: potential role in the pediatric population. J Child Neurol 35(2):155–165, 2020 31526168

Denckla MB: Attention deficit hyperactivity disorder: the childhood co-morbidity that most influences the disability burden in Tourette syndrome. Adv Neurol 99:17–21, 2006 16536349

Desta Z, Kerbusch T, Flockhart DA: Effect of clarithromycin on the pharmacokinetics and pharmacodynamics of pimozide in healthy poor and extensive metabolizers of cytochrome P450 2D6. Clin Pharmacol Ther 65(1):10–20, 1999 9951426

Dion Y, Annable L, Sandor P, Chouinard G: Risperidone in the treatment of Tourette syndrome: a double-blind, placebo-controlled trial. J Clin Psychopharmacol 22(1):31–39, 2002 11799340

Elia J, Borcherding BG, Rapoport JL, Keysor CS: Methylphenidate and dextroamphetamine treatments of hyperactivity: are there true nonresponders? Psychiatry Res 36(2):141–155, 1991 2017529

Erenberg G, Cruse RP, Rothner AD: Gilles de la Tourette's syndrome: effects of stimulant drugs. Neurology 35(9):1346–1348, 1985 2862607

Feigin A, Kurlan R, McDermott MP, et al: A controlled trial of deprenyl in children with Tourette's syndrome and attention deficit hyperactivity disorder. Neurology 46(4):965–968, 1996 8780073

Findling RL, McNamara NK: Atypical antipsychotics in the treatment of children and adolescents: clinical applications. J Clin Psychiatry 65(Suppl 6):30–44, 2004 15104524

Freeman RD, Fast DK, Burd L, et al: An international perspective on Tourette syndrome: selected findings from 3,500 individuals in 22 countries. Dev Med Child Neurol 42(7):436–447, 2000 10972415

Gadow KD, Sverd J, Sprafkin J, et al: Long-term methylphenidate therapy in children with comorbid attention-deficit hyperactivity disorder and chronic multiple tic disorder. Arch Gen Psychiatry 56(4):330–336, 1999 10197827

Gaffney GR, Perry PJ, Lund BC, et al: Risperidone versus clonidine in the treatment of children and adolescents with Tourette's syndrome. J Am Acad Child Adolesc Psychiatry 41(3):330–336, 2002 11886028

Geller DA, Biederman J, Stewart E, et al: Impact of comorbidity on treatment response to paroxetine in pediatric obsessive-compulsive disorder: is the use of exclusion criteria empirically supported in randomized controlled trials? J Child Adolesc Psychopharmacol 13(Suppl 1):s19–s29, 2003a

Geller DA, Biederman J, Stewart SE, et al: Which SSRI? A meta-analysis of pharmacotherapy trials in pediatric obsessive-compulsive disorder. Am J Psychiatry 160(11):1919–1928, 2003b 14594734

Ghanizadeh A, Haghighi A: Aripiprazole versus risperidone for treating children and adolescents with tic disorder: a randomized double blind clinical trial. Child Psychiatry Hum Dev 45(5):596–603, 2014 24343476

Gilbert DL, Batterson JR, Sethuraman G, Sallee FR: Tic reduction with risperidone versus pimozide in a randomized, double-blind, crossover trial. J Am Acad Child Adolesc Psychiatry 43(2):206–214, 2004 14726728

Goetz CG, Tanner CM, Klawans HL: Fluphenazine and multifocal tic disorders. Arch Neurol 41(3):271–272, 1984 6582810

Golden GS: Gilles de la Tourette's syndrome following methylphenidate administration. Dev Med Child Neurol 16(1):76–78, 1974 4521612

Green MW, Seeger JD, Peterson C, Bhattacharyya A: Utilization of topiramate during pregnancy and risk of birth defects. Headache 52(7):1070–1084, 2012 22724387

Gulisano M, Calì PV, Cavanna AE, et al: Cardiovascular safety of aripiprazole and pimozide in young patients with Tourette syndrome. Neurol Sci 32(6):1213–1217, 2011 21732066

Hammerman A, Dreiher J, Klang SH, et al: Antipsychotics and diabetes: an age-related association. Ann Pharmacother 42(9):1316–1322, 2008 18664607

Hedderick EF, Morris CM, Singer HS: Double-blind, crossover study of clonidine and levetiracetam in Tourette syndrome. Pediatr Neurol 40(6):420–425, 2009 19433274

Hirschtritt ME, Lee PC, Pauls DL, et al: Lifetime prevalence, age of risk, and genetic relationships of comorbid psychiatric disorders in Tourette syndrome. JAMA Psychiatry 72(4):325–333, 2015 25671412

Hunt RD, Minderaa RB, Cohen DJ: Clonidine benefits children with attention deficit disorder and hyperactivity: report of a double-blind placebo-crossover therapeutic trial. J Am Acad Child Psychiatry 24(5):617–629, 1985 3900182

Jankovic J: Botulinum toxin in the treatment of dystonic tics. Mov Disord 9(3):347–349, 1994 8041378

Jankovic J: Treatment of hyperkinetic movement disorders. Lancet Neurol 8(9):844–856, 2009 19679276

Jankovic J, Jimenez-Shahed J, Brown LW: A randomised, double-blind, placebo-controlled study of topiramate in the treatment of Tourette syndrome. J Neurol Neurosurg Psychiatry 81(1):70–73, 2010 19726418

Kelsey DK, Sumner CR, Casat CD, et al: Once-daily atomoxetine treatment for children with attention-deficit/hyperactivity disorder, including an assessment of evening and morning behavior: a double-blind, placebo-controlled trial. Pediatrics 114(1):e1–e8, 2004 15231966

King A, Harris P, Fritzell J, Kurlan R: Syncope in children with Tourette's syndrome treated with guanfacine. Mov Disord 21(3):419–420, 2006 16229000

Knight T, Steeves T, Day L, et al: Prevalence of tic disorders: a systematic review and meta-analysis. Pediatr Neurol 47(2):77–90, 2012 22759682

Kwak CH, Hanna PA, Jankovic J: Botulinum toxin in the treatment of tics. Arch Neurol 57(8):1190–1193, 2000 10927800

Law SF, Schachar RJ: Do typical clinical doses of methylphenidate cause tics in children treated for attention-deficit hyperactivity disorder? J Am Acad Child Adolesc Psychiatry 38(8):944–951, 1999 10434485

Leckman JF, Riddle MA, Hardin MT, et al: The Yale Global Tic Severity Scale: initial testing of a clinician-rated scale of tic severity. J Am Acad Child Adolesc Psychiatry 28(4):566–573, 1989 2768151

Leckman JF, Walker DE, Cohen DJ: Premonitory urges in Tourette's syndrome. Am J Psychiatry 150(1):98–102, 1993 8417589

Leckman JF, Grice DE, Barr LC, et al: Tic-related vs. non-tic-related obsessive compulsive disorder. Anxiety 1(5):208–215, 1994 9160576

Lewin AB, Chang S, McCracken J, et al: Comparison of clinical features among youth with tic disorders, obsessive-compulsive disorder (OCD), and both conditions. Psychiatry Res 178(2):317–322, 2010 20488548

Lin H, Yeh CB, Peterson BS, et al: Assessment of symptom exacerbations in a longitudinal study of children with Tourette's syndrome or obsessive-compulsive disorder. J Am Acad Child Adolesc Psychiatry 41(9):1070–1077, 2002 12218428

Lipkin PH, Goldstein IJ, Adesman AR: Tics and dyskinesias associated with stimulant treatment in attention-deficit hyperactivity disorder. Arch Pediatr Adolesc Med 148(8):859–861, 1994 8044265

Lowe TL, Cohen DJ, Detlor J, et al: Stimulant medications precipitate Tourette's syndrome. JAMA 247(12):1729–1731, 1982 6950128

Lyon GJ, Samar S, Jummani R, et al: Aripiprazole in children and adolescents with Tourette's disorder: an open-label safety and tolerability study. J Child Adolesc Psychopharmacol 19(6):623–633, 2009 20035580

Marras C, Andrews D, Sime E, Lang AE: Botulinum toxin for simple motor tics: a randomized, double-blind, controlled clinical trial. Neurology 56(5):605–610, 2001 11245710

Masi G, Gagliano A, Siracusano R, et al: Aripiprazole in children with Tourette's disorder and co-morbid attention-deficit/hyperactivity disorder: a 12-week, open-label, preliminary study. J Child Adolesc Psychopharmacol 22(2):120–125, 2012 22375853

Masi G, Pfanner C, Brovedani P: Antipsychotic augmentation of selective serotonin reuptake inhibitors in resistant tic-related obsessive-compulsive disorder in children and adolescents: a naturalistic comparative study. J Psychiatr Res 47(8):1007–1012, 2013 23664673

McDougle CJ, Goodman WK, Leckman JF, et al: Haloperidol addition in fluvoxamine-refractory obsessive-compulsive disorder: a double-blind, placebo-controlled study in patients with and without tics. Arch Gen Psychiatry 51(4):302–308, 1994 8161290

McGuire JF, Piacentini J, Brennan EA, et al: A meta-analysis of behavior therapy for Tourette syndrome. J Psychiatr Res 50:106–112, 2014 24398255

Meyer JM, Koro CE: The effects of antipsychotic therapy on serum lipids: a comprehensive review. Schizophr Res 70(1):1–17, 2004 15246458

Michelson D, Faries D, Wernicke J, et al: Atomoxetine in the treatment of children and adolescents with attention-deficit/hyperactivity disorder: a randomized, placebo-controlled, dose-response study. Pediatrics 108(5):E83, 2001 11694667

Michelson D, Allen AJ, Busner J, et al: Once-daily atomoxetine treatment for children and adolescents with attention deficit hyperactivity disorder: a randomized, placebo-controlled study. Am J Psychiatry 159(11):1896–1901, 2002 12411225

Mohammadi MR, Ghanizadeh A, Alaghband-Rad J, et al: Selegiline in comparison with methylphenidate in attention deficit hyperactivity disorder children and adolescents in a double-blind, randomized clinical trial. J Child Adolesc Psychopharmacol 14(3):418–425, 2004 15650498

Mølgaard-Nielsen D, Hviid A: Newer-generation antiepileptic drugs and the risk of major birth defects. JAMA 305(19):1996–2002, 2011 21586715

MTA Cooperative Group: Multimodal Treatment Study of Children with ADHD: a 14-month randomized clinical trial of treatment strategies for attention-deficit/hyperactivity disorder. Arch Gen Psychiatry 56(12):1073–1086, 1999 10591283

Mukaddes NM, Abali O: Quetiapine treatment of children and adolescents with Tourette's disorder. J Child Adolesc Psychopharmacol 13(3):295–299, 2003 14642017

Murphy TK, Mutch PJ, Reid JM, et al: Open label aripiprazole in the treatment of youth with tic disorders. J Child Adolesc Psychopharmacol 19(4):441–447, 2009 19702496

Murphy TK, Fernandez TV, Coffey BJ, et al: Extended-release guanfacine does not show a large effect on tic severity in children with chronic tic disorders. J Child Adolesc Psychopharmacol 27(9):762–770, 2017 28723227

Nicolson R, Craven-Thuss B, Smith J, et al: A randomized, double-blind, placebo-controlled trial of metoclopramide for the treatment of Tourette's disorder. J Am Acad Child Adolesc Psychiatry 44(7):640–646, 2005 15968232

Olvera C, Stebbins GT, Goetz CG, Kompoliti K. TikTok tics: a pandemic within a pandemic. Mov Disord Clin Pract 8(8): 1200–1205, 2021 34765687

Palumbo DR, Sallee FR, Pelham WE Jr, et al: Clonidine for attention-deficit/hyperactivity disorder, I: efficacy and tolerability outcomes. J Am Acad Child Adolesc Psychiatry 47(2):180–188, 2008 18182963

Pediatric OCD Treatment Study Team: Cognitive-behavior therapy, sertraline, and their combination for children and adolescents with obsessive-compulsive disorder: the Pediatric OCD Treatment Study (POTS) randomized controlled trial. JAMA 292(16):1969–1976, 2004 15507582

Peterson BS, Pine DS, Cohen P, Brook JS: Prospective, longitudinal study of tic, obsessive-compulsive, and attention-deficit/hyperactivity disorders in an epidemiological sample. J Am Acad Child Adolesc Psychiatry 40(6):685–695, 2001 11392347

Porta M, Maggioni G, Ottaviani F, Schindler A: Treatment of phonic tics in patients with Tourette's syndrome using botulinum toxin type A. Neurol Sci 24(6):420–423, 2004 14767691

Pringsheim T, Steeves T: Pharmacological treatment for attention deficit hyperactivity disorder (ADHD) in children with comorbid tic disorders. Cochrane Database Syst Rev (4):CD007990, 2011 21491404

Radhakrishnan L, Leeb RT, Bitsko RH, et al: Pediatric emergency department visits associated with mental health conditions before and during the COVID-19 pandemic—United States, January 2019–January 2022. MMWR Morb Mortal Wkly Rep 71(8):319–324, 2022 35202358

Riddle MA, Lynch KA, Scahill L, et al: Methylphenidate discontinuation and reinitiation during long-term treatment of children with Tourette's disorder and attention-deficit hyperactivity disorder. J Child Adolesc Psychopharmacol 5(3):205–214, 1995

Robertson MM: A personal 35 year perspective on Gilles de la Tourette syndrome: assessment, investigations, and management. Lancet Psychiatry 2(1):88–104, 2015 26359615

Roessner V, Rothenberger A, Rickards H, Hoekstra PJ: European clinical guidelines for Tourette syndrome and other tic disorders. Eur Child Adolesc Psychiatry 20(4):153–154, 2011 21445722

Ross MS, Moldofsky H: A comparison of pimozide and haloperidol in the treatment of Gilles de la Tourette's syndrome. Am J Psychiatry 135(5):585–587, 1978 347954

Rutter M, Tizard J, Whitmore K: Education, Health, and Behavior. London, Longman, 1970

Sallee FR, Nesbitt L, Jackson C, et al: Relative efficacy of haloperidol and pimozide in children and adolescents with Tourette's disorder. Am J Psychiatry 154(8):1057–1062, 1997 9247389

Sallee FR, Kurlan R, Goetz CG, et al: Ziprasidone treatment of children and adolescents with Tourette's syndrome: a pilot study. J Am Acad Child Adolesc Psychiatry 39(3):292–299, 2000 10714048

Sallee FR, Lyne A, Wigal T, McGough JJ: Long-term safety and efficacy of guanfacine extended release in children and adolescents with attention-deficit/hyperactivity disorder. J Child Adolesc Psychopharmacol 19(3):215–226, 2009 19519256

Sallee F, Kohegyi E, Zhao J, et al: Randomized, double-blind, placebo-controlled trial demonstrates the efficacy and safety of oral aripiprazole for the treatment of Tourette's disorder in children and adolescents. J Child Adolesc Psychopharmacol 27(9):771–781, 2017 28686474

Scahill L, Riddle MA, McSwiggin-Hardin M, et al: Children's Yale-Brown Obsessive Compulsive Scale: reliability and validity. J Am Acad Child Adolesc Psychiatry 36(6):844–852, 1997 9183141

Scahill L, Chappell PB, Kim YS, et al: A placebo-controlled study of guanfacine in the treatment of children with tic disorders and attention deficit hyperactivity disorder. Am J Psychiatry 158(7):1067–1074, 2001 11431228

Scahill L, Kano Y, King R, et al: Influence of age and tic disorders on obsessive compulsive disorder in a pediatric sample. J Child Adolesc Psychopharmacol 13(Suppl 1):s7–s17, 2003a

Scahill L, Leckman JF, Schultz RT, et al: A placebo-controlled trial of risperidone in Tourette syndrome. Neurology 60(7):1130–1135, 2003b 12682319

Scahill L, Erenberg G, Berlin CM Jr, et al: Contemporary assessment and pharmacotherapy of Tourette syndrome. NeuroRx 3(2):192–206, 2006 16554257

Scahill L, Specht M, Page C: The prevalence of tic disorders and clinical characteristics in children. J Obsessive Compuls Relat Disord 3(4):394–400, 2014 25436183

Scharf JM, Miller LL, Gauvin CA, et al: Population prevalence of Tourette syndrome: a systematic review and meta-analysis. Mov Disord 30(2):221–228, 2015 25487709

Schrock LE, Mink JW, Woods DW, et al: Tourette syndrome deep brain stimulation: a review and updated recommendations. Mov Disord 30(4):448–471, 2015 25476818

Shapiro AK, Shapiro E: Controlled study of pimozide vs. placebo in Tourette's syndrome. J Am Acad Child Psychiatry 23(2):161–173, 1984 6371107

Shapiro E, Shapiro AK, Fulop G, et al: Controlled study of haloperidol, pimozide and placebo for the treatment of Gilles de la Tourette's syndrome. Arch Gen Psychiatry 46(8):722–730, 1989 2665687

Singer HS, Brown J, Quaskey S, et al: The treatment of attention-deficit hyperactivity disorder in Tourette's syndrome: a double-blind placebo-controlled study with clonidine and desipramine. Pediatrics 95(1):74–81, 1995 7770313

Smith-Hicks CL, Bridges DD, Paynter NP, Singer HS: A double blind randomized placebo control trial of levetiracetam in Tourette syndrome. Mov Disord 22(12):1764–1770, 2007 17566124

Spencer T, Biederman J, Coffey B, et al: A double-blind comparison of desipramine and placebo in children and adolescents with chronic tic disorder and comorbid attention-deficit/hyperactivity disorder. Arch Gen Psychiatry 59(7):649–656, 2002 12090818

Stamenkovic M, Schindler SD, Aschauer HN, et al: Effective open-label treatment of Tourette's disorder with olanzapine. Int Clin Psychopharmacol 15(1):23–28, 2000 10836282

Stephens RJ, Bassel C, Sandor P: Olanzapine in the treatment of aggression and tics in children with Tourette's syndrome: a pilot study. J Child Adolesc Psychopharmacol 14(2):255–266, 2004 15319022

Sukhodolsky DG, Scahill L, Zhang H, et al: Disruptive behavior in children with Tourette's syndrome: association with ADHD comorbidity, tic severity, and functional impairment. J Am Acad Child Adolesc Psychiatry 42(1):98–105, 2003 12500082

Toren P, Weizman A, Ratner S, et al: Ondansetron treatment in Tourette's disorder: a 3-week, randomized, double-blind, placebo-controlled study. J Clin Psychiatry 66(4):499–503, 2005 15816793

Tourette's Syndrome Study Group: Treatment of ADHD in children with tics: a randomized controlled trial. Neurology 58(4):527–536, 2002 11865128

Varley CK, Vincent J, Varley P, Calderon R: Emergence of tics in children with attention deficit hyperactivity disorder treated with stimulant medications. Compr Psychiatry 42(3):228–233, 2001 11349243

Wang LJ, Chou WJ, Chou MC, Gau SS: The effectiveness of aripiprazole for tics, social adjustment, and parental stress in children and adolescents with Tourette's disorder. J Child Adolesc Psychopharmacol 26(5):442–448, 2016 27028456

Wang S, Wei YZ, Yang JH, et al: The efficacy and safety of aripiprazole for tic disorders in children and adolescents: a systematic review and meta-analysis. Psychiatry Res 254:24–32, 2017 28441584

Wijemanne S, Wu LJ, Jankovic J: Long-term efficacy and safety of fluphenazine in patients with Tourette syndrome. Mov Disord 29(1):126–130, 2014 24150997

Wonodi I, Reeves G, Carmichael D, et al: Tardive dyskinesia in children treated with atypical antipsychotic medications. Mov Disord 22(12):1777–1782, 2007 17580328

Woods DW, Piacentini J, Himle MB, Chang S: Premonitory Urge for Tics Scale (PUTS): initial psychometric results and examination of the premonitory urge phenomenon in youths with tic disorders. J Dev Behav Pediatr 26(6):397–403, 2005 16344654

Yamamuro K, Makinodan M, Ota T, et al: Paliperidone extended release for the treatment of pediatric and adolescent patients with Tourette's disorder. Ann Gen Psychiatry 13:13, 2014 24829608

Yang CS, Huang H, Zhang LL, Zhu CR, et al: Aripiprazole for the treatment of tic disorders in children: a systematic review and meta-analysis. BMC Psychiatry 15:179, 2015 26220447

Yang C, Yi Q, Zhang L, et al: Safety of aripiprazole for tics in children and adolescents: a systematic review and meta-analysis. Medicine (Baltimore) 98(22):e15816, 2019 31145316

Yoo HK, Lee JS, Paik KW, et al: Open-label study comparing the efficacy and tolerability of aripiprazole and haloperidol in the treatment of pediatric tic disorders. Eur Child Adolesc Psychiatry 20(3):127–135, 2011 21188439

Yoo HK, Joung YS, Lee JS, et al: A multicenter, randomized, double-blind, placebo-controlled study of aripiprazole in children and adolescents with Tourette's disorder. J Clin Psychiatry 74(8):e772–e780, 2013 24021518

Yu L, Yan J, Wen F, et al: Revisiting the efficacy and tolerability of topiramate for tic disorders: a meta-analysis. J Child Adolesc Psychopharmacol 30(5):316–325, 2020 32191124

Zheng W, Li XB, Xiang YQ, et al: Aripiprazole for Tourette's syndrome: a systematic review and meta-analysis. Hum Psychopharmacol 31(1):11–18, 2016 26310194

Zheng Y, Zhang Z-J, Han X-M, et al: A proprietary herbal medicine (5-Ling granule) for Tourette syndrome: a randomized controlled trial. J Child Psychol Psychiatry 57(1):74–83, 2016 26072932

9

Early-Onset Schizophrenia and Psychotic Illnesses

Ekaterina Stepanova, M.D., Ph.D.
David I. Driver, M.D.
Nitin Gogtay, M.D.
Judith L. Rapoport, M.D.

Childhood-onset schizophrenia (COS) or *very early-onset schizophrenia* is defined as the onset of psychotic symptoms before age 13 (Rapoport et al. 2012). Clinically, COS resembles the adult form in its positive and negative symptoms. Neurobiologically, it shares many of the same neuroanatomical anomalies, genetic risks, and neuropsychological deficits as adult-onset schizophrenia (for review, see Driver et al. 2020). The prevalence of COS is very low (Kleinhaus et al. 2011). In a National Institute of Mental Health (NIMH) study, the prevalence was less than 0.04% (Driver et al. 2020). Given the timing and nature of the onset, COS is associated with a particularly severe disruption of cognitive and social development, and the burden to the family can be devastating. The term *early-onset schizophrenia* (EOS) has been used to describe onset before age 18 years (American Academy of Child and Adolescent Psychiatry 2001). It is estimated that about 10% of patients with schizophrenia have onset before age 18 (Rabinowitz et al. 2006). Although many studies considered in this chapter include patients with symptom onset during adolescence, we emphasize studies of patients with COS (onset before age 13).

History and Classification of Psychosis in Children

Although the existence of childhood schizophrenia was recognized early in the twentieth century (Kraepelin 1919), the term *psychosis* was used broadly in children, and a spectrum of behavioral disorders and autism were also grouped under the category of childhood schizophrenia (Volkmar 1996). The landmark studies by Kolvin first established the clinical distinction between autism and other psychotic disorders of childhood (Kolvin 1971). Today, high rates of initial misdiagnosis remain because of symptom overlap, primarily in the context of the presence of hallucinations and delusions in nonpsychotic pediatric patients (Kelleher et al. 2012).

The prevalence of hallucinations in nonpsychotic youth is around 12% (Maijer et al. 2018). Negative life events and trauma leading to anxiety and stress have been suggested as the causes of hallucinations in preschool-age children, and the prognosis of these phenomena is usually benign. However, psychotic phenomena in school-age children may be more persistent and are associated with a significant increase in the prevalence and severity of illness (David and Rapoport 2012; David et al. 2011; Polanczyk et al. 2010). According to data from a large birth cohort, self-reported psychotic symptoms at age 11 predicted a high risk (OR 16.4) of schizophreniform diagnoses by age 26 (Poulton et al. 2000).

A heterogeneous but sizable group of children referred to as the NIMH Childhood-Onset Schizophrenia Study since 1991 show transient psychotic symptoms and multiple developmental abnormalities that cannot be adequately characterized by existing DSM-5 categories (American Psychiatric Association 2022; Gordon et al. 1994). Therefore, the term *multidimensionally impaired* has been used to capture the mix of stress-related transient episodes of psychosis, emotional instability, impaired interpersonal skills, and information-processing deficits exhibited by these children (Frazier et al. 1994; Kumra et al. 1998). Along with children with COS, children who are multidimensionally impaired have been followed up longitudinally, and they have provided a medication-matched contrast for various clinical and neuroimaging studies.

In this chapter, we highlight studies that focused on COS because of the unique psychiatric vantage point provided by this diagnostic subset (Rapoport et al. 2005a, 2005b).

Epidemiology

Due to the rarity of COS, large-scale epidemiological studies are not feasible. A study of hospital admissions of 312 psychotic youth over a 13-year period in Denmark found only four patients who were younger than 13 years at the time of symptom onset (Thomsen 1996). The NIMH study indicated that most children younger than 13 who are given a diagnosis of schizophrenia do not actually meet the criteria for schizophrenia (Driver et al. 2020; Rapoport and Gogtay 2011). After more than 3,500 screenings, only 217 children have been offered admission to our study (Driver et al. 2020). Of those, only 134 patients have received a diagnosis of COS.

Course and Outcome

Long-term follow-up of EOS cases indicates chronic illness and impairment. Hollis (2000) found that, compared with subjects with nonschizophrenic psychoses, a large cohort diagnosed with EOS (mean age at onset, 14 years) had significantly worse outcomes at a mean follow-up of 11 years. A follow-up at 42 years found that earlier age at onset among 44 patients retrospectively meeting diagnostic criteria for COS was associated with poorer clinical outcome and higher levels of disability (Eggers and Bunk 1997). Greenstein et al. (2006) reported on a prospective follow-up study over a mean of 5 years with 32 children in a NIMH cohort and noted that, despite optimal pharmacotherapy, high levels of disability and residual psychotic symptoms were evident. Data from these studies suggest a particularly disabling course of illness.

Although early age at onset was suggested to predict poorer outcomes (Remschmidt and Theisen 2012), a large longitudinal register-based study in Denmark did not support poorer long-term outcomes of EOS compared with adult onset (Vernal et al. 2020). Another study evaluated 10-year outcomes of youth with EOS and found that age at onset of psychotic symptoms was not associated with outcomes at follow-up (Xu et al. 2020). Interestingly, predictors of improved functioning in this cohort were an extroverted and suspicious personality as well as a high level of education.

Another factor that plays a large role in the course and outcome of EOS is treatment resistance, usually defined as a failure of symptoms to respond to at least two trials of antipsychotic medications (Keepers et al. 2020; Lehman et al. 2004). A large study examined predictors of treatment resistance in adolescents and young adults (Chan et al. 2021). The investigators showed that about 15% of patients with schizophrenia spectrum disorders developed treatment resistance. Predictors of treatment resistance were longer duration of the first episode, younger age at onset, poor premorbid functioning, and higher dose of antipsychotics.

Rationale for Psychopharmacological Treatment

Treatment of EOS is mostly focused on psychopharmacological intervention. Nevertheless, the role of psychological interventions should not be neglected, especially very early in the course of illness (Kendall et al. 2013; McClellan et al. 2013; Stafford et al. 2013).

The main treatment for schizophrenia is antipsychotic medications (McClellan et al. 2013). Most classifications of antipsychotics divide them into first-generation antipsychotics (FGAs; typical) and second-generation antipsychotics (SGAs; atypical). The FGAs are all high-affinity antagonists of dopamine D_2 receptors, a property that remains the most plausible explanation for their therapeutic effects. D_2 receptor antagonism also explains, in part, one of the other key features of FGAs: the high rate of movement-related side effects, particularly extrapyramidal side effects (EPS) and tardive dyskinesia (see "Extrapyramidal Side Effects" later in the chapter). SGAs differ pharmacologically from FGAs in their affinity for both D_2 and other neuroreceptors (Burstein et al. 2005). They are also thought to be associated with lower rates of EPS, tardive dyskinesia, and hyperprolactinemia, although they vary considerably in their side effect profiles (Abi-Dargham and Laruelle 2005; Miyamoto et al. 2005).

In clinical practice, SGAs have been more frequently prescribed. In a review of practices in the United States, SGA prescriptions increased by nearly 500% between 1995 and 2000 and accounted for most of the antipsychotic prescriptions among children and adolescents (Patel et al. 2002). The ratio of use for SGA to FGA antipsychotics is greater for children (2.7:1) and adolescents (3.8:1) than for adults (1.6:1) (Sikich et al. 2004). Similar trends are seen in European countries; however, psychotic disorders account for a minority of diagnoses in youth receiving antipsychotics (Varimo et al. 2020).

Pharmacotherapy

In evaluating the efficacy of antipsychotics in patients with COS, we focus on double-blind studies. In addition, we include summaries of the larger prospective open trials of SGAs that reflect current practices, and we share our experience with newer medications. It should be stressed here that antipsychotics are used for a wide range of disorders, and information about the use of both FGA and SGA formulations is presented throughout this manual.

First-Generation (Typical) Antipsychotics

Efficacy of First-Generation Antipsychotics Versus Placebo in EOS

Early studies of EOS used a placebo comparison to address the important question of whether antipsychotics had any treatment efficacy (Pool et al. 1976; Spencer et al. 1992) (Table 9–1). In one of the earliest such studies, Pool et al. (1976) conducted a double-blind, placebo-controlled trial comparing haloperidol (mean dosage, 9.8 mg/day), loxapine (mean dosage, 87.5 mg/day), and placebo in 75 hospitalized adolescents. All three groups showed significant improvement, as assessed with the Clinical Global Impression (CGI) scale, although patients rated as severely or very severely ill at baseline showed a trend toward greater improvement with the active treatments (88% for loxapine and 72% for haloperidol) than with placebo (38%).

The trial by Pool et al. (1976) had several limitations. First, the criteria for the diagnosis of schizophrenia rested on clinical consensus, and it is unclear

Table 9–1. Select controlled trials of antipsychotics in patients with COS or EOS

Study	Medication	Mean dosage	*N*	Mean age, *years*	Design	Criteria	Result
First-generation (typical) antipsychotics							
Engelhardt et al. 1973	Fluphenazine	10 mg/day	15	10	Randomized, DB	CGI much or very much improved	93% (14/15)
	Haloperidol	10 mg/day	15	10	Randomized, DB	CGI much or very much improved	87% (13/15)
Pool et al. 1976	Loxapine	87.5 mg/day	26	15	Randomized, DB	CGI much or very much improved	88% (23/26)
	Haloperidol	9.8 mg/day	25	15	Randomized, DB	CGI much or very much improved	72% (18/25)
	Placebo	NA	24	15	Randomized, DB	CGI much or very much improved	38% (9/24)
Paprocki and Versiani 1977	Loxapine	70 mg/day	25	16	Randomized, DB	CGI much or very much improved	64% (16/25)
	Haloperidol	8 mg/day	25	16	Randomized, DB	CGI much or very much improved	60% (15/25)

Table 9–1. Select controlled trials of antipsychotics in patients with COS or EOS *(continued)*

Study	Medication	Mean dosage	*N*	Mean age, *years*	Design	Criteria	Result
Realmuto et al. 1984	Thiothixene	0.26 mg/kg/day	13	15	Randomized, DB	CGI much or very much improved	54% (7/13)
	Thioridazine	2.57 mg/kg/day	8	15	Randomized, DB	CGI much or very much improved	63% (5/8)
Spencer et al. 1992	Haloperidol	8.8 mg/day	12	9	Randomized, DB crossover	Marked improvement on clinical judgment	75% (9/12)
	Placebo	NA	12	9	Randomized, DB crossover	Marked improvement on clinical judgment	0% (0/12)
Second-generation (atypical) antipsychotics							
Xiong 2004	Risperidone	2.6 mg/day	30	13.07	Randomized, DB	Responder stratified as remission, large improvement, or minor improvement based on BPRS	80% (24/30) responders
	Chlorpromazine	285.8 mg/day	30	93	Randomized, DB	Responder stratified as remission, large improvement, or minor improvement based on BPRS	82% (26/30) responders

Table 9–1. Select controlled trials of antipsychotics in patients with COS or EOS *(continued)*

Study	Medication	Mean dosage	*N*	Mean age, *years*	Design	Criteria	Result
McClellan et al. 2007; Sikich et al. 2008	Olanzapine	11.4 mg/day	35	8–19	Randomized, DB parallel groups, multisite	≥20% improvement of PANSS score and CGI score ≤2	34%
	Risperidone	2.8 mg/day	41	8–19	Randomized, DB parallel groups, multisite	≥20% improvement of PANSS score and CGI score ≤2	46%
	Molindone	59.9 mg/day (+1 mg/day benztropine)	40	8–19	Randomized, DB parallel groups, multisite	≥20% improvement of PANSS score and CGI score ≤2	50%
Kumra et al. 2008a	Olanzapine	26.2 mg/day	21[a]	15.6	Randomized, DB parallel groups, multisite	Decrease ≥30% in BPRS from baseline and CGI score ≤2	33% (7/21)
	Clozapine	403.1 mg/day	18[a]	15.6	Randomized, DB parallel groups, multisite	Decrease ≥30% in BPRS from baseline and CGI score ≤2	66% (12/18)

Table 9–1. Select controlled trials of antipsychotics in patients with COS or EOS *(continued)*

Study	Medication	Mean dosage	*N*	Mean age, *years*	Design	Criteria	Result
Jensen et al. 2008	Risperidone	3.4 mg/day	10[b]	15.6	Randomized, OL	Decrease ≥40% of PANSS total score and PANSS positive/negative subscale scores	70% (7/10)
	Olanzapine	14.0 mg/day	10[b]	15.3	Randomized, OL	Decrease ≥40% of PANSS total score and PANSS positive/negative subscale scores	50% (5/10)
	Quetiapine	611 mg/day	10[b]	14.8	Randomized, OL	Decrease ≥40% of PANSS total score and PANSS positive/negative subscale scores	30% (3/10)
Findling et al. 2012	Quetiapine (high)	800 mg/day	74	15.4	Randomized, DB, parallel groups, multisite	Decrease ≥30% in PANSS	36.5% (27/75)
	Quetiapine (low)	400 mg/day	73	15.4	Randomized, DB, parallel groups, multisite	Decrease ≥30% in PANSS	38.4% (28/73)

Table 9–1. Select controlled trials of antipsychotics in patients with COS or EOS *(continued)*

Study	Medication	Mean dosage	*N*	Mean age, *years*	Design	Criteria	Result
Findling et al. 2012 *(continued)*	Placebo	NA	73	15.4	Randomized, DB, parallel groups, multisite	Decrease ≥30% in PANSS	26.0% (19/73)
Findling et al. 2015	Asenapine (high)	5 mg/day bid	104	15.3	Randomized, DB, parallel groups, multisite	Decrease ≥20% in PANSS total score and PANSS positive/negative subscale scores	50% (52/104)
	Asenapine (low)	2.5 mg/day bid	96	15.3	Randomized, DB, parallel groups, multisite	Decrease ≥20% in PANSS total score and PANSS positive/negative subscale scores	49% (47/96)
	Placebo	NA	100	15.3	Randomized, DB, parallel groups, multisite	Decrease ≥20% in PANSS total score and PANSS positive/negative subscale scores	36% (36/100)

Table 9–1. Select controlled trials of antipsychotics in patients with COS or EOS *(continued)*

Study	Medication	Mean dosage	*N*	Mean age, *years*	Design	Criteria	Result
Savitz et al. 2015a	Paliperidone ER	6.75 mg/day	112	15.3	Randomized, DB, parallel groups, multisite	Maintained clinical stability[c] and ≥20% improvement on PANSS	52% (58/112) stable, 76.8% (86/112) PANSS
	Aripiprazole	11.56 mg/day	114	15.3	Randomized, DB parallel groups, multisite	Maintained clinical stability[c] and ≥20% improvement on PANSS	60% (47/114) stable, 81.6% (93/114) PANSS
Correll et al. 2017	Aripiprazole	10–30 mg/day	146	15.3	Randomized, DB, PC, withdrawal, multicenter	Time to symptom exacerbation	Longer time to exacerbation (HR 0.46)
Pagsberg et al. 2017a	Quetiapine ER	600 mg/day	55	15.8	DB, randomized, multicenter	PANSS positive score change	−5.05
	Aripiprazole	20 mg/day	58	15.7	DB, randomized, multicenter	PANSS positive score change	−6.21
Goldman et al. 2017	Lurasidone	40 mg/day	108	15.5	DB, randomized, PC	PANSS positive score change	−18.6
		80 mg/day	106	15.3	DB, randomized, PC	PANSS positive score change	−18.3

Table 9–1. Select controlled trials of antipsychotics in patients with COS or EOS *(continued)*

Study	Medication	Mean dosage	*N*	Mean age, *years*	Design	Criteria	Result
Goldman et al. 2017 *(continued)*	Placebo	NA	112	15.3	DB, randomized, PC	PANSS positive score change	−10.5

Note. BPRS=Brief Psychiatric Rating Scale; CGI=Clinical Global Impression Scale; COS=childhood-onset schizophrenia; DB=double-blind; EOS=early-onset schizophrenia; HR=hazard ratio; NA=not applicable; OL=open-label; PANSS=Positive and Negative Syndrome Scale; PC= placebo-controlled.

[a]This study was done with patients with treatment-refractory EOS.

[b]These populations included EOS and EOS spectrum disorders.

[c]*Clinical stability* is defined as >20% improvement from baseline PANSS, <4 on CGI by day 56, and no hospitalizations.

whether all of the subjects would meet contemporary DSM-5 criteria for schizophrenia. The exact age at onset of first symptoms was not given; subsequently, it may have been variable. Finally, the degree of treatment resistance was not provided. Despite these caveats, this remains a landmark study establishing the efficacy of FGAs in EOS. Additional trials of FGAs in EOS are summarized in Table 9–1, alongside the landmark atypical trial of the Treatment of Early-Onset Schizophrenia Spectrum Disorders (TEOSS) study (McClellan et al. 2007; Sikich et al. 2008). In a double-blind, placebo-controlled crossover study, Spencer et al. (1992) randomly assigned 12 children meeting DSM-III-R (American Psychiatric Association 1987) criteria for schizophrenia to either haloperidol for 4 weeks followed by placebo for 4 weeks or placebo for 4 weeks followed by haloperidol for 4 weeks. The exact details of prior antipsychotics response were not given. On the primary outcome measure (CGI) and ratings of positive psychotic symptoms, the haloperidol group alone showed significant improvement (decrease from a baseline score of 5.15 to 2.99; $P<0.001$), with no significant change in the placebo group. The authors noted that a relatively small dosage of haloperidol, with a range of 0.5–3.5 mg/day, was optimal.

Comparison of Efficacy of First-Generation Antipsychotics

Several studies have directly compared the efficacy of two FGAs in the absence of a placebo arm, including double-blind comparisons of fluphenazine and haloperidol (Engelhardt et al. 1973), thiothixene and thioridazine (Realmuto et al. 1984), and loxapine and haloperidol (Paprocki and Versiani 1977) (see Table 9–1). All studies reported high rates of response (based on the CGI), ranging from 54% to more than 90%, and the antipsychotics did not differ significantly from each other on nearly all outcome measures. However, these earlier studies all suffered from the same limitations: the criteria used to define schizophrenia were unclear, and changes in specific psychotic symptoms were not reported.

Indeed, given current prescribing practices, most comparisons of FGAs are of historical interest. However, the results of the NIMH Clinical Antipsychotic Trials of Intervention Effectiveness (CATIE) project, which demonstrated equal efficacy for the FGA perphenazine and four SGAs in adults with chronic schizophrenia, may renew interest in the use of FGAs for psychosis (Lieberman et al. 2005). Xiong (2004) extended this finding in a comparison of risperidone (response rate 80%) and chlorpromazine (response rate 82%). The TEOSS study (described in detail later in this chapter) found similar response rates between molindone and risperidone (Sikich et al. 2008).

Second-Generation (Atypical) Antipsychotics

Mechanisms of Action

The advent of SGAs appeared to herald an era of treatment for schizophrenia, with the possibility of more efficacious agents and more favorable side effect profiles (Kane et al. 1988). Several reviews have considered the issue of what makes an SGA atypical (e.g., Kapur and Remington 2001). Most agree on lowered risk of EPS and hyperprolactinemia, with some also reporting that SGAs are more effective in ameliorating the negative symptoms of schizophrenia, although this differential effect is likely to be small (effect size on the order of 0.1 [Cohen's *d*]).

In terms of pharmacological properties, most SGAs have a higher affinity for serotonin receptors, specifically the 5-HT_{2A} family, and, to a lesser extent, the dopamine D_4 receptor. However, neither property is necessary for atypicality. For example, amisulpride is a relatively pure D_2/D_3 antagonist lacking serotonin receptor antagonism, and several FGAs, including haloperidol, have high affinity for D_4 receptors. More recently, it has been proposed that SGAs may have a faster rate of dissociation from the D_2 receptor, allowing the drug to be more responsive to endogenous dopamine. This, in turn, allows an antipsychotic effect while avoiding EPS and prolactin elevation. Amato et al. (2011) discussed dynamic dopamine and serotonin responses in both treatment action and failure. Their work highlighted specific changes in dopaminergic response and their reversal as a possible fundamental underpinning for the action and failure of antipsychotics, respectively.

Efficacy of Second-Generation Antipsychotics

Several SGAs are currently FDA approved for the treatment of schizophrenia in youth ages 13–17, including olanzapine, risperidone, aripiprazole, lurasidone, and quetiapine. In addition, paliperidone has been approved by the FDA for the treatment of adolescents as young as 12 with schizophrenia. Most second-generation antipsychotics (aripiprazole, paliperidone, risperidone, quetiapine, olanzapine), with the exclusion of ziprasidone, show comparable efficacy based on Positive and Negative Syndrome Scale (PANSS) total symptom change (meta-analysis; Pagsberg et al. 2017b). Another meta-analysis suggested that only three antipsychotics (molindone, olanzapine, and risperidone) were associated with a statistically significant reduction in total PANSS score (Harvey et al. 2016). In the same study, only haloperidol, olanzapine, and risperidone showed significant change in positive PANSS scores, whereas none of the interventions was significant in improving negative PANSS scores. In this chapter, we look at SGAs individually to highlight understanding of their differences and respective strengths.

Risperidone. Among the SGAs, risperidone is prescribed more frequently than other antipsychotic medications for the treatment of EOS (Vernal et al. 2015). A 6-week open-label study of risperidone (mean dosage, 3.14 mg/day) in 11 treatment-naive adolescents who met DSM-IV (American Psychiatric Association 1994) criteria for schizophrenia reported significant improvements in ratings on the CGI and the Brief Psychiatric Rating Scale (BPRS) and positive, but not negative symptoms, rated on the PANSS (Zalsman et al. 2003). Another study reported a categorical response rate of 60% (response defined with the CGI) among 10 adolescents (Armenteros et al. 1997). The dosages of risperidone in this study were higher (mean, 6.6 mg/day), perhaps reflecting the inclusion of a large proportion of subjects with a history of treatment resistance.

In a 6-week, randomized, double-blind, placebo-controlled study, 160 adolescents ages 13–17 years with schizophrenia were given placebo, risperidone 1–3 mg/day, or risperidone 4–6 mg/day (Haas et al. 2009b). Both risperidone groups had significantly improved PANSS scores compared with the placebo group ($P<0.001$). Adverse effects were present at higher rates in both risperidone groups (75% and 76%) than in the placebo group (54%), with the higher-dosage group demonstrating increased rates of dizziness, hypertonia, and EPS than the lower-dosage group. Haas et al. (2009a) also published a study of adolescents with schizophrenia who were randomly assigned 1:1 to risperidone either 1.5–6.0 mg/day ($n=125$) or 0.15–0.6 mg/day ($n=132$). Although treatment was well tolerated overall, patients given the higher dosage experienced adverse events at a rate of 74%, whereas those given the lower dosage experienced adverse events at a rate of 65%. In consideration of the low overall incidence of EPS and lack of hyperprolactinemia, the authors recommended a dosage of risperidone 1–3 mg/day for adolescents with schizophrenia (Haas et al. 2009b).

Olanzapine. In some of the earliest work in COS, data from an open-label NIMH study suggested only modest improvement with olanzapine, with 17% improvement on the BPRS but only a 1% improvement in positive symptoms and no significant change in CGI Improvement subscale scores (Kumra et al. 1998). These modest gains are thought to reflect the treatment-refractory nature of the illness in most of the NIMH cohort.

In 12-week open-label olanzapine study involving a group of nine children with treatment-refractory schizophrenia, Mozes et al. (2003) found an overall response of significant improvement on all outcome measures. Studies that include a treatment-naive population or those involving youth with minimal prior exposure to antipsychotics show more robust effects. For example, among patients in an outpatient study, Findling et al. (2003) found responses in both negative and positive symptoms. Similarly, Ross et al. (2003) reported 37% full response and 32% partial response rates with olanzapine for school-age children with schizophrenia. Notably, this significant improvement was observed only at the 1-year mark, and there was evidence of an increasing amelioration of negative symptoms with time. This serves to emphasize the need for longer-term studies. The more recent literature echoes similar findings, although some researchers recommend considering olanzapine as a second-line agent for EOS because of its heightened risks for significant weight gain and lipid dysregulation (Deniau et al. 2008).

Shaw et al. (2006) performed an 8-week, double-blind randomized controlled trial (RCT) of olanzapine versus clozapine with a 2-year open-label follow-up in a large sample of children ages 7–16 years who met unmodified DSM-IV criteria for schizophrenia and whose schizophrenia was resistant to treatment. Compared with clozapine (see section "Use of Clozapine in Treating Childhood-Onset Schizophrenia"), olanzapine demonstrated a less consistent profile of clinical improvement. Although the results of this study do not definitively demonstrate the superiority of clozapine over olanzapine in treatment-refractory COS, the study suggests that in an independent, dichotomous comparison of the two antipsychotics, clozapine has a more favorable clinical response profile and is better balanced against associated adverse events.

In another randomized, single-blind, 6-month study conducted in 50 adolescents with early-onset psychosis, no changes were observed in patients' cognitive performance, and there was no evidence of differential efficacy of olanzapine or quetiapine on cognitive improvement (Robles et al. 2011).

More recent work has continued to highlight the complex relationship between olanzapine's potential for clinical response and its adverse side effects. One multisite, international, randomized (2:1), double-blind controlled trial assessed 117 adolescents with schizophrenia receiving flexible dosages of olanzapine 2.5–20.0 mg/day ($n=72$; mean age, 16.1 years) or placebo ($n=35$; mean age, 16.3 years) for up to 6 weeks (Kryzhanovskaya et al. 2009b). Participants given olanzapine showed significantly greater improvement in a comprehensive battery of measures: PANSS total ($P=0.005$) and positive ($P=0.002$) scores, BPRS total score ($P=0.003$), and CGI Severity of Illness subscale score ($P=0.004$). They also gained more weight (4.3 kg vs. 0.1 kg; $P<0.001$) and had higher mean prolactin and triglyceride levels compared with participants given placebo (Kryzhanovskaya et al. 2009b).

From a pooled analysis of olanzapine safety in adolescent schizophrenia populations and a comparison of these data with those of adults treated with olanzapine, Kryzhanovskaya et al. (2009a) reviewed the data from the acute phase of multiple olanzapine trials with a mean daily dose of 10.6 mg (exposure =48,946 patient-days). Among the adolescents ($N=454$) in this study, 2 (0.4%) attempted suicide and 13 (2.9%) experienced suicidal ideation. The most common adverse events were increased appetite (17.4%), increased weight (31.7%), and somnolence (19.8%). The adolescents gained significantly more weight than did the adults (7.4 kg vs. 3.2 kg; $P<0.001$). Specifically, within the placebo-controlled database, adolescents demonstrated significantly greater increases in prolactin levels (11.4 μg/L; $P<0.001$) from baseline to study end point (47.4% had high levels), and the overall magnitude of prolactin and weight increases was greater in adolescents than in adults (Kryzhanovskaya et al. 2009a).

In a continuation of the TEOSS study (see McClellan et al. 2007 and Sikich et al. 2008 rows in Table 9–1 and the discussion in "Efficacy of First-Generation Antipsychotics Versus Placebo in Early-Onset Schizophrenia"), participants ages 8–19 years with schizophrenia who had improved during an 8-week, randomized, double-blind acute trial of olanzapine, risperidone, or molindone (plus benztropine) were eligible to continue taking the same medication for up to 44 additional weeks under double-blind conditions. No particular agent was found to demonstrate superior efficacy; instead, patients taking any of the three medications exhibited typical weight gain and other metabolic side effects (Findling et al. 2010b; Sikich et al. 2008).

Aripiprazole. Aripiprazole has a unique receptor profile, with partial agonist action at the D_2 and 5-HT_{1A} receptors. According to Normala and Hamidin (2009), it has unique properties of fewer metabolic complications and EPS than are commonly observed with other SGAs used to treat children and adolescents with EOS.

One study evaluated the safety and pharmacokinetics of various dosages of aripiprazole in patients ages 10–17 years (Findling et al. 2008a). Patients received aripiprazole for up to 12 days by forced titration to achieve dosages of 20 mg/day, 25 mg/day, or 30 mg/day and then received the maximum dosage for 14 more days. Aripiprazole proved generally well tolerated; although all patients experienced at least one adverse side effect, none met criteria for a serious classification. The pharmacokinetics of aripiprazole administration in youth appeared linear across the dosage range and was comparable with previous pharmacokinetics observations in adults.

Another study by Findling et al. (2008b) enrolled youth ages 13–17 years with schizophrenia in a 6-week, multicenter, double-blind RCT comparing aripiprazole (10 mg/day and 30 mg/day) with placebo. Subjects given either aripiprazole dosage showed statistically significant improvement in PANSS total scores and improvement in PANSS Hostility factor scores compared with those given placebo. Although the medication was well tolerated overall, EPS, somnolence, and tremors emerged at twice the rate for placebo. However, both the aripiprazole 10-mg/day and 30-mg/day dosages proved to have superior efficacy to placebo in treating acute schizophrenia in this young population. The 30-mg/day dosage showed significant contrasts to placebo by week 3, whereas changes in the 10-mg/day dosage did not appear until week 6 (Findling et al. 2008b).

Aripiprazole's effectiveness in the treatment of EOS was evaluated in a multicenter, double-blind, placebo-controlled, randomized withdrawal trial of adolescents ages 13–17 years (Correll et al. 2017). In this study, participants' symptoms were stabilized on aripiprazole 10–30 mg/day for up to 21 weeks. Subsequently, they were randomly assigned either to continue the active medication or to placebo for 52 weeks. Those receiving aripiprazole had longer time to exacerbation of psychotic symptoms and had lower rates of discontinuation compared with the placebo group.

In light of this research, aripiprazole has been suggested as a possible initial choicc for the treatment of schizophrenia, with a better risk-benefit ratio than risperidone (Goeb et al. 2010), or as an augmentation option with alternative treatments such as repetitive transcranial magnetic stimulation (Normala and Hamidin 2009).

A head-to-head comparison of aripiprazole, olanzapine, and risperidone for the treatment of first-episode schizophrenia was conducted in a randomized open trial in China (Cheng et al. 2019). More people receiving risperidone had a reduction of 50% or greater in PANSS total score than did those receiving aripiprazole. However, all medications showed similar efficacy in reducing PANSS scores by 30% or more. Olanzapine was associated with the largest weight gain but with fewer neurological side effects.

Quetiapine. Quetiapine has a higher affinity for 5-HT_{2A} receptors relative to D_2 receptors and affinity for α_1-adrenergic and dopamine D_1 receptors but relatively little muscarinic action. Three open-label studies suggest that quetiapine has some efficacy in the treatment of a variety of psychotic disorders in children, including EOS (Findling et al. 2012; McConville et al. 2003; Shaw et al. 2001).

In a double-blind, randomized, fixed-dose study compared quetiapine 200 mg/day versus 400 mg/day in 141 drug-naive acutely ill patients ages 15–25 years with first-episode psychosis, both dosages were safe and well tolerated, although global and social functioning improved more in the 200-mg group than in the 400-mg group (Berger et al. 2008). The 200-mg group also had improvement on the Anhedonia-Asociality subscale of the Scale for the Assessment of Negative Symptoms, whereas the 400-mg group worsened slightly. The second phase of the study (a single-blind, naturalistic, flexible-dose, 8-week period) highlighted that, regardless of the initial dosage, the ability to flexibly modify the dosage resulted in similar quetiapine levels (average, 268 mg/day for both high- and low-dosage groups) after 12 weeks. The authors recommended conservative quetiapine dosing, beginning with 250–300 mg/day, for previously untreated patients with new-onset psychosis.

A head-to-head comparison of aripiprazole and extended-release quetiapine was described in a double-blind, multicenter, randomized trial in Denmark (Pagsberg et al. 2017a). In this study, youth ages 12–17 years diagnosed with psychotic disorder received treatment with either quetiapine 600 mg/day or aripiprazole 20 mg/day (both were titrated starting from smaller dosages) for 12 weeks. PANSS positive scores decreased from baseline but did not differ between the two groups. Treatment with quetiapine was associated with weight gain, whereas treatment with aripiprazole was associated with akathisia.

Ziprasidone and paliperidone. Ziprasidone has a complex pharmacology, acting as an agonist at 5-HT_{1A} receptors and an antagonist at 5-HT_{1D} and 5-HT_{2C} receptors—properties that may confer antidepressant effects. Published studies on the use of ziprasidone in patients with COS remain scarce, although its efficacy in open-label studies of youth with a variety of disorders has been reported (Barnett 2003). One industry-supported, double-blind, placebo-controlled, flexible-dose study failed to show any difference in efficacy between treatment with ziprasidone and placebo in 283 adolescents (Findling et al. 2010a).

Paliperidone is now approved for use in patients with schizophrenia as young as age 12 years, following recent additions to the literature of double-blind trials in adolescents. In a 6-week, double-blind, parallel-group study of 201 youth ages 12–17 years, three weight-based fixed doses of extended-release paliperidone were compared with placebo. Only the medium (3–6 mg) treatment resulted in a statistically significant improvement, and the authors concluded that this meant there was no need for weight-based dosing (Singh et al. 2011). Interestingly, Savitz et al. (2015a) compared extended-release paliperidone and aripiprazole in randomized, double-blind, parallel groups and found no difference between groups.

Long-term tolerability was assessed in 220 adolescents with schizophrenia in a large, 2-year, open-label study (Savitz et al. 2015b). The mean decrease in PANSS total scores was –19.1. Paliperidone was generally well tolerated. The most frequent side effects included somnolence, weight gain, headache, insomnia, akathisia, and tremor.

Amisulpride. Publications have discussed amisulpride as a possible alternative antipsychotic medication to treat adolescent schizophrenia (Varol Tas and Guvenir 2009), although the drug is not approved in the United States. Despite claims that amisulpride is associated with fewer EPS, case reports of induced tardive dyskinesia have surfaced in adult and adolescent patients. These findings have encouraged other analyses, and some results suggest that a combination of amisulpride and multiple other medications, especially antidepressants, may synergistically raise rates of tardive dyskinesia (Goyal and Sinha 2010). Other work suggests that amisulpride does not provide any efficacy advantage over other SGAs, but a possible reduction in weight gain risk is indicated (Martin et al. 2002; Rummel et al. 2003). Currently, the use of amisulpride in the treatment of COS has been found to be limited in scope; with the limited available research, no definitive conclusions can be drawn (Komossa et al. 2009).

Asenapine and lurasidone. Interest has arisen regarding the use of asenapine in adolescent patients. Findling et al. (2015) conducted a randomized, double-blind, parallel-group comparison of high- and low-dose asenapine versus placebo in a group of 300 adolescents. Although they noted a trend toward improvement both of the asenapine groups at day 56, this trend did not achieve statistical significance. Although there is no evidence that asenapine's efficacy is superior to that of currently available agents, its favorable weight and metabolic profiles are of clinical interest (Citrome 2009).

One study evaluated the efficacy and safety of lurasidone in adolescents ages 13–17 years with schizophrenia (Goldman et al. 2017). This 6-week, randomized placebo-controlled trial showed statistically significant reductions in PANSS scores compared with placebo at dosages of 40 mg/day (PANSS score change –18.6) or 80 mg/day (change –18.3). The most common side effects in this study were nausea, somnolence, akathisia, vomiting, and sedation.

Efficacy of Second-Generation Antipsychotics Versus First-Generation Antipsychotics in Childhood-Onset Schizophrenia

A direct comparison between two SGAs, olanzapine and risperidone, and the most commonly prescribed FGA, haloperidol, was made in a double-blind, parallel-treatment study (Sikich et al. 2004). The 8-week study included 75 children and adolescents with psychotic symptoms. All three treatments were associated with significant reductions in BPRS for Children total scores, which fell to 50% of the baseline score in the risperidone group, 44% of the baseline score in the olanzapine group, and 67% of the baseline score in the haloperidol group. The categorical response rates, like most outcome measures, did not differ significantly, but there was a trend toward better response rates with the SGAs: 74% (14 of 19) with risperidone, 88% (14 of 16) with olanzapine, and 53% (8 of 15) with haloperidol. However, there are important limitations to the generalizability of these findings. The trials included a diagnostically heterogeneous group, and only half of the subjects had a diagnosis of schizophrenia. A large proportion of the participants were receiving other psychotropic medications; however, no differences in response rates were found across treatment groups for those treated exclusively with an antipsychotic. These latter findings are congruent with an 8-week, open-label, nonrandomized comparison of olanzapine, risperidone, and haloperidol in 43 adolescents in which all three of the agents were found to be equally efficacious (Gothelf et al. 2003), as well as with a randomized, double-blind comparison of risperidone and chlorpromazine in 60 adolescents that found equal efficacy (Xiong 2004).

Kennedy et al. (2007) examined the Cochrane Schizophrenia Group Trials Register in 2006–2007 for antipsychotic effects in COS. Use of FGAs or SGAs emerged as the only significant distinction criterion in treatment groups. Although Kennedy et al. (2007) noted that any benefit from SGA use was offset by an increase in adverse effects, Halloran et al. (2010) found that SGAs were the common primary treatment choice for children with severe psychosis or multiple psychiatric diagnoses.

Sikich, McClellan, and colleagues conducted the TEOSS study (McClellan et al. 2007; Sikich et al. 2008), which was undertaken in an effort to bring clarity to the debate regarding the increased efficacy of SGAs. This double-blind multisite trial randomly assigned children with EOS and schizoaffective disorder to risperidone (0.5–6 mg/day), olanzapine (2.5–20 mg/day), or molindone (10–140 mg/day plus benztropine 1 mg/day) for 8 weeks. Results from the 116 pediatric patients receiving treatment indicated that there was no significant difference in response rate between treatment groups (see Table 9–1). The study also showed that risperidone and olanzapine were implicated in the risk of weight gain, with olanzapine causing greater changes than risperidone. Additionally, olanzapine was associated with an increased risk of raising total cholesterol and lipoprotein levels. The patients receiving molindone had higher rates of self-reported akathisia (a dysphoric sensation of restlessness associated with an intense need for movement).

In follow-up work from the TEOSS study, Findling et al. (2010b) found that patients who had shown improvement during the 8-week randomized trial continued taking the same medication (for up to 44 weeks under double-blind conditions). These data confirmed their earlier suppositions that no one medication had significantly improved efficacy compared with the others. In addition, although the olanzapine and risperidone groups experienced greater weight gain during the acute trial, maintenance treatment showed no significant differences, with increased weight gain and side effects seen in all groups. From these findings, the researchers questioned recent trends of nearly exclusive SGA use for schizophrenia treatment in youth, while pointing out the considerable metabolic complications resulting from their administration.

Age-Specific Pharmacotherapy Considerations

Factors such as age at onset, diagnosis subtype, premorbid adjustment, and cognitive functioning have a meaningful impact on treatment-response trajectories (Levine and Rabinowitz 2010). Vahia et al. (2010) observed nuances in treatment variations for patients with early- or late-onset schizophrenia. The EOS group differed from the late-onset group on all measures of psychopathology and cognitive functioning. Despite similarities on measures of depression severity, education, and negative symptoms, patients with EOS included more males, experienced more severe symptoms, and required higher antipsychotic dosages. The differences between the subgroups remained significant after adjustments for biological sex, age, illness duration, and negative symptom severity, highlighting treatment differences influenced by age at onset of psychosis. Similarly, in a study from Japan, Uchida et al. (2008) found age to be a vital factor in determining the appropriate antipsychotic dosages for patients with schizophrenia spectrum disorders, noting that dosage increases progressed with patient age through the third decade, and then they reached a plateau for two decades before decreasing.

Use of Clozapine in Treating Childhood-Onset Schizophrenia

Clozapine has emerged as the gold-standard antipsychotic for patients with treatment-refractory schizophrenia (Kane et al. 1988). Most but not all meta-analyses suggest clozapine is more efficacious than FGAs and possibly most SGAs in the short term in adults (Davis et al. 2003; Geddes et al. 2000; Kumra et al. 2008b; Leucht et al. 2003; Moncrieff 2003). Unfortunately, the data for youth are much more limited. However, one systematic review found that clozapine led to an average improvement of 69% on the BPRS in youth (Schneider et al. 2014). One study found that in 120 youth available for follow-up in a COS cohort, 72.5% remained adherent to long-term clozapine therapy, a rate likely reflective of the highly effective nature of clozapine as treatment (Kasoff et al. 2016). Unfortunately, despite the evidence in favor of clozapine, the benefits must be weighed carefully against its risks, often limiting its use.

Clinical trials of clozapine for COS have all incorporated the criteria of treatment resistance, which is a convention for current routine clinical use. Thus, no data are available on the efficacy of clozapine as a first-line agent for COS (unlike in adult schizophrenia; see Lieberman et al. 2003). A striking result is that all open trials found clear efficacy for clozapine in children with treatment-resistant COS. Frazier et al. (1994) found that 9 of 11 adolescents from the NIMH cohort showed a greater than 33% reduction in BPRS ratings. Turetz et al. (1997) demonstrated a reduction of approximately 50% on all measures and also noted that the response occurred relatively early in treatment, between weeks 2 and 8, and was sustained at a 4-month follow-up. Notably, data show that about 25%–70% of patients with treatment-resistant schizophrenia do not achieve response with clozapine (Chan et al. 2021; Siskind et al. 2017). However, long-term follow-up suggests that patients with treatment-resistant schizophrenia who were given clozapine had lower mortality rates compared with patients whose schizophrenia was not treatment resistant (Chan et al. 2021).

Clozapine has been compared with both SGAs and FGAs. In the first study, Kumra et al. (1996) compared haloperidol, probably the most widely used FGA at the time of the study (1990–1996), with clozapine. They randomly assigned 21 children to haloperidol or clozapine for 6 weeks. Clozapine was markedly superior on all components of the BPRS and ratings of clinical improvement—a striking finding, given the small sample and the severity of illness at baseline. The mean dosage of haloperidol was 16.8 mg/day, which is at the upper end of the contemporary treatment range. Such relatively high dosages have been implicated in an excess of side effects that mimic the negative symptoms of schizophrenia and lead to an underestimation of antipsychotic efficacy (Geddes et al. 2000). However, given the history of previous resistance to antipsychotics among the patients in this study, high dosages would have been expected and were guided by clinical judgment.

Shaw et al. (2006) compared the efficacy and safety of olanzapine with that of clozapine. In an 8-week, double-blind RCT with a 2-year follow-up, 25 patients with COS were randomly assigned to treatment with clozapine ($n=12$) or olanzapine ($n=13$). In this study, clozapine was associated with a significant reduction in all outcome measures, with olanzapine showing a rather less impressive improvement. A direct comparison of treatment efficacy showed generally no significant difference between the groups, but a significant advantage for clozapine did emerge in the alleviation of negative symptoms of schizophrenia (producing a 45% greater reduction in Scale for the Assessment of Negative Symptoms ratings; $P=0.04$; effect size, 0.89). The size of the differential effect on negative symptoms is therefore large and in marked contrast to studies of adults with schizophrenia, which report no significant difference between olanzapine and clozapine in treating negative symptoms, despite a larger sample size and power to detect smaller effects (Bitter et al. 2004; Tollefson et al. 2001; Volavka et al. 2002). The improvement in negative symptoms is unlikely to have been an epiphenomenon of improvement in mood or EPS, given the lack of correlation between change in these indices and change in negative symptoms.

Data on the effectiveness and tolerability of antipsychotics in the longer term are of importance. However, with some significant exceptions (Findling et al. 2004; Ross et al. 2003), such data are scarce in the pediatric literature. In the NIMH trial, Shaw et al. (2006) reported that by the 2-year stage, 15 of 18 patients were being treated with clozapine; olanzapine produced a moderately sustained treatment response for only 2 patients. Thus, clozapine appears to be a highly efficacious choice in a treatment-resistant population.

Considerable interest has been shown in determining what attributes afford clozapine its efficacy. A study of 54 patients with COS determined that outcome at 2 years (using the Children's Global Assessment Scale) was associated with less severe illness at baseline and a greater initial clinical response to clozapine during the first 6 weeks of treatment (Shaw et al. 2006), as reported in studies of adults with schizophrenia (Pickar et al. 1994; Sporn et al. 2007). Intriguingly, the ratio of one of the metabolites of clozapine, *N*-desmethylclozapine (NDMC), to clozapine was the only variable that was significantly associated with response at 6 weeks. This result replicated a finding in an adult-onset schizophrenia study that indicated that a greater NDMC-to-clozapine ratio, but not the concentrations of clozapine and NDMC themselves, is associated with better response (Weiner et al. 2004).

About the time the first edition of this manual was being prepared, Findling et al. (2007) discussed evidence in support of the FDA's eventual allowance for clozapine use in children and adolescents, based on controlled treatment trial data showing clozapine to be more effective for pediatric patients with treatment-refractory COS or other refractory EOS-spectrum disorders than at least two FGA medications, haloperidol and olanzapine (Kumra et al. 2008b; Shaw and Rapoport 2006). In addition, a 12-week controlled comparison of clozapine versus high-dose olanzapine (up to 30 mg/day) in youth ages 10–18 years with treatment-refractory schizophrenia supported clozapine as the agent of choice (Kumra et al. 2008a). Significantly more participants given clozapine met the response criteria (66%) than those given olanzapine (33%), and clozapine proved superior in the reduction (from baseline to end point of their analysis) of negative symptoms as well as psychosis cluster scores.

The course of COS is difficult, but the high overall response rates found among patients treated with clozapine are encouraging. Although not currently seen consistently in the NIMH COS study (Driver et al. 2020), a finding reported by some studies (e.g., Sholevar et al. 2000) is significantly *greater* improvement with clozapine in *younger* subjects. However, although clozapine is now better established for treatment-resistant schizophrenia, its use in pediatric populations continues to be rare, mainly due to lingering community concern about its potential adverse effects (Gogtay and Rapoport 2008).

Treatment of Comorbid Conditions

Patients with COS have a very high rate of comorbid conditions (Driver et al. 2013b; Nicolson et al. 2000). Among 76 children from the NIMH cohort, the most frequent comorbid diagnosis at screening was depression (54%), followed by OCD (21%) and generalized anxiety disorder (15%) (Gochman et al. 2011). A particularly challenging comorbid condition is ADHD (present in 15% of the NIMH sample). Psychiatrists have often been reluctant to treat these symptoms with stimulants for fear of worsening psychosis. However, Tossell et al. (2004) found that a case series of five children showed a significant improvement in Brief Conners' Teacher Rating Scale scores of inattentive symptoms with stimulant treatment following stabilization with an antipsychotic, without any initial worsening of psychosis. This reflects a more general principle of comorbidity treatment in children with psychosis: treatment of a coexisting condition should not be overlooked and should be modeled on the evidence for each disorder *following* the stabilization of psychosis.

Treatment of Side Effects

The available data from short-term studies suggest that youth might be more sensitive than adults to developing antipsychotic-related adverse side effects (e.g., EPS, prolactin elevation, weight gain) (Kumra et al. 2008b). Because the chronic course of COS necessitates long-term treatment, a thorough consideration of side effects and differential profile is vital in the treatment of pediatric and adolescent populations.

Extrapyramidal Side Effects

EPS are among the most troublesome and distressing unwanted sequelae of treatment with antipsychotic medications. Pathophysiologically, the blockade of nigrostriatal dopaminergic tracts mimics the neurochemical deficits seen in Parkinson's disease and exhibits a similar clinical profile. The mechanisms underlying tardive dyskinesias are less clear but may stem from the development of supersensitivity to dopamine resulting from chronic blockade. As mentioned in the subsection "Mechanisms of Action," SGAs have a high serotonin-to-dopamine receptor blockade ratio in the brain. The serotonergic blockade leads to increased dopamine release, which may partially offset the postsynaptic dopaminergic blockade, resulting in fewer EPS (Glazer 2000).

Abnormal movements that arise in the first few hours or days of treatment are typically acute dystonic reactions, which may manifest as spasms of the orofacial or oculogyric muscles. Adverse effects typically arising after a prolonged period of use include akathisia and pseudoparkinsonism (a form of dyskinetic movement distinguished from parkinsonism by the presence of apraxic slowness and gait, essential tremor, paratonic rigidity, and frontal ataxia). Several rating scales have been developed to assess abnormal movements, including the Abnormal Involuntary Movement Scale (Guy 1976), the Barnes

Akathisia Rating Scale (Barnes 1989), and the Simpson-Angus Rating Scale (Simpson and Angus 1970).

A comparison of rates of EPS across various studies suggests that FGAs are associated with high levels of EPS (26%–73%) in patients with COS (Table 9–2). These rates are higher than those typically reported in patients with adult-onset schizophrenia (32%–55%; Bobes et al. 2003; Novick et al. 2010).

By contrast, five open-label studies of olanzapine and quetiapine, involving patients with varying treatment histories and a range of ages at illness onset, found no significant change in ratings of EPS from baseline (Findling et al. 2003; McConville et al. 2003; Mozes et al. 2003; Ross et al. 2003; Shaw et al. 2001). One randomized, double-blind comparison of extended-release paliperidone and aripiprazole noted a low incidence of, and no statistically significant difference on, the occurrence of EPS (Savitz et al. 2015a).

Three open-label studies of risperidone suggest that this SGA is associated with EPS, akathisia, and acute dystonic reactions, especially at higher dosages (Armenteros et al. 1997; Grcevich et al. 1996; Zalsman et al. 2003). However, some studies comparing FGAs and SGAs did not see more severe EPS in patients treated with risperidone compared with other treatment groups (Findling et al. 2010b; Sikich et al. 2004).

The management of EPS in children follows the principles derived from adult populations. Strategies such as dosage reduction—with awareness that this reduction may be associated with a temporary increase in abnormal movements—and switching while using anticholinergics to provide immediate relief are commonly used. For tardive dyskinesia, two controlled studies in adults suggest that switching to clozapine may be the best overall option, given its ability to treat both the psychosis and the EPS, although the risks and intensive monitoring make this a less attractive option. Other agents carrying a low risk of adverse effects, such as vitamin E (Attard and Taylor 2012; Lieberman et al. 1991), can be used as part of an augmentation strategy.

Akathisia

Akathisia has been described mostly in association with typical neuroleptics but also with olanzapine and risperidone (at rates of about 13%) and clozapine (at rates of about 7%) (Chengappa et al. 1994; Leucht et al. 1999). In the NIMH cohort, 2 of 40 children treated with clozapine developed akathisia,

Table 9–2. Rates of extrapyramidal symptoms (EPS) in select controlled studies of antipsychotics in treatment of childhood-onset and/or early-onset schizophrenia

Study	Medication	Mean dosage, *mg/day*	Measures	Results
First-generation (typical) antipsychotics				
Engelhardt et al. 1973	Fluphenazine	10.4	Clinical	8/15 EPS, 1/15 acute dystonia, 0/15 akathisia
	Haloperidol	10.4		4/15 EPS, 0/15 acute dystonia, 1/15 akathisia
Pool et al. 1976	Loxapine	87.5	Clinical, EPS defined as muscular rigidity of parkinsonian type	19/26 EPS
	Haloperidol	9.8		18/25 EPS
	Placebo	NA		1/24 EPS
Spencer et al. 1992	Haloperidol	8.8	AIMS	3/12 parkinsonian, 2/12 orofacial dyskinesia, 2/12 acute dystonia
	Placebo	NA		No symptoms (0/12)
First-generation and second-generation (atypical) antipsychotics				
Kumra et al. 1996	Haloperidol	16	AIMS/SAS	No significant difference from baseline
	Clozapine	176		No significant difference from baseline
Gothelf et al. 2003	Olanzapine	12.9	AIMS/UKU	3/19 EPS, 0/19 dystonia, 0/19 akathisia
	Risperidone	3.3		4/17 EPS, 1/17 dystonia, 1/17 akathisia
	Haloperidol	8.3		4/7 EPS, 2/7 dystonia, 3/7 akathisia

Table 9–2. Rates of extrapyramidal symptoms (EPS) in select controlled studies of antipsychotics in treatment of childhood-onset and/or early-onset schizophrenia *(continued)*

Study	Medication	Mean dosage, *mg/day*	Measures	Results
Sikich et al. 2004	Olanzapine	12.3	AIMS, SAS	No significant difference from baseline, 56% given anticholinergics, no acute dystonia, 2/16 akathisia
	Risperidone	4		No significant difference from baseline, 53% given anticholinergics, no acute dystonia, no akathisia
	Haloperidol	5		Mean SAS significantly higher at end point than baseline, mean SAS score change significantly higher than olanzapine or risperidone groups, 67% receiving anticholinergics, 2/15 acute dystonia, 2/15 akathisia
Shaw et al. 2006	Olanzapine	18.1	AIMS, BARS, SAS	No significant difference from baseline
	Clozapine	327		No significant difference from baseline
Findling et al. 2010b[a]	Risperidone	1.4	NRS, BARS, AIMS	5% (1/21); no significant difference in mean changes between groups, no patient in any group had tardive dyskinesia
	Olanzapine	9.6		8% (1/13); no significant difference in mean changes between groups, no patient in any group had tardive dyskinesia

Table 9–2. Rates of extrapyramidal symptoms (EPS) in select controlled studies of antipsychotics in treatment of childhood-onset and/or early-onset schizophrenia *(continued)*

Study	Medication	Mean dosage, *mg/day*	Measures	Results
Findling et al. 2010b[a] (continued)	Molindone	76.5 (+1 benztropine for molindone group)		35% (7/20) experienced pacing or restlessness; no significant difference in mean changes between groups, no patient in any group had tardive dyskinesia
Findling et al. 2012	Quetiapine (high)	800	AIMS, BARS, SAS	13.5% mild to moderate EPS events
	Quetiapine (low)	400		12.4% mild to moderate EPS events
	Placebo	NA		5.3% mild to moderate EPS events; no significant difference in baseline to final between groups
Findling et al. 2015[b]	Asenapine (high)	5 (bid)	Clinical, narrow EPS[c]	10.4% (11/106) EPS, 6.6% (7/114) akathisia
	Asenapine (low)	2.5 (bid)		5.1% (5/98) EPS, 4.1% (4/98) akathisia
	Placebo	NA		3.9% (4/102) EPS, 1% (1/102) akathisia
Savitz et al. 2015a	Paliperidone ER	6.75	AIMS, BARS, SAS	11.5% (13/113) akathisia, 6.2% (7/113) muscle rigidity
	Aripiprazole	11.56		7.9% (9/114) akathisia, 2.6% (3/114) muscle rigidity

Table 9–2. Rates of extrapyramidal symptoms (EPS) in select controlled studies of antipsychotics in treatment of childhood-onset and/or early-onset schizophrenia *(continued)*

Study	Medication	Mean dosage, *mg/day*	Measures	Results
Correll et al. 2017	Aripiprazole	10–30	AIMS, BARS, SAS	6.1% (6/98) EPS, 3.1% (3/98) akathisia, 2% (2/98) muscle rigidity
Pagsberg et al. 2017a	Quetiapine ER	600	AIMS, SAS	32% (15/47) akathisia
	Aripiprazole	20		27% (13/48) akathisia

Note. AIMS = Abnormal Involuntary Movement Scale; BARS = Barnes Akathisia Rating Scale; ER = extended release; NRS = Neurological Rating Scale; SAS = Simpson-Angus Rating Scale; UKU = Udvalg for Kliniske Undersøgelser Side Effect Rating Scale.

[a]This is an extension trial of the Sikich et al. (2008) and McClellan et al. (2007) studies. These data are from week 52; earlier data were to week 8.

[b]Reported data are only from the double-blind portion of the trial (first 8 weeks).

[c]EPS included akathisia, dyskinesia, dystonia, and Parkinson's-like events.

which was misinterpreted as a worsening of psychotic symptoms in one case and led to a temporary increase in clozapine dosage and a concomitant worsening of symptoms (Gogtay et al. 2002). However, when the diagnosis was made, propranolol was initiated and ameliorated symptoms greatly, allowing continued treatment with clozapine. Other useful agents include benzodiazepines and perhaps anticholinergics.

Neuroleptic Malignant Syndrome

Neuroleptic malignant syndrome (NMS), a rare but potentially life-threatening complication of antipsychotics, typically arises in the early stages of treatment and has been attributed to the effects of dopamine blockade. Classic signs and symptoms of NMS include severe muscle rigidity or marked EPS; autonomic instability, including a high or sometimes fluctuating temperature and blood pressure; delirium; and laboratory findings of elevated creatine kinase and leukocytosis. SGAs are thought to have a lower incidence of and produce perhaps a milder form of NMS (Caroff et al. 2000). However, some dramatic case studies illustrate the potential for this side effect in adolescents who are only briefly exposed to even SGAs (Hanft et al. 2004). Treatment of NMS relies on prompt transfer to a medical setting, withdrawal of the neuroleptic, intensive supportive care, and, if indicated, treatment with dantrolene and/or bromocriptine. Psychotic exacerbations during this period of abrupt antipsychotic withdrawal have sometimes been treated successfully with electroconvulsive therapy.

Sedation

High rates of fatigue or sedation have been consistently reported in association with nearly all antipsychotics in patients with COS. Rates for haloperidol range from a low of 25% in a NIMH double-blind study (Shaw et al. 2006) to 50% and 66% in two earlier trials of the medication (Pool et al. 1976; Spencer et al. 1992). Other FGAs have been associated with even higher rates of sedation (Pool et al. 1976; Spencer et al. 1992).

SGAs are well known to produce the side effect of sedation, and rates higher than 50% have been reported for ziprasidone and clozapine, with risperidone occupying an intermediate position (31%) and olanzapine (20%) and quetiapine (20%) having lower, but still high, rates (for review, see Cheng-

Shannon et al. 2004). Interestingly, one study linked initial sedation when taking olanzapine with a better clinical response at 8 weeks, suggesting the need for perseverance with fatigue and sedation occurring early in treatment (Sholevar et al. 2000). The management of sedation is empirical and requires rigorous assessment to exclude underlying psychopathology, maintenance treatment with as low a dosage as possible, encouragement of activity scheduling, and constant motivation.

Weight Gain

Weight gain, reported in association with antipsychotics since their initial use, has become a focus of more interest given the increased awareness of morbidity and mortality accompanying obesity (Deckelbaum and Williams 2001). In their study of 50 children with psychotic symptoms, Sikich et al. (2004) found a weight gain of 7.1 kg over an 8-week period for children given olanzapine—a value greater than the gains of 4.9 kg and 3.5 kg reported for risperidone and haloperidol, respectively. In a double-blind comparison of clozapine and olanzapine, a similar weight gain of just under 4 kg over an 8-week period was associated with both agents, corresponding to an increase of 1.5 units in BMI (Shaw et al. 2006), with the most extreme weight gains occurring with clozapine. The TEOSS study reported average weight gain of 0.74 kg for molindone, 4.13 kg for risperidone, and 7.29 kg for olanzapine (Taylor et al. 2018). In that study, age, sex, socioeconomic status, baseline weight, and symptoms did not moderate weight changes.

Among the SGAs other than clozapine, open-label studies report the greatest weight gain with olanzapine (see Fedorowicz and Fombonne 2005). A systematic review of antipsychotic use in children, regardless of diagnoses, found weight gains of 4% with ziprasidone, 7% with clozapine, 17% with risperidone, and 22% with olanzapine and quetiapine (Cheng-Shannon et al. 2004). In another study, a significant link was found between early-onset diagnoses and the subsequent increase in BMI after 6 months of risperidone use (Goeb et al. 2010). We caution that there may be subtle biological sex and age confounds in such BMI conclusions, because the general dearth of pediatric studies does not allow for definitive conclusions (Goeb et al. 2010).

Actively avoiding the use of SGAs solely on the basis of weight gain concerns is debated in the literature. A recent study of EOS showed that although SGAs caused a significantly larger ($P=0.04$) gain in baseline weight compared with FGAs, this difference was not seen 6 weeks later (Hrdlicka et al. 2009). The results suggest that pediatric populations may demonstrate much more variability in weight responses than do adult patients. Because medication non-compliance may follow excessive weight gain, this should be a particular concern for physicians as they consider social withdrawal and stigma consequences (Goeb et al. 2010).

Similar weight gain concerns occur in adult studies, which should further encourage clinicians to explore this side effect holistically. A recent study of 400 patients recruited in the 52-week Comparison of Atypicals in First Episode of Psychosis trial evaluated olanzapine, quetiapine, and risperidone (Patel et al. 2009). The investigators found that 31% of patients were overweight and 18% were obese at baseline (Patel et al. 2009). In addition, 4.3% of patients met criteria for metabolic syndrome.

Mechanistically, the relative affinities of the SGAs for histamine H_1 receptors appear to be the most robust correlate of these clinical findings, although interactions with serotonergic and dopaminergic receptors are also likely to play a role (Wirshing et al. 1999). Elevated levels of leptin, a hormone secreted by adipocytes that partly regulates body weight, are also greater among the antipsychotics most closely linked with weight gain (Herrán et al. 2001).

The management of this side effect has typically relied on behavioral programs, which unfortunately have mixed evidence of success (Faulkner et al. 2003). One long-term trial of behavior counseling in adolescents receiving olanzapine did not show differences between intense behavior intervention and standard weight counseling (Detke et al. 2016). Pharmacological interventions are also unproven; some case reports suggest that amantadine, topiramate, and various anorectic agents attenuate antipsychotic-induced weight gain (Generali and Cada 2014; Reekie et al. 2015). Metformin has been investigated as a possible effective and safe therapy option to manage weight gain (Klein et al. 2006). Although literature on controlled trials still remains scarce (Canitano 2005; Gracious et al. 2002), a recent meta-analysis found significant weight loss in youth receiving metformin along with SGAs (Ellul et al. 2018). Adolescents taking antipsychotics and metformin lost an average of 3.23 kg after 16 weeks of treatment.

Studies focused on weight gain from antipsychotic treatment remain scarce. The use of antipsychotics is increasing, despite adverse side effects, with an increase in the use of SGA medications for off-label purposes (Hartung et al. 2008). The risk for weight gain, as well as metabolic side effects, should be weighed carefully when contemplating the use of any antipsychotic and should be monitored closely.

Glycemic Control

The link between impaired glycemic control and SGAs is well established in both children and adults. Sikich et al. (2004) found that olanzapine, but not risperidone or haloperidol, was associated with a trend toward increased fasting blood glucose. During direct comparison of clozapine and olanzapine (see "Use of Clozapine in Treating Childhood-Onset Schizophrenia"), little evidence was found for marked hyperglycemia, although comprehensive data were available only for the 8-week phase. The link with impaired glucose control could arise through hyperinsulinemia and the impaired sensitivity to insulin found with SGA use (Sowell et al. 2002). Antipsychotics may also have direct toxic effects on the pancreas. A final link between antipsychotics and type 2 diabetes mellitus could be through obesity and weight gain associated with both. Despite the lack of an association between antipsychotic use and impaired glycemic control in our cohort (Driver et al. 2020), given the limited evidence, regular blood monitoring is judicious (Jin et al. 2004).

Hyperlipidemia

Sikich et al. (2004) noted a deleterious increase in low-density lipoprotein and a decrease in high-density lipoprotein in patients randomly assigned to olanzapine but not those assigned to risperidone or haloperidol. In the NIMH cohort, high levels of hypercholesterolemia and hypertriglyceridemia were seen in 6 of 15 patients followed up for a 2-year period while receiving open-label clozapine (Shaw et al. 2006). Although all cases were detected early and managed through diet and lipid-lowering agents, the high rates underscore the need for regular monitoring (Melkersson et al. 2004).

Hyperprolactinemia

An increase in prolactin secondary to antipsychotics reflects the D_2 receptor blockade in the tuberoinfundibular pathway that releases the tonic inhibition from dopamine upon pituitary lactotrophs, leading to increased prolactin (for review, see Pappagallo and Silva 2004). As a result, elevated prolactin levels are typically produced by the antipsychotics with greatest D_2 affinity (Saito et al. 2004). The sequelae of hyperprolactinemia range from sexual dysfunction, menstrual irregularities, and lactation to decreased bone density and possible cardiovascular disease. Wudarsky et al. (1999) found increased prolactin levels in 36 children with early-onset psychosis after 6 weeks of treatment with either haloperidol or olanzapine but not with clozapine. The association may be modulated by biological sex; in the NIMH cohort, a correlation between olanzapine and prolactin levels was found among females only (Alfaro et al. 2002). In this study, all but one child remained asymptomatic; the female with the highest prolactin levels developed transient galactorrhea.

The most effective treatment for symptomatic hyperprolactinemia is to either reduce the dosage of the antipsychotic (Masi et al. 2001) or switch to an agent that is possibly less associated with the complication (Shaw et al. 2001). Dopamine agonists reinstitute the dopaminergic inhibition of prolactin release, and cabergoline has been used with success in male children with risperidone-induced hyperprolactinemia (Cohen and Biederman 2001), although bromocriptine has a more established role. Whether asymptomatic hyperprolactinemia requires intervention is more controversial, given evidence for the normalization of prolactin levels at 1-year follow-up in disruptive children being treated with risperidone (Findling et al. 2004).

Cardiovascular and Autonomic Side Effects

Several antipsychotics alter repolarization of cardiac muscle, as reflected in a prolonged QT interval. In turn, this change may act as a risk factor for more serious arrhythmias, such as torsades de pointes. In a double-blind study comparing clozapine and olanzapine (see subsection "Use of Clozapine in Treating Childhood-Onset Schizophrenia"), there were higher rates of supine tachycardia, but no serious arrhythmias, among patients treated with clozapine. However, seven patients in the clozapine arm became hypertensive during the trial, compared with only one patient treated with olanzapine.

Cardiometabolic effects of SGAs are of concern to the clinician but have not been sufficiently studied in pediatric and adolescent patients who were previously unexposed to antipsychotic medication. Correll et al. (2009) showed that first-time use of SGAs was associated with significant cardiometabolic risk. Biases regarding baseline weights and race and ethnicity were limitations to this study (Correll et al. 2009; Mangurian et al. 2010).

Side Effects Particularly Associated With Clozapine

The association between clozapine and neutropenia is well established. In a review of data on more than 1,100 patients treated with clozapine, the risk of agranulocytosis was greater in patients younger than 21 years than in those 21–40 years (Alvir et al. 1993). However, Cheng-Shannon et al. (2004) reported two cases of agranulocytosis occurring among 243 children and adolescents treated with clozapine, giving a rate more in line with that seen in the adult population. Because of this connection, clozapine requires intensive blood monitoring.

The high rates of neutropenia and agranulocytosis in children are particularly unfortunate given the severity of COS, for which clozapine is often the only effective treatment. As a result, there is considerable interest in developing strategies to maximize the opportunity for children to be treated with clozapine following initial withdrawal due to the development of neutropenia. Sporn et al. (2003) described the management of two cases of clozapine-induced neutropenia in which the addition of lithium carbonate was associated with a sustained elevation of the white blood cell count, allowing a successful rechallenge with clozapine. A common strategy is to ensure that blood is drawn after a 2-hour period of wakefulness/movement as well as in the afternoon, capitalizing on the diurnal variation in neutrophil levels (McKee et al. 2011). Another relatively new development is the FDA's modification of the monitoring parameters for neutropenia associated with clozapine use, introducing both the ability to consider benign ethnic neutropenia and the use of clinical judgment.

Epileptiform abnormalities are not uncommon in the electroencephalograms of children and adolescents taking clozapine. Clozapine also has the potential to reduce seizure threshold, and seizures occur in approximately 2% of children taking the medication. Most patients can continue clozapine along with an adjunctive anticonvulsant, and prophylactic anticonvulsants are justified when patients are given high dosages of clozapine. We recommend gabapentin as an anticonvulsant for clozapine-induced seizures, chosen because of its relatively benign side effect profile and its lack of significant medication interactions (Usiskin et al. 2000).

Hypersalivation is a distressingly common side effect of clozapine that has been reported only rarely with the use of other antipsychotics. Proposed mechanisms include the action of clozapine at the muscarinic M_4 receptor, blockade of α_2-adrenoceptors, or distortion of the swallowing reflex. Treatment options include using chewing gum, reducing the dosage of clozapine, or using pharmacological agents such as anticholinergics, α_2-adrenergic agonists, or, in extreme cases, botulinum toxin (Kahl et al. 2004). Some studies suggest that the addition of other antipsychotics, such as amisulpride, at low dosages may be efficacious, although a double-blind study found that pirenzepine, one of the most promising agents (based on results of open-label studies), was no more effective than placebo (Bai et al. 2001).

Fever, unrelated to neutropenia, agranulocytosis, or NMS, is a rare side effect of clozapine, with only one report of its occurrence in a child. In the adult literature, the incidence ranges from 2% to 55%. In both populations, the consensus is that continuing therapy and providing supportive care are recommended (Driver et al. 2013a).

Early Intervention Studies

Most of the existing literature focuses on improving treatment when a patient is already involved with psychiatric services. However, there are several other windows for intervention. From childhood, adults who develop schizophrenia have subtle motor and cognitive abnormalities similar to the constellation of deficits found in children who are at high risk of developing psychosis by virtue of having a parent with schizophrenia (Cornblatt 2002). Many other studies—most notably, Age, Beginning, and Course, the large epidemiological study on the course of psychosis—have established the existence of a prodromal phase lasting 2–5 years (Beiser et al. 1993; Häfner et al. 1998). During this time, an individual experiences a marked decline in overall functioning, and mental state is characterized by abnormalities of thought, perception, and action. Nearer the onset of established psychosis, many patients have fully developed positive psychotic symptoms, but these are transient, intermittent, and self-terminating. Finally, several studies have demonstrated that typically a long period of delay occurs between the onset of definite psychotic symptoms and the onset of treatment.

Research into interventions during the period between the development of a DSM-IV-TR (American Psychiatric Association 2000) psychotic disorder and the beginning of treatment was fueled by evidence that a longer duration of untreated psychosis is linked to poorer clinical outcome in many, but not all, studies (for review, see Ruhrmann et al. 2005). Additionally, there are concerns that untreated psychosis is not only intensely distressing for the patient but also possibly neurotoxic (Lieberman et al. 1997; Pantelis et al. 2003).

Another, more ambitious strategy attempts to identify people who are in a prepsychotic or prodromal phase and to intervene during this stage. Considering that the median age at onset of schizophrenia is 19 years, most subjects in the prodromal phase are adolescents, making the rise of preventive interventions of particular relevance to the psychiatrist working with youth.

The feasibility of such preventive intervention relies on the ability to accurately identify individuals at high risk of psychosis. The current dominant approach defines patients at ultrahigh risk of developing psychosis in the near future by combining the traditional definition of genetic high risk (having a first-degree relative with a psychotic disorder) with early symptomatic and functional changes. McGorry et al. (2003) led the field in developing criteria that suggest ultrahigh risk for the development of psychosis: genetic high risk and/or schizotypal personality disorder as well as a rapid, recent decline in global function. Other groups at ultrahigh risk are those with clusters of attenuated positive symptoms (including unusual thought content/delusional ideation, suspiciousness/persecutory ideas, grandiosity) and brief, limited, or intermittent psychotic symptoms. Overall, approximately 40% of patients meeting these criteria will transition to psychosis (not just schizophrenia) within 12 months, with *psychosis* defined as the presence of positive psychotic symptoms for longer than 1 week (Yung et al. 2003).

An alternative approach emphasizes so-called basic symptoms, which are subtle, self-experienced neuropsychological deficits such as thought pressure, perseverative thinking, derealization, and slight perceptual aberrations. In one study using this approach, the Cologne Early Recognition Study investigators correctly predicted a transition to schizophrenia (not only psychosis) in 78% of cases within 4 years (Klosterkötter et al. 2001), and their work has partly formed the basis of ongoing prevention studies in Germany.

One of the first studies on early intervention at the prodromal stage was conducted in the United Kingdom (Falloon 1992). In this study, all patients who were in the prodromal phase, as defined by DSM-III criteria (American Psychiatric Association 1980), were given psychoeducation, and some patients additionally received low-dose antipsychotics. The authors reported a 10-fold decrease in the incidence of schizophrenia in the region compared with a previous period, although the study was uncontrolled, and it is unclear which components of the intervention were efficacious.

In the first RCT, McGorry et al. (2003) found that significantly fewer patients who were treated with a mix of low-dose risperidone and psychotherapy progressed to first-episode psychosis by the end of the 6-month trial period compared with a group who received nonspecific "needs-based" interventions (9.7% vs. 35.7%, respectively; $P<0.05$). This and other RCTs are summarized in Table 9–3. The significant difference between the groups was not sustained at a 6-month follow-up after the active intervention, however, because of an increase in the number of patients in the specific-intervention group who became psychotic. A post hoc analysis suggested that, overall, subjects in the specific-intervention group who received low-dose risperidone had the lowest rates of transition to psychosis, although the numbers were small. Given the design of the study, it is difficult to determine the specific contribution of risperidone to the findings.

In the Prevention Through Risk Identification, Management, and Education trial comparing olanzapine with placebo, Woods et al. (2003) found that although olanzapine treatment reduced the rate of transition to psychosis by 50% (from 35% to 16%), the reduction was not statistically significant. Detailed reporting on the data 8 weeks after initial randomization suggested more improvement in psychopathology associated with olanzapine treatment, given at a mean dosage of 10 mg/day over the period (with a significant interaction of groups with scores on the PANSS and the Scale of Prodromal Symptoms in a linear, mixed-model regression). However, these results must be taken with caution. A larger, double-blind, placebo-controlled study of 1.4 g/day of omega-3 acids in young people at ultra-high risk for psychosis failed to detect significant difference between the intervention and placebo groups in rates of transition to psychosis (Nelson et al. 2018).

A descriptive, interim analysis of a German intervention trial comparing amisulpride with placebo indicates beneficial effects with amisulpride not only on attenuated positive symptoms but also on negative and depressive symptoms and global functioning (Ruhrmann et al. 2003). Whether these promising initial results will be sustained by future work with additional data is unclear.

Issues of intervention are contentious. There are several ethical and pragmatic issues related to using psychotropic drugs during the prepsychotic or

Table 9–3. Randomized trials of interventions for patients at ultrahigh risk of developing psychosis

Study	Interventions	*N*	Outcome measures	Results	Comments
McGorry et al. 2003	NBI vs. SPI (risperidone 1.3 mg/day + CBT)	59	Development of definite psychotic symptoms	10/28 NBI vs. 3/31 SPI developed psychosis at 6 months; difference not sustained at 12 months	Lower rate of development of psychosis in patients fully adherent to risperidone (2/17 adherent, 7/17 not)
Woods et al. 2003	Olanzapine (average 8 mg/day) vs. PBO	60	Development of psychosis (based on SOPS)	5/31 olanzapine vs. 10/29 PBO developed psychosis at 8 weeks	Significant group difference found at 8 weeks using linear mixed-models analyses
Morrison et al. 2004	TAU vs. CT	58	Development of definite psychotic symptoms (based on PANSS)	4/23 TAU vs. 2/35 CT developed psychosis at 12 months	96% reduction in odds of making a transition to psychosis in CT group*
Amminger and McGorry 2012; Amminger et al. 2010	ω-3 PUFA (1.2 g/day) vs. PBO	81	Development of definite psychotic symptoms (based on PANSS)	2/41 PUFA vs. 11/40 PBO developed psychosis at 12 months (12-week treatment period)	Study in process of being replicated on a larger scale by Markulev et al. 2015
van der Gaag et al. 2012	CBT + TAU vs. TAU	201	Development of psychosis (defined by CAARMS and verified by SCAN)	10/98 CBT + TAU vs. 22/103 TAU developed psychosis at 18 months (6-month treatment period)	Average age 22.9 years (range, 14–35); CBT specifically focused on normalization and awareness of cognitive biases

Table 9–3. Randomized trials of interventions for patients at ultrahigh risk of developing psychosis *(continued)*

Study	Interventions	*N*	Outcome measures	Results	Comments
Zarafonitis et al. 2012	IPI vs. SC	128	Transition to psychosis	12 months: 3.2% IPI vs. 16.9% SC 24 months: 6.3% IPI vs. 20% SC	Treatment for 12 months with follow-up at 24 months
McGorry et al. 2013	CT+risperidone vs. CT+PBO vs. ST+PBO	115	Transition to psychosis (assessed with CAARMS)	CT+risperidone: 10.7% CT+PBO: 9.6% ST+PBO: 21.8%	All three groups improved but no significant differences
Miklowitz et al. 2014	18 sessions FFT vs. 3 sessions PE	102	Development of psychotic conversion (change in 1+ SOPS positive symptoms for a score of 6)	1/55 of FFT vs. 5/47 PE developed psychosis	PE focused on symptom prevention, whereas FFT focused on early signs, stress management, communication, and problem-solving; PE was shorter, and neither group had 100% adherence

Table 9–3. Randomized trials of interventions for patients at ultrahigh risk of developing psychosis *(continued)*

Study	Interventions	*N*	Outcome measures	Results	Comments
Flach et al. 2015	CBT + MSM vs. MSM	288	Looked at CAARMS at several points in the study	On average, receiving all four of the necessary CBT components, symptom severity reduced by 20 points	CBT specifically included formulation and homework, and not everyone randomly assigned to CBT + MSM received all four necessary components of the CBT; significance of results depends on defining treatment effects for patients who received CBT with none of the four necessary components

Note. CAARMS = Comprehensive Assessment of At-Risk Mental States; CBT = cognitive-behavioral therapy; CT = cognitive therapy; FFT = family-focused therapy; IPI = integrated psychological intervention; MSM = medication self-management; NBI = needs-based intervention; PANSS = Positive and Negative Syndrome Scale; PBO = placebo; PE = psychoeducation; PUFA = polyunsaturated fatty acid; SC = supportive counseling; SCAN = Schedules for Clinical Assessment in Neuropsychiatry; SOPS = Scale of Prodromal Symptoms; SPI = specific preventive intervention; ST = supportive therapy; TAU = treatment as usual.

*After adjustment for potential moderating variables.

prodromal phase. The evidence base for psychotropic use is relatively scant. This is of particular concern because the best current criteria carry a high rate of false positives, which means that many patients will be exposed to medications without any clear evidence that they would have developed psychosis if left untreated.

The use of nonpharmacological interventions alone for patients in the prepsychotic and prodromal phrases has also proven to be a promising avenue (Flach et al. 2015; McGorry et al. 2013; van der Gaag et al. 2012). Morrison et al. (2004) found that 5.7% of patients receiving cognitive therapy developed psychosis over a 1-year period compared with 17.4% receiving treatment as usual. In addition to research on therapy and management styles, there is ongoing interest and controversy about the use of preventive omega-3 treatment, after one study showed results similar to those of antipsychotics or antidepressants: significantly fewer patients (0.05% vs. 27%; $n=81$) developed psychosis at 1 year following 3 months of omega-3 treatment (Amminger et al. 2010; Mischoulon and Freeman 2013; Mossaheb et al. 2013). Although promising, this result has not been replicated at this time, and a larger ($n=304$) replication study is ongoing (Markulev et al. 2015).

Moreover, whether antipsychotics are necessarily the only, or the best, pharmacological intervention remains unclear. In the Hillside Recognition and Prevention Program, adolescents first were identified as being at risk of developing psychosis based on specific combinations of neurocognitive deficits and then were treated (Cornblatt 2002). Unlike other studies, the youth did not have to display any attenuated positive symptoms. The 54 adolescents in this group were treated on an unrandomized, open-label basis with either antipsychotics or antidepressants (SSRIs). Interestingly, the antidepressants, often given in combination with mood stabilizers, were as effective as the antipsychotics in promoting clinical improvement.

One review agreed that randomized clinical trials may suggest a positive effect upon the completion of treatment (Masi and Liboni 2011). However, without significantly stronger results in the literature, continuing concerns about side effects and nonadherence preclude any validation to standardize prodromal intervention in a typical clinical setting (de Koning et al. 2009).

In theory, long-acting injectable antipsychotics (LAIs) could offer a solution for treating psychosis in children and adolescents who are noncompliant. This suggestion is extrapolated from data on the use of LAIs in adults with psychotic disorders, which show the benefit of LAIs in the prevention of hospitalization and relapse compared with oral antipsychotics (Kishimoto et al. 2018, 2021). One meta-analysis provided the best evidence data for a 3-month formulation of paliperidone and aripiprazole for relapse prevention in adult participants compared with placebo (Ostuzzi et al. 2021). Unfortunately, the use of LAIs in youth has not been empirically studied, and the literature is limited to a few case reports within a broader diagnostic cohort. The use of LAIs in the pediatric population is summarized in a review by Lytle et al. (2017). Nevertheless, the 2013 practice parameters of the American Academy of Child and Adolescent Psychiatry recommend that LAIs could be of value in adolescent patients with schizophrenia who show chronic psychotic symptoms in combination with poor medication compliance (McClellan et al. 2013).

Fàbrega et al. (2015) reported the use of LAI paliperidone palmitate in two adolescent patients. One patient received 50 mg per 28 days to treat EOS and showed significant improvement on the PANSS and the Global Assessment of Functioning (GAF) Scale after his initial dose. He sustained these improvements after 1 year of continued treatment and had no adverse effects. The other patient also received 50 mg per 28 days for psychotic disorder not otherwise specified. He had an oculogyric crisis but continued treatment with the addition of biperiden. Although the patient showed improvement on the PANSS and the GAF, he experienced drowsiness, concentration problems, and asthenia, causing him to refuse treatment (Fàbrega et al. 2015). In a case report, Kowalski et al. (2011) described the use of LAI paliperidone palmitate in an autistic 5-year-old with severe irritability and aggression that prevented daily medication use. After 3 months of treatment at 39 mg/0.25 mL/month, the patient's symptoms were rated as very much improved using the CGI Improvement subscale. The injections were well tolerated, and the only reported adverse effect was an increase in appetite.

These case reports suggest that although child and adolescent patients might benefit from LAI use, responses to treatment and the emergence of potentially harmful side effects are not fully understood. Given the lack of evidence, further research in pediatric populations is needed before LAIs can be recommended as a standard treatment course.

Conclusion

Considering the current body of evidence available to guide the child psychiatrist through this controversial field, further work to develop our understanding of primary and secondary prevention is key. Current reviews of the literature advocate judicious pharmacotherapy in combination with nonpharmacological intervention to greatly improve outcomes (Masi and Liboni 2011). Low pharmacological effect sizes, variable remission rates, and an overall high incidence of adverse effects, mainly metabolic, highlight the importance of future efficacy, effectiveness, and efficiency research incorporating randomized, placebo-controlled studies and long-term, naturalistic follow-up of large patient samples.

Clinical Pearls

- Childhood-onset schizophrenia (COS) is similar to the adult form of the disorder but is much more rare, usually more severe, and more challenging to treat.
- A good treatment plan includes multidisciplinary evaluations and treatment modalities because COS is associated with numerous deficits.
- Carefully consider the risks and benefits when choosing between first-generation (typical) and second-generation (atypical) antipsychotics.
- Consider a trial of clozapine as a third-line option because it remains the only antipsychotic, typical or atypical, with clear, superior efficacy for treatment-resistant forms of psychosis.
- All antipsychotics are associated with adverse side effects, including extrapyramidal symptoms and metabolic complications. Prudent monitoring is key, regardless of the agent used.
- It remains unclear whether treatment during the prepsychotic or prodromal phase is effective; this continues to be an area of focused research.

References

Abi-Dargham A, Laruelle M: Mechanisms of action of second generation antipsychotic drugs in schizophrenia: insights from brain imaging studies. Eur Psychiatry 20(1):15–27, 2005 15642439

Alfaro CL, Wudarsky M, Nicolson R, et al: Correlation of antipsychotic and prolactin concentrations in children and adolescents acutely treated with haloperidol, clozapine, or olanzapine. J Child Adolesc Psychopharmacol 12(2):83–91, 2002 12188977

Alvir JM, Lieberman JA, Safferman AZ, et al: Clozapine-induced agranulocytosis: incidence and risk factors in the United States. N Engl J Med 329(3):162–167, 1993 8515788

Amato D, Natesan S, Yavich L, et al: Dynamic regulation of dopamine and serotonin responses to salient stimuli during chronic haloperidol treatment. Int J Neuropsychopharmacol 14(10):1327–1339, 2011 21281560

American Academy of Child and Adolescent Psychiatry: Practice parameter for the assessment and treatment of children and adolescents with schizophrenia. J Am Acad Child Adolesc Psychiatry 40(7 Suppl):4S–23S, 2001 11434484

American Psychiatric Association: Diagnostic and Statistical Manual of Mental Disorders, 3rd Edition. Washington, DC, American Psychiatric Association, 1980

American Psychiatric Association: Diagnostic and Statistical Manual of Mental Disorders, 3rd Edition, Revised. Washington, DC, American Psychiatric Association, 1987

American Psychiatric Association: Diagnostic and Statistical Manual of Mental Disorders, 4th Edition. Washington, DC, American Psychiatric Association, 1994

American Psychiatric Association: Diagnostic and Statistical Manual of Mental Disorders, 4th Edition, Text Revision. Washington, DC, American Psychiatric Association, 2000

American Psychiatric Association: Diagnostic and Statistical Manual of Mental Disorders, 5th Edition, Text Revision. Washington, DC, American Psychiatric Association, 2022

Amminger GP, McGorry PD: Update on omega-3 polyunsaturated fatty acids in early stage psychotic disorders. Neuropsychopharmacology 37(1):309–310, 2012 22157875

Amminger GP, Schäfer MR, Papageorgiou K, et al: Long-chain omega-3 fatty acids for indicated prevention of psychotic disorders: a randomized, placebo-controlled trial. Arch Gen Psychiatry 67(2):146–154, 2010 20124114

Armenteros JL, Whitaker AH, Welikson M, et al: Risperidone in adolescents with schizophrenia: an open pilot study. J Am Acad Child Adolesc Psychiatry 36(5):694–700, 1997 9136505

Attard A, Taylor DM: Comparative effectiveness of atypical antipsychotics in schizophrenia: what have real-world trials taught us? CNS Drugs 26(6):491–508, 2012 22668246

Bai YM, Lin CC, Chen JY, Liu WC: Therapeutic effect of pirenzepine for clozapine-induced hypersalivation: a randomized, double-blind, placebo-controlled, cross-over study. J Clin Psychopharmacol 21(6):608–611, 2001 11763010

Barnes TR: A rating scale for drug-induced akathisia. Br J Psychiatry 154:672–676, 1989 2574607

Barnett M: Ziprasidone monotherapy in pediatric bipolar disorder. Poster presented at the annual meeting of the American Psychiatric Association, San Francisco, CA, May 2003

Beiser M, Erickson D, Fleming JA, Iacono WG: Establishing the onset of psychotic illness. Am J Psychiatry 150(9):1349–1354, 1993 8352345

Berger GE, Proffitt TM, McConchie M, et al: Dosing quetiapine in drug-naive first-episode psychosis: a controlled, double-blind, randomized, single-center study investigating efficacy, tolerability, and safety of 200 mg/day vs. 400 mg/day of quetiapine fumarate in 141 patients aged 15 to 25 years. J Clin Psychiatry 69(11):1702–1714, 2008 19036233

Bitter I, Dossenbach MR, Brook S, et al: Olanzapine versus clozapine in treatment-resistant or treatment-intolerant schizophrenia. Prog Neuropsychopharmacol Biol Psychiatry 28(1):173–180, 2004 14687871

Bobes J, Gibert J, Ciudad A, et al: Safety and effectiveness of olanzapine versus conventional antipsychotics in the acute treatment of first-episode schizophrenic inpatients. Prog Neuropsychopharmacol Biol Psychiatry 27(3):473–481, 2003 12691783

Burstein ES, Ma J, Wong S, et al: Intrinsic efficacy of antipsychotics at human D2, D3, and D4 dopamine receptors: identification of the clozapine metabolite N-desmethylclozapine as a D2/D3 partial agonist. J Pharmacol Exp Ther 315(3):1278–1287, 2005 16135699

Canitano R: Clinical experience with topiramate to counteract neuroleptic induced weight gain in 10 individuals with autistic spectrum disorders. Brain Dev 27(3):228–232, 2005 15737706

Caroff SN, Mann SC, Campbell EC, et al: Atypical APs and neuroleptic malignant syndrome. Psychiatr Ann 30:314–321, 2000

Chan SKW, Chan HYV, Honer WG, et al: Predictors of treatment-resistant and clozapine-resistant schizophrenia: a 12-year follow-up study of first-episode schizophrenia-spectrum disorders. Schizophr Bull 47(2):485–494, 2021 33043960

Cheng Z, Yuan Y, Han X, et al: An open-label randomised comparison of aripiprazole, olanzapine and risperidone for the acute treatment of first-episode schizophrenia: eight-week outcomes. J Psychopharmacol 33(10):1227–1236, 2019 31487208

Chengappa KN, Shelton MD, Baker RW, et al: The prevalence of akathisia in patients receiving stable doses of clozapine. J Clin Psychiatry 55(4):142–145, 1994 7915271

Cheng-Shannon J, McGough JJ, Pataki C, McCracken JT: Second-generation antipsychotic medications in children and adolescents. J Child Adolesc Psychopharmacol 14(3):372–394, 2004 15650494

Citrome L: Asenapine for schizophrenia and bipolar disorder: a review of the efficacy and safety profile for this newly approved sublingually absorbed second-generation antipsychotic. Int J Clin Pract 63(12):1762–1784, 2009 19840150

Cohen LG, Biederman J: Treatment of risperidone-induced hyperprolactinemia with a dopamine agonist in children. J Child Adolesc Psychopharmacol 11(4):435–440, 2001 11838826

Cornblatt BA: The New York High Risk Project to the Hillside Recognition and Prevention (RAP) program. Am J Med Genet 114(8):956–966, 2002 12457393

Correll CU, Manu P, Olshanskiy V, et al: Cardiometabolic risk of second-generation antipsychotic medications during first-time use in children and adolescents. JAMA 302(16):1765–1773, 2009 19861668

Correll CU, Kohegyi E, Zhao C, et al: Oral aripiprazole as maintenance treatment in adolescent schizophrenia: results from a 52-week, randomized, placebo-controlled withdrawal study. J Am Acad Child Adolesc Psychiatry 56(9):784–792, 2017 28838583

David CN, Rapoport JL: A neurodevelopmental perspective on hallucinations, in The Neuroscience of Hallucinations. Edited by Jardris R. New York, Springer, 2012, pp 203–230

David CN, Greenstein D, Clasen L, et al: Childhood onset schizophrenia: high rate of visual hallucinations. J Am Acad Child Adolesc Psychiatry 50(7):681–686, 2011 21703495

Davis JM, Chen N, Glick ID: A meta-analysis of the efficacy of second-generation antipsychotics. Arch Gen Psychiatry 60(6):553–564, 2003 12796218

Deckelbaum RJ, Williams CL: Childhood obesity: the health issue. Obes Res 9(Suppl 4):239S–243S, 2001 11707548 de Koning MB, Bloemen OJ, van Amelsvoort TA, et al: Early intervention in patients at ultra high risk of psychosis: benefits and risks. Acta Psychiatr Scand 119(6):426–442, 2009 19392813

Deniau E, Bonnot O, Cohen D: Drug treatment of early onset schizophrenia. Presse Med 37(5 Pt 2):853–858, 2008 18356007

Detke HC, DelBello MP, Landry J, et al: A 52-week study of olanzapine with a randomized behavioral weight counseling intervention in adolescents with schizophrenia or bipolar I disorder. J Child Adolesc Psychopharmacol 26(10):922–934, 2016 27676420

Driver D, Gogtay N, Greenstein D, et al: Premorbid impairments in childhood-onset schizophrenia. Schizophr Res 153(14):70883-70887, 2013a

Driver DI, Gogtay N, Rapoport JL: Childhood onset schizophrenia and early onset schizophrenia spectrum disorders. Child Adolesc Psychiatr Clin N Am 22(4):539–555, 2013b 24012072

Driver DI, Thomas S, Gogtay N, et al: Childhood-onset schizophrenia and early-onset schizophrenia spectrum disorders: an update. Child Adolesc Psychiatr Clin N Am 29(1):71–90, 2020 31708054

Eggers C, Bunk D: The long-term course of childhood-onset schizophrenia: a 42-year followup. Schizophr Bull 23(1):105–117, 1997 9050117

Ellul P, Delorme R, Cortese S: Metformin for weight gain associated with second-generation antipsychotics in children and adolescents: a systematic review and meta-analysis. CNS Drugs 32(12):1103–1112, 2018 30238318

Engelhardt DM, Polizos P, Waizer J, Hoffman SP: A double-blind comparison of fluphenazine and haloperidol in outpatient schizophrenic children. J Autism Child Schizophr 3(2):128–137, 1973 4583792

Fàbrega M, Sugranyes G, Baeza I: Two cases of long-acting paliperidone in adolescence. Ther Adv Psychopharmacol 5(5):304–306, 2015 26557986

Falloon IR: Early intervention for first episodes of schizophrenia: a preliminary exploration. Psychiatry 55(1):4–15, 1992 1557469

Faulkner G, Soundy AA, Lloyd K: Schizophrenia and weight management: a systematic review of interventions to control weight. Acta Psychiatr Scand 108(5):324–332, 2003 14531752

Fedorowicz VJ, Fombonne E: Metabolic side effects of atypical antipsychotics in children: a literature review. J Psychopharmacol 19(5):533–550, 2005 16166191

Findling RL, McNamara NK, Youngstrom EA, et al: A prospective, open-label trial of olanzapine in adolescents with schizophrenia. J Am Acad Child Adolesc Psychiatry 42(2):170–175, 2003 12544176

Findling RL, Aman MG, Eerdekens M, et al: Long-term, open-label study of risperidone in children with severe disruptive behaviors and below-average IQ. Am J Psychiatry 161(4):677–684, 2004 15056514

Findling RL, Frazier JA, Gerbino-Rosen G, et al: Is there a role for clozapine in the treatment of children and adolescents? J Am Acad Child Adolesc Psychiatry 46(3):423–428, 2007 17314729

Findling RL, Kauffman RE, Sallee FR, et al: Tolerability and pharmacokinetics of aripiprazole in children and adolescents with psychiatric disorders: an open-label, dose-escalation study. J Clin Psychopharmacol 28(4):441–446, 2008a 18626272

Findling RL, Robb A, Nyilas M, et al: A multiple-center, randomized, double-blind, placebo-controlled study of oral aripiprazole for treatment of adolescents with schizophrenia. Am J Psychiatry 165(11):1432–1441, 2008b 18765484

Findling RL, Cavus I, Pappadopulos E, et al: A placebo-controlled trial to evaluate the efficacy and safety of flexibly dosed oral ziprasidone in adolescent subjects with schizophrenia. Presented at the Biannual Schizophrenia International Research Conference, Florence, Italy, 2010a

Findling RL, Johnson JL, McClellan J, et al: Double-blind maintenance safety and effectiveness findings from the Treatment of Early Onset Schizophrenia Spectrum (TEOSS) study. J Am Acad Child Adolesc Psychiatry 49(6):583–594, quiz 632, 2010b 20494268

Findling RL, McKenna K, Earley WR, et al: Efficacy and safety of quetiapine in adolescents with schizophrenia investigated in a 6-week, double-blind, placebo-controlled trial. J Child Adolesc Psychopharmacol 22(5):327–342, 2012 23083020

Findling RL, Landbloom RP, Mackle M, et al: Safety and efficacy from an 8 week double-blind trial and a 26 week open-label extension of asenapine in adolescents with schizophrenia. J Child Adolesc Psychopharmacol 25(5):384–396, 2015 26091193

Flach C, French P, Dunn G, et al: Components of therapy as mechanisms of change in cognitive therapy for people at risk of psychosis: analysis of the EDIE-2 trial. Br J Psychiatry 207(2):123–129, 2015 25999337

Frazier JA, Gordon CT, McKenna K, et al: An open trial of clozapine in 11 adolescents with childhood-onset schizophrenia. J Am Acad Child Adolesc Psychiatry 33(5):658–663, 1994 8056728

Geddes J, Freemantle N, Harrison P, Bebbington P: Atypical antipsychotics in the treatment of schizophrenia: systematic overview and meta-regression analysis. BMJ 321(7273):1371–1376, 2000 11099280

Generali JA, Cada DJ: Topiramate: antipsychotic-induced weight gain. Hosp Pharm 49(4):345–347, 2014 24958940

Glazer WM: Extrapyramidal side effects, tardive dyskinesia, and the concept of atypicality. J Clin Psychiatry 61(Suppl 3):16–21, 2000 10724129

Gochman P, Miller R, Rapoport JL: Childhood-onset schizophrenia: the challenge of diagnosis. Curr Psychiatry Rep 13(5):321–322, 2011 21713647

Goeb JL, Marco S, Duhamel A, et al: Metabolic side effects of risperidone in early onset schizophrenia. Encephale 36(3):242–252, 2010 20620267

Gogtay N, Rapoport J: Clozapine use in children and adolescents. Expert Opin Pharmacother 9(3):459–465, 2008 18220495

Gogtay N, Sporn A, Alfaro CL, et al: Clozapine-induced akathisia in children with schizophrenia. J Child Adolesc Psychopharmacol 12(4):347–349, 2002 12625995

Goldman R, Loebel A, Cucchiaro J, et al: Efficacy and safety of lurasidone in adolescents with schizophrenia: a 6-week, randomized placebo-controlled study. J Child Adolesc Psychopharmacol 27(6):516–525, 2017 28475373

Gordon CT, Frazier JA, McKenna K, et al: Childhood-onset schizophrenia: an NIMH study in progress. Schizophr Bull 20(4):697–712, 1994 7701277

Gothelf D, Apter A, Reidman J, et al: Olanzapine, risperidone and haloperidol in the treatment of adolescent patients with schizophrenia. J Neural Transm (Vienna) 110(5):545–560, 2003 12721815

Goyal N, Sinha VK: Amisulpride-induced tardive dyskinesia in childhood onset schizophrenia. Prog Neuropsychopharmacol Biol Psychiatry 34(4):728–729, 2010 20347912

Gracious BL, Krysiak TE, Youngstrom EA: Amantadine treatment of psychotropic-induced weight gain in children and adolescents: case series. J Child Adolesc Psychopharmacol 12(3):249–257, 2002 12427299

Grcevich SJ, Findling RL, Rowane WA, et al: Risperidone in the treatment of children and adolescents with schizophrenia: a retrospective study. J Child Adolesc Psychopharmacol 6(4):251–257, 1996 9231318

Greenstein D, Lerch J, Shaw P, et al: Childhood onset schizophrenia: cortical brain abnormalities as young adults. J Child Psychol Psychiatry 47(10):1003–1012, 2006 17073979

Guy W: Clinical Global Impressions, in ECDEU Assessment Manual for Psychopharmacology, Revised (NIMH Publ No 76-338). Rockville, MD, National Institute of Mental Health, 1976, pp 218–222

Haas M, Eerdekens M, Kushner S, et al: Efficacy, safety and tolerability of two dosing regimens in adolescent schizophrenia: double-blind study. Br J Psychiatry 194(2):158–164, 2009a 19182179

Haas M, Unis AS, Armenteros J, et al: A 6-week, randomized, double-blind, placebo-controlled study of the efficacy and safety of risperidone in adolescents with schizophrenia. J Child Adolesc Psychopharmacol 19(6):611–621, 2009b 20035579

Häfner H, Maurer K, Löffler W, et al: The ABC Schizophrenia Study: a preliminary overview of the results. Soc Psychiatry Psychiatr Epidemiol 33(8):380–386, 1998 9708025

Halloran DR, Swindle J, Takemoto SK, Schnitzler MA: Multiple psychiatric diagnoses common in privately insured children on atypical antipsychotics. Clin Pediatr (Phila) 49(5):485–490, 2010 20118088

Hanft A, Eggleston CF, Bourgeois JA: Neuroleptic malignant syndrome in an adolescent after brief exposure to olanzapine. J Child Adolesc Psychopharmacol 14(3):481–487, 2004 15650507

Hartung DM, Wisdom JP, Pollack DA, et al: Patterns of atypical antipsychotic subtherapeutic dosing among Oregon Medicaid patients. J Clin Psychiatry 69(10):1540–1547, 2008 19192436

Harvey RC, James AC, Shields GE: A systematic review and network meta-analysis to assess the relative efficacy of antipsychotics for the treatment of positive and negative symptoms in early-onset schizophrenia. CNS Drugs 30(1):27–39, 2016 26801655

Herrán A, García-Unzueta MT, Amado JA, et al: Effects of long-term treatment with antipsychotics on serum leptin levels. Br J Psychiatry 179:59–62, 2001 11435270

Hollis C: Adult outcomes of child- and adolescent-onset schizophrenia: diagnostic stability and predictive validity. Am J Psychiatry 157(10):1652–1659, 2000 11007720

Hrdlicka M, Zedkova I, Blatny M, Urbanek T: Weight gain associated with atypical and typical antipsychotics during treatment of adolescent schizophrenic psychoses: a retrospective study. Neuroendocrinol Lett 30(2):256–261, 2009 19675512

Jensen JB, Kumra S, Leitten W, et al: A comparative pilot study of second-generation antipsychotics in children and adolescents with schizophrenia-spectrum disorders. J Child Adolesc Psychopharmacol 18(4):317–326, 2008 18759641

Jin H, Meyer JM, Jeste DV: Atypical antipsychotics and glucose dysregulation: a systematic review. Schizophr Res 71(2–3):195–212, 2004 15474892

Kahl KG, Hagenah J, Zapf S, et al: Botulinum toxin as an effective treatment of clozapine-induced hypersalivation. Psychopharmacology (Berl) 173(1–2):229–230, 2004 14747903

Kane J, Honigfeld G, Singer J, Meltzer H: Clozapine for the treatment-resistant schizophrenic: a double-blind comparison with chlorpromazine. Arch Gen Psychiatry 45(9):789–796, 1988 3046553

Kapur S, Remington G: Atypical antipsychotics: new directions and new challenges in the treatment of schizophrenia. Annu Rev Med 52:503–517, 2001 11160792

Kasoff LI, Ahn K, Gochman P, et al: Strong treatment response and high maintenance rates of clozapine in childhood-onset schizophrenia. J Child Adolesc Psychopharmacol 26(5):428–435, 2016 26784704

Keepers GA, Fochtmann LJ, Anzia JM, et al: The American Psychiatric Association practice guideline for the treatment of patients with schizophrenia. Am J Psychiatry 177(9):868–872, 2020 32867516

Kelleher I, Connor D, Clarke MC, et al: Prevalence of psychotic symptoms in childhood and adolescence: a systematic review and meta-analysis of population-based studies. Psychol Med 42(9):1857–1863, 2012 22225730

Kendall T, Hollis C, Stafford M, Taylor C: Recognition and management of psychosis and schizophrenia in children and young people: summary of NICE guidance. BMJ 346:f150, 2013 23344308

Kennedy E, Kumar A, Datta SS: Antipsychotic medication for childhood-onset schizophrenia. Cochrane Database Syst Rev (3):CD004027, 2007 17636744

Kishimoto T, Hagi K, Nitta M, et al: Effectiveness of long-acting injectable vs oral antipsychotics in patients with schizophrenia: a meta-analysis of prospective and retrospective cohort studies. Schizophr Bull 44(3):603–619, 2018 29868849

Kishimoto T, Hagi K, Kurokawa S, et al: Long-acting injectable versus oral antipsychotics for the maintenance treatment of schizophrenia: a systematic review and comparative meta-analysis of randomised, cohort, and pre-post studies. Lancet Psychiatry 8(5):387–404, 2021 33862018

Klein DJ, Cottingham EM, Sorter M, et al: A randomized, double-blind, placebo-controlled trial of metformin treatment of weight gain associated with initiation of atypical antipsychotic therapy in children and adolescents. Am J Psychiatry 163(12):2072–2079, 2006 17151157

Kleinhaus K, Harlap S, Perrin M, et al: Age, sex and first treatment of schizophrenia in a population cohort. J Psychiatr Res 45(1):136–141, 2011 20541769

Klosterkötter J, Hellmich M, Steinmeyer EM, Schultze-Lutter F: Diagnosing schizophrenia in the initial prodromal phase. Arch Gen Psychiatry 58(2):158–164, 2001 11177117

Kolvin I: Studies in the childhood psychoses I: diagnostic criteria and classification. Br J Psychiatry 118(545):381–384, 1971 5576635

Komossa K, Rummel-Kluge C, Schmid F, et al: Aripiprazole versus other atypical antipsychotics for schizophrenia. Cochrane Database Syst Rev (4):CD006569, 2009 19821375

Kowalski JL, Wink LK, Blankenship K, et al: Paliperidone palmitate in a child with autistic disorder. J Child Adolesc Psychopharmacol 21(5):491–493, 2011 22040196

Kraepelin E: Dementia Praecox and Paraphrenia. Huntington, NY, Robert E. Krieger, 1919

Kryzhanovskaya LA, Robertson-Plouch CK, Xu W, et al: The safety of olanzapine in adolescents with schizophrenia or bipolar I disorder: a pooled analysis of 4 clinical trials. J Clin Psychiatry 70(2):247–258, 2009a 19210948

Kryzhanovskaya L, Schulz SC, McDougle C, et al: Olanzapine versus placebo in adolescents with schizophrenia: a 6-week, randomized, double-blind, placebo-controlled trial. J Am Acad Child Adolesc Psychiatry 48(1):60–70, 2009b 19057413

Kumra S, Frazier JA, Jacobsen LK, et al: Childhood-onset schizophrenia: a double-blind clozapine-haloperidol comparison. Arch Gen Psychiatry 53(12):1090–1097, 1996 8956674

Kumra S, Jacobsen LK, Lenane M, et al: Childhood-onset schizophrenia: an open-label study of olanzapine in adolescents. J Am Acad Child Adolesc Psychiatry 37(4):377–385, 1998 9549958

Kumra S, Kranzler H, Gerbino-Rosen G, et al: Clozapine and "high-dose" olanzapine in refractory early onset schizophrenia: a 12-week randomized and double-blind comparison. Biol Psychiatry 63(5):524–529, 2008a 17651705

Kumra S, Oberstar JV, Sikich L, et al: Efficacy and tolerability of second-generation antipsychotics in children and adolescents with schizophrenia. Schizophr Bull 34(1):60–71, 2008b 17923452

Lehman AF, Lieberman JA, Dixon LB, et al: Practice guideline for the treatment of patients with schizophrenia, second edition. Am J Psychiatry 161(2 Suppl):1–56, 2004 15000267

Leucht S, Pitschel-Walz G, Abraham D, et al: Efficacy and extrapyramidal side-effects of the new antipsychotics olanzapine, quetiapine, risperidone, and sertindole compared to conventional antipsychotics and placebo: a meta-analysis of randomized controlled trials. Schizophr Res 35(1):51–68, 1999 9988841

Leucht S, Wahlbeck K, Hamann J, et al: New generation APs versus low-potency conventional antipsychotics: a systematic review and meta-analysis. Lancet 361(9369):1581–1589, 2003 12747876

Levine SZ, Rabinowitz J: Trajectories and antecedents of treatment response over time in early episode psychosis. Schizophr Bull 36(3):624–632, 2010 18849294

Lieberman JA, Saltz BL, Johns CA, et al: The effects of clozapine on tardive dyskinesia. Br J Psychiatry 158:503–510, 1991 1675900

Lieberman JA, Sheitman BB, Kinon BJ: Neurochemical sensitization in the pathophysiology of schizophrenia: deficits and dysfunction in neuronal regulation and plasticity. Neuropsychopharmacology 17(4):205–229, 1997 9326746

Lieberman JA, Phillips M, Gu H, et al: Atypical and conventional antipsychotic drugs in treatment-naive first-episode schizophrenia: a 52-week randomized trial of clozapine vs chlorpromazine. Neuropsychopharmacology 28(5):995–1003, 2003 12700715

Lieberman JA, Stroup TS, McEvoy JP, et al: Effectiveness of antipsychotic drugs in patients with chronic schizophrenia. N Engl J Med 353(12):1209–1223, 2005 16172203

Lytle S, McVoy M, Sajatovic M: Long-acting injectable antipsychotics in children and adolescents. J Child Adolesc Psychopharmacol 27(1):2–9, 2017 28112539

Maijer K, Begemann MJH, Palmen SJMC, et al: Auditory hallucinations across the lifespan: a systematic review and meta-analysis. Psychol Med 48(6):879–888, 2018 28956518

Mangurian C, Fuentes-Afflick E, Newcomer JW: Risks from antipsychotic medications in children and adolescents. JAMA 303(8):729–730, author reply 730, 2010 20179279

Markulev C, McGorry PD, Nelson B, et al: NEURAPRO-E study protocol: a multicentre randomized controlled trial of omega-3 fatty acids and cognitive-behavioural case management for patients at ultra high risk of schizophrenia and other psychotic disorders. Early Interv Psychiatry 11(5):418–428, 2015 26279065

Martin S, Ljo H, Peuskens J, et al: A double-blind, randomised comparative trial of amisulpride versus olanzapine in the treatment of schizophrenia: short-term results at two months. Curr Med Res Opin 18(6):355–362, 2002 12442883

Masi G, Liboni F: Management of schizophrenia in children and adolescents: focus on pharmacotherapy. Drugs 71(2):179–208, 2011 21275445

Masi G, Cosenza A, Mucci M: Prolactin levels in young children with pervasive developmental disorders during risperidone treatment. J Child Adolesc Psychopharmacol 11(4):389–394, 2001 11838821

McClellan J, Sikich L, Findling RL, et al: Treatment of Early Onset Schizophrenia Spectrum Disorders (TEOSS): rationale, design, and methods. J Am Acad Child Adolesc Psychiatry 46(8):969–978, 2007 17667476

McClellan J, Stock S, American Academy of Child and Adolescent Psychiatry Committee on Quality Issues: Practice parameter for the assessment and treatment of children and adolescents with schizophrenia. J Am Acad Child Adolesc Psychiatry 52(9):976–990, 2013 23972700

McConville B, Carrero L, Sweitzer D, et al: Long-term safety, tolerability, and clinical efficacy of quetiapine in adolescents: an open-label extension trial. J Child Adolesc Psychopharmacol 13(1):75–82, 2003 12804128

McGorry PD, Yung AR, Phillips LJ: The "close-in" or ultra high-risk model: a safe and effective strategy for research and clinical intervention in prepsychotic mental disorder. Schizophr Bull 29(4):771–790, 2003 14989414

McGorry PD, Nelson B, Phillips LJ, et al: Randomized controlled trial of interventions for young people at ultra-high risk of psychosis: twelve-month outcome. J Clin Psychiatry 74(4):349–356, 2013 23218022

McKee JR, Wall T, Owensby J: Impact of complete blood count sampling time change on white blood cell and absolute neutrophil count values in clozapine recipients. Clin Schizophr Relat Psychoses 5(1):26–32, 2011 21459736

Melkersson KI, Dahl ML, Hulting AL: Guidelines for prevention and treatment of adverse effects of antipsychotic drugs on glucose-insulin homeostasis and lipid metabolism. Psychopharmacology (Berl) 175(1):1–6, 2004 15221198

Miklowitz DJ, O'Brien MP, Schlosser DA, et al: Family focused treatment for adolescents and young adults at high risk for psychosis: results of a randomized trial. J Am Acad Child Adolesc Psychiatry 53(8):848–858, 2014 25062592

Mischoulon D, Freeman MP: Omega-3 fatty acids in psychiatry. Psychiatr Clin North Am 36(1):15–23, 2013 23538073

Miyamoto S, Duncan GE, Marx CE, Lieberman JA: Treatments for schizophrenia: a critical review of pharmacology and mechanisms of action of antipsychotic drugs. Mol Psychiatry 10(1):79–104, 2005 15289815

Moncrieff J: Clozapine v. conventional antipsychotic drugs for treatment-resistant schizophrenia: a re-examination. Br J Psychiatry 183:161–166, 2003 12893670

Morrison AP, French P, Walford L, et al: Cognitive therapy for the prevention of psychosis in people at ultra-high risk: randomised controlled trial. Br J Psychiatry 185:291–297, 2004 15458988

Mossaheb N, Schäfer MR, Schlögelhofer M, et al: Effect of omega-3 fatty acids for indicated prevention of young patients at risk for psychosis: when do they begin to be effective? Schizophr Res 148(1–3):163–167, 2013 23778032

Mozes T, Greenberg Y, Spivak B, et al: Olanzapine treatment in chronic drug-resistant childhood-onset schizophrenia: an open-label study. J Child Adolesc Psychopharmacol 13(3):311–317, 2003 14642019

Nelson B, Amminger GP, Yuen HP, et al: NEURAPRO: a multi-centre RCT of omega-3 polyunsaturated fatty acids versus placebo in young people at ultra-high risk of psychotic disorders-medium-term follow-up and clinical course. NPJ Schizophr 4(1):11, 2018 29941938

Nicolson R, Lenane M, Singaracharlu S, et al: Premorbid speech and language impairments in childhood-onset schizophrenia: association with risk factors. Am J Psychiatry 157(5):794–800, 2000 10784474

Normala I, Hamidin A: The use of aripiprazole in early onset schizophrenia: safety and efficacy. Med J Malaysia 64(3):240–241, 2009 20527278

Novick D, Haro JM, Bertsch J, Haddad PM: Incidence of extrapyramidal symptoms and tardive dyskinesia in schizophrenia: thirty-six-month results from the European Schizophrenia Outpatient Health Outcomes Study. J Clin Psychopharmacol 30(5):531–540, 2010 20814320

Ostuzzi G, Bertolini F, Del Giovane C, et al: Maintenance treatment with long-acting injectable antipsychotics for people with nonaffective psychoses: a network meta-analysis. Am J Psychiatry 178(5):424–436, 2021 33596679

Pagsberg AK, Jeppesen P, Klauber DG, et al: Quetiapine extended release versus aripiprazole in children and adolescents with first-episode psychosis: the multicentre, double-blind, randomised Tolerability and Efficacy of Antipsychotics (TEA) trial. Lancet Psychiatry 4(8):605–618, 2017a 28599949

Pagsberg AK, Tarp S, Glintborg D, et al: Acute antipsychotic treatment of children and adolescents with schizophrenia-spectrum disorders: a systematic review and network meta-analysis. J Am Acad Child Adolesc Psychiatry 56(3):191–202, 2017b 28219485

Pantelis C, Velakoulis D, McGorry PD, et al: Neuroanatomical abnormalities before and after onset of psychosis: a cross-sectional and longitudinal MRI comparison. Lancet 361(9354):281–288, 2003 12559861

Pappagallo M, Silva R: The effect of atypical antipsychotic agents on prolactin levels in children and adolescents. J Child Adolesc Psychopharmacol 14(3):359–371, 2004 15650493

Paprocki J, Versiani M: A double-blind comparison between loxapine and haloperidol by parenteral route in acute schizophrenia. Curr Ther Res Clin Exp 21(1):80–100, 1977 12922

Patel JK, Buckley PF, Woolson S, et al: Metabolic profiles of second-generation antipsychotics in early psychosis: findings from the CAFE study. Schizophr Res 111(1–3):9–16, 2009 19398192

Patel NC, Sanchez RJ, Johnsrud MT, Crismon ML: Trends in antipsychotic use in a Texas Medicaid population of children and adolescents: 1996 to 2000. J Child Adolesc Psychopharmacol 12(3):221–229, 2002 12427295

Pickar D, Litman RE, Hong WW, et al: Clinical response to clozapine in patients with schizophrenia. Arch Gen Psychiatry 51(2):159–160, 1994 8297214

Polanczyk G, Moffitt TE, Arseneault L, et al: Etiological and clinical features of childhood psychotic symptoms: results from a birth cohort. Arch Gen Psychiatry 67(4):328–338, 2010 20368509

Pool D, Bloom W, Mielke DH, et al: A controlled evaluation of loxitane in seventy-five adolescent schizophrenic patients. Curr Ther Res Clin Exp 19(1):99–104, 1976 812671

Poulton R, Caspi A, Moffitt TE, et al: Children's self-reported psychotic symptoms and adult schizophreniform disorder: a 15-year longitudinal study. Arch Gen Psychiatry 57(11):1053–1058, 2000 11074871

Rabinowitz J, Levine SZ, Häfner H: A population based elaboration of the role of age of onset on the course of schizophrenia. Schizophr Res 88(1–3):96–101, 2006 16962742

Rapoport JL, Gogtay N: Childhood onset schizophrenia: support for a progressive neurodevelopmental disorder. Int J Dev Neurosci 29(3):251–258, 2011 20955775

Rapoport JL, Addington A, Frangou S: The neurodevelopmental model of schizophrenia: what can very early onset cases tell us? Curr Psychiatry Rep 7(2):81–82, 2005a 15802082

Rapoport JL, Addington AM, Frangou S, Psych MR: The neurodevelopmental model of schizophrenia: update 2005. Mol Psychiatry 10(5):434–449, 2005b 15700048

Rapoport JL, Giedd JN, Gogtay N: Neurodevelopmental model of schizophrenia: update 2012. Mol Psychiatry 17(12):1228–1238, 2012 22488257

Realmuto GM, Erickson WD, Yellin AM, et al: Clinical comparison of thiothixene and thioridazine in schizophrenic adolescents. Am J Psychiatry 141(3):440–442, 1984 6367494

Reekie J, Hosking SP, Prakash C, et al: The effect of antidepressants and antipsychotics on weight gain in children and adolescents. Obes Rev 16(7):566–580, 2015 26016407

Remschmidt H, Theisen FP: Early-onset schizophrenia. Neuropsychobiology 66(1):63–69, 2012 22797279

Robles O, Zabala A, Bombín I, et al: Cognitive efficacy of quetiapine and olanzapine in early onset first-episode psychosis. Schizophr Bull 37(2):405–415, 2011 19706697

Ross RG, Novins D, Farley GK, Adler LE: A 1-year open-label trial of olanzapine in school-age children with schizophrenia. J Child Adolesc Psychopharmacol 13(3):301–309, 2003 14642018

Ruhrmann S, Schultze-Lutter F, Klosterkötter J: Early detection and intervention in the initial prodromal phase of schizophrenia. Pharmacopsychiatry 36(Suppl 3):S162–S167, 2003 14677074

Ruhrmann S, Schultze-Lutter F, Maier W, Klosterkötter J: Pharmacological intervention in the initial prodromal phase of psychosis. Eur Psychiatry 20(1):1–6, 2005 15642437

Rummel C, Hamann J, Kissling W, Leucht S: New generation antipsychotics for first episode schizophrenia. Cochrane Database Syst Rev (4):CD004410, 2003 14584012

Saito E, Correll CU, Gallelli K, et al: A prospective study of hyperprolactinemia in children and adolescents treated with atypical antipsychotic agents. J Child Adolesc Psychopharmacol 14(3):350–358, 2004 15650492

Savitz AJ, Lane R, Nuamah I, et al: Efficacy and safety of paliperidone extended release in adolescents with schizophrenia: a randomized, double-blind study. J Am Acad Child Adolesc Psychiatry 54(2):126–137, 2015a 25617253

Savitz A, Lane R, Nuamah I, et al: Long-term safety of paliperidone extended release in adolescents with schizophrenia: an open-label, flexible dose study. J Child Adolesc Psychopharmacol 25(7):548–557, 2015b 26218669

Schneider C, Corrigall R, Hayes D, et al: Systematic review of the efficacy and tolerability of clozapine in the treatment of youth with early onset schizophrenia. Eur Psychiatry 29(1):1–10, 2014 24119631

Shaw JA, Lewis JE, Pascal S, et al: A study of quetiapine: efficacy and tolerability in psychotic adolescents. J Child Adolesc Psychopharmacol 11(4):415–424, 2001 11838824

Shaw P, Rapoport JL: Decision making about children with psychotic symptoms: using the best evidence in choosing a treatment. J Am Acad Child Adolesc Psychiatry 45(11):1381–1386, 2006 17075361

Shaw P, Sporn A, Gogtay N, et al: Childhood-onset schizophrenia: a double-blind, randomized clozapine-olanzapine comparison. Arch Gen Psychiatry 63(7):721–730, 2006 16818861

Sholevar EH, Baron DA, Hardie TL: Treatment of childhood-onset schizophrenia with olanzapine. J Child Adolesc Psychopharmacol 10(2):69–78, 2000 10933117

Sikich L, Hamer RM, Bashford RA, et al: A pilot study of risperidone, olanzapine, and haloperidol in psychotic youth: a double-blind, randomized, 8-week trial. Neuropsychopharmacology 29(1):133–145, 2004 14583740

Sikich L, Frazier JA, McClellan J, et al: Double-blind comparison of first- and second-generation antipsychotics in early onset schizophrenia and schizo-affective disorder: findings from the Treatment of Early Onset Schizophrenia Spectrum Disorders (TEOSS) study. Am J Psychiatry 165(11):1420–1431, 2008 18794207

Siskind D, Siskind V, Kisely S: Clozapine response rates among people with treatment-resistant schizophrenia: data from a systematic review and meta-analysis. Can J Psychiatry 62(11):772–777, 2017 28655284

Simpson GM, Angus JW: A rating scale for extrapyramidal side effects. Acta Psychiatr Scand Suppl 212:11–19, 1970 4917967

Singh J, Robb A, Vijapurkar U, et al: A randomized, double-blind study of paliperidone extended-release in treatment of acute schizophrenia in adolescents. Biol Psychiatry 70(12):1179–1187, 2011 21831359

Sowell MO, Mukhopadhyay N, Cavazzoni P, et al: Hyperglycemic clamp assessment of insulin secretory responses in normal subjects treated with olanzapine, risperidone, or placebo. J Clin Endocrinol Metab 87(6):2918–2923, 2002 12050274

Spencer EK, Kafantaris V, Padron-Gayol MV, et al: Haloperidol in schizophrenic children: early findings from a study in progress. Psychopharmacol Bull 28(2):183–186, 1992 1513922

Sporn A, Gogtay N, Ortiz-Aguayo R, et al: Clozapine-induced neutropenia in children: management with lithium carbonate. J Child Adolesc Psychopharmacol 13(3):401–404, 2003 14642024

Sporn AL, Vermani A, Greenstein DK, et al: Clozapine treatment of childhood-onset schizophrenia: evaluation of effectiveness, adverse effects, and long-term outcome. J Am Acad Child Adolesc Psychiatry 46(10):1349–1356, 2007 17885577

Stafford MR, Jackson H, Mayo-Wilson E, et al: Early interventions to prevent psychosis: systematic review and meta-analysis. BMJ 346:f185, 2013 23335473 (Erratum BMJ 346:f762, 2013)

Taylor JH, Jakubovski E, Gabriel D, Bloch MH: Predictors and moderators of antipsychotic-related weight gain in the Treatment of Early Onset Schizophrenia Spectrum Disorders study. J Child Adolesc Psychopharmacol 28(7):474–484, 2018 29920116

Thomsen PH: Schizophrenia with childhood and adolescent onset: a nationwide register-based study. Acta Psychiatr Scand 94(3):187–193, 1996 8891086

Tollefson GD, Birkett MA, Kiesler GM, Wood AJ: Double-blind comparison of olanzapine versus clozapine in schizophrenic patients clinically eligible for treatment with clozapine. Biol Psychiatry 49(1):52–63, 2001 11163780

Tossell JW, Greenstein DK, Davidson AL, et al: Stimulant drug treatment in childhood-onset schizophrenia with comorbid ADHD: an open-label case series. J Child Adolesc Psychopharmacol 14(3):448–454, 2004 15650502

Turetz M, Mozes T, Toren P, et al: An open trial of clozapine in neuroleptic-resistant childhood-onset schizophrenia. Br J Psychiatry 170:507–510, 1997 9330014

Uchida H, Suzuki T, Mamo DC, et al: Effects of age and age of onset on prescribed antipsychotic dose in schizophrenia spectrum disorders: a survey of 1,418 patients in Japan. Am J Geriatr Psychiatry 16(7):584–593, 2008 18591578

Usiskin SI, Nicolson R, Lenane M, Rapoport JL: Gabapentin prophylaxis of clozapine-induced seizures. Am J Psychiatry 157(3):482–483, 2000 10698845

Vahia IV, Palmer BW, Depp C, et al: Is late-onset schizophrenia a subtype of schizophrenia? Acta Psychiatr Scand 122(5):414–426, 2010 20199491

van der Gaag M, Nieman DH, Rietdijk J, et al: Cognitive behavioral therapy for subjects at ultrahigh risk for developing psychosis: a randomized controlled clinical trial. Schizophr Bull 38(6):1180–1188, 2012 22941746

Varimo E, Saastamoinen LK, Rättö H, et al: New users of antipsychotics among children and adolescents in 2008–2017: a nationwide register study. Front Psychiatry 11:316, 2020 32390885

Varol Tas F, Guvenir T: Amisulpride treatment of adolescent patients with schizophrenia or schizo-affective disorders. Eur Child Adolesc Psychiatry 18(8):511–513, 2009 19267176

Vernal DL, Kapoor S, Al-Jadiri A, et al: Outcome of youth with early phase schizophrenia-spectrum disorders and psychosis not otherwise specified treated with second-generation antipsychotics: 12 week results from a prospective, naturalistic cohort study. J Child Adolesc Psychopharmacol 25(7):535–547, 2015 26375767

Vernal DL, Boldsen SK, Lauritsen MB, et al: Long-term outcome of early-onset compared to adult-onset schizophrenia: a nationwide Danish register study. Schizophr Res 220:123–129, 2020 32299717

Volavka J, Czobor P, Sheitman B, et al: Clozapine, olanzapine, risperidone, and haloperidol in the treatment of patients with chronic schizophrenia and schizoaffective disorder. Am J Psychiatry 159(2):255–262, 2002 11823268

Volkmar FR: Childhood and adolescent psychosis: a review of the past 10 years. J Am Acad Child Adolesc Psychiatry 35(7):843–851, 1996 8768343

Weiner DM, Meltzer HY, Veinbergs I, et al: The role of M1 muscarinic receptor agonism of N-desmethylclozapine in the unique clinical effects of clozapine. Psychopharmacology (Berl) 177(1–2):207–216, 2004 15258717

Wirshing DA, Wirshing WC, Kysar L, et al: Novel antipsychotics: comparison of weight gain liabilities. J Clin Psychiatry 60(6):358–363, 1999 10401912

Woods SW, Breier A, Zipursky RB, et al: Randomized trial of olanzapine versus placebo in the symptomatic acute treatment of the schizophrenic prodrome. Biol Psychiatry 54(4):453–464, 2003 12915290 (Erratum: Biol Psychiatry 54:497, 2003)

Wudarsky M, Nicolson R, Hamburger SD, et al: Elevated prolactin in pediatric patients on typical and atypical antipsychotics. J Child Adolesc Psychopharmacol 9(4):239–245, 1999 10630453

Xiong Y: Comparison study of childhood schizophrenia treated with risperidone and chlorpromazine. Guizhou Med J 28:697–698, 2004

Xu L, Guo Y, Cao Q, et al: Predictors of outcome in early onset schizophrenia: a 10-year follow-up study. BMC Psychiatry 20(1):67, 2020 32059664

Yung AR, Phillips LJ, Yuen HP, et al: Psychosis prediction: 12-month follow up of a high-risk ("prodromal") group. Schizophr Res 60(1):21–32, 2003 12505135

Zalsman G, Carmon E, Martin A, et al: Effectiveness, safety, and tolerability of risperidone in adolescents with schizophrenia: an open-label study. J Child Adolesc Psychopharmacol 13(3):319–327, 2003 14642020

Zarafonitis S, Wagner M, Putzfeld V, et al: Psychoeducation for persons at risk of psychosis. Psychotherapeut (German) 57(4):326–334, 2012

10

Eating Disorders

Roxanne Demarest, P.A.-C.
Griffin Stout, M.D.

Eating disorders are a complex and multifaceted group of diagnoses that have high rates of morbidity and mortality, and they are often difficult to treat. Eating disorders are prevalent among adolescents, and onset often occurs from adolescence to young adulthood. Treatment options for eating disorders are limited, often requiring the patient's acceptance of the diagnosis to make a change and do what is feared most: gain weight and adjust their dietary intake. The treatments that are most studied include psychosocial therapies, including family-based therapy (FBT), cognitive-behavioral therapy (CBT), and adolescent-focused therapy (Herpertz-Dahlmann 2017). There is limited research on psychopharmacological treatment of eating disorders, especially in childhood and adolescence. Clinicians should use medications cautiously because of the lack of strong evidence and because no medications have been FDA-approved for treating eating disorder symptoms in youth. Medications, if used, should be accompanied by multimodal treatment (e.g., nutrition, psychosocial, medical) (Reinblatt et al. 2008). Owing to the dearth of data, the World Federation of Societies of Biological Psychiatry (WFSBP) instituted a task force that systematically reviewed psychopharmacological treatments of eating disorders from 1977 to 2010 (Aigner et al. 2011), which is frequently referred to in this chapter along with the American Psychiatric Association (APA), American Academy of Child and Adolescent Psychiatry (AACAP), and National Institute for Health and Care Excellence (NICE) guidelines.

In this chapter, we discuss the current evidence base for psychopharmacological treatment of eating disorders. Published randomized controlled trials (RCTs) of medications conducted specifically with children and adolescents are very limited (Golden and Attia 2011); therefore, we also discuss the results of adult studies so that the background evidence can be understood. However, it is difficult to extrapolate evidence from the adult data for many reasons, including differing pharmacodynamics and pharmacokinetics, lack of FDA approval of medication treatments for youth, and the varying developmental needs of youth versus adults (Gowers et al. 2010).

Eating disorders are characterized in DSM-5 (American Psychiatric Association 2022) as a persistent disturbance of eating that alters consumption or absorption of food and leads to impairment of physical or psychosocial functioning. This is an expanded view from DSM-IV-TR (American Psychiatric Association 2000), which focused on anorexia nervosa (AN), bulimia nervosa (BN), and eating disorder not otherwise specified (EDNOS). The Eating Disorders Work Group made criteria clearer and more inclusive across the life span and the sexes, accounting for developmental changes in childhood and adolescence. They combined the two separate feeding and eating disorders of infancy or early childhood and eating disorders sections in DSM-IV-TR and created the "Feeding and Eating Disorders" chapter, which now includes pica, rumination disorder, avoidant/restrictive food intake disorder (ARFID), AN, BN, and binge-eating disorder (BED). Other changes include elimination of amenorrhea as a required criterion for AN because males and premenarchal females cannot meet this criterion, expansion of the frequency requirement of compensatory behaviors for BN, and the addition of BED. Using DSM-IV (American Psychiatric Association 1994) criteria, more than 50% of children and adolescents with eating disorders were diagnosed with EDNOS (Fisher et al. 2014). With the new DSM-5 criteria, discussed for each diagnosis, the goal is making more specific diagnoses in children and adolescents and therefore employing more focused and appropriate treatment.

Anorexia Nervosa

Diagnosis

AN is a serious illness involving the persistent restriction of food intake, fear of gaining weight, and behavior that interferes with weight gain (Box 10–1). The severity of AN is determined by the patient's current BMI; extreme AN is diagnosed in individuals with a BMI below 15 (calculated as height in kilograms divided by meters squared). Developmentally, this leads to a body weight that is below what is appropriate based on the person's age, sex, physical health, and developmental trajectory, which can lead to life-threatening medical conditions. Medically, starvation can affect most major organ systems and can cause amenorrhea, bradycardia, QTc prolongation, loss of bone mineral density, loss of hair, blood count abnormalities, and so on (Moore and Bokor 2022). The malnourished brain often displays symptoms of worsened mood, depression, irritability, and obsession with food. Some patients with AN have extreme guilt when they eat, leading to behaviors such as binge eating and subsequent purging and excessive exercising. The suicide risk is high for those with AN, with rates of completed suicide of 12 per 100,000 per year (American Psychiatric Association 2013). The mortality rate is approximately 5.6% per decade from either medical complications or suicide (Moore and Bokor 2022). It is important to highlight how debilitating and deadly this diagnosis can be.

Box 10–1. Anorexia Nervosa

A. Restriction of energy intake relative to requirements, leading to a significantly low body weight in the context of age, sex, developmental trajectory, and physical health. *Significantly low weight* is defined as a weight that is less than minimally normal or, for children and adolescents, less than that minimally expected.
B. Intense fear of gaining weight or of becoming fat, or persistent behavior that interferes with weight gain, even though at a significantly low weight.
C. Disturbance in the way in which one's body weight or shape is experienced, undue influence of body weight or shape on self-evaluation, or

persistent lack of recognition of the seriousness of the current low body weight.

Coding note: The ICD-10-CM code depends on the subtype (see below).

Specify whether:

F50.01 Restricting type: During the last 3 months, the individual has not engaged in recurrent episodes of binge-eating or purging behavior (i.e., self-induced vomiting or the misuse of laxatives, diuretics, or enemas). This subtype describes presentations in which weight loss is accomplished primarily through dieting, fasting, and/or excessive exercise.

F50.02 Binge-eating/purging type: During the last 3 months, the individual has engaged in recurrent episodes of binge-eating or purging behavior (i.e., self-induced vomiting or the misuse of laxatives, diuretics, or enemas).

Specify if:

In partial remission: After full criteria for anorexia nervosa were previously met, Criterion A (low body weight) has not been met for a sustained period, but either Criterion B (intense fear of gaining weight or becoming fat or behavior that interferes with weight gain) or Criterion C (disturbances in self-perception of weight and shape) is still met.

In full remission: After full criteria for anorexia nervosa were previously met, none of the criteria have been met for a sustained period of time.

Specify current severity:

The minimum level of severity is based, for adults, on current body mass index (BMI) (see below) or, for children and adolescents, on BMI percentile. The ranges below are derived from World Health Organization categories for thinness in adults; for children and adolescents, corresponding BMI percentiles should be used. The level of severity may be increased to reflect clinical symptoms, the degree of functional disability, and the need for supervision.

Mild: BMI $\geq$17 kg/m^2.
Moderate: BMI 16–16.99 kg/m^2.
Severe: BMI 15–15.99 kg/m^2.
Extreme: BMI $<$15 kg/m^2.

Source. Reprinted from American Psychiatric Association: *Diagnostic and Statistical Manual of Mental Disorders*, 5th Edition, Text Revision. Washington, DC, American Psychiatric Association, 2022.

Epidemiology

AN commonly begins during adolescence or young adulthood (Moore and Bokor 2022), and the average prevalence is 0.5%–1.5% in young females. The female-to-male ratio for AN is estimated to be 10:1 (Lock 2019; Lock et al. 2015). Data regarding its racial and ethnic distribution are sparse; however, AN can occur in all racial, socioeconomic, and gender groups (Lock 2019; Lock et al. 2015).

Treatment

In the past decade, no significant strides have been made in effective treatment for AN, and no new psychopharmacological treatments have been identified for adolescents (Lock 2019). According to a 2020 meta-analysis, no evidence has been published for the use of any psychotropic medication for weight recovery, anxiety, or depression in acute-phase AN (Cassioli et al. 2020). High-quality evidence supporting specific pharmacological interventions for AN at any age is very limited (Frank and Shott 2016). Thus, medication should not be used as the sole or primary treatment (National Collaborating Centre for Mental Health 2004; Treasure and Schmidt 2003). Often, depressive and obsessive-compulsive symptoms can resolve with weight restoration alone. Medications that may have a negative cardiac effect, especially QTc prolongation, orthostatic hypotension, or cardiac arrhythmias (Pacher and Kecskemeti 2004), should be used with caution in those with AN because of the cardiac complications associated with the starvation state. The primary goal of initial treatment is to restore weight through nutritional rehabilitation. FBT is the most well-studied therapeutic treatment, with repeated positive results in youth.

Psychotropic medications for AN are greatly needed, especially in adolescents. Research studies in this field are difficult due to high dropout and refusal rates as well as the minority of patients who accept a treatment that will lead to weight gain or who have the resources to participate in an intensive treatment (Halmi 2008). This may affect the outcome of studies because the individuals who are most willing to take part in a study already have some motivation to recover.

Nutritional Rehabilitation

Treatment for any eating disorder requires a multidisciplinary team including a medical physician, therapist, dietitian, and, if necessary, a psychiatrist. Individuals struggling with AN are at higher risk for medical and psychiatric comorbidities; therefore, involving other disciplines is key. Weight restoration is of utmost importance because many symptoms may resolve once weight is restored. Outpatient treatment is recommended, with a weight restoration goal of 0.5–1 kg/week, which may require consuming an additional 3,500–7,000 calories per week. Hospitalization may be necessary and is most frequently recommended when there is vital sign instability, including bradycardia, orthostatic hypotension, QTc prolongation, electrolyte abnormalities, or suicidality (National Collaborating Centre for Mental Health 2004).

Family-Based Therapy

FBT, or Maudsley family therapy, is one of the most effective treatments for youth with AN. The philosophy of FBT is that the parent's involvement is essential in the treatment because the adolescent is unable to make good decisions about food due to their eating disorder cognitions. FBT has three main phases: 1) weight restoration, 2) transition of control of eating back to the adolescent, and 3) resolution of typical adolescent issues and termination (Lock and LeGrange 2013).

Studies of FBT involve varying ages of adolescents up to young adults; therefore, it is difficult to separate the evidence pertaining to adults from that pertaining to youth. Some RCTs have supported the efficacy of FBT for AN in adolescents. Patients increased their BMI, improved their scores on eating disorder assessments, and overall experienced improved psychopathological symptoms (Lock 2015). FBT has been recommended as the initial treatment of choice for adolescents with AN (Carr 2000; Eisler et al. 2005; Wilson and Fairburn 1998; Yager et al. 2014). Individual therapy can be offered for patients in places where FBT is not feasible. Adolescent-focused therapy is another evidence-based treatment option for AN when FBT is not appropriate; this approach encourages the patient to work individually on eating and weight gain with their therapist (Lock 2019). CBT for eating disorders (CBT-E) is often used in individual therapy for eating disorders, and multiple studies have shown efficacy of CBT-E for adolescents with AN (Dalle Grave et al. 2019, 2020; Lock et al. 2015).

Atypical Antipsychotics

Initially, there was significant interest in antipsychotics for helping those with AN for many reasons. Antipsychotics block both serotonergic and dopaminergic pathways and have been shown to improve anxiety, agitation, depression, and obsessions in patients with psychosis. Individuals with AN often have significant fixed and near-delusionary thoughts about body image and a distorted self-image. Weight gain is also one of the most commonly noted side effects of atypical antipsychotics, which could medically benefit patients but worsen their emotional distress.

Adult studies. The WFSBP found that olanzapine had grade-B evidence (i.e., "limited positive evidence from controlled studies") for weight gain, and other atypical antipsychotics received a grade C (i.e., "evidence from uncontrolled studies or case reports/expert opinion") (Aigner et al. 2011). Olanzapine is the most studied antipsychotic in patients with AN and shows modest efficacy, with more rapid weight gain and improvement in disordered thoughts/obsessions versus placebo. It has also been shown to improve depression, anxiety, OCD, and aggression (Aigner et al. 2011; Flament et al. 2012; Mitchell et al. 2013). RCTs of olanzapine include a trial of 34 adults with AN that indicated improvement in obsessive thoughts and weight gain (Bissada et al. 2008). However, a more recent study found no benefit of olanzapine for psychological symptoms (Attia et al. 2019). With atypical antipsychotics, concerns have been raised about increasing fasting glucose and insulin levels in olanzapine treatment groups as well as increased thyroid-stimulating hormone and prolactin in those with AN (Swenne and Rosling 2011).

Among other antipsychotics, risperidone, quetiapine, amisulpride, and aripiprazole have case studies and small trials that show modest efficacy in improving core AN depression and anxiety symptoms (Aigner et al. 2011; Flament et al. 2012; Marzola et al. 2015). Evidence is unclear regarding weight gain in this population while taking antipsychotics (Aigner et al. 2011; Flament et al. 2012; McKnight and Park 2010). In systematic reviews and meta-analyses, minimal evidence has been found for the benefit of antipsychotics (Kishi et al. 2012; Lebow et al. 2013). Typical antipsychotics (e.g., pimozide, sulpiride, haloperidol, chlorpromazine) have been studied; however, they were found to be not efficacious and to have a high side effect burden (Aigner et al. 2011; Flament et al. 2012; Mitchell et al. 2013).

Youth studies. Although studies in children and adolescents are limited, olanzapine and quetiapine have been used safely in these populations (Boachie et al. 2003; Mehler et al. 2001; Mehler-Wex et al. 2008). The handful of open-label and case studies of olanzapine for AN in youth have had mixed results. One open-label study demonstrated an improvement in BMI (Leggero et al. 2010). Some case reports have shown improved anxiety and agitation before and after meals at a dosage of 2.5 mg/day (Boachie et al. 2003), and decreased body concerns, anxiety, and sleep disturbances at dosages of 1.255–7.5 mg/day (Dennis et al. 2006). However, an RCT conducted by Kafantaris et al. (2011) found no benefit in weight gain or psychological functioning to adding olanzapine to intensive behavioral treatment for adolescent females with restricting-type AN.

Case reports of the benefits and safety of risperidone (Fisman et al. 1996; Mehler-Wex et al. 2008; Newman-Toker 2000) are also very limited. In a recent RCT pilot trial of risperidone (dosage up to 2.5 mg/day for 4 weeks) given to 40 hospitalized adolescents, no advantage was seen in psychological measures, including the Eating Disorder Inventory–2, the Color-A-Person Body Dissatisfaction Test, and the Multidimensional Anxiety Scale for Children, or in weight gain with the treatment arm versus placebo (Hagman et al. 2011). Hyperprolactinemia with risperidone remains a concern because this is a previously associated medical complication of AN (Strike et al. 2012).

In general, side effects with atypical antipsychotics in individuals with eating disorders were similar to side effects in those without eating disorders (Swenne and Rosling 2011). Overall, these medications exhibit insufficient evidence to support their use in the treatment of AN, but they may be helpful for comorbid conditions. Although the evidence remains limited, providers commonly use atypical antipsychotics off-label clinically, most frequently olanzapine (Beykloo et al. 2019).

Antidepressants

In a literature review of case studies, RCTs, and open-label studies in adolescents and adults with AN, Marvanova and Gramith (2018) showed that antidepressants do not benefit AN pathology but may improve symptoms of comorbid anxiety and depression.

Adult studies. Antidepressants have limited proven efficacy in studies of individuals with AN. In a Cochrane review of four RCTs, it was determined that information was of limited quality, and none of the evidence supported the use of antidepressants for weight gain or eating disorder pathology (Claudino et al. 2006). There are many theories about why antidepressants are not helpful for those with AN. Flament et al. (2012) found that patients who are severely underweight may not experience a response to antidepressants. Malnourished patients have depleted levels of tryptophan due to nutritional deficiencies and therefore have lower peripheral serotonin levels and profound depletion of central serotonin due to weight loss, which can limit the antidepressant's efficacy (Brewerton 2012; Kaye 2008). Therefore, guidelines do not advocate for the use of antidepressants in patients with AN without premorbid anxiety or depressive illnesses (National Collaborating Centre for Mental Health 2004).

Two studies of fluoxetine have attempted to determine any benefit regarding relapse prevention in adults. Kaye et al. (2001) found improvement in weight gain and a reduction in eating disorder symptoms as well as depression/anxiety symptoms. However, Walsh et al. (2006) found no difference between fluoxetine and placebo in time to relapse, BMI, or symptoms of depression 1 year after weight restoration in a large, well-designed multisite study. One preliminary study showed that antidepressants used in conjunction with transcranial magnetic stimulation (TMS) may improve eating disorder symptoms more than TMS alone (Dalton et al. 2021).

Tricyclic antidepressants (TCAs) were among the first antidepressants to be studied; however, no evidence of weight gain in patients was found, and side effects were significant. Of primary concern are cardiac arrhythmias and toxicity in overdose (Flament et al. 2012; Mitchell et al. 2013). Monoamine oxidase inhibitors are also not recommended because of safety concerns (Marvanova and Gramith 2018).

Youth studies. For children and adolescents with AN, several studies have shown no significant benefit with antidepressant treatment on underlying AN pathology (Attia et al. 1998; Holtkamp et al. 2005; Kaye et al. 2001). In one case report, a 16-year-old with AN and depression showed clinical improvement with mirtazapine (Jaafar et al. 2007). Ebeling et al. (2003) studied youth in recovery who had weight restored and who showed a reduction in eating-related anxiety when treated with fluoxetine and short-acting benzodiazepines. Antidepressants may negatively influence bone marrow density in adolescents with AN (DiVasta et al. 2017).

Overall, antidepressants can be used to treat comorbid disorders in youth with AN. Gowers et al. (2010) found that clinically selective serotonin reuptake inhibitors (SSRIs) are used to treat comorbid depression and obsessive-compulsive symptoms in patients with AN.

Other Agents

Low levels of zinc have been thought to contribute to reduced dietary intake. It has also been hypothesized that zinc deficiency worsens anorexia symptoms because it affects the areas of the brain involved in food seeking, serotonin metabolism, and weight regulation (Birmingham et al. 1994). The use of zinc supplementation has been supported by the APA and been given a grade B in the WFSBP guidelines (Aigner et al. 2011; American Psychiatric Association 2006); however, these effects were less beneficial in children and adolescents (Lask et al. 1993). Oxytocin may play a role in the AN disease process due to altered social-emotional functioning (Giel et al. 2018). Results of the benefits of oxytocin are mixed at this time, and more research is needed. In a study by Halmi et al. (1986), cyproheptadine was shown to have promise for improvement in weight gain and reduced depressive symptoms in patients who were not purging; however, there is insufficient evidence for the routine use of antihistamines for weight gain with AN (Aigner et al. 2011). Cannabinoids have not been found to be effective and were shown to have frequent side effects (Contreras et al. 2017; Rosager et al. 2021). Studies on benzodiazepines, lithium, naltrexone, Δ-9-tetrahydrocannabinol, and D-cycloserine are limited; therefore, their use cannot be recommended (Aigner et al. 2011; Flament et al. 2012).

Bulimia Nervosa

Diagnosis

BN is a complex illness involving periods of binge eating along with maladaptive, compensatory behaviors to prevent weight gain and address poor body image. Severity is based on the frequency of these behaviors (American Psychiatric Association 2022). Being of significantly low body weight is not a criterion for a BN diagnosis (Box 10–2) as it is for AN (see Box 10–1) (American Psychiatric Association 2022). Compensatory behaviors can include vomiting, laxative and diuretic abuse, other medication misuse, fasting, and excessive exercise (Gorrell and Le Grange 2019). The numerous medical complications of BN include electrolyte imbalances, cardiac arrhythmias, parotid gland enlargement, and, rarely, esophageal tears. Individuals who abuse laxatives are susceptible to an array of gastrointestinal symptoms and disorders (Castillo and Weiselberg 2017).

Box 10–2. Bulimia Nervosa

A. Recurrent episodes of binge eating. An episode of binge eating is characterized by both of the following:
    1. Eating, in a discrete period of time (e.g., within any 2-hour period), an amount of food that is definitely larger than what most individuals would eat in a similar period of time under similar circumstances.
    2. A sense of lack of control over eating during the episode (e.g., a feeling that one cannot stop eating or control what or how much one is eating).

B. Recurrent inappropriate compensatory behaviors in order to prevent weight gain, such as self-induced vomiting; misuse of laxatives, diuretics, or other medications; fasting; or excessive exercise.

C. The binge eating and inappropriate compensatory behaviors both occur, on average, at least once a week for 3 months.

D. Self-evaluation is unduly influenced by body shape and weight.

E. The disturbance does not occur exclusively during episodes of anorexia nervosa.

Specify if:

In partial remission: After full criteria for bulimia nervosa were previously met, some, but not all, of the criteria have been met for a sustained period of time.

In full remission: After full criteria for bulimia nervosa were previously met, none of the criteria have been met for a sustained period of time.

Specify current severity:

The minimum level of severity is based on the frequency of inappropriate compensatory behaviors (see below). The level of severity may be increased to reflect other symptoms and the degree of functional disability.

Mild: An average of 1–3 episodes of inappropriate compensatory behaviors per week.
Moderate: An average of 4–7 episodes of inappropriate compensatory behaviors per week.
Severe: An average of 8–13 episodes of inappropriate compensatory behaviors per week.
Extreme: An average of 14 or more episodes of inappropriate compensatory behaviors per week.

Source. Reprinted from American Psychiatric Association: *Diagnostic and Statistical Manual of Mental Disorders*, 5th Edition, Text Revision, Washington, DC, American Psychiatric Association, 2022.

Epidemiology

The median age at onset of BN is 16–17 years. The lifetime prevalence is between 0.9% and 3%, with a female-to-male ratio of 10:1 to 3:1. Rates of BN are highest in the Hispanic/Latino population, second highest in the Black population, and lowest in the white population, in contrast with AN, for which the 12-month and lifetime prevalence is consistent among ethnic groups (Castillo and Weiselberg 2017; Lock et al. 2015; Marques et al. 2011).

Treatment

Per AACAP practice parameters (Lock et al. 2015), CBT is the recommended treatment for BN in adolescents; however, FBT has also been shown to be an evidence-based treatment for this population (Gorrell and Le Grange 2019). Current clinical guidelines for treating BN in youth do not recommend psychiatric medication due to the limited amount of published positive studies (Gorrell and Le Grange 2019). As discussed later in this section (see "Medication Treatment"), fluoxetine (60 mg/day) has an FDA indication for treatment of purging and binge-eating urges in adults (Sohel et al. 2022).

Psychological Treatment

CBT and FBT have been shown to be effective treatments for adolescents with BN (Gorrell and Le Grange 2019; Lock et al. 2015). CBT focuses first on normalizing eating patterns. Once this is accomplished, the patient's beliefs, fears, and cognitive distortions are challenged via behavioral experiments (Lock et al. 2015). Two RCTs of FBT for BN versus supportive psychotherapy and CBT for adolescents have demonstrated statistical and clinical improvements with FBT in binge eating and purging that were maintained up to 12 months posttreatment (Gorrell and Le Grange 2019).

CBT-E for eating disorders is recommended if FBT is not indicated (Gorrell and Le Grange 2019). There is emerging evidence that CBT can be effective for older adults and older adolescents with BN, and multiple subtypes of CBT are currently being studied (Atwood and Friedman 2019; Gorrell and Le Grange 2019). In one subtype, CBT-E, stage 1 includes psychoeducation and preparing the patient for change, weekly weighing, and regular eating (three meals and two or three snacks per day). Stage 2 is a brief check-in with progress, involving either praise for positive movement or refocusing if there is a lack of change. Stage 3 focuses on cognitions associated with eating disorders, including body image, dietary rules, perfectionism, and low self-esteem. Finally, stage 4 includes relapse prevention and termination of therapy (Murphy et al. 2010). A meta-analysis by Wade (2019) showed that CBT-E outperformed other psychological treatment comparisons, including interpersonal therapy (IPT) and psychoanalytic therapy. This meta-analysis also showed that CBT-E can be effective when used as guided self-help. IPT is a second-line therapeutic option for the treatment of BN in adults (Hagan and Walsh 2021).

Medication Treatment

Antidepressants. New evidence for medication efficacy in BN has been limited. Therapy continues to be the recommended first-line treatment, and very few RCTs for BN in adolescents exist (Hagan and Walsh 2021).

Adult studies. The most well-studied antidepressant is fluoxetine, which has an FDA indication for the acute and maintenance treatment of binge eating and self-induced vomiting behaviors in adults with moderate to severe BN. Its use consistently has been shown to improve BN psychopathology and to help with relapse prevention (Goldstein et al. 1999; Gorrell and Le Grange 2019; McElroy et al. 2019). Fluoxetine is supported as the first-line medication treatment for adults with BN at a dosage of 60 mg/day over 8–16 weeks (Aigner et al. 2011; Bacaltchuk and Hay 2003; Flament et al. 2012). In a trial of 387 adults with BN, fluoxetine medication response, as measured by at least a 60% decrease in binge eating or vomiting, was predictable at 3 weeks; however, 8 weeks were required to see a full response (Sysko et al. 2010; Walsh et al. 2006). The positive effects of antidepressants in bingeing/purging symptoms are independent of their positive effects on mood (Goldstein et al. 1995; Shapiro et al. 2007; Walsh et al. 1984). In one study, citalopram showed a positive effect for reducing depressive feelings in adults with BN (Leombruni et al. 2006).

Bupropion is contraindicated in patients with BN due to its increased risk of seizures (McElroy et al. 2019). In a 1988 study, 4 of 55 patients with no previous history of seizures who received bupropion experienced grand mal seizures. The study was discontinued because of the perceived danger to patients (Horne et al. 1988).

In their review, the WFSBP looked at 36 RCTs of medications for the treatment of BN. Looking for an overall decrease in bulimic behaviors, Aigner et al. (2011) gave grade A to fluoxetine, with a good risk-benefit ratio. TCAs and topiramate were also given grade A, but with a moderate risk-benefit ratio (Aigner et al. 2011).

Youth studies. One uncontrolled, open trial suggested that antidepressants may be helpful for adolescents with BN. Kotler et al. (2003) studied 10 adolescents ages 12–18 years who received fluoxetine 60 mg/day along with supportive psychotherapy for 8 weeks. Weekly binge-and-purge episodes decreased to zero and "almost none," respectively, as rated by the youth. Although TCAs have shown efficacy, their use is discouraged in children and adolescents due to concerns about their side effect profile and toxicity in overdose (Aigner et al. 2011; Flament et al. 2012; Mitchell et al. 2013).

Other Agents

Topiramate has shown efficacy in adults at reducing core BN symptoms, bingeing, and purging. However, topiramate has frequent side effects that impact tolerability (Aigner et al. 2011; Hedges et al. 2003; Hoopes et al. 2003; Nickel et al. 2005). One RCT of extended-release phentermine-topiramate that included four adults with BN found this medication to be well tolerated and more effective at reducing binge eating than placebo (Safer et al. 2020). Case studies in adults treated with aripiprazole and methylphenidate have shown positive effects for treatment-resistant BN; however, their use is not supported because of the potential risk of seizures (Aigner et al. 2011). Currently, no studies have shown efficacy for lisdexamfetamine in BN, although it has been shown to be safe in adults with BN (Keshen et al. 2021). In an open-label trial that included seven adults with BN, a reduction in objective and subjective binge episodes was seen when polaprezinc was added to antidepressant treatment (Sakae et al. 2020). In a double-blind, placebo-controlled crossover study in Korea, a single dose of intranasal oxytocin in college-age women with BN led to enhanced emotional sensitivity and decreased caloric intake over 24 hours (Kim et al. 2015).

Binge-Eating Disorder

Diagnosis

BED is a serious illness associated with significant stigma (Hollett and Carter 2021; Phelan et al. 2015). Symptoms can be debilitating; however, patients often do not seek treatment due to shame. They also rarely self-disclose binge behaviors; therefore, physicians should screen for BED (Maguen et al. 2018). Embarrassment related to the binge episode is a diagnostic criterion of BED, so providers must gather information sensitively and with compassion. BED was first defined in DSM-5 (Box 10–3; American Psychiatric Association 2013) and the primary symptoms include eating an objectively large amount of food (more than what most would eat) and the sense that one has lost control of their eating.

Box 10–3. Binge-Eating Disorder

A. Recurrent episodes of binge eating. An episode of binge eating is characterized by both of the following:

   1. Eating, in a discrete period of time (e.g., within any 2-hour period), an amount of food that is definitely larger than what most people would eat in a similar period of time under similar circumstances.
   2. A sense of lack of control over eating during the episode (e.g., a feeling that one cannot stop eating or control what or how much one is eating).

B. The binge-eating episodes are associated with three (or more) of the following:

   1. Eating much more rapidly than normal.
   2. Eating until feeling uncomfortably full.

3. Eating large amounts of food when not feeling physically hungry.
4. Eating alone because of feeling embarrassed by how much one is eating.
5. Feeling disgusted with oneself, depressed, or very guilty afterward.

C. Marked distress regarding binge eating is present.
D. The binge eating occurs, on average, at least once a week for 3 months.
E. The binge eating is not associated with the recurrent use of inappropriate compensatory behavior as in bulimia nervosa and does not occur exclusively during the course of bulimia nervosa or anorexia nervosa.

Specify if:

In partial remission: After full criteria for binge-eating disorder were previously met, binge eating occurs at an average frequency of less than one episode per week for a sustained period of time.
In full remission: After full criteria for binge-eating disorder were previously met, none of the criteria have been met for a sustained period of time.

Specify current severity:
The minimum level of severity is based on the frequency of episodes of binge eating (see below). The level of severity may be increased to reflect other symptoms and the degree of functional disability.

Mild: 1–3 binge-eating episodes per week.
Moderate: 4–7 binge-eating episodes per week.
Severe: 8–13 binge-eating episodes per week.
Extreme: 14 or more binge-eating episodes per week.

Source. Reprinted from American Psychiatric Association: *Diagnostic and Statistical Manual of Mental Disorders*, 5th Edition, Text Revision, Washington, DC, American Psychiatric Association, 2022.

Although research for treatments of BED often uses weight loss and BMI as a primary outcome measure, it is crucial to recognize that weight is not a criterion of BED. There are significant concerns with using weight and BMI as a measure. The measure of BMI is not an effective tool in measuring adiposity, and near the start of the obesity epidemic, the National Institutes of Health reclassified the BMI categories, thus classifying millions of Americans as "overweight" overnight. The medical community often recommends that patients be within normal weight; however, a meta-analysis showed that individuals in the overweight category (BMI 25–30) had significantly lower mortality compared with all other categories, including those with normal weight. Individuals with grade 1 obesity did not have higher mortality compared with individuals with normal weight (Flegal et al. 2013). There are significant concerns about misclassifying a patient's cardiac health based on their BMI. Tomiyama et al. (2016) found that more than half of patients in the overweight BMI category were metabolically healthy, and 30% of those in the normal-weight category were metabolically unhealthy. Therefore, clinicians should exercise caution when using BMI as a measure of overall health and not assume that a lower BMI means improved health.

In children and adolescents, BED may be even more difficult to diagnose because children may struggle with describing the subjective feeling of loss of control. Also, the amount of food a growing youth eats may vary depending on multiple factors, including pubertal development, growth trajectory, activity, and others (Tanofsky-Kraff et al. 2007).

Epidemiology

BED is the most prevalent eating disorder, with a lifetime prevalence of 2.6% in the United States (Guerdjikova et al. 2017; Kessler et al. 2013). Data from the World Health Organization Mental Survey Study show a lifetime prevalence of 1.4% across 14 countries (Yilmaz et al. 2015). The male-to-female ratio (4:6) is higher for BED than for other eating disorders based on the current literature (Bohon 2019). BED has been found to be a highly heritable illness, with studies suggesting 41%–57% heritability, independent of obesity (Yilmaz et al. 2015). The prevalence of BED in children and adolescents is estimated to be between 1% and 3% (Smink et al. 2014).

Clinical Presentation

A common clinical presentation of a patient with BED is a person of higher weight who has attempted to lose weight several times in the past and has often been told by medical professionals that they need to lose weight to improve their health. In an attempt to do so, they often underfuel their bodies during the day, intentionally restricting their dietary intake for as long as they can. Toward the end of the day, their hunger and physical drive for food often overpowers their "willpower," and they participate in one or multiple binges in secrecy. They experience significant shame and remorse around their loss of control and their perception of "failing" their diet. They promise to stick with their diet the next day, and the cycle repeats. Dietary restraint has been consistently shown to be the most direct cause of binge eating (Lowe et al. 2011). A 5-year longitudinal study of adolescents found that dieting and unhealthful weight control predicted obesity and eating disorders for both males and females (Neumark-Sztainer et al. 2011). A prospective study of adolescent girls showed that elevated dieting, pressure to be thin, modeling of eating disturbances, appearance overvaluation, body dissatisfaction, depressive symptoms, emotional eating, body mass, and low self-esteem predicted binge-eating onset with 92% accuracy (Stice et al. 2002).

Patients with BED often have comorbid psychiatric illness. For example, a previous study reported that 79% of those with BED have at least one other psychiatric disorder (most frequently anxiety, PTSD, or alcohol abuse or dependence) (Kessler et al. 2013). Binges are often triggered by a negative affect. Neuropathway changes in dopaminergic reward processing and poor inhibitory control have also been proposed as potential avenues for treatment, targeting the dopamine pathway (Dingemans et al. 2017; Goracci et al. 2015).

Treatment

Similar to other eating disorders, a multidisciplinary team is crucial to helping patients achieve full recovery from BED. Nutritional rehabilitation focusing on consistent, adequate fueling is necessary for full recovery. One potential limitation of current research is weight loss as a common outcome. Although individuals with BED often have larger bodies, it is important to consider whether long-term weight loss is an appropriate measure. Questions have been raised as to whether long-term weight loss, beyond 5 years, is achievable (Anderson et al. 2001; Melby et al. 2017; Sumithran et al. 2013). This may be hindering current research, and treatments may already exist that are effective in decreasing binge-eating behaviors but not in decreasing weight, especially in long-term studies (Mann et al. 2007). Therefore, it could be beneficial for future research to focus more on behaviors rather than explicit weight loss. The Women's Health Initiative studied more than 20,000 women with behavioral weight loss and moderately decreasing intake; at 8-year follow-up, participants demonstrated no change in weight, and their waist circumference actually increased (Howard et al. 2006).

Therapy

CBT and self-help programs have been shown to be helpful for those with BED. A meta-analysis of nearly 8,000 patients across 114 studies looked at outcomes over 12 months, and the authors found that CBT and self-help psychotherapy showed improvements in binge-eating episodes and abstinence and in overall psychopathology (Hilbert et al. 2014, 2020). CBT is the best-established therapeutic treatment and, per NICE guidelines, has been identified as grade A. CBT and IPT have shown improvements with eating disorder psychopathology through 24 and 48 months (Hilbert et al. 2012; Wilson et al. 2010). Behavioral weight loss has also been studied in females; however, despite participants maintaining a reduced calorie/fat intake, no change in weight was recorded (Howard et al. 2006).

Psychopharmacology

There has been increasing research on the neurobiological targets, including reward center and dopaminergic systems, to address BED behaviors. Studies of BED in adolescents and children are limited; therefore, the focus of the following discussion is on adult studies.

Stimulants

Lisdexamfetamine dimesylate (LDX) is the only FDA-approved medication for adults with moderate to severe BED. The drug received approval after one large Phase-II RCT and two Phase-III RCTs (McElroy et al. 2015). LDX was found to separate from placebo at a dosage of 50–70 mg/day in measures of decreasing binge-eating symptoms and obsessive-compulsive features of binge eating (Citrome 2015). Side effects reported included decreased appetite, insomnia, dry mouth, and headache (McElroy et al. 2015). Citrome (2015) completed a meta-analysis and determined that the number needed to treat to remission was 4, and the number needed to harm was 44. Overall, these findings indicate that LDX is safe; studies showed low dropout and adverse effects. Given that LDX is a stimulant, clinicians should keep in mind the general safety considerations with this controlled medication, including its potential for misuse and precipitation of mania. Currently, no studies of LDX for BED have been performed in children and adolescents.

Antiepileptics

Topiramate has been tested in three RCTs and was shown to be significantly superior to placebo in decreasing binge-eating episodes (Claudino et al. 2007; McElroy et al. 2003, 2007). It was also found to have clinically significant benefit as augmentation in patients with BED whose symptoms had not responded to CBT alone (Claudino et al. 2007). However, topiramate has been shown to have significant adverse events, most notably cognitive dulling and difficulty with word finding. Previous studies had high dropout rates, with 68% discontinuing topiramate due to adverse events (Claudino et al. 2007; McElroy et al. 2003, 2007). Zonisamide was shown in one RCT to decrease binge eating (McElroy et al. 2006). In an open-label study, zonisamide was also found to decrease eating disorder behaviors and depression when it was added to CBT at 24 weeks and 12 months (Ricca et al. 2009). Lamotrigine was not found to separate from placebo (Guerdjikova et al. 2009). Therefore, although some antiepileptics have shown some early promise, adverse effects are noted more frequently for these agents than for other medications.

Antidepressants

SSRIs have been the most frequently studied medications for BED in adults. They have not consistently shown to decrease binge-eating episodes either independently or in combination with CBT or behavioral weight loss. There have been open-label studies of fluoxetine, desipramine, and fluvoxamine (Agras et al. 1994; Ricca et al. 2001). Imipramine and fluoxetine have been studied in several double-blind RCTs, and results have been inconclusive (Devlin et al. 2005, 2007; Grilo et al. 2005, 2012; Laederach-Hofmann et al. 1999). These studies have demonstrated some benefits for depressive symptoms with fluoxetine, but otherwise no significant improvements in eating disorder symptoms or weight loss were observed, compared with CBT or behavioral weight loss. One positive study looked at patients with comorbid depression and BED. Participants receiving duloxetine showed improvements in binge-eating episodes and depression symptoms after 12 weeks, compared with those receiving placebo (Guerdjikova et al. 2012).

Avoidant/Restrictive Food Intake Disorder

Diagnosis and Epidemiology

ARFID is an expansion of the DSM-IV diagnosis of feeding disorders of infancy or early childhood. ARFID involves the restriction of food, leading to a failure to meet appropriate nutritional requirements, weight loss, and nutritional deficiencies that require enteral feedings and affect psychosocial functioning (Box 10–4). A key feature that differentiates ARFID from other eating disorder diagnoses is the lack of body image disturbance. ARFID etiology is heterogeneous, including fear of food contamination, fear of choking, lack of interest in food, or sensory concerns (Zimmerman and Fisher 2017). Further research is needed into this heterogeneous etiology to best understand and guide treatment.

Box 10–4. Avoidant/Restrictive Food Intake Disorder

A. An eating or feeding disturbance (e.g., apparent lack of interest in eating or food; avoidance based on the sensory characteristics of food; concern about aversive consequences of eating) associated with one (or more) of the following:
   1. Significant weight loss (or failure to achieve expected weight gain or faltering growth in children).
   2. Significant nutritional deficiency.
   3. Dependence on enteral feeding or oral nutritional supplements.
   4. Marked interference with psychosocial functioning.

B. The disturbance is not better explained by lack of available food or by an associated culturally sanctioned practice.

C. The eating disturbance does not occur exclusively during the course of anorexia nervosa or bulimia nervosa, and there is no evidence of a disturbance in the way in which one's body weight or shape is experienced.

D. The eating disturbance is not attributable to a concurrent medical condition or not better explained by another mental disorder. When the eating disturbance occurs in the context of another condition or disorder, the severity of the eating disturbance exceeds that routinely associated with the condition or disorder and warrants additional clinical attention.

Specify if:

In remission: After full criteria for avoidant/restrictive food intake disorder were previously met, the criteria have not been met for a sustained period of time.

Source. Reprinted from American Psychiatric Association: *Diagnostic and Statistical Manual of Mental Disorders*, 5th Edition, Text Revision, Washington, DC, American Psychiatric Association, 2022.

ARFID can be diagnosed across the age spectrum but is more frequently diagnosed in childhood. The average age of youth diagnosed with ARFID is 11–14 years, and it is most common in females; however, the male-to-female ratio is higher for ARFID than for AN or BN (Mammel and Ornstein 2017; Zimmerman and Fisher 2017). Prevalence of ARFID has varied across studies from less than 1% to 15.5% (Bourne et al. 2020). Patients are more likely to have comorbid medical and psychiatric conditions. The most common comorbid psychiatric illnesses are anxiety disorders, but mood disorders, autism spectrum disorder, ADHD, and learning disorders or cognitive impairment can also be present. Medically, the most common comorbid conditions are malnutrition, bradycardia, QT prolongation, and electrolyte abnormalities (Katzman et al. 2019).

Treatment

Currently, no empirically validated treatments are available for patients with ARFID, in part due to the heterogeneous etiology of the diagnosis. In treatment, the underlying origin of the food restriction must be addressed. As with other eating disorders, it is important to treat the malnutrition and medical complications by increasing the variety or amount of food. Because of the severity of malnutrition that can occur, clinicians should monitor vital signs, order laboratory tests to check for electrolyte imbalances, consider a dual x-ray absorptiometry bone density scan, and assess for cardiac effects. ARFID has been successfully treated in outpatient, day-program, and inpatient settings. An interdisciplinary approach that includes medical care, behavioral health, and nutrition can be beneficial. In cases involving sensory issues, occupational therapy also can be helpful. Case studies of CBT and FBT for ARFID have shown promising results; however, more rigorous studies are needed (Bourne et al.

2020; Mammel and Ornstein 2017). Monitoring and treating any underlying comorbid psychiatric illnesses, specifically anxiety, neurocognitive, or depressive disorders, is recommended. Medications that have been studied to target anxiety and appetite in ARFID, including olanzapine, mirtazapine, and buspirone, have had mixed results. A small, double-blind, placebo-controlled study was performed with D-cycloserine, and preliminary findings suggest that this may be an effective adjunct to behavioral intervention (Bourne et al. 2020). Considerably more research is needed to substantiate the use of medications for treating ARFID.

Pica

Diagnosis and Epidemiology

Pica is defined as the eating of nonnutritive, nonfood substances that are not developmentally appropriate or related to cultural practices (Box 10–5). Pica is generally seen in individuals diagnosed with autism spectrum disorder, intellectual developmental disorder (intellectual disability), schizophrenia, or OCD and, more rarely, during pregnancy. It is necessary to assess whether the oral intake is developmentally appropriate; therefore, pica is not diagnosed in children younger than age 2 years, for whom teething and oral exploration have not yet ceased (Bohon 2015). The patient's and family's cultural beliefs should also be assessed; some cultures support eating nonnutritive substances because they are believed to have some value. Pica tends to be initially recognized and identified by primary care practitioners, gastroenterologists, or dentists. The eating of nonnutritive substances can lead to damaging metabolic abnormalities, parasitic infections, gastrointestinal complications (from obstruction to perforations), iron deficiency, or lead poisoning as well as damage to the teeth (Leung and Hon 2019; Liu et al. 2015). Thus, early identification and intervention are important.

Box 10–5. Pica

A. Persistent eating of nonnutritive, nonfood substances over a period of at least 1 month.
B. The eating of nonnutritive, nonfood substances is inappropriate to the developmental level of the individual.

C. The eating behavior is not part of a culturally supported or socially normative practice.
D. If the eating behavior occurs in the context of another mental disorder (e.g., intellectual developmental disorder [intellectual disability], autism spectrum disorder, schizophrenia) or medical condition (including pregnancy), it is sufficiently severe to warrant additional clinical attention.

Coding note: The ICD-10-CM codes for pica are (F98.3) in children and (F50.89) in adults.

Specify if:

In remission: After full criteria for pica were previously met, the criteria have not been met for a sustained period of time.

Source. Reprinted from American Psychiatric Association: *Diagnostic and Statistical Manual of Mental Disorders*, 5th Edition, Text Revision, Washington, DC, American Psychiatric Association, 2022.

Pica can be associated with ARFID, especially in patients with strong sensory avoidance issues, and can be comorbid with AN. However, if the goal of ingesting nonfood items is to decrease appetite and thus weight, then the diagnosis is purely AN. Pica may be comorbid with factitious disorder if the nonfood is ingested to induce symptoms of illness. Pica may also be associated with nonsuicidal self-injury, in which the individual may swallow objects such as utensils or pens in order to self-harm (Bohon 2015).

Overall, the prevalence of pica is unclear due to the different populations studied, cultural and regional differences, and underreporting. It also can often be overlooked by physicians. Pica occurs worldwide, and prevalence studies in German, Swiss, and Australian children have shown prevalence rates between 10% and 22.4%. The prevalence of pica has been found to be highest in Africa and higher in children from lower-income backgrounds as well as in refugees and immigrants (Leung and Hon 2019).

Treatment

Individuals with a diagnosis of pica for whom it is cognitively appropriate should seek a therapist to explore the reasoning behind the eating of nonnutritive substances because attention to emotional stressors and needs are of high importance to recovery (Leung and Hon 2019). In the case of a child with autism spectrum disorder or an intellectual disability, environmental restrictions, including increasing supervision and removing objects that may be eaten from the environment, are necessary. Iron deficiency, lead poisoning, or gastrointestinal obstruction should be treated if present (Leung and Hon 2019). Currently, no evidence exists for medication management in the treatment of pica.

Rumination Disorder

Diagnosis and Epidemiology

Rumination disorder is characterized by the regurgitation of food that has occurred for at least 1 month (Box 10–6). Generally, the food is regurgitated, then rechewed and reswallowed or spit out. In rumination disorder, intense fear of weight gain is not present as with other eating disorders. However, rumination symptoms can be comorbid with other eating disorders (Murray et al. 2019). Rumination can be used as a self-soothing mechanism, similar to head banging in those with neurocognitive disorders (American Psychiatric Association 2022). Rumination behaviors can cause shame and embarrassment; thus, many individuals are secretive and do not report symptoms, making identification of the disorder difficult. Medically, patients may experience weight loss, malnutrition, gastrointestinal issues, and dental problems. Before diagnosing rumination disorder, clinicians should rule out any gastrointestinal or medical issues, including gastroesophageal reflux or pyloric stenosis. Rumination disorder is diagnosed exclusively via clinical history (Murray et al. 2019). The causes of rumination behaviors are not fully clear; however, high anxiety or a stressful/neglectful environment may be contributing factors. Habitual abdominal wall contraction through a conditioned response to stimuli is the most widely recognized primary etiology (Murray et al. 2019).

Box 10–6. Rumination Disorder

A. Repeated regurgitation of food over a period of at least 1 month. Regurgitated food may be re-chewed, re-swallowed, or spit out.
B. The repeated regurgitation is not attributable to an associated gastrointestinal or other medical condition (e.g., gastroesophageal reflux, pyloric stenosis).

C. The eating disturbance does not occur exclusively during the course of anorexia nervosa, bulimia nervosa, binge-eating disorder, or avoidant/restrictive food intake disorder.
D. If the symptoms occur in the context of another mental disorder (e.g., intellectual developmental disorder [intellectual disability] or another neurodevelopmental disorder), they are sufficiently severe to warrant additional clinical attention.

Specify if:

In remission: After full criteria for rumination disorder were previously met, the criteria have not been met for a sustained period of time.

Source. Reprinted from American Psychiatric Association: *Diagnostic and Statistical Manual of Mental Disorders*, 5th Edition, Text Revision, Washington, DC, American Psychiatric Association, 2022. Copyright © 2022 American Psychiatric Association. Used with permission.

Rumination disorder is more prevalent in individuals with intellectual disabilities, and there is a higher incidence among those with anxiety disorders. Rumination can occur in infancy, childhood, adolescence, or adulthood; however, it is most commonly present around ages 3–12 months. There is no clear sex bias (American Psychiatric Association 2022).

Treatment

The first-line treatment for rumination disorder is diaphragmatic breathing (Kusnik and Vaqar 2022). This is an easy-to-learn treatment that can be implemented in the outpatient setting and has substantial evidence for efficacy (Robles et al. 2020). Diaphragmatic breathing is the most effective behavioral intervention that has been studied, most likely because it operates as a competing response to habitual abdominal wall contractions. Baclofen, TCAs, and various gastrointestinal medications have been studied in this disorder; however, no significant evidence of benefit has been found for any medication, and more research is needed (Murray et al. 2019).

Conclusion

Although eating disorders are prevalent, with a high rate of morbidity and mortality, evidence and research around their treatment are limited, especially for children and adolescents. The current standard of treatment is a combination of therapy, dietary interventions, and psychopharmacological management of comorbid psychiatric illnesses. Due to the dearth of current research, few treatment options are available; however, with future studies, eating disorders may be better understood, thus prompting better treatments and outcomes.

Clinical Pearls

- Treatment of children and adolescents with eating disorders requires a multidisciplinary team including a therapist, dietitian, and medical and psychiatric practitioners.
- Anorexia nervosa (AN) has the second highest mortality rate of any psychiatric illness due to its medical complications and increased rate of suicide.
- Nutritional rehabilitation is the best treatment for numerous psychiatric symptoms related to AN.
- Olanzapine has the most evidence for the treatment of AN symptoms.
- Initial treatment for bulimia nervosa should include cognitive-behavioral therapy (CBT); individuals whose symptoms do not respond to CBT may benefit from the addition of fluoxetine.
- Initial treatment for binge-eating disorder should focus on nutritional rehabilitation and behavioral therapies, including CBT and interpersonal therapy.
- A key feature of avoidant/restrictive food intake disorder is the lack of an abnormal body image.
- Pica is the eating of nonfood substances that are inappropriate to a person's developmental age and that are not culturally appropriate for that person.
- Rumination syndrome is the repeated regurgitation of food, and workup should include ruling out any organic gastrointestinal causes.

References

Agras WS, Telch CF, Arnow B, et al: Weight loss, cognitive-behavioral, and desipramine treatments in binge eating disorder: an additive design. Behav Ther 25(2):225–238, 1994

Aigner M, Treasure J, Kaye W, Kasper S: World Federation of Societies of Biological Psychiatry (WFSBP) guidelines for the pharmacological treatment of eating disorders. World J Biol Psychiatry 12(6):400–443, 2011 21961502

American Psychiatric Association: Diagnostic and Statistical Manual of Mental Disorders, 4th Edition. Washington, DC, American Psychiatric Association, 1994

American Psychiatric Association: Diagnostic and Statistical Manual of Mental Disorders, 4th Edition, Text Revision. Washington, DC, American Psychiatric Association, 2000

American Psychiatric Association: Practice Guideline for the Treatment of Patients With Eating Disorders, 3rd Edition. Arlington, VA, American Psychiatric Association, 2006

American Psychiatric Association: Diagnostic and Statistical Manual of Mental Disorders, 5th Edition. Arlington, VA, American Psychiatric Association, 2013

American Psychiatric Association: Diagnostic and Statistical Manual of Mental Disorders, 5th Edition, Text Revision. Washington, DC, American Psychiatric Association, 2022

Anderson JW, Konz EC, Frederich RC, Wood CL: Long-term weight-loss maintenance: a meta-analysis of US studies. Am J Clin Nutr 74(5):579–584, 2001 11684524

Attia E, Haiman C, Walsh BT, Flater SR: Does fluoxetine augment the inpatient treatment of anorexia nervosa? Am J Psychiatry 155(4):548–551, 1998 9546003

Attia E, Steinglass JE, Walsh BT, et al: Olanzapine versus placebo in adult outpatients with anorexia nervosa: a randomized clinical trial. Am J Psychiatry 176(6):449–456, 2019 30654643

Atwood ME, Friedman A: A systematic review of enhanced cognitive behavioral therapy (CBT-E) for eating disorders. Int J Eat Disord 53(3):311–330, 2020 31840285

Bacaltchuk J, Hay P: Antidepressants versus placebo for people with bulimia nervosa. Cochrane Database Syst Rev (4):CD003391, 2003 14583971

Beykloo MY, Nicholls D, Simic M, et al: Survey on self-reported psychotropic drug prescribing practices of eating disorder psychiatrists for the treatment of young people with anorexia nervosa. BMJ Open 9(9):e031707, 2019 31542765

Birmingham CL, Goldner EM, Bakan R: Controlled trial of zinc supplementation in anorexia nervosa. Int J Eat Disord 15(3):251–255, 1994 8199605

Bissada H, Tasca GA, Barber AM, Bradwejn J: Olanzapine in the treatment of low body weight and obsessive thinking in women with anorexia nervosa: a randomized, double-blind, placebo-controlled trial. Am J Psychiatry 165(10):1281–1288, 2008 18558642

Boachie A, Goldfield GS, Spettigue W: Olanzapine use as an adjunctive treatment for hospitalized children with anorexia nervosa: case reports. Int J Eat Disord 33(1):98–103, 2003 12474205

Bohon C: Feeding and eating disorders, in Study Guide to DSM-5. Edited by Roberts LW, Louie AK. Arlington, VA, American Psychiatric Publishing, 2015, pp 233–250

Bohon C: Binge eating disorder in children and adolescents. Child Adolesc Psychiatr Clin N Am 28(4):549–555, 2019 31443873

Bourne L, Bryant-Waugh R, Cook J, Mandy W: Avoidant/restrictive food intake disorder: a systematic scoping review of the current literature. Psychiatry Res 288:112961, 2020 32283448

Brewerton TD: Antipsychotic agents in the treatment of anorexia nervosa: neuropsychopharmacologic rationale and evidence from controlled trials. Curr Psychiatry Rep 14(4):398–405, 2012 22628000

Carr A: Evidence-based practice in family therapy and systemic consultation. J Fam Ther 22(1):29–60, 2000

Cassioli E, Sensi C, Mannucci E, et al: Pharmacological treatment of acute-phase anorexia nervosa: evidence from randomized controlled trials. J Psychopharmacol 34(8):864–873, 2020 32448045

Castillo M, Weiselberg E: Bulimia nervosa/purging disorder. Curr Probl Pediatr Adolesc Health Care 47(4):85–94, 2017 28532966

Citrome L: Lisdexamfetamine for binge eating disorder in adults: a systematic review of the efficacy and safety profile for this newly approved indication—what is the number needed to treat, number needed to harm and likelihood to be helped or harmed? Int J Clin Pract 69(4):410–421, 2015 25752762

Claudino AM, Hay P, Lima MS, et al: Antidepressants for anorexia nervosa. Cochrane Database Syst Rev (1):CD004365, 2006 16437485

Claudino AM, de Oliveira IR, Appolinario JC, et al: Double-blind, randomized, placebo-controlled trial of topiramate plus cognitive-behavior therapy in binge-eating disorder. J Clin Psychiatry 68(9):1324–1332, 2007 17915969

Contreras T, Bravo-Soto GA, Rada G: Do cannabinoids constitute a therapeutic alternative for anorexia nervosa? Medwave 17(9):e7095, 2017 29194432

Dalle Grave R, Sartirana M, Calugi S: Enhanced cognitive behavioral therapy for adolescents with anorexia nervosa: outcomes and predictors of change in a real-world setting. Int J Eat Disord 52(9):1042–1046, 2019 31199022

Dalle Grave R, Conti M, Calugi S: Effectiveness of intensive cognitive behavioral therapy in adolescents and adults with anorexia nervosa. Int J Eat Disord 53(9):1428–1438, 2020 32691431

Dalton B, McClelland J, Bartholdy S, et al: A preliminary exploration of the effect of concurrent antidepressant medication on responses to high-frequency repetitive transcranial magnetic stimulation (rTMS) in severe, enduring anorexia nervosa. J Eat Disord 9(1):16, 2021 33509288

Dennis K, Le Grange D, Bremer J: Olanzapine use in adolescent anorexia nervosa. Eat Weight Disord 11(2):e53–e56, 2006 16809970

Devlin MJ, Goldfein JA, Petkova E, et al: Cognitive behavioral therapy and fluoxetine as adjuncts to group behavioral therapy for binge eating disorder. Obes Res 13(6):1077–1088, 2005 15976151

Devlin MJ, Goldfein JA, Petkova E, et al: Cognitive behavioral therapy and fluoxetine for binge eating disorder: two-year follow-up. Obesity (Silver Spring) 15(7):1702–1709, 2007 17636088

Dingemans A, Danner U, Parks M: Emotion regulation in binge eating disorder: a review. Nutrients 9(11):E1274, 2017 29165348

DiVasta AD, Feldman HA, O'Donnell JM, et al: Effect of exercise and antidepressants on skeletal outcomes in adolescent girls with anorexia nervosa. J Adolesc Health 60(2):229–232, 2017 27939877

Ebeling H, Tapanainen P, Joutsenoja A, et al: A practice guideline for treatment of eating disorders in children and adolescents. Ann Med 35(7):488–501, 2003 14649331

Eisler I, le Grange D, Asen E: Family interventions, in The Essential Handbook of Eating Disorders, edited by Treasure J, Schmidt U, van Furth E. New York, John Wiley 2005, pp 163–182

Fisher MM, Rosen DS, Ornstein RM, et al: Characteristics of avoidant/restrictive food intake disorder in children and adolescents: a "new disorder" in DSM-5. J Adolesc Health 55(1):49–52, 2014 24506978

Fisman S, Steele M, Short J, et al: Case study: anorexia nervosa and autistic disorder in an adolescent girl. J Am Acad Child Adolesc Psychiatry 35(7):937–940, 1996 8768355

Flament MF, Bissada H, Spettigue W: Evidence-based pharmacotherapy of eating disorders. Int J Neuropsychopharmacol 15(2):189–207, 2012 21414249

Flegal KM, Kit BK, Orpana H, Graubard BI: Association of all-cause mortality with overweight and obesity using standard body mass index categories: a systematic review and meta-analysis. JAMA 309(1):71–82, 2013 23280227

Frank GK, Shott ME: The role of psychotropic medications in the management of anorexia nervosa: rationale, evidence and future prospects. CNS Drugs 30(5):419–442, 2016 27106297

Giel K, Zipfel S, Hallschmid M: Oxytocin and eating disorders: a narrative review on emerging findings and perspectives. Curr Neuropharmacol 16(8):1111–1121, 2018 29189166

Golden NH, Attia E: Psychopharmacology of eating disorders in children and adolescents. Pediatr Clin North Am 58(1):121–138, 2011 21281852

Goldstein DJ, Wilson MG, Thompson VL, et al: Long-term fluoxetine treatment of bulimia nervosa. Br J Psychiatry 166(5):660–666, 1995 7620754

Goldstein DJ, Wilson MG, Ascroft RC, al-Banna M: Effectiveness of fluoxetine therapy in bulimia nervosa regardless of comorbid depression. Int J Eat Disord 25(1):19–27, 1999 9924649

Goracci A, di Volo S, Casamassima F, et al: Pharmacotherapy of binge-eating disorder: a review. J Addict Med 9(1):1–19, 2015 25629881

Gorrell S, Le Grange D: Update on treatments for adolescent bulimia nervosa. Child Adolesc Psychiatr Clin N Am 28(4):537–547, 2019 31443872

Gowers S, Claxton M, Rowlands L, et al: Drug prescribing in child and adolescent eating disorder services. Child Adolesc Ment Health 15(1):18–22, 2010 32847208

Grilo CM, Masheb RM, Wilson GT: Efficacy of cognitive behavioral therapy and fluoxetine for the treatment of binge eating disorder: a randomized double-blind placebo-controlled comparison. Biol Psychiatry 57(3):301–309, 2005 15691532

Grilo CM, Crosby RD, Wilson GT, Masheb RM: 12-month follow-up of fluoxetine and cognitive behavioral therapy for binge eating disorder. J Consult Clin Psychol 80(6):1108–1113, 2012 22985205

Guerdjikova AI, McElroy SL, Welge JA, et al: Lamotrigine in the treatment of binge-eating disorder with obesity: a randomized, placebo-controlled monotherapy trial. Int Clin Psychopharmacol 24(3):150–158, 2009 19357528

Guerdjikova AI, McElroy SL, Winstanley EL, et al: Duloxetine in the treatment of binge eating disorder with depressive disorders: a placebo-controlled trial. Int J Eat Disord 45(2):281–289, 2012 21744377

Guerdjikova AI, Mori N, Casuto LS, McElroy SL: Binge eating disorder. Psychiatr Clin North Am 40(2):255–266, 2017 28477651

Hagan KE, Walsh BT: State of the art: the therapeutic approaches to bulimia nervosa. Clin Ther 43(1):40–49, 2021 33358256

Hagman J, Gralla J, Sigel E, et al: A double-blind, placebo-controlled study of risperidone for the treatment of adolescents and young adults with anorexia nervosa: a pilot study. J Am Acad Child Adolesc Psychiatry 50(9):915–924, 2011 21871373

Halmi KA: The perplexities of conducting randomized, double-blind, placebo-controlled treatment trials in anorexia nervosa patients. Am J Psychiatry 165(10):1227–1228, 2008 18829874

Halmi KA, Eckert E, LaDu TJ, Cohen J: Anorexia nervosa: treatment efficacy of cyproheptadine and amitriptyline. Arch Gen Psychiatry 43(2):177–181, 1986 3511877

Hedges DW, Reimherr FW, Hoopes SP, et al: Treatment of bulimia nervosa with topiramate in a randomized, double-blind, placebo-controlled trial, part 2: improvement in psychiatric measures. J Clin Psychiatry 64(12):1449–1454, 2003 14728106

Herpertz-Dahlmann B: Treatment of eating disorders in child and adolescent psychiatry. Curr Opin Psychiatry 30(6):438–445, 2017 28777106

Hilbert A, Bishop ME, Stein RI, et al: Long-term efficacy of psychological treatments for binge eating disorder. Br J Psychiatry 200(3):232–237, 2012 22282429

Hilbert A, Pike KM, Goldschmidt AB, et al: Risk factors across the eating disorders. Psychiatry Res 220(1-2):500–506, 2014 25103674

Hilbert A, Petroff D, Herpertz S, et al: Meta-analysis on the long-term effectiveness of psychological and medical treatments for binge-eating disorder. Int J Eat Disord 53(9):1353–1376, 2020 32583527

Hollett KB, Carter JC: Separating binge-eating disorder stigma and weight stigma: a vignette study. Int J Eat Disord 54(5):755–763, 2021 33480447

Holtkamp K, Konrad K, Kaiser N, et al: A retrospective study of SSRI treatment in adolescent anorexia nervosa: insufficient evidence for efficacy. J Psychiatr Res 39(3):303–310, 2005 15725429

Hoopes SP, Reimherr FW, Hedges DW, et al: Treatment of bulimia nervosa with topiramate in a randomized, double-blind, placebo-controlled trial, part 1: improvement in binge and purge measures. J Clin Psychiatry 64(11):1335–1341, 2003 14658948

Horne RL, Ferguson JM, Pope HG Jr, et al: Treatment of bulimia with bupropion: a multicenter controlled trial. J Clin Psychiatry 49(7):262–266, 1988 3134343

Howard BV, Manson JE, Stefanick ML, et al: Low-fat dietary pattern and weight change over 7 years: the Women's Health Initiative Dietary Modification Trial. JAMA 295(1):39–49, 2006 16391215

Jaafar NR, Daud TI, Rahman FN, Baharudin A: Mirtazapine for anorexia nervosa with depression. Aust N Z J Psychiatry 41(9):768–769, 2007 17687663

Katzman DK, Norris ML, Zucker N: Avoidant restrictive food intake disorder. Psychiatr Clin North Am 42(1):45–57, 2019 30704639

Kafantaris V, Leigh E, Hertz S, et al: A placebo-controlled pilot study of adjunctive olanzapine for adolescents with anorexia nervosa. J Child Adolesc Psychopharmacol 21(3):207–212, 2011 21663423

Kaye W: Neurobiology of anorexia and bulimia nervosa. Physiol Behav 94(1):121–135, 2008 18164737

Kaye WH, Nagata T, Weltzin TE, et al: Double-blind placebo-controlled administration of fluoxetine in restricting- and restricting-purging-type anorexia nervosa. Biol Psychiatry 49(7):644–652, 2001 11297722

Keshen AR, Dixon L, Ali SI, et al: A feasibility study evaluating lisdexamfetamine dimesylate for the treatment of adults with bulimia nervosa. Int J Eat Disord 54(5):872–878, 2021 33534199

Kessler RC, Berglund PA, Chiu WT, et al: The prevalence and correlates of binge eating disorder in the World Health Organization World Mental Health Surveys. Biol Psychiatry 73(9):904–914, 2013 23290497

Kim YR, Eom JS, Yang JW, et al: The impact of oxytocin on food intake and emotion recognition in patients with eating disorders: a double blind single dose within-subject cross-over design. PLoS One 10(9):e0137514, 2015 26402337

Kishi T, Kafantaris V, Sunday S, et al: Are antipsychotics effective for the treatment of anorexia nervosa? Results from a systematic review and meta-analysis. J Clin Psychiatry 73(6):e757–e766, 2012 22795216

Kotler LA, Devlin MJ, Davies M, Walsh BT: An open trial of fluoxetine for adolescents with bulimia nervosa. J Child Adolesc Psychopharmacol 13(3):329–335, 2003 14642021

Kusnik A, Vaqar S: Rumination disorder, in StatPearls [Internet]. Treasure Island, FL, StatPearls Publishing, 2022

Laederach-Hofmann K, Graf C, Horber F, et al: Imipramine and diet counseling with psychological support in the treatment of obese binge eaters: a randomized, placebo-controlled double-blind study. Int J Eat Disord 26(3):231–244, 1999 10441239

Lask B, Fosson A, Rolfe U, Thomas S: Zinc deficiency and childhood-onset anorexia nervosa. J Clin Psychiatry 54(2):63–66, 1993 8444822

Lebow J, Sim LA, Erwin PJ, Murad MH: The effect of atypical antipsychotic medications in individuals with anorexia nervosa: a systematic review and meta-analysis. Int J Eat Disord 46(4):332–339, 2013 23001863

Leggero C, Masi G, Brunori E, et al: Low-dose olanzapine monotherapy in girls with anorexia nervosa, restricting subtype: focus on hyperactivity. J Child Adolesc Psychopharmacol 20(2):127–133, 2010 20415608

Leombruni P, Amianto F, Delsedime N, et al: Citalopram versus fluoxetine for the treatment of patients with bulimia nervosa: a single-blind randomized controlled trial. Adv Ther 23(3):481–494, 2006 16912031

Leung AKC, Hon KL: Pica: a common condition that is commonly missed. An update review. Curr Pediatr Rev 15(3):164–169, 2019 30868957

Liu YH, Pesch MH, Lumeng JC, Stein MT: Pica in a four-year-old girl with global developmental delay. J Dev Behav Pediatr 36(9):758–760, 2015 26468937

Lock J: Updates on treatments for adolescent anorexia nervosa. Child Adolesc Psychiatr Clin N Am 28(4):523–535, 2019 31443871

Lock J, LeGrange D: Treatment Manual for Anorexia Nervosa, 2nd Edition: A Family-Based Approach. New York, Guilford, 2013

Lock J, La Via MC, American Academy of Child and Adolescent Psychiatry (AACAP) Committee on Quality Issues (CQI): Practice parameter for the assessment and treatment of children and adolescents with eating disorders. J Am Acad Child Adolesc Psychiatry 54(5):412–425, 2015 25901778

Lowe MR, Berner LA, Swanson SA, et al: Weight suppression predicts time to remission from bulimia nervosa. J Consult Clin Psychol 79(6):772–776, 2011 22004302

Maguen S, Hebenstreit C, Li Y, et al: Screen for disordered eating: improving the accuracy of eating disorder screening in primary care. Gen Hosp Psychiatry 50:20–25, 2018 28987918

Mammel KA, Ornstein RM: Avoidant/restrictive food intake disorder: a new eating disorder diagnosis in the Diagnostic and Statistical Manual 5. Curr Opin Pediatr 29(4):407–413, 2017 28537947

Mann T, Tomiyama AJ, Westling E, et al: Medicare's search for effective obesity treatments: diets are not the answer. Am Psychol 62(3):220–233, 2007 17469900

Marques L, Alegria M, Becker AE, et al: Comparative prevalence, correlates of impairment, and service utilization for eating disorders across US ethnic groups: implications for reducing ethnic disparities in health care access for eating disorders. Int J Eat Disord 44(5):412–420, 2011 20665700

Marvanova M, Gramith K: Role of antidepressants in the treatment of adults with anorexia nervosa. Ment Health Clin 8(3):127–137, 2018 29955558

Marzola E, Desedime N, Giovannone C, et al: Atypical antipsychotics as augmentation therapy in anorexia nervosa. PLoS One 10(4):e0125569, 2015 25922939

McElroy SL, Arnold LM, Shapira NA, et al: Topiramate in the treatment of binge eating disorder associated with obesity: a randomized, placebo-controlled trial. Am J Psychiatry 160(2):255–261, 2003 12562571

McElroy SL, Kotwal R, Guerdjikova AI, et al: Zonisamide in the treatment of binge eating disorder with obesity: a randomized controlled trial. J Clin Psychiatry 67(12):1897–1906, 2006 17194267

McElroy SL, Hudson JI, Capece JA, et al: Topiramate for the treatment of binge eating disorder associated with obesity: a placebo-controlled study. Biol Psychiatry 61(9):1039–1048, 2007 17258690

McElroy SL, Hudson JI, Mitchell JE, et al: Efficacy and safety of lisdexamfetamine for treatment of adults with moderate to severe binge-eating disorder: a randomized clinical trial. JAMA Psychiatry 72(3):235–246, 2015 25587645

McElroy SL, Guerdjikova AI, Mori N, Romo-Nava F: Progress in developing pharmacologic agents to treat bulimia nervosa. CNS Drugs 33(1):31–46, 2019 30523523

McKnight RF, Park RJ: Atypical antipsychotics and anorexia nervosa: a review. Eur Eat Disord Rev 18(1):10–21, 2010 20054875

Mehler C, Wewetzer C, Schulze U, et al: Olanzapine in children and adolescents with chronic anorexia nervosa: a study of five cases. Eur Child Adolesc Psychiatry 10(2):151–157, 2001 11469288

Mehler-Wex C, Romanos M, Kirchheiner J, et al: Atypical antipsychotics in severe anorexia nervosa in children and adolescents: review and case reports. Eur Eat Disord Rev 16(2):100–108, 2008 18000964

Melby CL, Paris HL, Foright RM, et al: Attenuating the biologic drive for weight regain following weight loss: must what goes down always go back up? Nutrients 9(5):468, 2017 28481261

Mitchell JE, Roerig J, Steffen K: Biological therapies for eating disorders. Int J Eat Disord 46(5):470–477, 2013 23658094

Moore CA, Bokor BR: Anorexia nervosa, in StatPearls. Treasure Island, FL, StatPearls Publishing, 2022

Murphy R, Straebler S, Cooper Z, Fairburn CG: Cognitive behavioral therapy for eating disorders. Psychiatr Clin North Am 33(3):611–627, 2010 20599136

Murray HB, Juarascio AS, Di Lorenzo C, et al: Diagnosis and treatment of rumination syndrome: a critical review. Am J Gastroenterol 114(4):562–578, 2019 30789419

National Collaborating Centre for Mental Health: Eating Disorders: Core Interventions in the Treatment and Management of Anorexia Nervosa, Bulimia Nervosa and Related Eating Disorders. London, National Institute for Health and Care Excellence, 2004

Neumark-Sztainer D, Wall M, Larson NI, et al: Dieting and disordered eating behaviors from adolescence to young adulthood: findings from a 10-year longitudinal study. J Am Diet Assoc 111(7):1004–1011, 2011 21703378

Newman-Toker J: Risperidone in anorexia nervosa. J Am Acad Child Adolesc Psychiatry 39(8):941–942, 2000 10939220

Nickel C, Tritt K, Muehlbacher M, et al: Topiramate treatment in bulimia nervosa patients: a randomized, double-blind, placebo-controlled trial. Int J Eat Disord 38(4):295–300, 2005 16231337

Pacher P, Kecskemeti V: Trends in the development of new antidepressants: is there a light at the end of the tunnel? Curr Med Chem 11(7):925–943, 2004 15078174

Phelan SM, Burgess DJ, Yeazel MW, et al: Impact of weight bias and stigma on quality of care and outcomes for patients with obesity. Obes Rev 16(4):319–326, 2015 25752756

Reinblatt SP, Redgrave GW, Guarda AS: Medication management of pediatric eating disorders. Int Rev Psychiatry 20(2):183–188, 2008 18386210

Ricca V, Mannucci E, Mezzani B, et al: Fluoxetine and fluvoxamine combined with individual cognitive-behaviour therapy in binge eating disorder: a one-year follow-up study. Psychother Psychosom 70(6):298–306, 2001 11598429

Ricca V, Castellini G, Lo Sauro C, et al: Zonisamide combined with cognitive behavioral therapy in binge eating disorder: a one-year follow-up study. Psychiatry (Edgmont) 6(11):23–28, 2009 20049147

Robles A, Romero YA, Tatro E, et al: Outcomes of treating rumination syndrome with a tricyclic antidepressant and diaphragmatic breathing. Am J Med Sci 360(1):42–49, 2020 32381269

Rosager EV, Møller C, Sjögren M: Treatment studies with cannabinoids in anorexia nervosa: a systematic review. Eat Weight Disord 26(2):407–415, 2021 32240516

Safer DL, Adler S, Dalai SS, et al: A randomized, placebo-controlled crossover trial of phentermine-topiramate ER in patients with binge-eating disorder and bulimia nervosa. Int J Eat Disord 53(2):266–277, 2020 31721257

Sakae K, Suka M, Yanagisawa H: Polaprezinc (zinc-L-carnosine complex) as an add-on therapy for binge eating disorder and bulimia nervosa, and the possible involvement of zinc deficiency in these conditions: a pilot study. J Clin Psychopharmacol 40(6):599–606, 2020 33044355

Shapiro JR, Berkman ND, Brownley KA, et al: Bulimia nervosa treatment: a systematic review of randomized controlled trials. Int J Eat Disord 40(4):321–336, 2007 17370288

Smink FR, van Hoeken D, Oldehinkel AJ, Hoek HW: Prevalence and severity of DSM-5 eating disorders in a community cohort of adolescents. Int J Eat Disord 47(6):610–619, 2014 24903034

Sohel AJ, Shutter MC, Molla M: Fluoxetine, in StatPearls. Treasure Island, FL: StatPearls Publishing, 2022

Stice E, Presnell K, Spangler D: Risk factors for binge eating onset in adolescent girls: a 2-year prospective investigation. Health Psychol 21(2):131–138, 2002 11950103

Strike MK, Norris S, Kearney S, et al: More than just milk: a review of prolactin's impact on the treatment of anorexia nervosa. Eur Eat Disord Rev 20(1):e85–e90, 2012 21774041

Sumithran P, Prendergast LA, Delbridge E, et al: Ketosis and appetite-mediating nutrients and hormones after weight loss. Eur J Clin Nutr 67(7):759–764, 2013 23632752

Swenne I, Rosling A: No unexpected adverse events and biochemical side effects of olanzapine as adjunct treatment in adolescent girls with eating disorders. J Child Adolesc Psychopharmacol 21(3):221–227, 2011 21663424

Sysko R, Sha N, Wang Y, et al: Early response to antidepressant treatment in bulimia nervosa. Psychol Med 40(6):999–1005, 2010 20441691

Tanofsky-Kraff M, Goossens L, Eddy KT, et al: A multisite investigation of binge eating behaviors in children and adolescents. J Consult Clin Psychol 75(6):901–913, 2007 18085907

Tomiyama AJ, Hunger JM, Nguyen-Cuu J, Wells C: Misclassification of cardiometabolic health when using body mass index categories in NHANES 2005–2012. Int J Obes 40(5):883–886, 2016 26841729

Treasure J, Schmidt U: Anorexia nervosa. Clin Evid (9):986–996, 2003 12967403

Wade TD: Recent research on bulimia nervosa. Psychiatr Clin North Am 42(1):21–32, 2019 30704637

Walsh BT, Stewart JW, Roose SP, et al: Treatment of bulimia with phenelzine: a double-blind, placebo-controlled study. Arch Gen Psychiatry 41(11):1105–1109, 1984 6388524

Walsh BT, Kaplan AS, Attia E, et al: Fluoxetine after weight restoration in anorexia nervosa: a randomized controlled trial. JAMA 295(22):2605–2612, 2006 16772623

Wilson G, Fairburn C: Treatments for eating disorders, in A Guide to Treatments That Work, Edited by Nathan PE, Gorman JM. New York, Oxford University Press, 1998, pp 501–530

Wilson GT, Wilfley DE, Agras WS, Bryson SW: Psychological treatments of binge eating disorder. Arch Gen Psychiatry 67(1):94–101, 2010 20048227

Yager J, Devlin MJ, Halmi KA, et al: Guideline Watch (August 2012): Practice Guideline for the Treatment of Patients With Eating Disorders, 3rd Edition. Focus 12(4):416–431, 2014

Yilmaz Z, Hardaway JA, Bulik CM: Genetics and epigenetics of eating disorders. Adv Genomics Genet 5:131–150, 2015 27013903

Zimmerman J, Fisher M: Avoidant/restrictive food intake disorder (ARFID). Curr Probl Pediatr Adolesc Health Care 47(4):95–103, 2017 28532967

Index

Page numbers printed in **boldface** type refer to tables or figures.

HOW DID WE ALL BEGIN
WHERE IS GOD IN ALL THAT?

Religion and Spirituality

Additional books in this series can be found on Nova's website under the Series tab.

Additional E-books in this series can be found on Nova's website under the E-book tab.

RELIGION AND SPIRITUALITY

HOW DID WE ALL BEGIN: WHERE IS GOD IN ALL THAT?

CALVIN S. KALMAN

Nova Science Publishers, Inc.
New York

For permission to use material from this book please contact us:
Telephone 631-231-7269; Fax 631-231-8175
Web Site: http://www.novapublishers.com

LIBRARY OF CONGRESS CATALOGING-IN-PUBLICATION DATA

Kalman, C. S. (Calvin S.)
How did we all begin : where is God in all that? / author, Calvin S. Kalman.
p. cm.
Includes index.
ISBN 978-1-61668-364-1 (softcover)
1. Cosmology. 2. God--Proof, Cosmological. I. Title.
QB981.K135 2010
523.1--dc22

2010016708

Published by Nova Science Publishers, Inc. ✢ New York

Dedication

To my wife Marilyn Cooperman,
my two sons, Samuel Adam de Sola Kalman, Benjamin Modecai Mendes Kalman, my daughter-in-law Brenda Brown and my grandson Joshua John de Sola Kalman

CONTENTS

PREFACE

This new and insightful book promotes a better understanding of how each person, and God, fit into a vast universe composed of billions of galaxies. The book explains that the universe follows very clearly defined laws and that we can describe the unfolding of the universe almost from the very beginning - a tiny fraction of a second after it started. Furthermore, the book examines the fact that there is never any certainty in science and that a true scientist must be willing to accept any hypothesis. Similarly, although s/he cannot comprehend God, a scientist can maintain a personal belief in God.

ABSTRACT

An insightful and copiously illustrated work of non-fiction, this 27,000 word manuscript allows readers to better understand how they, and God, fit into a vast universe composed of billions of galaxies.

While unfolding the framework of the structure and origin of the universe, How did we all begin: Where is God in all that? delivers the author's thoughts and feelings about his belief in God. He explains that the universe follows very clearly defined laws and that we can describe the unfolding of the universe almost from the very beginning- a tiny fraction of a second after it started.

Furthermore, the book examines the fact that there is never any certainty in science and that a true scientist must be willing to accept any hypothesis. Although he, as a Physicist, cannot quite comprehend electrons and light, his experiments and knowledge allow him to believe in them. Similarly, although he cannot comprehend God, he maintains his beliefs.

Author Calvin S. Kalman's illustrious career includes having held a faculty position at Concordia University, being chair of the physics department, and working as a full professor. He has been the chair and editor-in chief of the International Series of Conferences on Hyperons, Charm and Beauty Hadrons, held worldwide. Calvin won the Canadian Association of Physicists Gold Medal for excellence in undergraduate teaching, the Concordia University Council on Student Life Teaching Excellence award and the Concordia University faculty of Arts and Science Dean's Award for Teaching Excellence. He is presently principal of Science College at Concordia University.

Additionally, Calvin's book on Preon Models was published in 1992 by World Scientific, Invitation to Successful Science/Engineering Teaching was published by Jossey-Bass/Wiley in 2006 and Theoretical and Learning Perspective on Science Teaching was published by Springer April 2008. He is presently Editor-in Chief of the Prestigious Book Series; Science and Engineering Education Sources.

INTRODUCTION

Atheists cannot prove that God does not exist. Arguments based upon the description by Physicists of the origin of the universe imply a chance event among many previous and future events that occur over and over again. With infinite occurrences, at least once a universe is created with exactly the physical laws needed for our present universe. This is a matter of belief for an atheist.

There are many religions among humankind. Does that mean that we should reject God because they can't all be true. What if they are all true- or at least most of them? God must have a nature that is vastly different from that of humankind.

JOB CHAPTER 40

[6] Then the LORD replied to Job out of the tempest and
said:
[7] Gird your loins like a man;
I will ask, and you will inform Me.
[8] Would you impugn My justice?
Would you condemn Me that you may be right?
[9] Have you an arm like God's?
Can you thunder with a voice like His?
[10] Deck yourself now with grandeur and eminence;
Clothe yourself in glory and majesty.
[11] Scatter wide your raging anger;
See every proud man and bring him low.
[12] See every proud man and humble him,
And bring them down where they stand.
[13] Bury them all in the earth;
Hide their faces in obscurity.
[14] Then even I would praise you

For the triumph your right hand won you.

God may have chosen to reveal the Godhead to different people in different ways. We are all very different and the different revelations might have a Divine purpose. Are religions to be blamed because people war in their name? The root cause of war is found in people and cannot be ascribed to religion.

To believe in God does not mean a belief that every word in a Holy Book is true. Galileo told us that the bible is written in the language of humankind. Holy Books are inspired by God and written to provide moral guidance for humankind. They are guidebooks for living a moral life and not intended to be history books or descriptions of the Physical universe and its creation. Religion shows us how to live a moral life. The choice of what we do with our lives is ours.

Moral Imperative

> [5] Now Jonah had left the city and found a place east
> of the city. He made a booth there and sat under it in
> the shade, until he should see what happened to the city.
> [6] The LORD God provided a ricinus plant, which grew up
> over Jonah, to provide shade for his head and save him
> from discomfort. Jonah was very happy about the plant.
> [7] But the next day at dawn God provided a worm, which
> attacked the plant so that it withered.
> [8] And when the sun rose, God provided a sultry east wind;
> the sun beat down on Jonah's head, and he became faint. He begged for
> death, saying, "I would rather die than live."
> [9] Then God said to Jonah, "Are you so deeply grieved about the
> plant?" "Yes," he replied, "so deeply that I want to die."
> [10] Then the LORD said: "You cared about the plant,
> which you did not work for and which you did not grow,
> which appeared overnight and perished overnight.

There is a second message in these verses aside from the usual interpretation. You cannot take ownership of something that you have not put any effort into acquiring.

For me, although the finder has the legal right to keep the items, there is a moral imperative to return the items. We are given the freedom to keep the items, but it is necessary for harmony in the world, that we return them. The characteristic of the case is that we never expected to find the item, and we have no vested interest in the item. Let me give you one of many of my own experiences:

Many years ago I bought an American Motors car. The dealership was highly unusual. It was owned by three brothers. One ran the new car sales, one the used car sales, and the last one repairs and parts. When I saw the salesman, he told me that their policy was never to bargain with anyone. Instead he presented the invoice from American motors and asked for $150 more than the invoice. I added a car radio and accepted. When I came to pick up the car, the salesman told me that of course the dealership would honour the signed contract and I could have the car immediately including the radio. He did, however show me that through his negligence the cost of the radio had been omitted from the signed contract. I decided immediately to pay for the radio and said:

> "Since your dealings with me were totally honourable, I will pay for the radio on one condition. Namely, that whenever you hear people talk about how Jews only care for money, you will tell them this story about my giving you the money for the radio."

Giving the money for the radio was not a mitzvah [a good deed done from religious duty] and if I acquired any merit, it could only be for my condition. Nonetheless, I feel that I acted in the only way possible.

Here is a story where a mitzvah is involved: To help me deal with my first wife's death June 2006, I saw a Jewish gentleman, whose wife died in similar circumstances in 2000. He told me that the one wish his wife had when she was dying was to be buried near her parents. Her parents were buried in the Papermans' owned cemetery in Beaconsfield. He was told that there were two unused double plots near her parents' graves, but that they had been purchased. The Papermans would speak to the owners of the real estate. As luck would have it, one of the owners was willing to relinquish the double plot. He spoke to the owner and suggested that he would pay him a premium for the real estate. "Nonsense" said the owner. "It's a mitzvah." Here indeed is a mitzvah [good deed]. The double plot was owned and the owner had undoubtedly chosen the location with care.

When my first wife taught a course on Holocaust literature, she tried to teach students the moral imperative. That she succeeded with some of her students is clear from the following story: My wife was asked on more than one occasion to talk about the course to groups of holocaust survivors. On this particular occasion, she brought two non-Jewsih students with her. (The majority of students were always non-Jewish and many students were Moslem.) One student told of how before the course she had been saving money for a car. After taking the course, she decided to take the money she had saved and use it to visit her grandmother in

England. After she described the course and told her story, the holocaust survivors all burst into tears.

My first wife died at the untimely age of 60. She still had much to offer. I am not angry with God because of her death. We cannot blame God because cancer exists. Rather I thank God that I had the opportunity of spending 40 years with a very remarkable woman. I thank God for my two wonderful children, my exceptional daughter-in-law (who is a daughter to me in every way) and a terrific grandson.

Are we to be upset because people in Holy Books do horrible deeds? If the people in these books were all saints, we would feel that we could never be like them. They mostly have failings just like you and me. We can relate to them and their moral struggles.

Religion is not just a blind acceptance of anything. In the bible Abraham and Moses argue with God. They do not accept God's determinations. If Abraham and Moses were totally perfect, we would not see that we too can argue with God. Abraham was wrong to tell Pharaoh that Sarah was his sister. Moses was ordered to bring water for the people by speaking to a rock. Instead he struck the rock. Moses was not denied accompanying the people to the promised land because he argued with God at the time of the making of the molten calf, but because he disobeyed Gods commandment.

As a physicist, I have found a remarkable amount of order to the universe. Our universe is vast almost beyond belief, but it is not chaotic. It follows very clearly defined laws. It also seems that by an examination of these laws, we can describe the unfolding of the universe almost from the very beginning- a tiny fraction of a second after it started. These facts cannot prove the existence or nonexistence of God. For the believer, they are, nonetheless a source of awe.

PART I. PHYSICS OF THE STRUCTURE OF THE UNIVERSE

Chapter 1

OUR VIEW OF THE UNIVERSE CHANGES

Humankind moved from a belief that our Earth was the centre of the universe to a belief that our Sun was the centre of the universe to a belief that the universe was composed of only one Galaxy to the discovery that there are billions of Galaxies and humankind has only a tiny place in the universe. God is not the God of a single Human tribe or nation. God is likely not just the God of Humans but of a vast panoply of species, whom we have yet to meet.

The earth has long been known to be a sphere. The ancient Greeks had calculated its radius and found a value that is not far off from Modern observations. Nonetheless, Aristotle was sure that the earth was the centre of the universe because of simple observation.

If you mount a high tower and drop a stone, it falls straight down beside the tower. If the earth were rotating, Aristotle reasoned that you would rotate away from the stone at high speed leaving the stone far behind. Since this doesn't happen, the earth is not moving. Because of Aristotle's reasoning, attempts by Aristarchus and others in ancient Greek times to suggest that the Earth moved around the sun failed to gain much support. Galileo in his early works had argued against the motion of the earth; "… objects which one lets fall from high places to the ground such as a stone from the top of a tower would not fall towards the foot of the tower; for during the time which the stone coming rectilinearly towards the ground spends in the air, the earth escaping it, and moving towards the east would receive it in a part far removed from the foot of the tower in exactly the same manner in which a stone that is dropped from the mast of a rapidly moving ship will not fall towards its foot, but move towards the stern" When Galileo began to change his mind, he needed to have a scientific principle that would justify the Copernican point of view.

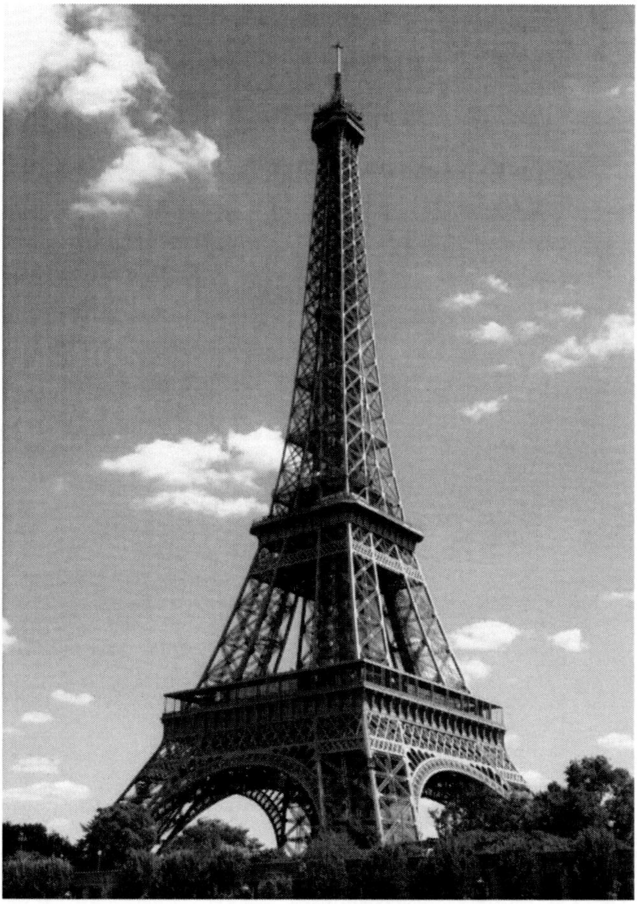

Figure 1. Eiffel Tower Paris, Photographer: Tina Phillips.

Galileo had to have experimental backing for his hypothesis. To reinterpret the high tower experiment in terms of an Earth that rotates around its North South axis, bodies had to have the property of *inertia*. Once the body is dropped from the high tower, it had to continue moving with the same rotational speed as the rotating Earth even though it is moving freely in the air. This property, *inertia* of the body had to be general. Thus a body moving on an infinite perfectly smooth plane must move forever at the same speed. Such an ideal would be acceptable to Plato, but rejected by Aristotle. Only observable situations were acceptable to Aristotle and such a plane is an idealization.

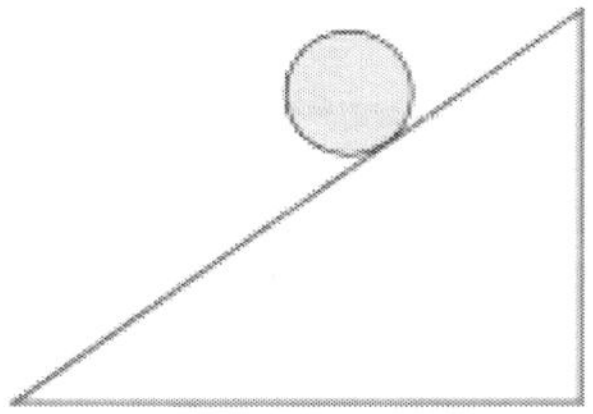

Figure 2.

This hypothesis had consequences, which Galileo could test. To Galileo once you have a working theory, all possible developments based on the theory must be correct. Once the law is sufficiently well established, all predictions based on the law are assumed to be correct. Thus the value of the demonstration is to open the mind to further possibilities (facts) "without the need of recourse to experiment". Galileo reasoned that objects rolling down an inclined plane behave exactly like a freely falling body, but with the effect of gravity greatly reduced.

Start a ball rolling up a highly polished inclined plane If the plane is tilted up, the ball while rolling uphill, will go more and more slowly. If it is tilted down, the ball will go faster and faster. Based upon this result, Galileo reasoned that if the plane is perfect and horizontal, the ball will neither slow down nor speed up but continue forever. This hypothesis is called the principle of inertia. Galileo used this principle to refute Aristotle. If the ball is dropped from the high tower, and the Earth is rotating, the ball would continue rotating with the Earth after it was dropped and land beside the tower. Galileo's hypothesis is grounded in the high tower experiment, but the obvious solution to the high tower experiment is the Aristotelian solution. The invention of inertia requires an examination of what would be needed to have the Earth rotate around its axis and a ball fall straight down beside the high tower. The experiment on the inclined plane is not used to arrive at the principle of inertia. Rather the principle of inertia is deduced as the necessary hypothesis needed to refute Aristotle. The experiment is then performed to demonstrate that the principle works in practice.

Curiously Galileo never endorsed the discovery by Kepler that the planets moved in elliptical orbits. For some this wretched distortion of the god-like circle was worse than the change to a sun-centred solar system:

From "An Anatomy of the World" by John Donne

'Tis all in pieces, all cohaerence gone
All just supply, and all relation:
Prince, Subject, Father, Son are things forgot,
For every man alone thinks he hath got
To be a Phoenix, and that there can be
None of that kind, of which he is but he.
...
Nor can the Sun
Perfit a circle, or maintain his way
One inch direct; but where he rose today
He comes no more, but with a cousening line
Steals by that part and so is Serpentine.

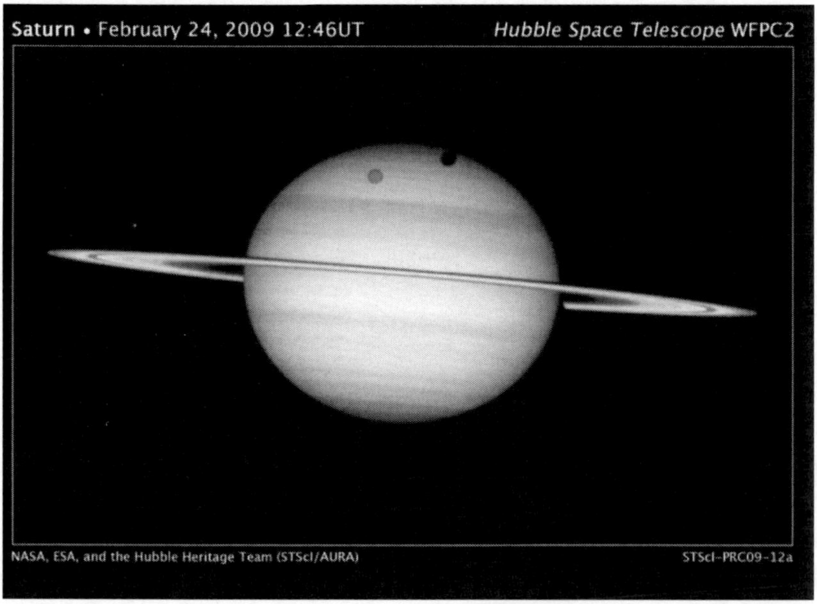

Figure 3.

Newton used Galileo's notion of inertia as the basis of his first law of motion: In the absence of external forces, an object at rest remains at rest and an object in motion continues in motion with constant speed in a straight line. Newton's philosophy was that "from the phenomenon of motions to investigate the forces of nature and then from these to demonstrate[deduce] the other phenomenon...I derive from the celestial phenomenon the forces of gravity with which bodies tend to the sun and the planets. Then from the forces, …I deduce the motions of planets, the comets, the moon and the sea [tides]…" To us it is enough that gravity does exist, and acts according to the laws which we have explained, and abundantly serves to account for all the motions of the celestial bodies and of our sea." It is easy to see how Newton's idea of philosophizing arises from Galileo's method in deducing the principle of inertia.

Newton and Leibnitz were equally credited with inventing the calculus. It is an invaluable tool to understanding basic notions of motion. From the point of view of both physics and philosophy, Leibniz and Newton stand out as the preeminent personalities of the 17th century. Each believed in God, but their viewpoints were so radically different that the followers of one would refer to the other as an atheist. It is interesting to note that the bible has two creation stories and the ideas of Newton and Leibnitz correspond to the two different notions of divinity found in the two stories. For Newton, God was like the ideal English King. Indeed God to be God had to have a kingdom to rule over.

> On account of his dominion, He is wont to be called Lord God Pantokrator. For god is a relative word and refers to servants. The Supreme God is a Being eternal, infinite, absolutely perfect; but a Being however perfect without dominion is not the Lord God. For we say my God, your God, the God of Israel, but we do not say my Eternal, your Eternal, the Eternal of Israel; we do not say my Infinite, your Infinite, the Infinite of Israel; we do not say my Perfect, your Perfect, the Perfect of Israel. These titles have no relation to servants. [1713 edition of Newton's Principia].

"For a God without dominion, providence and final causes is nothing more than Fate and Nature." [General Scholium 1713 edition of Newton's Principia] God perpetually interfered in the world to set it aright. For this purpose God used Angels. With Newton, a century after John Donne, Alexander Pope finds order again restored:

> Say first, of God above, or Man below,
> What can we reason, but from what we know?
> Of Man what see we, but his station here,
> From which to reason, or to which refer?
> Thro' worlds unnumber'd tho' the God be known,
> 'Tis ours to trace him only in our own.

> He, who thro' vast immensity can pierce,
> See worlds on worlds compose one universe,
> Observe how system into system runs,
> What other planets circle other suns,
> What vary'd being peoples ev'ry star,
> May tell why Heav'n has made us as we are.
> [Essay on Man: The First Epistle]

Indeed, although Newton was the first to successfully show how Physics could explain how the planets moved around the sun, he felt that that motion would decay without the continuous interference of Gods angels:

> Blind fate could never make all the planets move one and the same way in orbits concentric, some inconsiderable irregularities excepted which may have arisen from the mutual action of comets and planets upon one another and which will be apt to increase, till this system wants a reformation.[Newton: end of query 31 Opticks, 1706.]

Newton's views are in line with the second creation story, starting half way through verse 4 of chapter 2, YHWH, our God plants a garden in Eden and places Adam (literal translation the Man) , to look after the garden. YHWH, our God walks about the garden checking up on Adam and his wife. The second creation story is the view of, YHWH, our God, who constantly interferes in the world.

Leibnitz ridiculed this position:

> As to dynamics or the doctrine of forces, I am astonished that M. Newton and his followers believe that God has made his machine so badly that unless he affects it by extraordinary means, the watch will very soon cease to go. [Leibnitz: Letter to Abbé Conti, Nov or Dec 1715.]
>
> "He [Clarke acting as Newton's spokesman] and his like do not properly understand that great principle, that nothing happens without a sufficient reason and, what follows, that even God cannot choose without having a reason for this choice. [Leibnitz to Princess Caroline, June 2, 1716.]

This view of Leibnitz is in line with the first creation story found at the beginning of Genesis, God creates humankind to "rule over the fish of the sea, the birds of the sky, the cattle, the whole earth, and all the creeping things." [1:26] God leaves the earth to man.

Does God interfere with Human affairs? God is an inspiration for living. We are uplifted in spirit by our faith in God. But we cannot expect God to act in our stead. A story is told that when the people Israel left Egypt and arrived at the Sea of Reeds, Moses began praying to God. The Egyptian Army is fast approaching and Moses is praying. At this critical point, the prince of the tribe of Judah jumps into the sea. He can't swim and is thrashing about. Now God speaks to Moses. What are you doing praying, when the Prince of Judah is about to drown. Finally Moses steps into the sea and it parts leaving dry land for the people Israel to walk on. Action on the part of the prince of Judah saved the people.

We cannot know who is right (Newton or Leibnitz), because God's nature is at a plane far beyond our nature. With increasing democratization, political society came to be conceived to be composed of independent individuals just as matter is composed of atoms. Society is held in balance by the conflicting forces of the executive, the legislature and the vested interests of the crown, the aristocracy and the corporation. It is of course necessary that such a society should not inevitably collapse. We do know that Newton was wrong about the stability of the solar system. Ironically, by developing and applying the calculus of variations as it had been formulated by Leibniz, Laplace in his five-volume Traité de mécanique céleste (1798–1827; Celestial Mechanics) was able to show that the whole solar system is a dynamically stable, Newtonian gravitational system. It would seem that God does not need to interfere with the day to day running of the universe. Yet in some people's minds this led to a perfect all knowing God, who had foreseen everything. Evil will of necessity have consequences. It is out of this new "clockwork" universe that works such as Thomas Hardy's Mayor of Casterbridge arise. The retribution for Michael Henchard's youthful selling of his wife is as inevitable as the path of a classical projectile once its initial conditions are specified.

Chapter 2

THE END OF CLASSICAL DETERMINISM

Is the universe immutable or is it constantly changing? Parmenides deduced the nature of reality from logical arguments. He rejected the idea of what is not, as inconceivable. He said the universe is uniform, immovable, and unchanging, with no generation or destruction. Change and motion, are unreal because they require the existence of what is not.

In response to Parmenides, Leucippus, and Democritus developed the idea of atomism. The Greek word atomos means "not to be cut". To Democritus, atoms were small, hard identical particles of different shapes and sizes. The universe consists of tiny, *constantly moving* solid, indivisible atoms, which cluster together to form the larger objects of common experience.

In opposition, Plato argued that change in this world is illusory. If we can see past the illusions of the material world, we could see that our world is really based on mathematics, because only mathematics has the eternal nature that reflects Parmenides requirement of an unchanging nature.

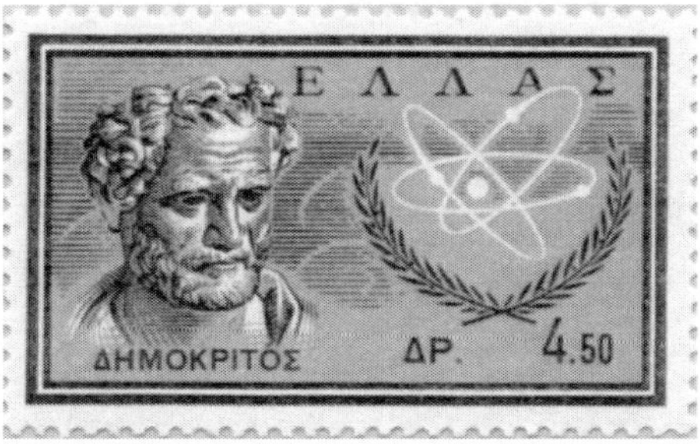

Figure 4. Greek stamp showing Democritus and an idealized atom.

The ideals: the truly permanent structures and relationships behind the apparent ever-changing world could only be found in a physical theory built on a numerical and geometrical framework. Astronomy and the theory of matter were, in Plato's view, fields in which such a mathematical framework within which this mathematical methodology could be immediately applied. The movements of the planets and the stars could be explained by constructions drawn from three-dimensional geometry and the physics of matter could be described by atoms with shapes reflecting the geometry of the five regular solids (the tetrahedron, dodecahedron, etc.).

Aristotle's scientific preoccupations were centred on marine biology rather than astronomy and motion, and so he developed a very different scientific methodology. He felt that the many particular real situations could not be covered by mathematical entities and relations. The ultimate elements of nature had to be specific entities, recognizable within the familiar sequences of experience. Basic prototypes could be discovered in the typical life cycles of different creatures. Thus, for example, the morphogenesis of a seed exemplifies the "coming into being" of the corresponding type of animal or plant, of which the mature specific form—as defined by its prototype—is the natural destination of its development. Having recognized the natural destinations toward which natural processes of different kinds were directed, it was then possible to construct a comprehensive classification of prototypes, in terms of which, the whole natural world could, in principle, be understood. Such a classification scheme, would also account directly for the specific qualitative characters of different observed substances and processes. Only what is directly observable matters.

The themes stated by Plato and Aristotle are still represented today by two rival approaches to the philosophy of science—one (Platonic) based on ideals such as the infinite perfectly smooth plane used by Galileo to examine inertia, and the other (Aristotelian) based on the idea that science must be grounded in particular observations. As Aristotle put it: "How can an idealization of nature help a weaver or a carpenter in the practice of his craft, or how can anyone, by contemplating the pure archetype, become a better physician or a better general? The physician studies the health of some particular man, for it is individuals that he has to cure."

In the nineteenth century, there was a schism in science between those who favoured the modern atomic hypothesis as developed by John Dalton (1766 – 1844) and those (the positivist movement) who felt that since atoms could not be directly observed, they were of no importance in Science. Can

Science describe only the world that we can see with our eyes or can it also accurately describe the world that cannot be seen?

Dalton's atomic hypothesis states that matter is composed of indestructible particles, which are unique to and characteristic of each element. Scientists were able to give a description of many different physical phenomena using the language of Dalton's atomic hypothesis. This internal motion of underlying particles began to take on meaning as the concept of energy became established during the nineteenth century. It was only at the end of the eighteenth century that it was recognized that heat represents a flow of energy.

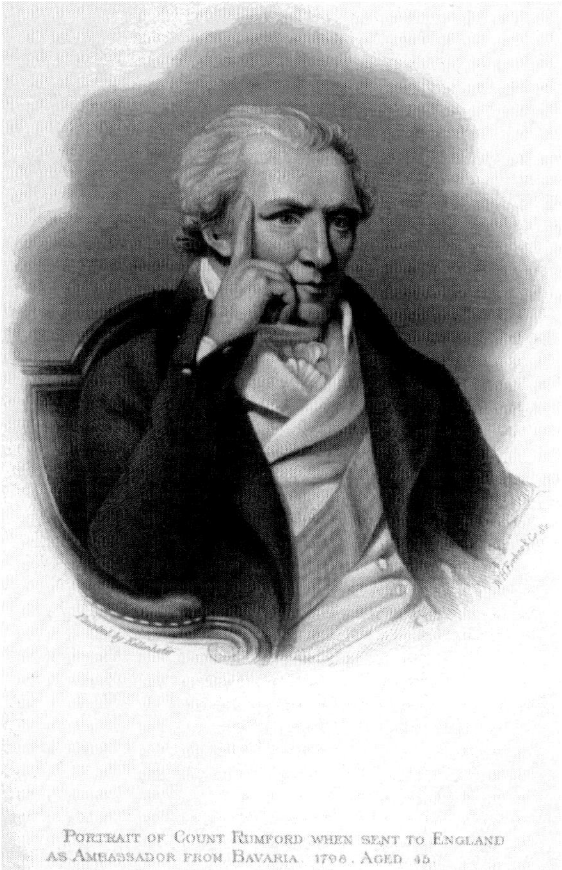
Portrait of Count Rumford when sent to England
as Ambassador from Bavaria. 1798. Aged 45.

Figure 5. Painted by Kellenhofer, W. H. Forbes and Co. Ss., courtesy AIP Emilio Segres Visual Archives, Brittle Books Collection.

In 1798 Benjamin Thompson, an American from Woburn, Massachusetts, who later became Count Rumford of Bavaria, did an experiment which produced the first conclusive evidence for this notion. This experiment consisted of measuring the change in temperature of the brass chips produced during the boring of cannon. Rumford surrounded his apparatus with cold water and to the great astonishment of himself and many bystanders actually boiled the water after 2 1/2 hours. Rumford concluded that the mechanical motion of the drill is converted to heat and that heat is simply a different form of motion. Though at the time this work met with a hostile reception, it was subsequently important in establishing the laws of conservation of energy later in the 19th century. Ultimately this rise in temperature became associated with an increase in energy of the atoms in the brass.

To Dalton and many others atoms were real. To the positivists, "atoms" were only a tool to describe the real world with no meaning of its own. In a way this is a continuation of the debate that Galileo had opened with his emphasis on models. Why talk about a perfectly smooth flat infinite plane when such a thing does not exist. Letters between Guidobaldo del Monte and Galileo illustrate this point. Galileo claimed that motion in a semicircle was tautochronous meaning that any body on the curve – a tautochrone will reach the bottom in exactly the same time no matter which point on the curve the body is started from. Galileo was actually wrong in this claim. The tautochrone is actually a curve called a cycloid. However, what is of interest is the different approaches to the claim by Galileo and del Monte. Del Monte was basically an Aristotelian and believed that tests against experience were the ultimate criteria for judging the worth of a scientific claim. He rolled iron balls inside a semicircular curve and found that they did not behave in the manner that Galileo had anticipated. This in no way dissuaded Galileo:

> The experiment you tell me you made in the sieve may be inconclusive, perhaps by reason of the surface not being perfectly circular, and again because in a single passage one cannot well observe the precise beginning of motion.
>
> (Letter of Galileo to del Monte 1602.)

Galileo's opponents felt that the universe was created for man. Anything not observable to anyone without the use of instruments cannot exist. They would not even look through a telescope. Francisco Sizzi stated with respect to Galileo's finding that Jupiter had moons (satellites): "satellites are invisible to the naked eye and therefore would be useless and therefore don't exist." The attitudes of the positivists are an extension of this. The instruments used to "see" atoms are not telescopes, but they collect data just as the telescope collects light. Atheists state: "I don't see God, nor measure him. So if I can't measure God, does God not exist?" *If I as a scientist believe that the satellites of Jupiter that I cannot see with my naked eye are real and atoms that I cannot observe directly with microscopes exist, I can also believe that God, whom I also cannot observe directly exists and I do.*

As the twentieth century approached, times changed once more. Darwinism became acceptable and in Thomas Hardy's last book we find Jude Fauley, beholding "scores of coupled earthworms lying half their length on the surface of the damp ground … It was impossible to advance in regular steps without crushing some of them at each tread." Which earthworm lives and which one dies? Do events happen to *us* in such a totally arbitrary manner? This is a great problem indeed. My son developed cancer at age 20. (As I write this he is now 33.) Is God responsible for this? Is God responsible for my first wife's death June 29, 2006 just after her 60th birthday, full of life and doing important things that no one else could do? My family members were not saints, but hardly sinners deserving of such treatment. I do not believe that God causes such events or the Shoah or World Wars. God does act in the World at times when God chooses to do so. I do not feel that God's essence is comprehensible to the human mind. But if we are open to God, we will be inspired by God. We also can experience at times a great feeling of awe, wonder and peace that I believe emanates from God.

Chapter 3

REMARKABLE DISCOVERIES AT AT THE END OF THE 19TH CENTURY

At the end of the nineteenth century, Darwin's theory was followed by many remarkable independent discoveries in Physics including the discovery of the electron, of x-rays and of Planck's Radiation Law. (This last was the first great step towards the development of Quantum Mechanics.)

To everyone, the positivists and the followers of Dalton, the free electron was a radical hypothesis in serious contradiction to the classical view of the structure of matter: The idea of atomism was that the smallest part of each chemical element is an atom. J. J. Thomson (referring to his discovery of the electron in 1897): "I had come to this explanation of my experiment with the greatest reluctance, and it was only after I was convinced that the experiment left no exception from it that I published my belief in the existence of bodies smaller than atoms."

Although it is impossible for an electron to be seen even with the aid of instruments such as microscopes, the electron possess a reality that had not been observed in the case of atoms. The electron is the component of Cathode rays. Julius Plücker discovered cathode rays in 1858 by sealing two electrodes inside the tube, evacuating the air, and forcing an electric current between the electrodes.

In 1869, Johann W. Hittorf, Plücker's pupil was able to discovered the existence of rays originating from the cathode when he observed a shadow cast by an object placed in front of the cathode bend away from the center when a magnet is held near the tube. The Cathode Ray Deflecting tube demonstrates the influence of a magnetic field on the electron beam. The visible beam that

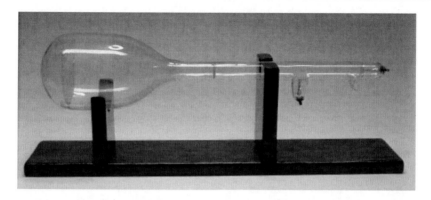

Figure 6. Early Cathode ray tube.

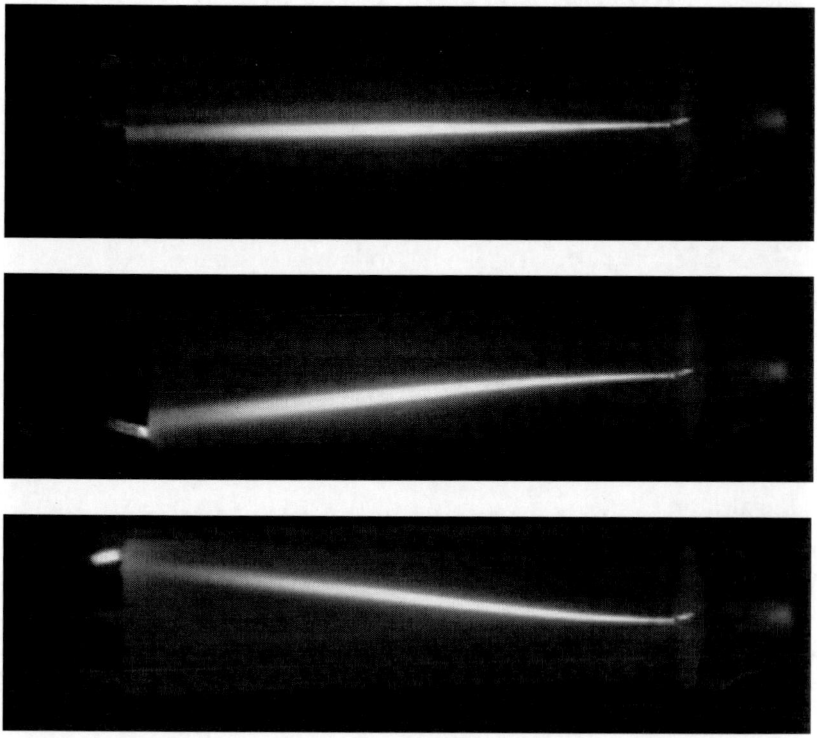

Figure 7. Rays traveling in a cathode ray tube.

The four images are reprinted with permission of Henk Dijkstra. The first of an early cathode ray tube is from http://members.chello.nl/~h.dijkstra19/index.html and the other three are from http://members.chello.nl/~h.dijkstra19/page7.html

appears on an aluminum sheet covered with phosphor, will bend away from the center when a magnet is held near the tube. This phenomenon was discovered by Julius Plücker and Johann Wilhelm Hittorf. Plücker published it in the Poggendorffs Annalen der Physik und Chemie 1858.

In 1897, Thomson showed that cathode rays were negatively charged particles and that the mass of these particles was very small, merely 1/1836 that of a hydrogen ion. Thus Thomson's newly discovered electron was more than 1,000 times lighter than the smallest atom.

Although individual electrons cannot be seen, the reality of a beam of such tiny particles had been established even before the nature of the electrons themselves had been understood. Understanding of the actual nature of the role of the electrons within the atom began with another development at the turn of the nineteenth century; Planck's radiation law.

To discuss the significance of Planck's law, we first have to know something about the nature of light. Since the middle of the nineteenth century, it had been agreed that light was composed of waves. Until the nineteenth century, physicists had favoured Newton's particle theory of light over the wave theory of Huyghens. At the beginning of that century, Thomas Young performed an experiment which introductory textbooks claim to be the deciding (crucial experiment) to show that light was indeed made of waves.

The idea of the crucial experiment goes back to Bacon. Francis Bacon used the phrase instantia crucis, "crucial instance," to refer to something in an experiment that proves one of two hypotheses and disproves the other. Bacon's phrase was based on a sense of the Latin word crux, "cross," which had come to mean "a guidepost that gives directions at a place where one road becomes two," and hence was suitable for Bacon's metaphor. Both Robert Boyle, often called the father of modern chemistry, and Isaac Newton used the similar Latin phrase experimentum crucis, "crucial experiment." When these phrases were translated into English, they became crucial instance and crucial experiment. (The American Heritage® Dictionary of the English Language: Fourth Edition. 2000.) Sir John Herschel was a distinguished scientist working in the first half of the nineteenth century. His "discourse on the study of natural philosophy" (1830) was widely read in the nineteenth century. Darwin read it and after completing this work, it is said that Darwin gained a burning zeal for science. Although Herschel respected the Baconian tradition, he was certain that advancement in science did not always proceed along the lines that Bacon had advocated. He maintained that theoretical statements derived inductively from experiments and wild guesses are equally acceptable provided that their deductive consequences are confirmed by observation. Thus it is the context of justification; the agreement with observations that is the most important criterion for scientific laws and theories to be acceptable. Indeed, Herschel emphasized the role of the "crucial experiment" in confirming theories. In his view an experiment is crucial in confirming a theory only if every other possible theory is incapable of explaining this particular experiment. The difference between Herschel and Bacon is in the origin of theory. For Bacon, theory had to be inductively derived from experiment. For Herschel, even a wild guess could result in a successful theory.

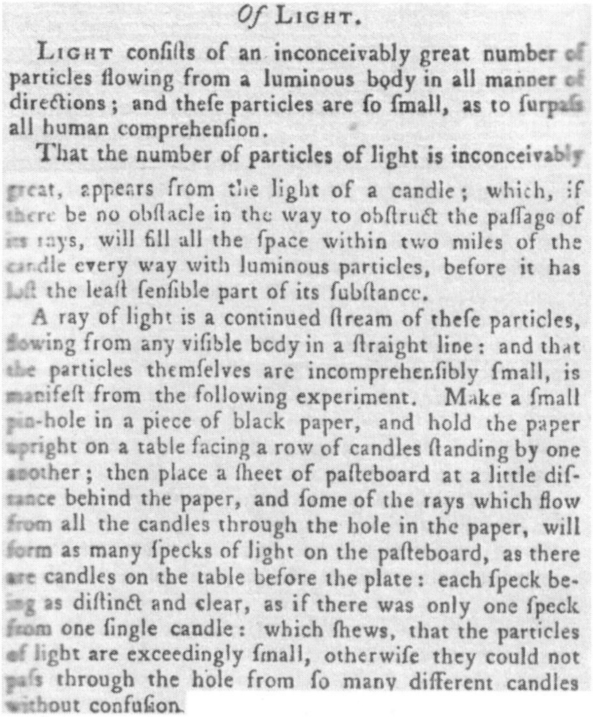

Of LIGHT.

LIGHT conſiſts of an inconceivably great number of particles flowing from a luminous body in all manner of directions; and theſe particles are ſo ſmall, as to ſurpaſs all human comprehenſion.

That the number of particles of light is inconceivably great, appears from the light of a candle; which, if there be no obſtacle in the way to obſtruct the paſſage of its rays, will fill all the ſpace within two miles of the candle every way with luminous particles, before it has loſt the leaſt ſenſible part of its ſubſtance.

A ray of light is a continued ſtream of theſe particles, flowing from any viſible body in a ſtraight line: and that the particles themſelves are incomprehenſibly ſmall, is manifeſt from the following experiment. Make a ſmall pin-hole in a piece of black paper, and hold the paper upright on a table facing a row of candles ſtanding by one another; then place a ſheet of paſteboard at a little diſtance behind the paper, and ſome of the rays which flow from all the candles through the hole in the paper, will form as many ſpecks of light on the paſteboard, as there are candles on the table before the plate: each ſpeck being as diſtinct and clear, as if there was only one ſpeck from one ſingle candle: which ſhews, that the particles of light are exceedingly ſmall, otherwiſe they could not paſs through the hole from ſo many different candles without confuſion.

Figure 8. Excerpt from the 1st edition of the Encyclopedia Brittanica published 1771.

However, the physics community as a whole at the time of Thomas Young did not accept the view that Young's experiment was a crucial experiment. Thus we find the following statement by Henry Bougham (Edinburgh Review 1, 451 (Jan 1803): The wave theory of Thomas Young (1801) "can have no other effect than to check the progress of science and renew all those wild phantoms of the imagination which ... Newton put to flight from her temple." Why then should students wholeheartedly accept the ex cathedra statement of their textbook that Young's experiment is a crucial experiment? It actually took further experiments to convince the community.

Atheists argue that there is no evidence for the existence of God. However, there is no experiment to tell us that God does not exist either. Belief in God does not contradict Science.

In 1818 Augustin Fresnel presented to the Prize Essay Committee of the French Academy an improved version of the Hook – Huyghens wave theory that would account for diffraction; the bending of light around obstacles.. Simeon Poisson, a member of the committee, dismissed Fresnel's theory as implausible. He reasoned that according to Fresnel's theory if light would shine on a circular obstacle, there would be an illumination at the center of the obstacle nearly as intense as if on obstacle were present.

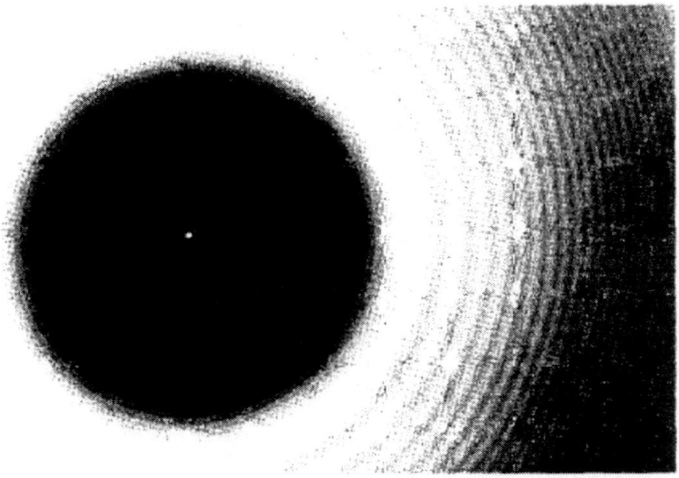

This photograph shows the appearance of the diffraction pattern due to a penny on a screen which is 20 m from the penny. The source of light is also 20 m from the penny. The Poisson spot is clearly shown in the center of the circular pattern and the distance from this spot to the farthest edge of the photograph is about 5 cm.

Figure 9. Reprinted with permission from P. M. Rinard. American Journal of Physics 44:70,1976. Copyright 1976, American Association of Physics Teachers.

A short time later, Domique Arago performed the experiment and found that such a bright spot as shown above actually occurred. (Maraldi had done the experiment 50 years earlier, but his result had been lost. See J. Strong. 1958, pp 181, 186)). Ironically, this effect is now known as the Poisson bright spot.

The experimental verification of this unexpected result gave confidence in Fresnel's wave theory of diffraction. According to Herschel the actual crucial experiment was performed by the French scientists Armand H. L. Fizeau and Jean B. L. Foucault during the mid-1800's. As first noted by Descartes, if light is composed of particles, the speed of light in a transparent medium (such as glass or water) is greater than the speed of light in empty space. According to the wave theory, it must be less than the speed of light in a vacuum. On the basis of this difference, François Arago proposed a "crucial experiment" which would compare the two speeds, thus deciding once and for all whether light is a particle or a wave. Around 1850, Fizeau and Foucault separately measured the speed of light in water and established conclusively that the speed of light in water is less than the speed of light in a vacuum.

Since we are comparing science and religion, it would be a good idea at this point to try and establish a demarcation criterion between science and other human endeavours. Herschel's views on the crucial experiment was disputed by the French theoretical physicist Pierre Duhem in the early 1900's. Duhem's viewpoint is that a single hypothesis by itself whether induced by observation or postulated by a guess is not really science. The essential difference between science and other human endeavours is that a scientific theory should provide coherent, consistent, and wide-ranging theoretical organizations. Observations are only scientifically relevant to the extent that they give guidance to how theories should be formulated and how they should be refined. Thus, no single observation can ever serve as a crucial experiment to confirm or refute any one specific hypothesis conclusively, taken apart from the whole complex of theory and interpretation. Scientists are always free to add new auxiliary hypotheses to the existing theory rather than to accept any single counter-example as a challenge to the general validity.

To illustrate his point, Duhem reexamined the "crucial experiment" of Fizeau and Foucault on the speed of light in water. In his view, the experiments of Fizeau and Foucault did not decide between two isolated hypotheses, but between two complete theoretical systems. True, the particle theory of light as formulated by pre 19th-century Newtonians is falsified, but in Duhem's opinion, it is not inconceivable that a future theory might be built upon the hypothesis that light is made up of particles, with the aid of some new auxiliary hypotheses which would be different from those comprising the Newtonian system. In such a theory, the refraction of light might be explained in a different manner, so that it would be possible to account for the results of the experiments of Fizeau and Foucault while still maintaining that light is a particle. Second, it is not at all certain that the current concepts "wave" and "particle" are the only possible ones; perhaps a new concept might be formulated, which would go beyond this dichotomy, possibly by combining some aspects of both concepts. Indeed events beginning with Planck's Radiation law were to result in the latter framework being formulated.

How can any scientist then eliminate (sic) God from the universe. There is never any certainty in science. A true scientist must be willing to accept any hypothesis. No hypothesis can ever be falsified. *That does not mean that I think that versions of God as the designer of the universe should be incorporated in any "theory" of science.* Far from it. *Religion and science should be separate.* Religion deals with ethics and should not be taken as an explanation of the structure nor of the origin of life, nor of the universe. Thus I have no use for study of the so-called anthropic principle: the cosmological principle that theories of the universe are constrained by the necessity to allow human existence. In its 'weak' form the principle affirms that a universe in which living observers cannot exist is inherently unobservable. 'Strong' forms take this line of reasoning further, seeking to explain features of the universe as being so because they are necessary for human existence. (Oxford dictionary). *If like me you believe in God, then the beauty of the complex ordered structure of the mature scientific theories of the structure and origin of life and the universe are a source of joy.* How could God have acted otherwise than to establish a coherent set of laws that guide the universe? The converse, however is not true. The existence of a structured universe cannot prove the existence of God. *Nothing can either prove, nor disprove God's existence.*

Properties of Radiation Emitted by All Bodies

All bodies radiate visible light, infrared, ultraviolet, microwaves and radiowaves in a continuous spectrum. All emitters at the same temperature have the same spectra. As the temperature increases, the peak in the spectral curve shifts towards shorter wavelengths. This is familiar to anyone turning on an electric stove. At first the peak is infrared and the element feels warm if you place your hand above the burner. As the burner warms up, the peak shifts towards the visible spectra and you can see that the element is now red hot. If we could raise the temperature higher, it would first become white hot and then blue hot.

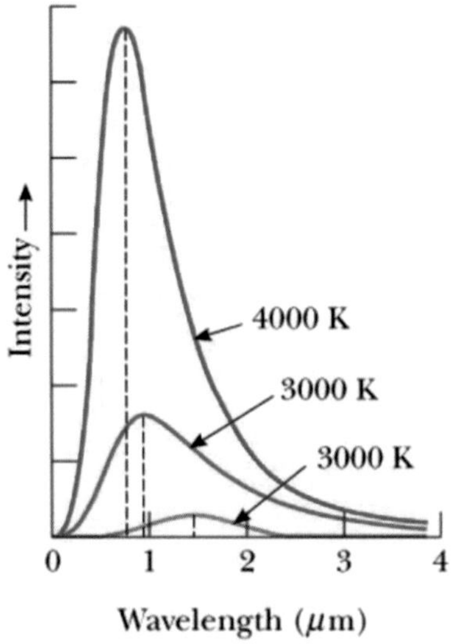

Figure 10. From Serway/Jewett. Physics for Scientists and Engineers, Volume 2, Chapters 23-46, 7E. © 2008 Brooks/Cole, a part of Cengage Learning, Inc. Reproduced by permission.

The problem in the late nineteenth century was to fit the spectral curve. There were several attempts to fit the correct form of this function. Finally Lord Rayleigh and Sir James Jeans produced a theory which does not require a detailed picture of the origin of the radiation and which has been shown to be a necessary consequence of Classical Physics.

The Rayleigh – Jeans result is a complete disaster. The total energy emitted by a body is infinite and the spectral curve is completely unrealistic at short wavelengths. Physicists called it the “ultraviolet catastrophe”. The problem appealed to Max Planck because the continuous spectra of ideal emitters is entirely independent of the emitting body. Emission “represents something absolute and I have always regarded the search for the absolute as the loftiest goal of all scientific activity.”

Most scientists expect that nature is based on absolute principles. And it always seems to be true. If you are an atheist, why would you think that there are any absolutes?

Planck found that he could only fit the experimental data by assuming that there were natural oscillators in the emitting body and that the body radiated only at integral multiples of the oscillator frequency, f; the energy radiated = hf, where h is a constant now called Planck's constant. But if as had been shown throughout the 19th century, the radiation consisted of waves, the radiation should be continuous, not in integral multiples of the oscillator frequency.

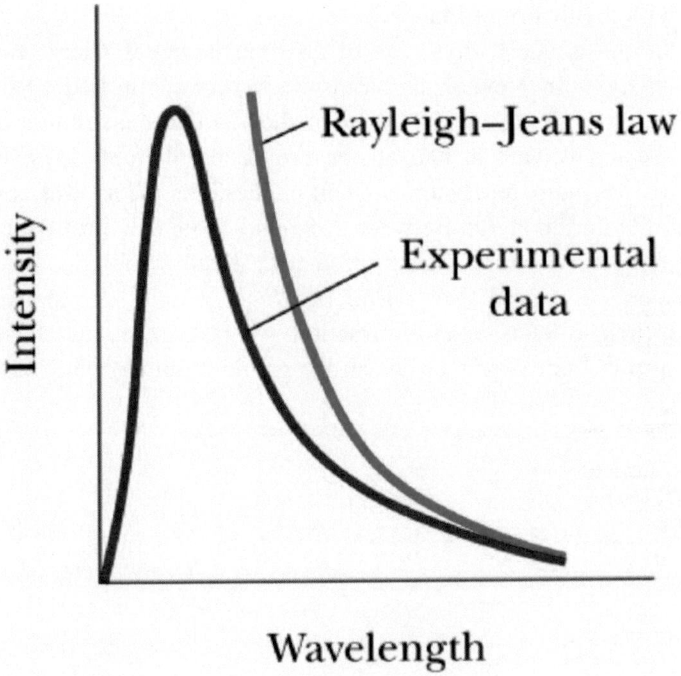

Figure 11. From SERWAY/JEWETT. Physics for Scientists and Engineers, Volume 2, Chapters 23-46 (with CengageNOW 2-Semester, Personal Tutor Printed Access Card), 7E. © 2008 Brooks/Cole, a part of Cengage Learning, Inc. Reproduced by permission. www.cengage.com/permissions.

The experimental validity of Planck's radiation law seemed apparent to many immediately, but because of the theoretical implications, doubts about the law continued for a while. In 1908, Hendrik Antoon Lorentz, winner of the 1902 Nobel Prize in Physics, gave a lecture in Rome in which he indicated a hope that the experiments were wrong. At this time, it may be said that Lorentz was regarded by all theoretical physicists as the world's leading spirit.

In reply to Lorentz, Wilhelm Wien, led a crescendo of criticism: “If we examine the Jeans-Lorentz formula [usually referred to as Rayleigh-Jeans as above.], we see at first glance that it leads to completely impossible consequences, which are in crass conflict, not only with the results of the observations of radiation, but also with everyday experience. We might therefore dismiss this formula without further examination were it not for the eminence and authority of the two theoretical physicists, who defend it.”

Two months later, in a letter to Wien, Lorentz reluctantly retracts: “We are left only with the theory of Planck.”

One of the greatest physicists of all time is James Clerk Maxwell. He ranks up there with Newton and Einstein. Maxwell unified Electricity and Magnetism into a single subject and then showed that the solution of his basic equations was a wave that had all the properties of light. Maxwell laid the groundwork for radio, television and cell phones. His theory was confirmed by the work of Heinrich Hertz. Between 1885 and 1889, as a professor of physics at Karlsruhe Polytechnic, Hertz produced electromagnetic waves in the laboratory and measured their wavelength and velocity. He showed that the nature of their reflection and refraction was the same as those of light, confirming that light waves are electromagnetic radiation obeying Maxwell’s equations.

Chapter 4

THE QUANTUM HYPOTHESIS

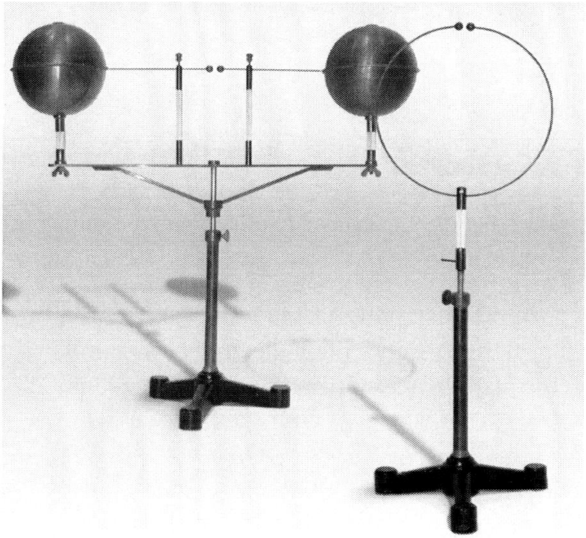

Figure 12. Hertz resonator and detector. Reproduced with permission from "Where Discovery Sparks Imagination - A Pictorial History of Radio and Electricity." By John Jenkins www.sparkmuseum.com.

The connection with light turned out to be more remarkable than Maxwell had anticipated. In the experiment (see above figure) electrons jump across a gap resulting in a large spark. According to Maxwell's theory the electrons emit radio waves as they jump across the gap. The radio waves are absorbed by electrons in a receiving loop (resonator). Hertz discovered that the spark was stronger if ultraviolet light is shone on the resonator. In 1899, JJ Thomson, the discoverer of the electron was able to show that ultraviolet light was absorbed by the electrons giving them the energy to jump the gap causing sparking.

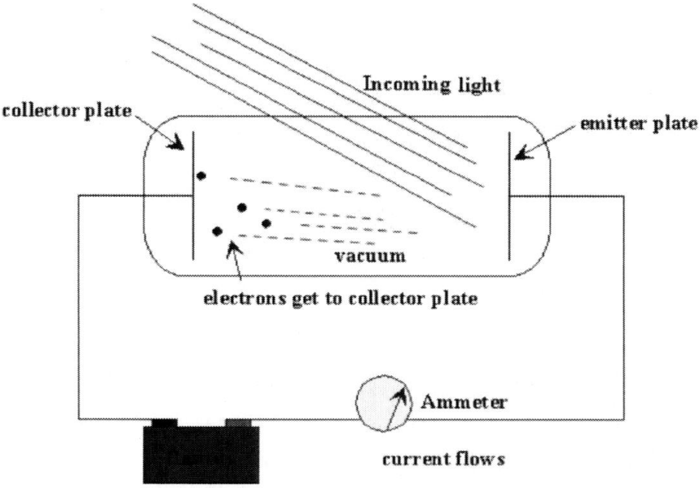

Figure 13. http://galileo.phys.virginia.edu/classes/252/photoelectric_effect.html reproduced with permission of the originator : Michael Fowler.

In 1902, Lenard began a study of the emission of electrons from metals, when the electrons absorb light (photoelectrons). Lenard had the electrons travel to a collector plate, where they could then complete a circuit as shown in the above diagram. The battery in the figure is used to charge the collector plate negatively to repel the negatively charged electrons coming towards it. Only electrons ejected with enough energy to overcome this repulsion contribute to the current. Lenard discovered that there was a well defined minimum voltage (called the stopping potential) that stopped any electrons getting through. To his surprise, Lenard found that the stopping potential did not depend at all on the intensity of the light! Doubling the light intensity doubled the number of electrons emitted, but did not affect the energies of the emitted electrons. Then Lenard tried illuminating the emitting plate with different colours. This time Lenard found that the maximum energy of the ejected electrons did depend on the colour. Shorter wavelengths caused electrons to be ejected with more energy.

In 1905, Einstein wrote a number of memorable papers. One of them was his paper on Special relativity. In 1921 Einstein won the Nobel Prize "for his services to Theoretical Physics, and especially for his discovery of the law of the photoelectric effect". The citation refers to Einstein's explanation in 1905 of the experiment by Lenard on photoelectrons. Basically, Einstein builds upon Planck's radiation law and goes further. He supposes that the Maxwellian equations hold only for time averages, and that the process of emitting light described by Planck's radiation law and of absorption of light as found in Lenard's experiments may be of a discontinuous nature, closer to particle than a wave. Light radiation is then understood to be composed of "light quanta" (photons). Each photon has the energy, previously described by Planck hf. When you shine light on the emitter plate, each photoelectron absorbs one photon. The electrons are bound to the metal and require an energy P to break their bond. The remaining energy is the kinetic energy K of the free electron. Thus hf = P + K. Einstein then points out that no matter how intense the beam of light shining on the metal, *no* electrons can escape the metal if the frequency of the light is such that hf is less than P. This is because an electron does not absorb energy from the beam but rather absorbs single photons. The energy gained by absorbing one photon in such a case is not enough to permit the electron to escape the metal. On the other hand, if the frequency of the light is high enough so that hf is larger than P, even the feeblest light shone on the emitting plate will produce some photoelectrons *without any delay*. Now suppose a stopping potential V is applied. Since the electrons now just barely reach the collector plate, $V = K = hf_0 - P$. Again no matter how intense the beam of light, if light of frequency smaller than f_0 is shone on the emitter plate, the photoelectron will not have enough energy to reach the collector plate.

The last two points cannot be explained by the "light as a wave" theory. Using the wave theory, if light is absorbed uniformly over the whole wavefront, we would have to wait a few seconds for the emission of an electron upon illumination by a weak beam of light. Also an intense beam must result in some absorption of light by the electrons from the wavefront. It is not possible that no electrons would be emitted.

It is not surprising that after all the experiments in the nineteenth century that seem to have conclusively established that "light is a wave" theory that Einstein's ideas were viewed with astonishment. 1910 Planck mentioned only Einstein, Stark, Larmor and Thomson as adherents of the light quantum hypothesis. Planck at this time stated that by the acceptance of Einstein's photons "the theory of light would be thrown back centuries."

Recall the statement made one hundred years earlier by Henry Bougham (Edinburgh Review 1, 451 (Jan 1803): The wave theory of Thomas Young

(1801) “can have no other effect than to check the progress of science and renew all those wild phantoms of the imagination which ... Newton put to flight from her temple.” There is always a resistance in Science to change. But the whole industry of science had markedly changed over that one hundred years. Recall Pierre Duhem’s discussion of science: The essential difference between science and other human endeavours is that a scientific theory should provide coherent, consistent, and wide-ranging theoretical organizations. Observations are only scientifically relevant to the extent that they give guidance to how theories should be formulated and how they should be refined.

Thus, no single observation can ever serve as a crucial experiment to confirm or refute any one specific hypothesis conclusively, taken apart from the whole complex of theory and interpretation.

Scientists are always free to add new auxiliary hypotheses to the existing theory rather than to accept any single counter-example as a challenge to the general validity.

Indeed Duhem’s speculation that the current concepts "wave" and "particle" are the only possible ones; perhaps a new concept might be formulated, which would go beyond this dichotomy, possibly by combining some aspects of both concepts was now to come to fruition. In an address to the 81st Assembly of German Natural Scientists and Physicians, Salzburg, 1909.,Einstein put forward exactly this point. Evaluating energy fluctuations exhibits two terms: one following from a quantum, the other from the wave theory of light. The second term corresponds to Maxwell’s electrodynamics and would necessarily follow from the Rayleigh Jeans formula. The first term is obtained “if the radiation were composed of independently moving point quanta of energy hf”.

Eventually, after much research into the structure of atoms, Einstein’s ideas became the basis of a new theory of physics. In 1924 in Paris, Prince Louis-Victor Pierre Raymond de Broglie wrote a PhD thesis, which was based upon the idea that particles like the electron could have wavelike properties as well as particle properties. The examiners were unsure of what to do with this thesis and referred it to Einstein, who happened to be visiting Paris at the time. He was in favour of approving the thesis.

Two years later 1926 Davisson and Germer and G. P. Thomson demonstrated electron diffraction. That is they showed that a beam of electrons aimed at a crystal exhibited exactly the same wave behaviour as X rays, which according to de Broglie’s hypothesis had the wavelengths identical to electrons. (see figures showing pictures of electron and X ray diffraction from a crystal.)

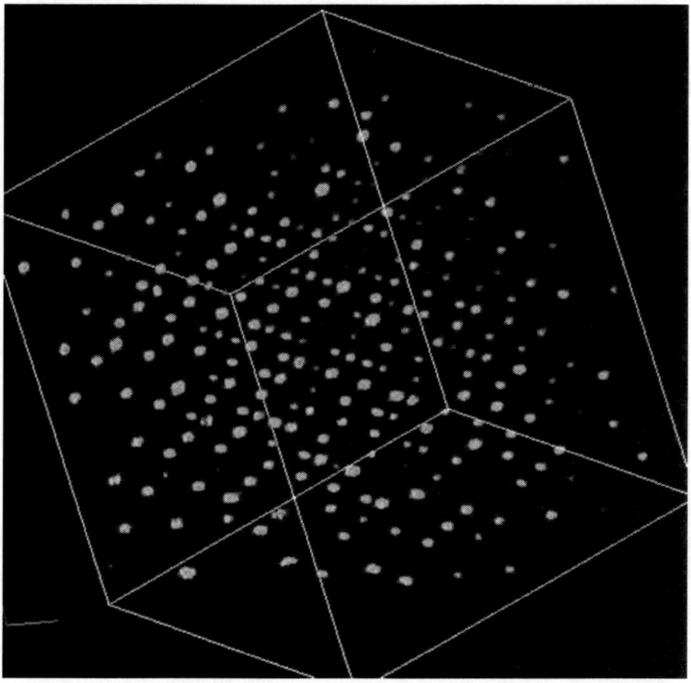

Figure 14. X ray diffraction from a crystal Jim Britten, Chemistry department, McMaster University.

Shortly afterwards, Erwin Schroedinger and Werner Heisenberg independently developed the theory of "Quantum Mechanics. Max Born: "We are compelled to use words of common language ... a picture appealing to the imagination. Classical physics has restricted itself to ... analyzing visible motions [by] ... moving particles and waves. There is no other way of giving a pictorial description of motion - we have to apply it even in the region of atomic processes where classical physics breaks down. Every process can be interpreted either in terms of corpuscles [particles] or in terms of waves ... We can therefore say that the waves and corpuscles descriptions are only to be regarded as complementary ways of viewing one and the same objective process, a process which only in definite limiting cases admit of complete pictorial interpretation..". Bohr's Complementarity Principle: The wave and particle theories are examples of complementary modes of description, each valid by itself though (in terms of Newtonian Physics) incompatible with each other.

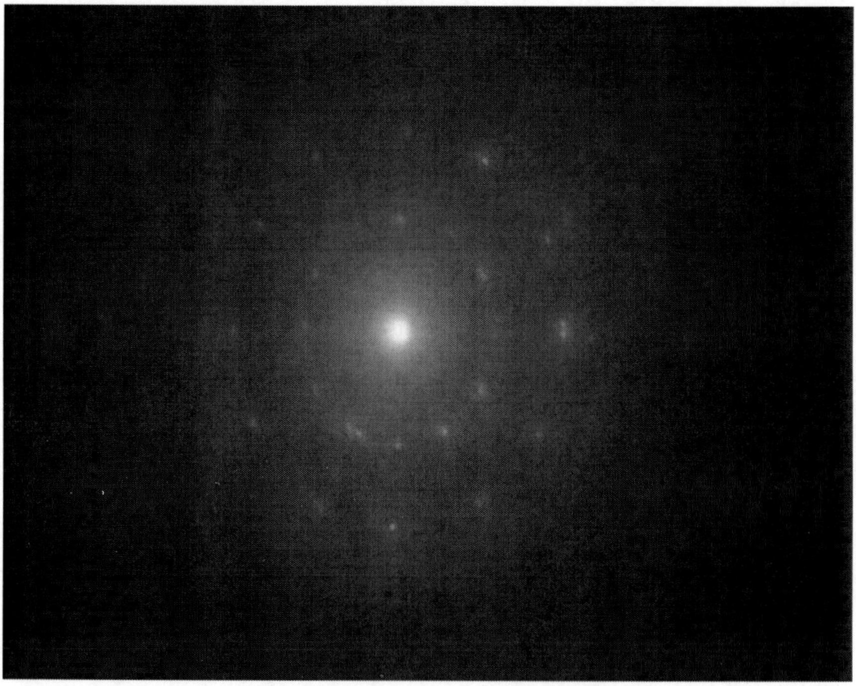

Figure 15. Electron diffraction from a crystal courtesy Jeff Rudd, Physics department Simon Fraser University.

Niels Bohr: "To the physicist it will at first seem deplorable that in atomic physics problems we have apparently met with such a limitation of our usual means of visualization. This regret will however, have to give way to thankfulness that mathematicians in this field too present us with tools to prepare the way for further progress."

Copenhagen interpretation: The physical world has just those properties that are revealed by experts including the wave and particle aspects and that the theory can only deal with the results of observation, not with a hypothetical underlying reality that may or may not lie beneath the appearance. The Copenhagen interpretation is used in all present day Chemistry and Physics textbooks. At the time (1930's), quantum mechanics with the Copenhagen interpretation met with strong objections from de Broglie, Einstein and Schroedinger because it drops deterministic predictions of events. It predicts the probability of the appearance of a particle in a given location instead of determining the particle's exact motion. [See chapter 5 for more details on the use of probability in Quantum Mechanics.] David Bohm has constructed an alternate theory that is intrinsically deterministic, but is not generally accepted.

So physicists faced the same problem with the "book of nature" that theologians have with the bible. We can only read it in a language that we can understand. People in ancient times could only understand their experiences in terms of a world that stood still while the sun revolved around it. Physicists as people can only understand waves and particles. *The electron and light are neither waves nor particles. What they are is beyond human comprehension.* In a given experiment we observe a wave or a particle, because that is what we are able to comprehend. *I accept the physics view of an electron, which is a thing I cannot comprehend. I believe in God, whom I also cannot comprehend.*

Chapter 5

READING THE BOOK OF NATURE

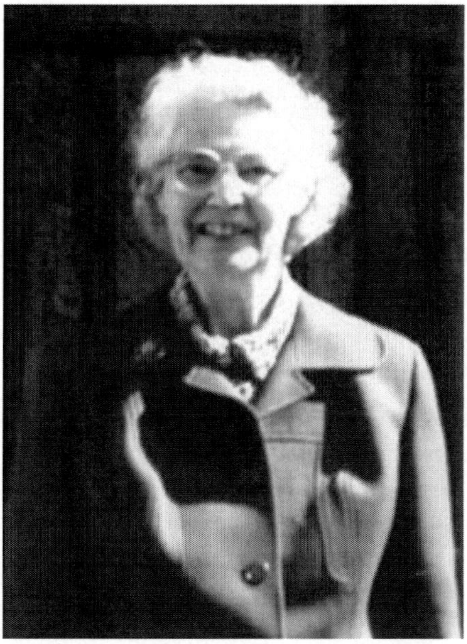

Figure 16. Mary Hess, courtesy Department of History and Philosophy of Science, University of Cambridge..

Richard Manson in the Biographical Dictionary of Twentieth-Century Philosophers, gives a brief introduction to the philosophical work of Mary Hesse: Hesse has been one of the most important figures in the philosophy of science from the 1960s, particularly because of her emphasis on the place of analogy, models and metaphors in the development of the sciences. … She shares with Kuhn and Feyerabend a use of examples from the history of science to undermine empiricist and deductivist theories of scientific development and method. The starting-point for her own critique of empiricism has been the thesis of the underdetermination of (scientific) theories by (observational) data. This had been stated by Duhem and understood by Quine, but Hesse appreciated its critical significance for truth-as-correspondence as a possible objective for scientific theories (or even as an end-point for their convergence). She has recognized that relativism is a consequence of this thesis, but has said that her aim has been to "steer a course between the extremes of metaphysical realism and relativism".

Of particular interest to us is her work on hermeneutics. She builds on the modern theory of hermeneutics developed by Hans-Georg Gadamer based upon notions put forth by his teacher Heidegger. Gadamer argued that it is through language that the world is opened up for us. Our prejudices, whatever aspects of our cultural horizon that we take for granted, are brought into the open in the encounter with the past. As a part of the tradition in which we stand, historical texts have an authority that precedes our own.

Gadamer refers to this movement of understanding as the fusion of horizons. As we come, through the work of interpretation, to understand what at first appears alien, we participate in the production of a richer, more encompassing context of meaning. The resulting interaction of text and reader is Gadamer's version of the hermeneutic circle. The interplay between the parts and the whole of a text is the way in which our reading adds to the complexity and depth of its meaning. Jürgen Habermas emphasized that the hermeneutic circle view, must involve critical judgment and reflection.

Mary Hesse accepts Jürgen Habermas proposition that science cannot be considered as neutral imquiry. But unlike Habermas, she feels that hermeneutics has a role to play in all the sciences:

It is convenient to take as starting - point a perceptive discussion by Jurgen Habermas of similarities and differences between empirical and hermeneutic method in his book published in English as Knowledge and Human Interests. I shall consider first a group of distinctions concerning traditional problems of the language and epistemology of science taken from his exposition of Wilhelm Dilthey. These are distinctions that I believe are made largely untenable by recent more accurate analyses of natural science. (Hesse, 1980, p. 169).

There follows a detailed description of five points . Mary Hesse's feeling is that the distinctions that Habermas was making are based on the instrumentalist perspective promoted by the Vienna circle prior to World War 1:

> What is immediately striking to readers versed in recent literature in philosophy of science is that almost every point made about the human sciences has recently been made about the natural sciences, and that the five points made about the natural sciences presupposes a traditional empiricist view of natural science that is almost universally discredited. In this traditional view it is assumed that the sole basis of scientific knowledge is the given in experience, that descriptions of this given are available in a theory-independent and stable language, whether of sense data or of common sense observations, that theories make no ontological claims about the real world except in so far as they are reducible to mere external correlations of observables. It is no novelty that all these empiricist theses have been subject to much philosophic controversy. It has been accepted since Kant that experience is partly constituted by theoretical categories, and more recently than Kant it has generally that these categories are not a priori, but are conjectured by creative imagination, having a mental source different from experiential stimuli. Moreover the work of Wittgenstein, Quine, Kuhn, Feyerabend and others has in various ways made it apparent that the descriptive language of observables is 'theory-laden', that is to say, in every empirical assertion that can be used as a starting-point of scientific investigation and theory, we employ concepts that interpret the data in terms of some general view of the world or other, and this is true however rooted in 'ordinary language' the concepts are. There are no stable observational descriptions, whether of sense data, or protocol sentences, in which the empirical reference of science can be directly captured.
>
> ...
>
> It follows, so it is held, that the logic of science is necessarily circular: data are interpreted and sometimes corrected by coherence with theory, and, at least in less extreme versions of the account, theory is also somehow constrained by empirical data. (Hesse, 1980, pp. 171, 172).

Martin Eger (2006) points out that this point is provocative, because hermeneutics had been taken by many philosophers to be the demarcation criterion between the human and natural sciences. In reaching her conclusions, Mary Hesse makes a distinction between the low-level deductions arrived at by Baconian induction and high-level theories of the type propounded by Maxwell and Einstein. A high-level theory can never be derived from experiment by induction in part because it is underdetermined by empirical evidence. Eger points out that high-level theories should be regarded "as metaphors of the environment, not as pictures, not even as partial, always to be improved, correspondences with some underlying but pre-existing domain of natural kinds."

A low-level description of the fall of an object by a formula relating time and distance is a direct testable statement. A high-level description of the fall using Einstein's General theory of Relativity by means of a metric tensor is according to Eger as much of a metaphorical manner of speaking "as those who use the popular phrase 'space-warp.' "

Since metaphors are intrinsically a part of high-level theories, then hermeneutics are needed for the study of these theories. "Scientific theory is a reading of the 'book of nature,' requiring circular reinterpretations between theory and observation and also theory and theory, and also requiring 'dialogue' about the meaning of theoretical language within the scientific community" (Hesse 1986,181). The examination by Maxwell of the state of Electricity and magnetism in his day and his discovery of an inconsistency between the treatment of the electric and magnetic fields is likewise a hermeneutical circle between theory and theory.

In quantum theories, not only do light and electrons have both particle and wave aspects, but events can only be determined statistically. In the nineteenth century, it was understood that with the vast numbers of molecules in a gas , motion could only be understood statistically – a subject called the Kinetic Theory of Gases. However that subject is built on the foundation that the motion of every molecule is completely determined by Newton's equations of motion. Probability is only used to deal with the vast number of molecules in a macroscopic system. In Quantum Mechanics probability is intrinsic. It is impossible to determine even in principle the motion of an individual particle. The mechanistic viewpoint advocated by Descartes and Boyle in the 17th century has been overthrown.

One consequence of the inherent uncertainty at microscopic levels is that in radioactive decay, it is impossible to know which atom will decay at any given time. We can say that half the atoms in the sample will decay in a given known time, but we cannot predict which atoms will decay in that time.

Figure 17 on page 39 exhibits Heisenberg's uncertainty principle, which relates pairs of physical properties: The more accurately we try to measure one property in the pair, the less accurate will be our measurement of the other one. Performing an experiment to find an electrons position (x) converts our knowledge of it's position into a certainty, but results in a complete loss of any knowledge of it's momentum (p).

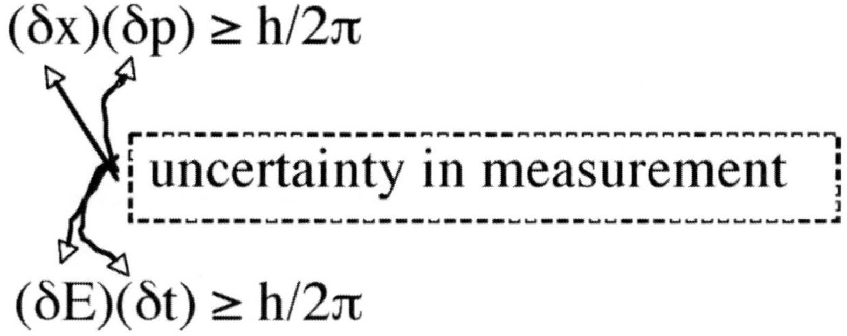

Figure 17.

The corresponding energy relation implies that our knowledge of the total energy (E) in a process is uncertain. Over macroscopic times, energy is conserved, but within times (t) that cannot be observed, energy fluctuations can occur. The possibility of such fluctuations has experimental consequences that have been verified. According to current theory, this feature is, as we shall see, crucial to the creation of the universe.

Chapter 6

THE MODERN ATOM

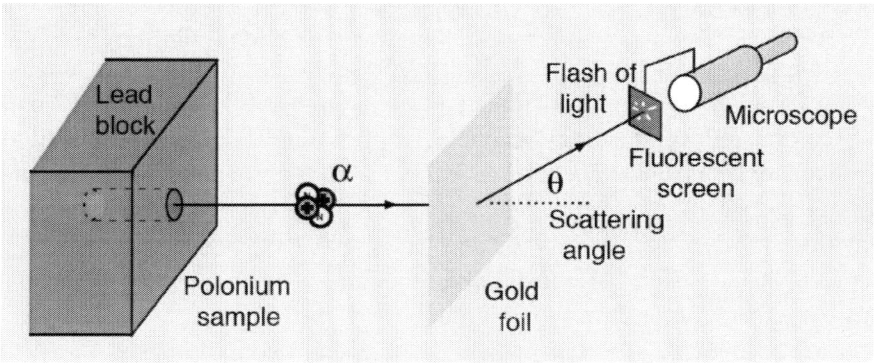

Figure 18. With permission - Rod Nave Department of Physics and Astronomy Georgia State University.

During the period of 1909-1911 Rutherford conducted scattering experiments firing alpha particles (now known to be the nucleus of the Helium atom) at heavy metals. To minimize alpha loss by scattering from air molecules, the experiments as shown above were carried out in a fairly good vacuum. The alphas came from a few milligrams of radium (to be precise, its decay product radon 222) as indicated in the figure above. According to the original paper, " a pencil of alpha particles was directed normally on to the scattering foil. By rotating the microscope the alpha particles scattered in different directions could be observed on the screen." Actually, this was more difficult than it sounds. A single alpha caused a slight fluorescence on the zinc sulphide screen at the end of the microscope. This could only be reliably seen by dark-adapted eyes (after half an hour in complete darkness) and one person could only count the flashes accurately for one minute before needing a break, and counts above 90 per minute were too fast for reliability. The experiment accumulated data from hundreds of thousands of flashes.

Rutherford states that "Dr. Geiger ... found in thin pieces of heavy metal, that the scattering was usually small of the order of one degree... 'Why not let him [Marsden] see if any alpha -particles can be scattered through a large angle?' ... I did not believe that they would be ... two or three days later Geiger [old me that] ... 'We have been able to get some alpha -particles coming backwards...'...

It was almost as incredible as if you could fire a 15-inch [38 cm] shell at a piece of tissue paper and it came back and hit you. ... It was then that I had the idea of an atom with a minute massive center carrying a charge."

Charges originate in the constituents of the basic building blocks of matter, the atom. Atoms contain a central heavy nucleus and comparatively light negatively charged electrons circulating outside of it. Typically, a nucleus has a diameter of the order of 10^{-14}m compared to a diameter of the order of 10^{-10}m for an atom. That is, the diameter of an atom is one tenth of a billionth of a meter and the diameter of the nucleus of the atom is one ten thousandth of the diameter of an atom. The nucleus contains electrically neutral neutrons and positively charged protons; each almost 2000 times heavier than an electron. Franklin's notion that matter contains equal parts of negative and positive charge is due to the electrical neutrality of atoms; each atom normally contains equal numbers of electrons and protons and the absolute charge of each electron is identical to the absolute charge on each proton.

Such an atom could not be stable. The electrons traveling around such a central nucleus would be constantly accelerated. Such an acceleration, according to Maxwell's theory, would cause the electron to emit energy in the form of electromagnetic waves (photons). As the electron loses energy, its orbit continuously changes to distances closer to the nucleus. Within a millionth of a second such an atom would collapse.

Niels Bohr elaborated a model that would take incorporate Rutherford's findings and resolve the conflict with Maxwell's theory:

1) Classical electrodynamics is inadequate to describe the behaviour of systems of atomic size.
2) The electrons are in orbits around the nucleus and radiate discontinuously.
3) The electrons only radiate or absorb energy when moving from one stable orbit to another.

4) Ordinary mechanics and electricity might be used to discuss the motion of the electron in a stable and nonradiating orbit but the passing of the electron between orbits cannot be treated on this basis.

Furthermore Bohr used his theory to derive an empirical formula due to Balmer,. Balmer's formula came about as follows-

Absorption lines had been observed in sunlight. Each line was assigned to some specific gas. In this way Helium was first identified in the sun [named after the Greek word for the sun-helios].

Kirchoff: noted that after absorbing radiation at the characteristic frequency of the gas, the gas may reradiate it at the same frequency. There were the following problems:

1) The absorption and emission of radiation is different in gases than in liquids and solids. Recall on liquids and solids, the spectrum is the same for all elements.
2) The electrons corresponding to the radiation had been expected to to produce one line for each electron, but many elements exhibit far too many lines.
3) Every absorption line corresponds to the same emission line but the reverse doesn't hold: there are many lines in the emission spectrum without equivalents in the absorption spectra.
4) If an absorption line corresponds to a vibration state of the atom, this represents a degree of freedom of the atom and the corresponding energy should increase the specific heat of the gas, but the degrees of freedom, without including these vibration states already corresponds to a theoretical value above the experimental value.

Holton: "This was a period of almost obsessed searching for some hint of numerical relation among the tantalizing lines, for some mathematical key to decode the message that surely had to be behind the appearances. It is almost as if we watched again the pupils of Plato trying to reduce the offensive disordiliness of planetary motion to a series of circular motions."

Balmer produced a formula that fit four lines in the visible Hydrogen spectrum. After publication, many other lines predicted by the use of this formula were found in the visible and in the ultraviolet spectrum. Balmer speculated that there were many other series of lines, which were indeed found later.

Bohr's model also accounted for all the lines in all the series.

With the advent of Quantum Mechanics, the problems of the contradictions between Bohr's model and Maxwell's theory of Electrodynamics disappeared. As the constituent of the Cathode rays, the electron manifests itself as a particle. In an atom, the electron manifests itself as a wave.

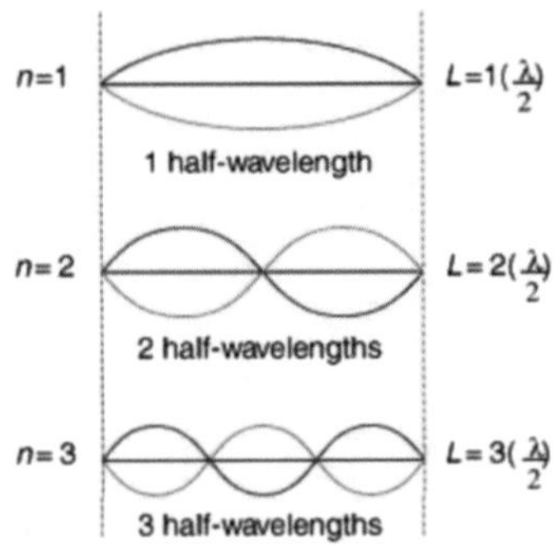

Figure 19. Waves on a guitar string of length L. Musical notes are produced by a guitar when any multiple of half the wavelength corresponding to the note can fit on the length of the string.

In an analogous manner, to the wave on a guitar string in the above figure, the wavelength of the electron must fit around the nucleus of an atom:

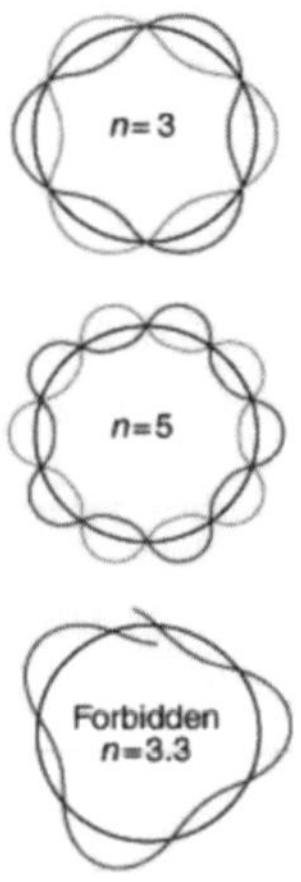

Figure 20. Fitting an electron wavelegth around the nucleus of an atom.

(Figure 20 should actually be three-dimensional.) This picture not only accounts for the structure of the atom, but also means that the electron actually forms a *stationary* standing wave around the atom (a cloud of charge). Since we no longer have an accelerating electron, there is no longer a violation of Maxwell's theory.

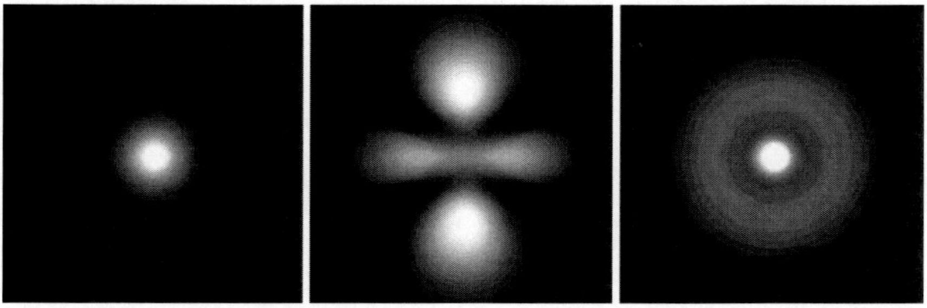

Figure 21.The electron appearing in s wavelike cloud in an atom.

Figure 21 shows examples of the appearance of the electron cloud around the atom (for the ground state and two excited states – corresponding to fundamental and harmonics for notes on a guitar string.

The fact that an atom has a discrete set of possible states and a discrete set of corresponding energy values emerges automatically as a mathematical property of Schroedinger's equation; the set of rules for constructing the Schroedinger equation replaces the previous postulates about allowed orbits in the Bohr atom. These rules apply to all conceivable atomic and molecular systems, whereas in Bohr's theory, the postulates had to be constructed by trial and error for each case, with only the physicists intuition and experience to guide her.

Moseley: "There is in the atom a fundamental quantity, which increases by regular steps as we pass from one element to the next. This quantity can only be the charge on the central positive nucleus." The positive charge of the nucleus is the same as the atomic number, Z, which identifies each of the atomic elements. In 1919, Rutherford reported that the nucleus of the Hydrogen atom is emitted when Nitrogen is bombarded by alpha -particles. In 1920: the nucleus of the Hydrogen atom was given the name "proton" For the atom to be electrically neutral, the number of positively charged protons in the nucleus must equal the number of electrons surrounding the nucleus. "Only the progressively increasing charge on the nucleus gives us a truly secure foundation for the arrangement of elements in a unique order."

For a time, it appeared that the world was based upon just two elements-electrons and protons. This was remarkable. It outmatched the ancient Greek atomic idea, which was based upon four elements. To account for the weight of the chemical elements, it was thought that there were additional protons *and* electrons in the nucleus. This seemed to be confirmed by the known forms of radioactivity. Unstable chemical elements decay in three ways; emission of alpha rays – the nuclei of the Helium nucleus, emission of gamma rays or photons and emission of beta rays – electrons. In the case of beta rays, the electron was known to come out of the nucleus. In the early 1920's a proton-electron combination was called a neutron. By 1930, theory showed that electrons could not be contained in the nucleus. Then in 1932: Chadwick discovered " radiation [that] consisted of particles of mass nearly equal to that of a proton and with no net charge, or neutrons" This would have to be a fundamental particle and not a (p-e) combination. Moreover, free neutrons can decay into a proton and an electron. All chemical elements with the identical chemical properties are called isotopes. Isotopes contain the same number of protons but different numbers of neutrons. Isotopic masses are not exactly integral multiples of the Hyrogen nucleus (1proton) because neutrons are slightly heavier. Proton mass (938.27 MeV) Neutron mass (939.57MeV).

Chapter 7

THE PARTICLE ZOO

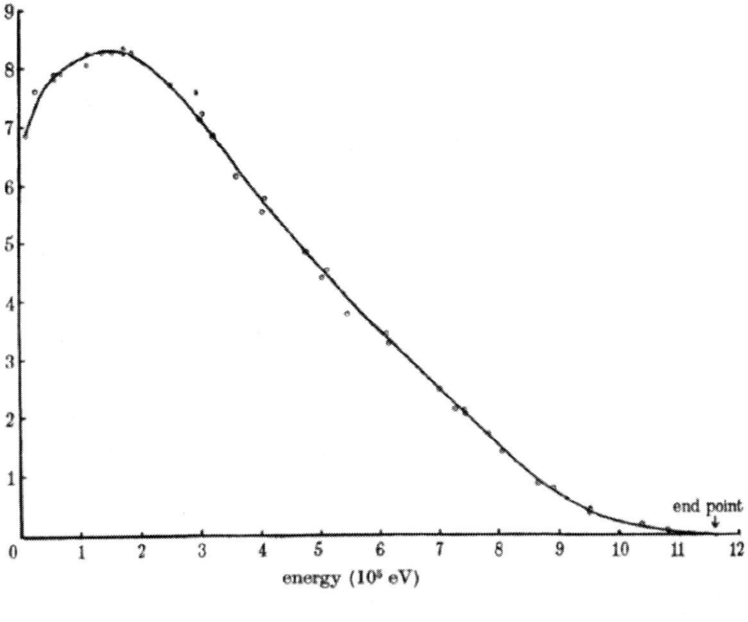

Figure 22. Energy spectrum of β rays ejected from p. 79 from G. J. Neary, Proceedings of the Royal Society of London. Series A, Mathematical and Physical Sciences, Vol. 175, No. 960 (Mar. 28, 1940), p 71-87.

In the above figure, the nucleus of an atom A decays to the nucleus of another atom B. In the decay process, a beta (β) ray is emitted. Since A is at rest, the total energy of A is always the same. It is found that the energy of B is independent of the energy of the emitted electron (*e*), but the energy of *e*the electron varies!!

Was a neutral particle emitted?

When calorimetry measurements were made. (A calorimeter is an apparatus for measuring the amount of heat involved in a chemical reaction or other process.) **the photon was ruled out. The neutron is too heavy**

Figure 23.

A definitive experiment was made by Charles Ellis and showed that the average energy released is always less than difference in energy between the nuclei A and B. Subsequently, Niels Bohr speculated that energy is not conserved in the nuclear domain. In 1930 Pauli suggested that a hereto unknown neutral particle, the neutrino (ν) is produced in this process.

- The reaction is then of the form: $A \rightarrow B+e+\nu$
- The neutrino (ν) must have little reaction with matter to escape detection

From only two elementary particles, the number had now grown to electrons, positrons (antielectrons- if a positon and an electron encounter each other they both are annihilated and a pair of photons are produced) neutrinos, protons, and neutrons.. (Presumably all particles have antimatter counter parts – indeed there are antiprotons and antineutrons which were ultimately discovered). And many more so-called elementary particles were still to come.

In 1936 Anderson and Neddermeyer discovered the muon. It's mass is roughly 200 times greater than that of an electron. In all other aspects, it had exactly the same properties as that of an electron. The response of response of I. I.. Rabi to this discovery was "who ordered that?".

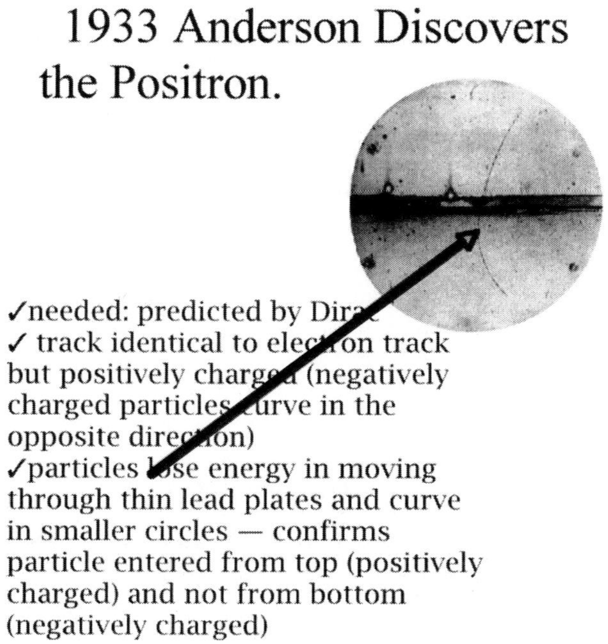

1933 Anderson Discovers the Positron.
✓needed: predicted by Dirac
✓ track identical to electron track but positively charged (negatively charged particles curve in the opposite direction)
✓particles lose energy in moving through thin lead plates and curve in smaller circles — confirms particle entered from top (positively charged) and not from bottom (negatively charged)

Figure 24. Figure 1 p. 493 of Carl D. Anderson Phys. Rev. 43, 491 - 494 (1933) Copyright (1933) by The American Physical Society.

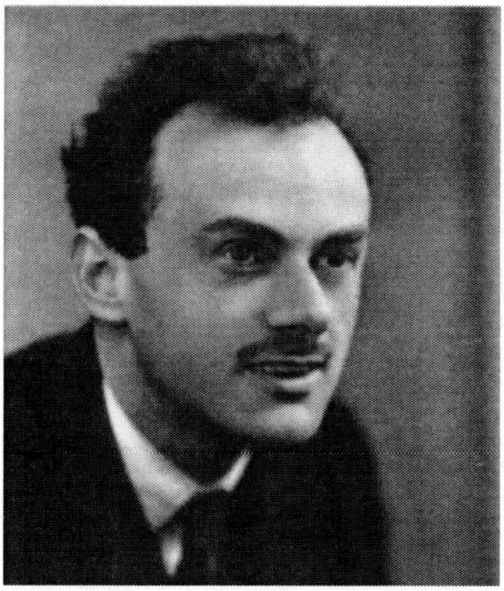

Figure 25. Paul Dirac *Photograph by A. Bortzells Tryckeri, courtesy AIP Emilio Segre Visual Archives.*

We will eventually see that there is indeed a reason for the existence of the muon. The design of the world is indeed very intricate. Now you can argue that God does not exist and this universe exists the way it is because the universe can only exist in the way it is. I cannot argue with you if that is the way you see things. ***But for me the intricate plan of the universe is a manifestation of God's plan for it. It is awesome and beautiful. We are one world of billions, but no matter. The ways of God are beyond human understanding:***

JOB CHAPTER 38

[1] Then the LORD replied to Job out of the tempest and said:
[2] Who is this who darkens counsel,
Speaking without knowledge?
[3] Gird your loins like a man;
I will ask and you will inform Me.
[4] Where were you when I laid the earth's foundations?
Speak if you have understanding.
[5] Do you know who fixed its dimensions
Or who measured it with a line?
[6] Onto what were its bases sunk?
Who set its cornerstone
[7] When the morning stars sang together
And all the divine beings shouted for joy?

On this note, it is good to return to the neutrino (ν). For a long time the concept was very spooky. It was only accepted to exist because of the missing momentum and energy that occurred during certain reactions. Neutrinos hardly ever react with matter. On the average a neutrino would travel in water about 10 times the distance from the Earth to the Sun before reacting with any protons in the molecules of water. In 1955, Fred Reines (Nobel prize 1995) and Clyde Cowan (Very sadly, Clyde Cowan, Jr. was not alive and so could not share the award with Fred Reines, but his equal contribution are recognized by all) mounted an experiment at the new Savannah River nuclear reactor to try and detect neutrinos. Reactors produce immense amounts of neutrinos. Something like 10000000000000 per square centimeter per second. With this number of neutrinos, a small number of them would interact with water in a detector.

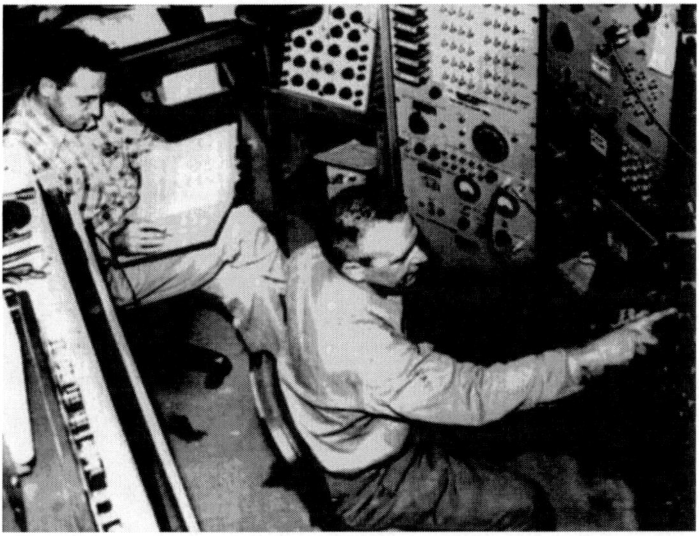

Figure 26. Fred Reines and Clyde Cowan at the Control Center of the Hanford Experiment (1953). (http://www.ps.uci.edu/physics/news/nuexpt.html).

The neutrinos produced in the beta-decay of fission fragments[3] in a powerful chain reacting pile are to be allowed to pass through a large volume (10-ft^3) liquid scintillator. The protons in the scintillator have a cross section of about 10^{-44} cm^2 for conversion by the fission fragment neutrinos to neutrons with the emission of a positron. It seems feasible to obtain some tenths such events per minute in the detector. Loading the scintillator solution with boron or cadmium compounds and counting the neutron capture gamma-pulse in delayed coincidence with the positron and annihilation radiation pulse assists in an important way in the reduction of background. Also necessary to the reduction of background in our experiment is the use of thick boron paraffin shielding, massive composite lead-steel shields, and Geiger tube anticoincidence umbrellas, the latter to discriminate against double pulses arising from μ-meson decay, stars, etc.

Figure 27. A Proposed Experiment to Detect the Free Neutrino by F. Reines and C. L. Cowan, Jr. The Physical Review volume 90, pages 492 - 493 (1953) Copyright (1953) by The American Physical Society."

The other problem is to ensure that the water in the detector is shielded so that almost the only kind of particle that reaches the detector are the neutrinos.

Otherwise reactions of other kinds of particles could be mistaken for reactions of neutrinos with protons in the molecules of water.

> A covering GM blanket which reduced the μ-meson counting rate by 75 percent when turned on in anticoincidence reduced this delayed pair rate insignificantly. A six-foot thick water shield installed above the detector and capable of absorbing at least 30 percent of the cosmic-ray nucleonic component also failed to change the delayed-pair rate significantly. Subsequent work in an underground location in which the cosmic-ray background is greatly diminished indicates that the Hanford background is probably due to cosmic rays, for example, neutrons arising from μ^- capture in shield materials, stars which include neutrons and gamma rays energetic enough to create electron-positron pairs, showers, etc.

Figure 28. Detection of the Free Neutrino by F. Reines and C. L. Cowan, Jr. Phys. Rev. 92, 830 - 831 (1953) Copyright (1953) by The American Physical Society."

In this experiment Reines and Cowan had a well-shielded location for the experiment, 11 meters from the reactor center and 12 meters underground. The neutrinos would then interact with protons in a tank of water, creating neutrons and positrons. Each positron would create a pair of gamma rays when it annihilated with an electron.

The exceedingly few neutrinos that do react with the water combine with the protons producing a neutron and a positron. The positrons quickly find electrons and produce two gamma rays by pair-annihilation. This very distinctive event is evident if you can simultaneously detect two gammas of energy precisely two 0.5 MeV in opposite directions.

The gamma rays were detected by placing scintillator material in a tank of water. The scintillator material gives off flashes of light in response to the gamma rays and the light flashes are detected by photomultiplier tubes. To ensure that there is absolutely no error in the coincident detection of the pair annihilation, Reines and Cowan arranged to detect the neutron that is also produced in the reaction.

They would detect the neutrons by placing cadmium chloride into the tank. Cadmium is a highly effective neutron absorber (and so finds use in nuclear control rods) and gives off a gamma ray when it absorbs a neutron. The arrangement was such that a gamma ray produced by after absorption of the neutron by the cadmium would be detected 5 microseconds after detection of the gamma rays from the annihilation of the positron with an electron.

Muons also produce neutrinos. Physicists wondered whether these neutrinos were the same as the neutrinos observed by Reines and Cowan. To test this you need an extremely large number of neutrinos produced pion decay and then everything has to pass through a large amount of matter to block everything except the neutrinos. The neutrinos then enter a detector where a very small number of them interact with matter. If only muons emerge, then these neutrinos are distinct from the neutrinos observed in the Reines and Cowan experiment.

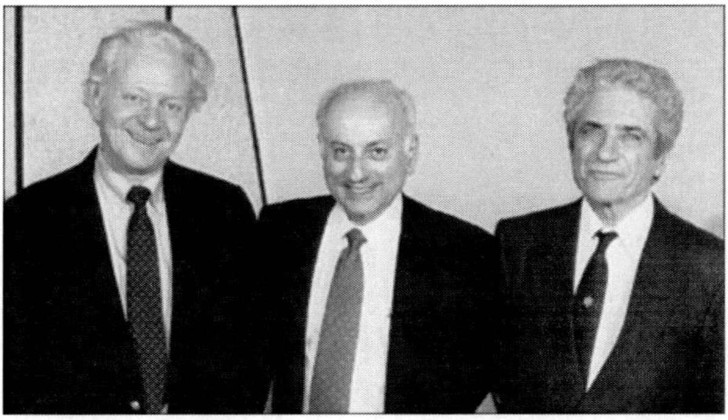

Figure 29. Leon Lederman, Melvin Schwartz and Jack Steinberger directed an experiment at the Alternating Gradient Synchrotron (AGS).

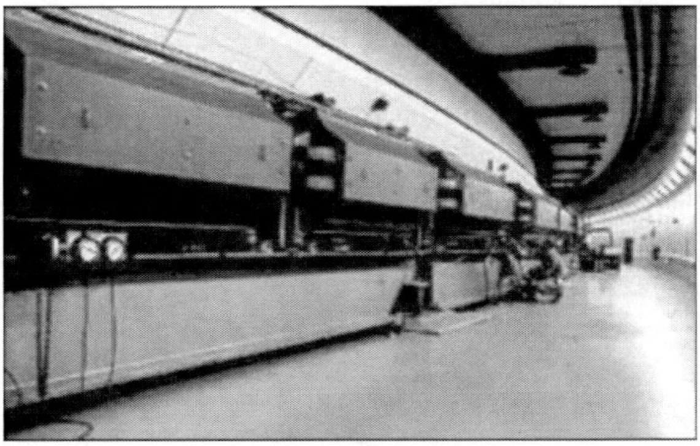

Figure 30. The Alternating Gradient Synchrotron (AGS) at the Brookhaven National Laboratory.

Yukawa's conjecture is discussed in chapter 7.

In the experiment, the AGS produced a beam of protons, which collided with a beryllium target. A major component after the collision is a shower of pi mesons, which traveled 70 feet toward a 5,000-ton steel wall made of plates taken from surplus World War II battleships. Pions deacy rapidly. So before the pions reach the plates, they decayed into muons and neutrinos The steel wall stops the muons and anything else coming out of the target except for neutrinos. The resulting neutrino beam passed through a neon-filled aluminum detector called a spark chamber.

56 of these neutrinos are observed to interact with aluminum atoms in the 10 ton detector in a 10 month period. In every interactions muons are produced and no electron. The neutrinos produced in the Brookhaven experiment are therefore muon neutrinos a distinctly different particle than the neutrinos produced in the Reines and Cowan experiment, which are electron neutrinos. The mystery of "who ordered that" deepens.

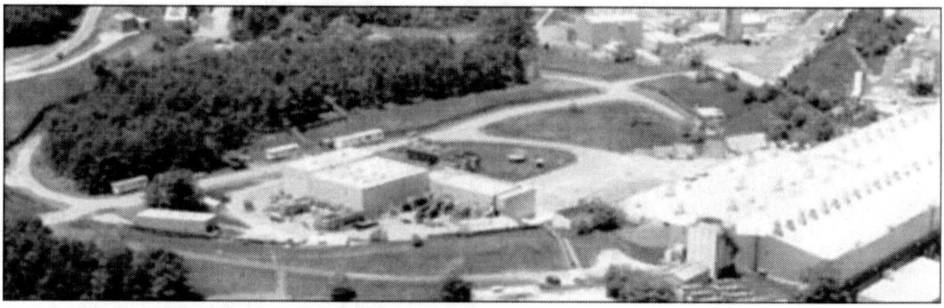

Figure 31. The Brookhaven National Laboratory.

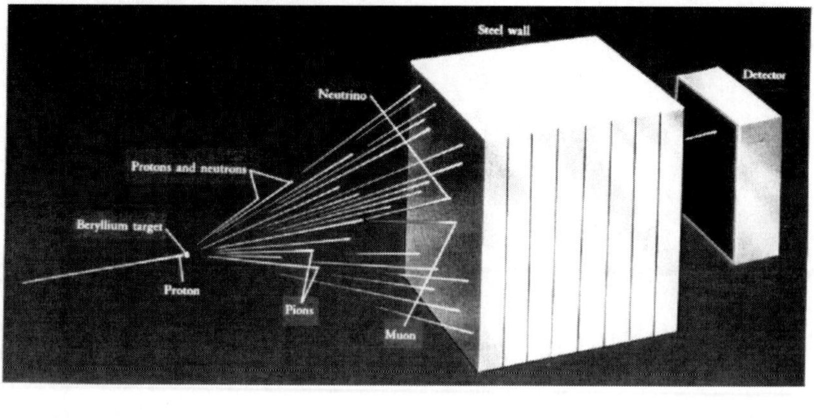

Figure 32. Illustration: "The neutrino experiment at the Brookhaven AGS" from the book, From Quarks To the Cosmos by Leon Lederman and David Schramm. Copyright © 1989, 1995 by Scientific American Library. Reprinted by arrangement with Henry Holt and Company, LLC.

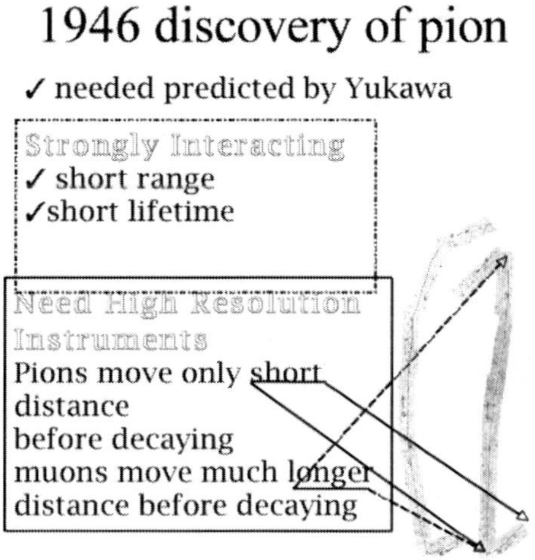

1946 discovery of pion
✓ needed predicted by Yukawa
Strongly Interacting
✓ short range
✓short lifetime
Need High Resolution Instruments
Pions move only short distance before decaying
muons move much longer distance before decaying

Figure 33. Decays of pions produce muons and neutrinos.

Chapter 8

NEUTRINOS AND SUPERNOVAE

At this point let us for the moment interrupt the story of the structure of the universe and neutrinos tell us about the cosmos:

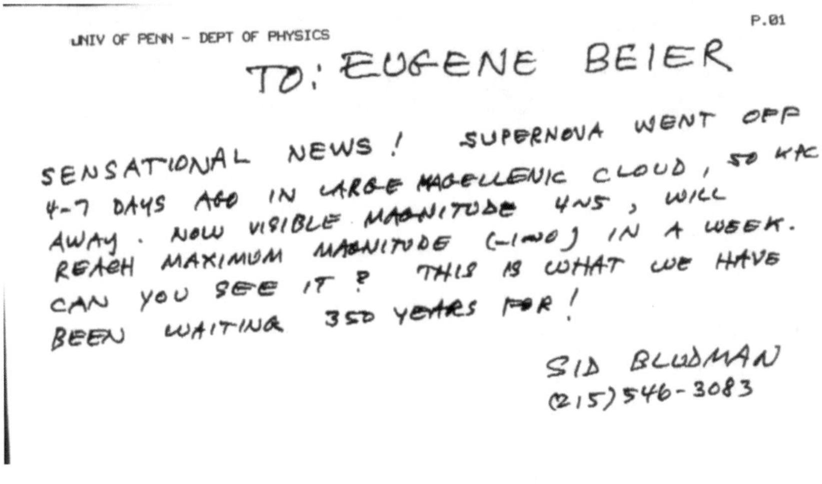
P.01

UNIV OF PENN - DEPT OF PHYSICS

TO: EUGENE BEIER

SENSATIONAL NEWS! SUPERNOVA WENT OFF 4-7 DAYS AGO IN LARGE MAGELLENIC CLOUD, 50 KPC AWAY. NOW VISIBLE MAGNITUDE 4NS, WILL REACH MAXIMUM MAGNITUDE (-1 to 0) IN A WEEK. CAN YOU SEE IT? THIS IS WHAT WE HAVE BEEN WAITING 350 YEARS FOR!

SID BLUDMAN
(215)546-3083

Figure 34. Reproduced by permission of Professor Sidney Bludman.

On Feb 23, 1983 (my first wife's birthday!) a supernova was seen. The closest a supernova has appeared since Kepler's Supernova of 1604, which occurred before the invention of the telescope.

At the time of the observation of the supernova, there were two neutrino observatories iat opposite ends of the Earth. The SuperKamioka detector consists of a huge 50,000 ton double layered tank of ultra pure water, observed by 11,146 twenty inch diameter photomultiplier tubes (a photomultiplier is a device which converts light, photons, into useable electrical signals). This amounts to a total of about 1 acre of photocathodes, more than a factor of ten more light detection area than heretofore assembled. It is located in a specially carved out cavity in an old zinc mine 2000 feet under Mount Ikena in the Japanese Alps, near the town of Kamioka.

Figure 35. © 1989-2002, Anglo-Australian Observatory, photograph by David Malin. On the right, the star that is to become a supernova. On the left, the same star after it became a supernova.

The Irvine-Michingan-Brookhaven (IMB) detector was located in a purpose-built cavern located 2000 ft underground in the Morton Salt mine at Fairport Harbor (near Cleveland), Ohio. The IMB proton decay detector shown above was a 60-foot cube of ultra-pure water surrounded by 2048 light-sensitive phototubes to detect the distinctive patterns of light given off by proton decays or neutrino interactions in the water volume.

Looking back at the data collected on Feb 23, it was seen that at 7:35 AM the SuperKamioka detector had recorded 11 separate neutrino events. The IMB had detected eight. All events occurred within 10 seconds. Not surprisingly, given how rarely neutrinos interact with matter, never before had more than two events been recorded within 10 seconds. The last observation of the large Magellanic cloud (a dwarf galaxy that orbits our own galaxy, the Milky Way) was at 9 AM. By 11 AM supernova 1987A was observed in this

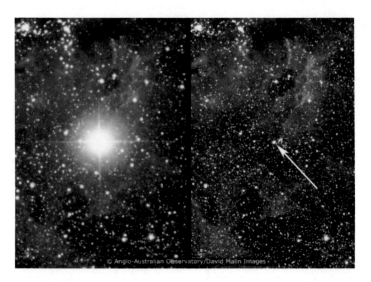

galaxy as seen above. An intense beam of neutrinos were observed at least two hours before the light from the supernova. How could this have happened?

More than twenty years earlier, theoretical astrophysicists had argued that a supernova explosion should release a huge number of neutrinos. Neutrinos travel at or near the speed of light. Since they interact so weakly with matter, neutrinos emitted at the very center of the exploding star would pass right through the material of the star. The shock wave from the central explosion would take a few hours or days to make its way to the surface of the star and only then would a blast of light be emitted. All of the action actually took place 170,000 years ago in the large Megallanic Cloud, when the wave of neutrinos and light began their journeys.

Events that took place 170,000 years ago are suddenly seen here on Earth. The action takes place in a few hours. The drama of a supernova explosion is preceded by the observation of the smallest known particles on opposite ends of the Earth. *If I were writing science fiction, I would never have dreamed of such implausible coincidences. The universe constantly amazes me. There is always that absolutely perfect fit. An atheist would argue that only the universe as it is could exist. An infinite number of universes are potential and only this one is successful. I prefer to look at the universe as God's handiwork.*

Chapter 9

QUARKS AND LEPTONS

Electrons, muons, and their neutrinos do not experience the force that binds neutrons and protons in the nucleus. That force is called the "strong interaction". Electrons, and muons, experience the gravitational, electromagnetic and weak interactions. Gravitational interactions are so small among basic particles that they can be ignored. Neutrinos only experience the weak interaction and it is because the weak interaction is so much weaker than the strong and the electromagnetic forces that neutrinos hardly ever interact with matter. Particles of matter that do not experience the strong interaction are called *leptons*. In 1975, Martin Perl discovered a third electron-like particle the tau. For this discovery, he shared the 1995 Nobel prize. (Fred Reines shared the prize, in his case for his work with neutrinos.) An international collaboration of scientists at the Department of Energy's Fermi National Accelerator Laboratory announced on July 21, 2000 the first direct evidence for the tau neutrino. They reported five instances of a neutrino interacting with an atomic nucleus to produce a tau lepton. Physicists needed about three years of painstaking work to identify the tracks revealing that the neutrinos were interacting to produce tau leptons and thus showing the existence of a unique particle – the tau neutrino. In the experiment a 900-GeV proton beam (until recently, the highest beam energy in the world) at Fermilab was steered into a tungsten target, where particles are produced that quickly decay into taus and tau neutrinos. Everything coming from the beam then passes through magnets to deflect the charged particles away and then the remnants pass through shielding material to absorb most of the other particles except for rarely interacting neutrinos. The neutrinos then enter a sequence of emulsion targets in which they can interact. The evidence for a tau neutrino in the emulsion is the creation of a tau lepton, which itself quickly decays (after traveling about 1 mm) into other particles. About 100000000000000 tau neutrinos entered the emulsion, of which perhaps 100 interacted therein.

The particles that do not experience the strong interaction; the electrons, muons tauons and their associated neutrinos are called leptons. Physicists speak about three generations of leptons:

	Flavor	Mass (GeV/c²)	Electric Charge (e)	
1st Generation		electron neutrino	<7 x 10-9	0
		electron	0.000511	-1
2nd Generation		muon neutrino	<0.0003	0
		muon (mu-minus)	0.106	-1
3rd Generation		tau neutrino	<0.03	0
		tau (tau-minus)	1.7771	-1

Figure 36. The "generations" of leptons.

The particles that experience the force that binds neutrons and protons in the nucleus, the strong interaction are called "hadrons". Hadrons are divided into two kinds of particles –baryons, and mesons. Baryons are particles similar to the nucleons. Baryons that occupy the same structure – for example nucleons in a nucleus, must all have different quantum numbers. Mesons on the other hand can all have the same quantum numbers.

Even more dramatic discoveries occurred concerning hadrons than in the case of the leptons. In 1952 there was observation of a new baryon, the Δ(1230 MeV). It occurred in four forms including one, which has double the charge of the proton. Even more exotic forms of particles had been observed earlier:

Between 1947and1954 particles were seen that:

- are produced copiously (looks like strong interaction)
- are always produced in pairs
- have long lifetimes (looks like weak interaction)

- Doctrine of Associated production (Pais 1952) These new strange particles interact by the strong interaction only in pairs. In isolation they can only decay via the weak interaction

- These particles are described by a new quantity, the "strangeness" S, which is conserved by the strong interaction and violated by the weak interaction.

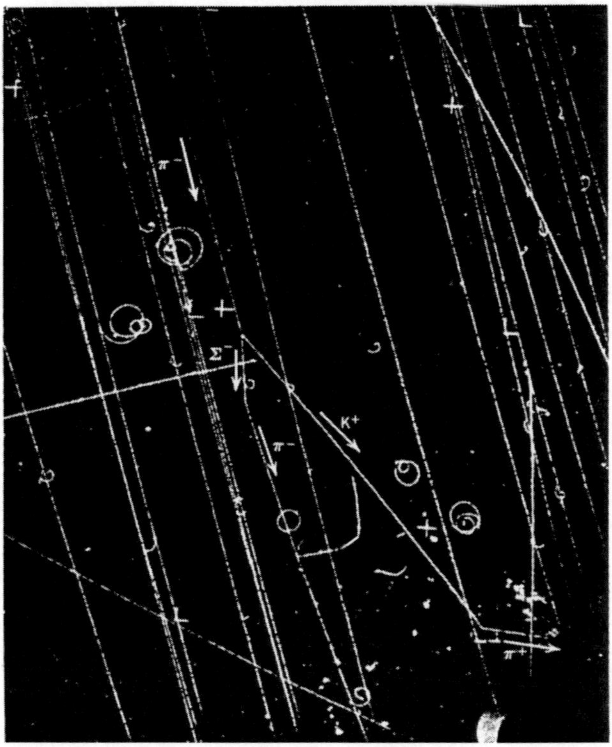

Figure 37. Associated Production of $\Sigma^- + K^+$. AA negative pion traveling through liquid hydrogen strikes a proton and produces the Σ^- baryon and the K^+ meson, both of which subsequently decay. Photograph taken by Prof. Hugh Bradner of the 10-in. liquid hydrogen bubble chamber at the Radiation Laboratory of the University of California.

Strongly interacting particles such as the neutron, the proton, the Δ and the pion have zero strangeness. Five strange particles were found initially, labeled Λ (S = 1), Σ (S = -1), Ξ (S= -2), and K (S = ±1). The proton, Δ, Λ, Σ and Ξ are all baryons. The pion and the K are mesons. This discovery gradually led to an understanding of the nucleon (proton or neutron) as an atom for the strong interaction.

The essential notion of Atomism was set out in 1750 by Rudjer Boscovich: atoms contain smaller parts, which in turn contain still smaller parts, and so on down to the fundamental building blocks of matter. These fundamental particles are indivisible bits of matter that are ungenerated and indestructible. The atoms, corresponding to the chemical elements found in Mendele'ev's table of the elements, as pictured in the Quantum Mechanics of the late 1920's involves a negatively charged electron cloud surrounding a positively charged central nucleus. In the 1930's as it became clear that the nucleons could only be held together in the nucleus by a strong interaction, Yukawa postulated that just as the electromagnetic force between the electrons and the nucleus is mediated by photons, the strong force between nucleons is mediated by pions. Experiments in scattering electrons off nucleons by Hofstadter at the Stanford Linear accelerator Center [SLAC] in 1961 seemed to confirm this notion. The electrons were of high enough energy that they penetrated inside the proton and the neutron. The scattering revealed the distribution of charges in the nucleons:

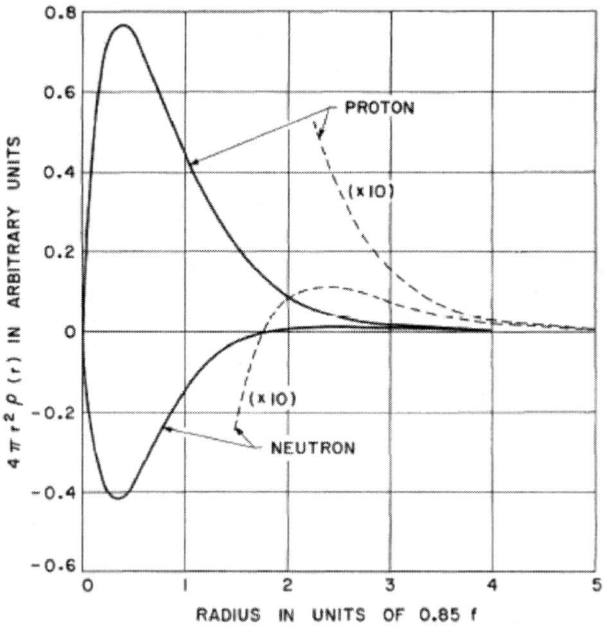

Figure 38. The proton and neutron charge density distributions. At the origin an additional vary narrow peak (practically a delta function) has been omitted. It contains about 0.3 of the total charge for the proton and neutralizes the total charge for the neutron. Figure 38 from R. Hofstadter and R. Herman, Phys. Rev. Letts. 92, 830 - 831 (1961) Copyright (1961) by The American Physical Society."

Following Yukawa's basic notion, the nucleon is viewed as containing a pionic cloud surrounding a nucleonic essence. Note that the core (postulated nucleonic essence) has no discernable size [the meaning of the statement very narrow peak (practically a delta function)] has charge 1/3 [0.3] . This will relate to developments that occurred later on.

At about the same time as Hofstadter's experiment, Gell-Mann and Ne'eman separately in 1961 developed a scheme that was analogous to Mendele'ev's table of the elements. Mendele'v had organized the chemical elements according to their chemical properties and their weight. Gell-Mann and Ne'eman used properties such as the strangeness to organize the known particles. When Mendele'ev had completed his task, he had noticed that there were gaps in his table. It was predicted that these gaps corresponded to chemical elements that had not yet been discovered. In 1962 Gell-Mann used this new table to predict the existence of a new particle which he called the Ω^-. This particle would have strangeness value of -3. At an international conference, Gell-Mann told the experimental community exactly how to perform an experiment to find this new particle. A couple of years later, the particle was found.

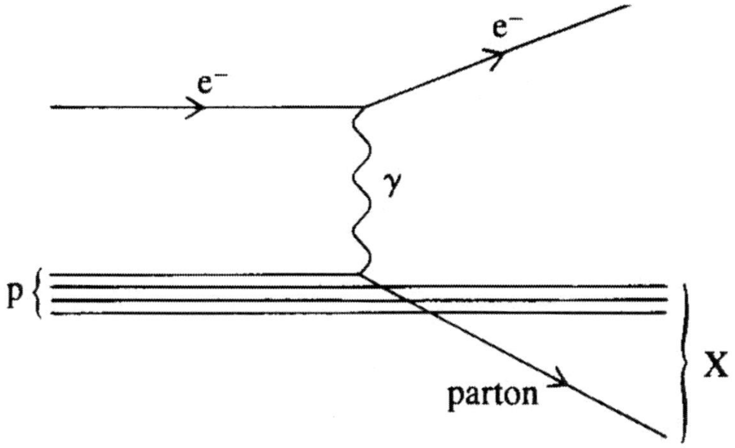

Deep-inelastic scattering in the parton model.

Figure 39. From "Quarks and Leptons" by Francis Halzen and Alan D, Martin © 1984 "This material is reproduced with permission of John Wiley and Sons, Inc."

Subsequently experiments continued to be performed at SLAC. More and more, it became clear through the analyses of Bjorken and Feynman that electrons were scattering off particles contained inside the nucleons. Until the status of these particles became clear, these particles were provisionally dubbed "partons". These partons could have been pions in the conjectured cloud inside the protons, but soon it was established that the properties of these partons did not match those of pions. There was another possibility. Viewing the nucleon as containing a pionic cloud surrounding a nucleonic essence did not correspond to the classification scheme devised by Gell-Mann and Ne'eman. Gell- Mann and Zweig had earlier pointed out that this classification scheme could be replicated if the strongly interacting baryons contained three point-like particles, which Gell-Mann named "quarks".

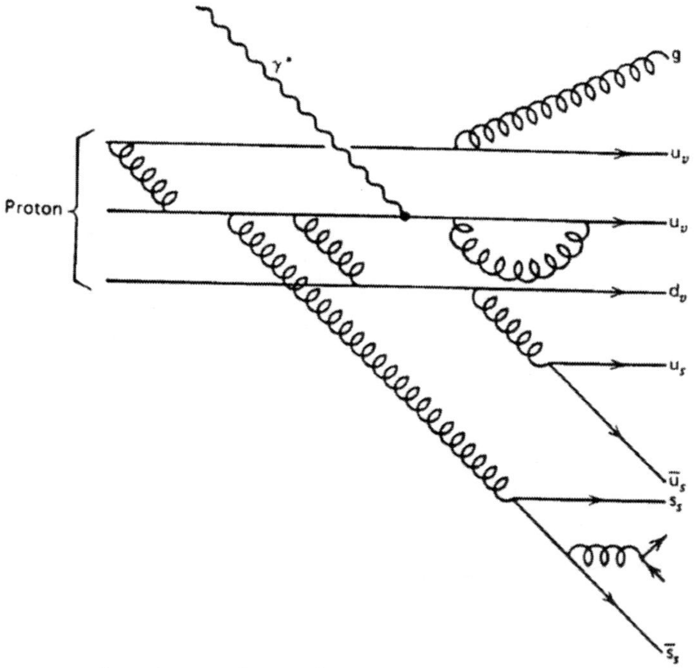

A proton made up of valence quarks, gluons, and slow debris consisting of quark–antiquark pairs.

Figure 40. From "Quarks and Leptons" by Francis Halzen and Alan D, Martin © 1984 "This material is reproduced with permission of John Wiley and Sons, Inc."

Non strange particles would contain u quarks (electric charge 2/3) and d quarks (electric charge -1/3) and strange particles would contain an s quark (electric charge -1/3). If the partons were not pions, could they be quarks? In such a model the analogy to the electrons interacting with the nucleus through the electromagnetic force mediated by photons would not be nucleons interacting with each other mediated by pions, but instead quarks interacting with each other mediated by new entities called gluons:

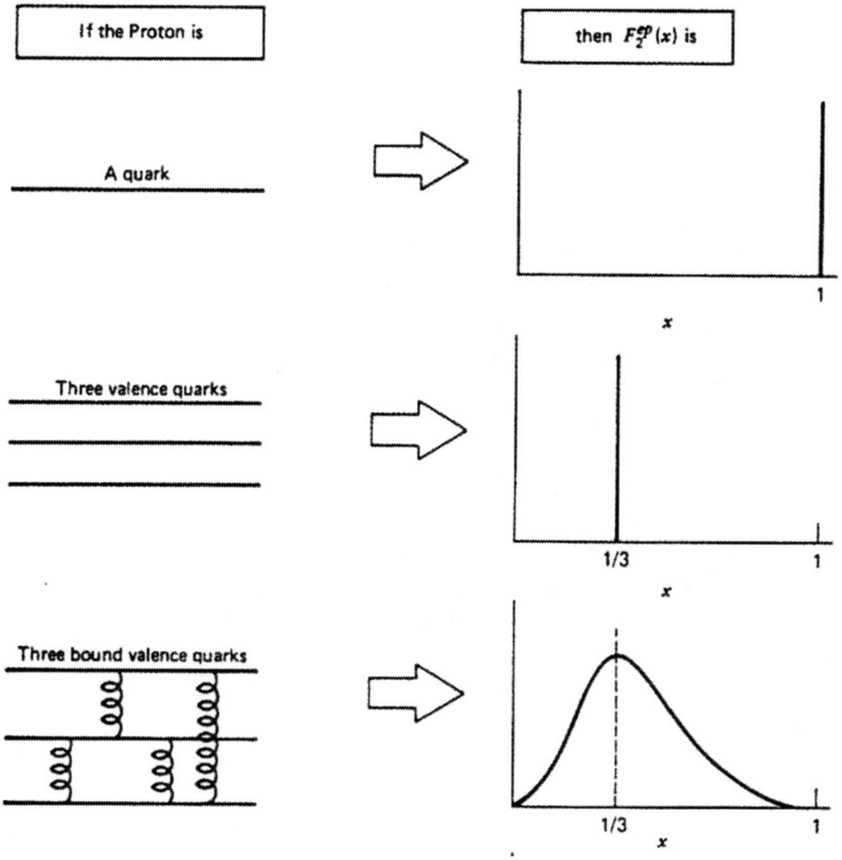

Figure 41. From “Quarks and Leptons” by Francis Halzen and Alan D, Martin © 1984 "This material is reproduced with permission of John Wiley and Sons, Inc.”

The actual experiments yielded:

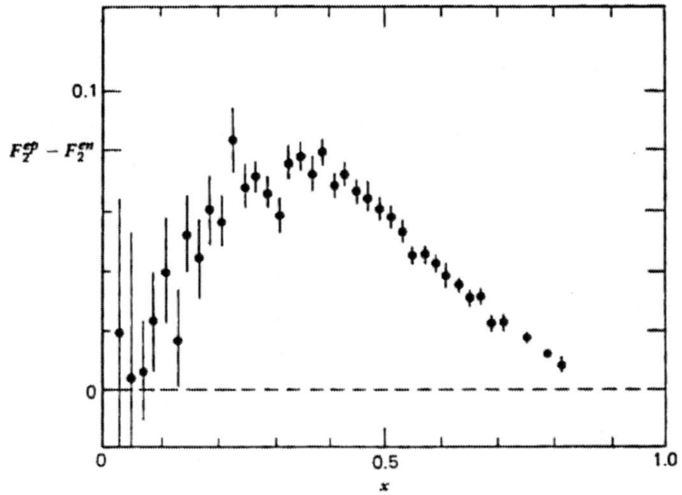

The difference $F_2^{ep} - F_2^{en}$ as a function of x, as measured in deep inelastic scattering. Data are from the Stanford Linear Accelerator.

Figure 42. From "Quarks and Leptons" by Francis Halzen and Alan D, Martin © 1984 "This material is reproduced with permission of John Wiley and Sons, Inc."

To have a complete analogy with the chemical atom, the only missing item is an analogy for electric charge. Based on work done by Greenberg in 1965, Han and Nambu proposed "colour" as the charge of the strong interaction.The complete analogy beween the chemical elements as atoms for the electromagnetic interaction and the nucleon, Δ. Λ, Σ, Ξ and Ω^- as atoms for the strong interaction is then:

The term "colour" is used for the charge corresponding to the strong interaction for the following reasons: A baryon contains three quarks each of a different "colour" charge. That is a baryon will contain a "red" charged quark, a "blue" charged quark and a "green" charged quark. Just as red light, blue light and green light (primary colours) combine to yield white light. The analogous combination of a "red" charged quark, a "blue" charged quark and a "green" charged quark is a baryon that is neutrally charge as far as the strong interaction is concerned. Mesons contain a quark and an anti-quark. The analogy is black – absence of colour. Mesons are also neutral as far as the strong interaction is concerned.

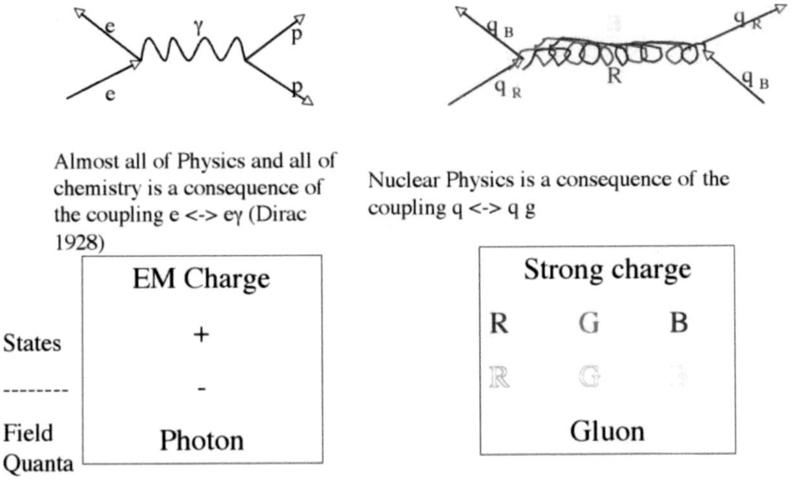

Figure 43.

It should be noted that a fourth quark, the "charm" or c quark [charge 2/3] had been proposed in 1964 separately by Hara; Amati; Bjorken and Glashow but largely ignored. The first serious reason for the existence of such a oarticle, the GIM (Glashow,Illiopoulos, Maiani mechanism. Without the GIM mechanism, a calculation for the decay of the K meson (which contains a d quark and an anti s quark) into two muons as given by:

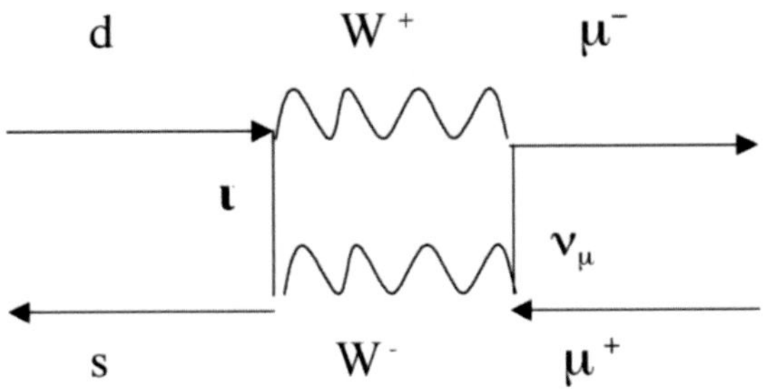

Figure 44.

Is 4 orders of magnitude too large. If there is, however a c quark, the u quark can be replaced by its counterpart the c quark. The K meson can then also decay according to the diagram:

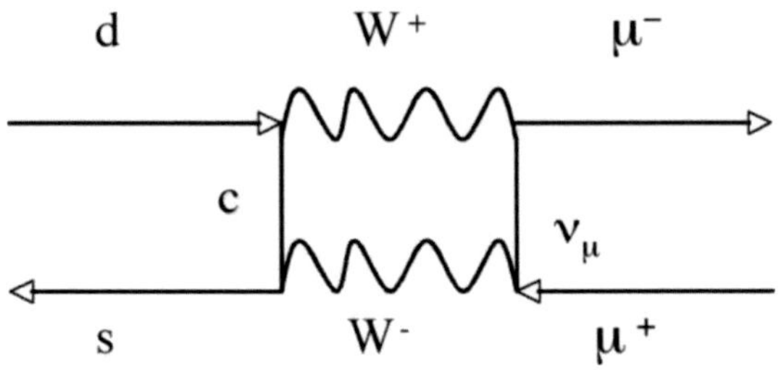

Figure 45.

This second diagram almost entirely cancels the original diagram yielding a result in accordance with the experimental value.

In the summer of 1974 Mary Gaillard, Ben Lee, and Jonathan Rosner circulated a preprint on charm. One possibility considered was the production of a vector (spin=1) particle with "hidden charm" (composition is c**c**, **c** is the antiparticle of the c quark). In the published version in Reviews of Modern Physics a "note added in proof" as long as the original paper discusses the J/ψ particle as this predicted particle.

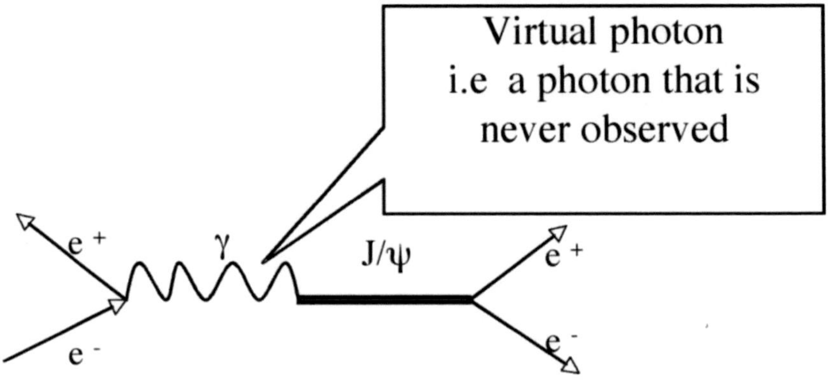

Figure 46.

The J/ψ particle had been discovered in the fall of 1974. It had unusual properties. It was very massive, but it took a long time to decay. A massive particle has many possible particles that it can decay into. Consequently, it normally would rapidly decay into one of these many possible particles by the strong interaction. Thus the Δ containing u and d quarks just like the nucleon rapidly decays into the nucleon. The least massive particles carrying the strange quark cannot decay by the strong interaction into the nucleon which contains only u and d quarks. Eventually, the strange quark decays by the weak interaction into a d quark.

The experimentalists were dubious of the notion of charm. Jerry Rosen of Northwestern stated "nature does not repeat itself". (The notion was that the charm quark was a repeat of the strange quark.) Panofsky, president of the American Physics Society and Director of SLAC stated end of January 1975 "there is no one interpretation that is remotely convincing…The charm quark interpretation is the simplest and perhaps the least defective…it is likely that the correct interpretation will be something else" [This was a very exciting meeting. I like the other theorists had been trying my best to understand this new development. On my way to the meeting, I had stopped at Indiana University where I had been invited to give a seminar by Don Lichtenberg. Continuing my journey with Don, I worked out some calculations, which I discussed with Don at our hotel rooms. On the way home, I completed a paper on the airplane, which was subsequently published.] The mystery had deepened as a repetition of the ψ, the ψ' had been discovered.

Subsequent to this meeting, De Rujula and Glashow, Appelquist, De Rujula, Politzer and Glashow, and Eichten et. al. made further use of the analogy between the chemical atom and the an atom based upon the strong interaction containing quarks. The Hydrogen atom contains a negatively-charged electron and a positively-charged proton. If instead of the proton, you have a positron, the combination called "positronium" will exist as long as the wave corresponding to the electron and the wave corresponding to the positron are sufficiently distant from each other. This occurs if positronium has extra energy. (It is said to be in an excited state.) The positronium "atom" will shed it's extra energy by emitting photons. The spectrum of states for positronium had been long known. The idea of De Rujula and Glashow, Appelquist, De Rujula, PolitzerandGlashow, and Eichten et. al. was to use the analogy of c**c** to $e^+ e^-$ (positronium) to predict 5 states between ψ and ψ'. When these were subsequently found, the consensus was that the ψ particle was indeed made up of a charm quark and an anticharm quark.

Chapter 10

SYMMETRIES AND FIELDS

.

Quantum Mechanically, interactions between matter are described by a mathematical entity called a Lagrangian. Conserved quantities are associated with symmetries of the Lagrangian.

To preserve local symmetry you must introduce a photon (Electricity and Magnetism) W or Z (weak interaction) gluon (strong interaction) or graviton (gravity). See Noether's theorem described below. The quantum version of Maxwell's Classical theory of electricity and Magnetism utilizing particles such as electrons and photons is called Quantum Electrodynamics. (QED)

The analogy between an atom based upon electrodynamics and an atom based upon Quantum Chromodynamics (QCD) [the name that began to be used for the physics of the strong interaction] is not exact. Chemical atoms contain very light electrons and a heavy nucleus sort of like a powerful central government and lightweight citizens.

The nucleon (proton or neutron) contains three equally massive pointlike quarks (democracy). The electrons are bound to the nucleus through an exchange of photons with the protons in the nucleus. The quarks are bound to each other through an exchange of gluons with each other. Photons have no charge and there is only one type of photon.

Gluons have combinations of three charges ("colours"). There are in all eight kinds of charged gluons. Because of their charges the gluons interact with each other.

It is the charge on a particle that gives rise to the photons and gluons.

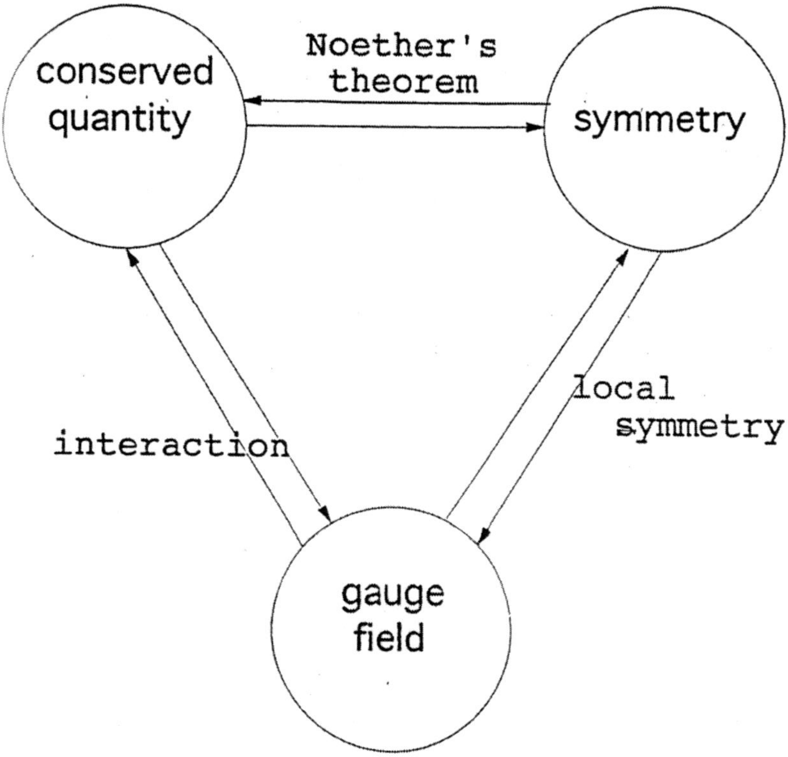

Figure 47.

The conserved quantity in the above diagram is the charge. According to a beautiful theorem of Emmy Noether, a conserved quantity always corresponds to a symmetry of nature.

1) Quarks and Leptons have various charges
2) Due to these charges they exchange gauge fields
3) The exchange of gauge fields between two particles produces a force between the particles

At the age of 18, Emmy Noether wanted to take classes in mathematics at the University of Erlangen, but because she was a woman, the university was only willing to give her permission to audit classes. She entered the University of Göttingen in 1903, again as an auditor, and transferred back to Erlangen in 1904 when the university finally let women enroll. She then took the exam that would permit her to be a doctoral student in mathematics. She passed the test, and after five more years of study, she became only the second woman to be granted a degree in the field of mathematics. The first woman had graduated a year earlier.

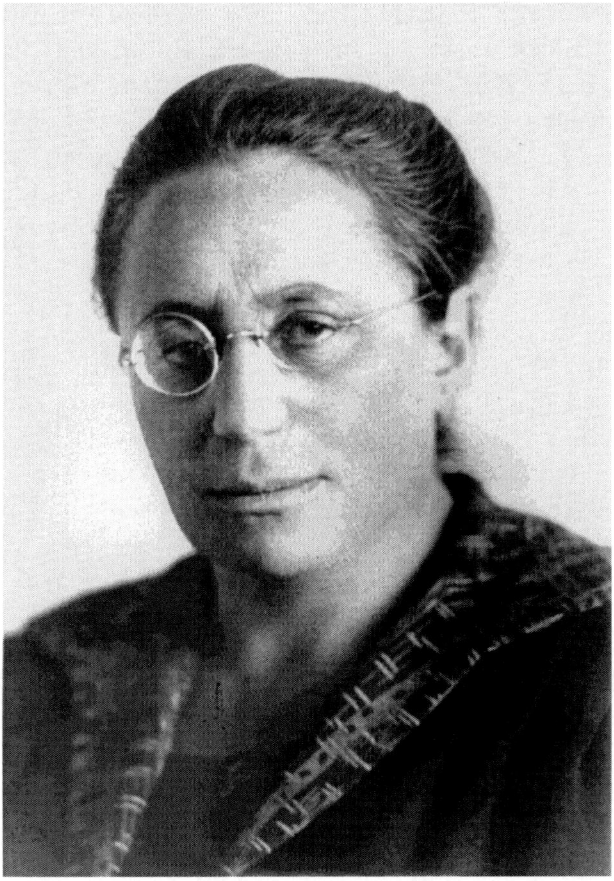

Figure 48. Emmy Noether permission Bryn Mawr College Library.

Noether worked at the Mathematical Institute of Erlangen, without pay or title, from 1908 to 1915. It was during this time that she collaborated with the algebraist Ernst Otto Fischer and started work on the more general, theoretical algebra for which she would later be recognized. In 1915 Felix Klein and David Hilbert at the University of Gottingen were working on refining the mathematics of Einstein's general theory of relativity. They felt that Emmy Noether's expertise could help them in their work and they asked her to come and join then. Since there were no women on the faculty, Noether was unsure if she would be welcome. Indeed, many of the faculty did not want her there, but in the end, she came. In 1918 she proved two theorems that were basic for both general relativity and elementary particle physics. One is the one referred to above as "Noether's Theorem." For a time, Noether was only allowed to lecture under Hilbert's name, as his assistant. Hilbert and Albert Einstein interceded for her, and in 1919 she obtained permission to lecture in her own right. Her reputation grew and soon students traveled from as far as Russia to study with her. Many went on to become great mathematicians themselves and they credited Noether for her part in teaching them to teach themselves.

In 1928-29 she was a visiting professor at the University of Moscow. In 1930, she taught at Frankfurt. The International Mathematical Congress in Zurich asked her to give a plenary lecture in 1932, and in the same year she was awarded the prestigious Ackermann-Teubner Memorial Prize in mathematics. In 1933, Hitler and the Nazis came into power in Germany. The Nazis demanded that all Jews be thrown out of the universities. Noether moved to the United States, accepting a position at Bryn Mawr College. She also lectured at the Institute for Advanced Study in Princeton. In April 1935 she had surgery to remove a uterine tumor and died from a postoperative infection at the age of 53.

Einstein's obituary notice of Emmy Noether in the New York Times (May 5, 1935):

To the Editor of The New York Times:

The efforts of most human-beings are consumed in the struggle for their daily bread, but most of those who are, either through fortune or some special gift, relieved of this struggle are largely absorbed in further improving their worldly lot. Beneath the effort directed toward the accumulation of worldly goods lies all too frequently the illusion that this is the most substantial and desirable end to be achieved; but there is, fortunately, a minority composed of those who recognize early in their lives that the most beautiful and satisfying experiences open to humankind are not derived from the outside, but are bound up with the development of the individual's own feeling, thinking and acting. The genuine artists, investigators and thinkers have always been persons of this kind. However inconspicuously the life of these individuals runs its course, none the less the fruits of their endeavors are the most valuable contributions which one generation can make to its successors.

Within the past few days a distinguished mathematician, Professor Emmy Noether, formerly connected with the University of Göttingen and for the past two years at Bryn Mawr College, died in her fifty-third year. In the judgment of the most competent living mathematicians, Fräulein Noether was the most significant creative mathematical genius thus far produced since the higher education of women began. In the realm of algebra, in which the most gifted mathematicians have been busy for centuries, she discovered methods which have proved of enormous importance in the development of the present-day younger generation of mathematicians. Pure mathematics is, in its way, the poetry of logical ideas. One seeks the most general ideas of operation which will bring together in simple, logical and unified form the largest possible circle of formal relationships. In this effort toward logical beauty spiritual formulas are discovered necessary for the deeper penetration into the laws of nature.

Born in a Jewish family distinguished for the love of learning, Emmy Noether, who, in spite of the efforts of the great Göttingen mathematician, Hilbert, never reached the academic standing due her in her own country, none the less surrounded herself with a group of students and investigators at Göttingen, who have already become distinguished as teachers and investigators. Her unselfish, significant work over a period of many years was rewarded by the new rulers of Germany with a dismissal, which cost her the means of maintaining her simple life and the opportunity to carry on her mathematical studies. Farsighted friends of science in this country were fortunately able to make such arrangements at Bryn Mawr College and at Princeton that she found in America up to the day of her death not only colleagues who esteemed her friendship but grateful pupils whose enthusiasm made her last years the happiest and perhaps the most fruitful of her entire career.

ALBERT EINSTEIN. Princeton University, May 1, 1935.

The life of Emmy Noether exemplifies what is beautiful and also what is sad about life on Earth. We struggle sometimes against incredible odds. If we are lucky, we accomplish something of worth. Nonetheless, when we finally feel we are safe death can unexpectedly take us. My first wife (Judy Kalman) did not have to struggle against Nazi Germany. Indeed she was a teacher of the holocaust, but she also had her problems. When she was a teenager (18), she wrote that it would be terrible to have reached 55 and not have something meaningful to do. Only at age 40 was she able to begin teaching and then only part time.. Around this time, she wrote an imagined piece based upon her experiences that included the following:

> Sit down,", he said, with a smile that barely showed his teeth. He was a short man, on the verge of rotundity in face and form, but his face belied the accepted conviction that a round face betokened a jolly temperament; his small eyes glittered meanly, and his mouth, corners curved upward, suggesting more a sense of self-satisfied power than a benign view of and generosity toward the world around him.
>
> "Thank you, but I prefer to stand," I answered, while positioning myself as upright as possible, in the middle of his line of vision.
>
> "As you will. I brought you here this morning (not too early, was it?) to discuss your resumé. You've been here in this department as part-time faculty for some time. You've taught our very basic writing courses, and I see you've given some sort of workshops occasionally at some teaching conference which you seem to have attended religiously. You have, of course, received your Masters degree, but I see you are having a little trouble working on your doctorate. You've switched universities, haven't you? Not a good sign, not a good sign at all, I'm afraid. And then, there is the matter of your student evaluations. Your students do seem to like your style; they mention your sense of humour a number of times, and also your mothering instinct, but of course, that doesn't seem to translate into higher marks, does it? I mean, being a mother is fine, but it isn't all that is needed to teach in an academic setting, is it?

Eventually at age 50 she received a full time position and was tenured before her death at age 60. During these last ten years of her life, she achieved her goal of doing something meaningful, teaching a holocaust literature course that touched many lives. The course was reported in major features in The Momtreal Gazette, The Canadian Jewish News, The Suburban and The Westmount Examiner.

One thing that the premature death of my first wife taught me is that you should never postpone anything important. So after a summer, when I felt absolutely numb and an autumn, where I felt alone and unneeded (despite my six month old grandson, and the kind efforts of my two sons, daughter-in-law and many friends and family) I decided that I could not wait any longer to start this book. If you put off a task, you may never complete it.

Chapter 11

HOW DOES THE FORCE BETWEEN PARTICLES TAKE PLACE THROUGH THE EXCHANGE OF PHOTONS OR GLUONS?

You exert a force to stop a moving tennis ball causing the ball to reverse directions according to the received acceleration

F=ma (Newton's 2nd law)

Simultaneously, the ball pushes back on the racquet and the racquet in turn pushes back on your hand.

(Newton's 3rd law)

What keeps a body moving at constant speed in the absence of a force? It is a combination of the body's mass (m) and its speed (v). This combination is called the momentum (p):

Momentum $p = mv$

Newton originally wrote his second law saying that a change in momentum produces a force. Photons and gluons carry momentum with them. This produces an effective force on both the particle that emits the photon or gluon and the particle that receives it.

Think of it this way. Suppose you and a partner decide to exercise by throwing a heavy medicine ball to each other. What happens when you throw the ball? (You stagger backwards – the medicine ball has a mass and you give it a speed- thus the ball moves away from you carrying off an amount of momentum.

Momentum is conserved so that you lose an amount of momentum equal to the amount carried off by the ball. The force you experience arises according to Newton from your loss of momentum.) What happens when your partner catches the ball? (Your partner is thrown backwards. According to Newton, this arises because of the momentum in the ball, which you acquire when you catch the ball.)

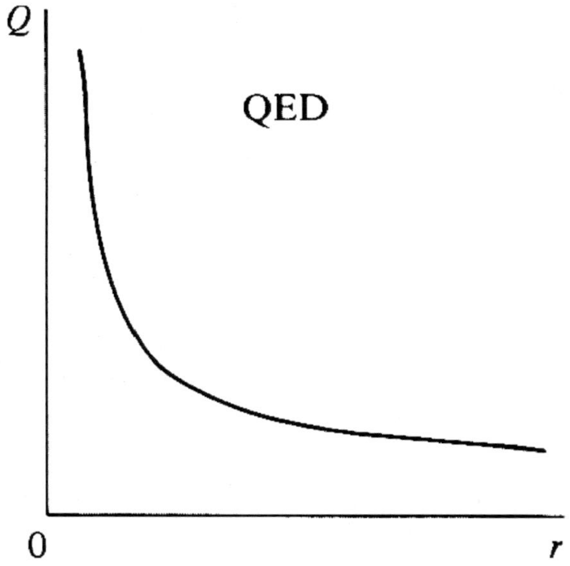

Figure 49.

Looking at the above diagram we see that the effective charge of a particle increases as you get closer to the particle. The size of the charge governs the strength of the interaction. So the forcc between two positively charged protons increases as they get closer to each other.

Politzer. Gross and Wilczek won the Nobel prize for the discovery of asymptotic freedom – that the effective colour charge in quantum chromodynamics (QCD) changes in a very different manner to the electric charge in QED:

Recollections of Ne'eman 1981

I was doing my best to find derivations that would not depend on an understanding of the dynamics of quarks, since these appeared incomprehensible. Quarks had to be very weakly bound·

but they also had to be very tightly bound, since they wouldn't come out even at very high energies!

Until 1968, I tended to regard quarks as a basic field that on the other hand had no direct manifestation. The SLAC "deep-inelastic" electron scattering experiments on nucleons revealed scaling, indicating the actual existence of point-charges within the extended nucleon. With more experiments, those "partons" looked moore and more like quarks. Quarks are thus observable, provided you "look" inside the nucleon. However, it was only after the renormalization of Yang-Mills theory, that G. 't Hooft himself, H. D. Politzer, and D. J. Gross and F. Wilczek discovered asymptotic freedom. This was just the kind of dynamics we now required: actual quarks, bound by a spring-like force roughly proportional to distance. Close quarks are thus weakly bound,

Figure 50.

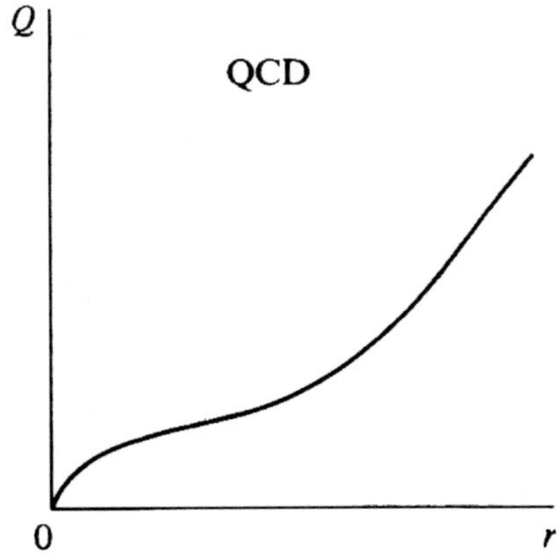

Figure 51.

When quarks are very close to each other, the force between quarks is small. As the quarks move away from each other the force between the gluons alters the nature of the force.

The force now resembles that of a spring. When the quarks are close together, the quarks experience very little force between each other, a phenomena called asymptotic freedom.

At large distance the quarks strain against a springy force that pushes them back with ever increasing strength. Paradoxically, the further a quark moves away from another quark, the stronger the force pushing the quark back towards the other quark.

The effective "colour" charge drops to zero as two quarks come close together. It is this phenomenon that is called asymptotic freedom. Quarks that are very close together act like free particles. In QED as particles move apart, the force diminishes. In QCD as the quarks move apart, the force markedly increases. For this reason, quarks can never escape outside of the nucleon. Free quarks can never be observed outside of a baryon or a meson.

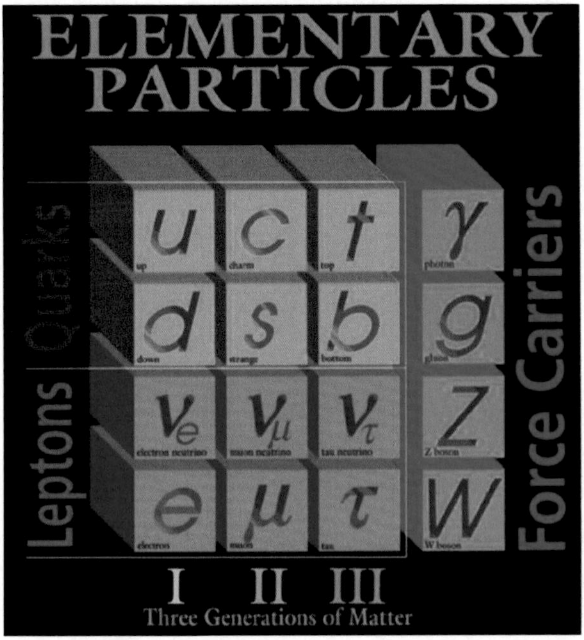

Figure 52.

Eventually two more quarks were observed – the b quark and the t quark. With these discoveries, quarks occurred in three generations just like the leptons. Cosmologists predicted that there are no more than three generations of quarks and leptons. In 1980, experiments with accelerators led high energy physicists to the same conclusion. Just as in the case of the neutrino observations and the telescopic observations of supernovae, we again see a close connection between the very small and the large scale in the universe. Such connection are at the heart of our understanding of how the universe unfolds. To learn more, it is time that we look at our understanding of the universe itself. We had left our examinations of astronomy with the change from our view of the solar system as Earth centred to a view that the Earth and all the planets orbit around the Sun.

Part II. The Cosmos

Chapter 12

ON GALAXIES

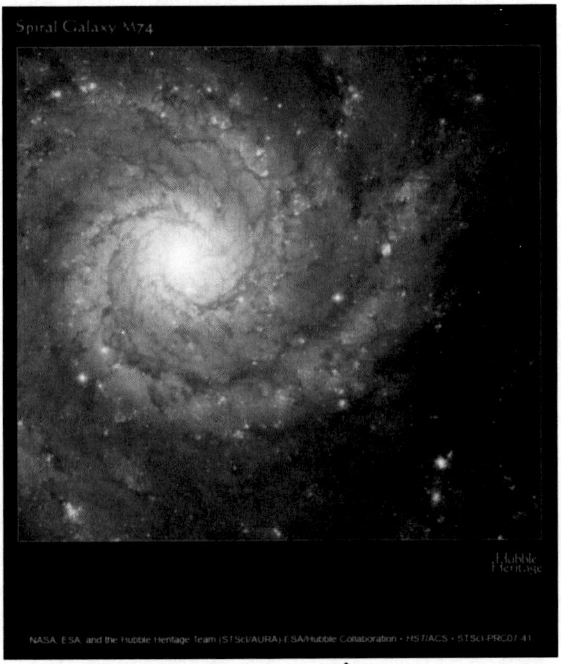

Figure 53.

The first reliable measurement of the size of the Milky Way Galaxy was made in 1917 by Harlow Shapley. Instead of a relatively small system with the Sun near its centre, as had previously been thought, Shapley found that our galaxy was immense, with the Sun nearer the edge than the centre. He determined that it has a radius of about 50,000 light-years and that the Sun lies about 30,000 light-years from the centre. His values have held up remarkably well over the years.

Not only is our planet, Earth, not the centre of the universe, but our star, the Sun, is not anywhere near the centre of our galaxy, the Milky Way. Our galaxy is an immense spiral system consisting of about 100 billion stars. It takes its name from the Milky Way, the irregular luminous band of stars and gas clouds at the center of our galaxy that stretches across the sky.

In 1920 the National Academy of Sciences at the Smithsonian Institution in Washington, D.C. organized a "Great Debate" featuring talks by Shapley and Heber Curtis. Shapley argued his view about the size of our galaxy, a view confirmed by later evidence.

Curtis argued for a smaller Milky Way Galaxy, and for the extragalactic nature of the spiral nebulas. Although Curtis was wrong about the size of our galaxy, he was right and Shapley was wrong about the nebulae.

Shapley argued that the apparent faint novas in M31 (the Andromeda Galaxy), were ordinary novas, for otherwise they would have been extremely luminous. Actually, these indeed are examples of supernovae, whose existence were to become clear a few years later

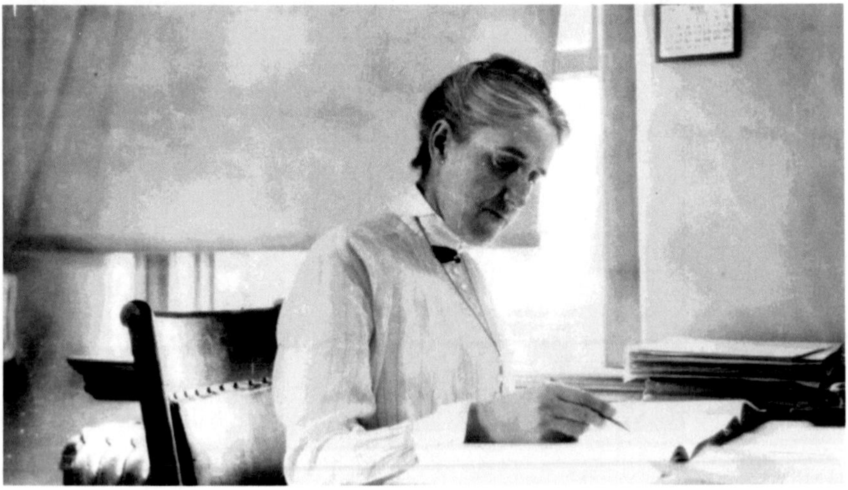

Figure 54. Henrietta Swan Leavitt. The photo is part of the Shapley Collection of the AIP Emilio Segrè Visual Archives.

During her career, Henrietta Leavitt discovered more than 2,400 variable stars, about half of the known total in her day. These stars change from bright to dim and back fairly regularly. Leavitt's work with variable stars led to her most important contribution to the field: the Cepheid variable period-luminosity relationship. Using this, astronomers only needed to know the period of a Cepheid variable to figure out how bright, and therefore how far away it was.

The existence of other galaxies became clear through the work of Edwin Hubble in examining 15 stars in the small, irregular cloudlike object NGC 6822 that varied in luminosity. After considerable effort, Hubble determined that 11 of the stars that he was examining were in fact Cepheid variables, with properties indistinguishable from those of normal Cepheids in the Milky Way Galaxy and in the Magellanic Clouds. Their periods ranged from 12 to 64 days, and they were all very faint, much fainter than their Magellanic counterparts. Using Leavitt's relationship, Hubble determined that NGC 6822 was well outside the limits of the Milky Way Galaxy and must be a galaxy on its own.

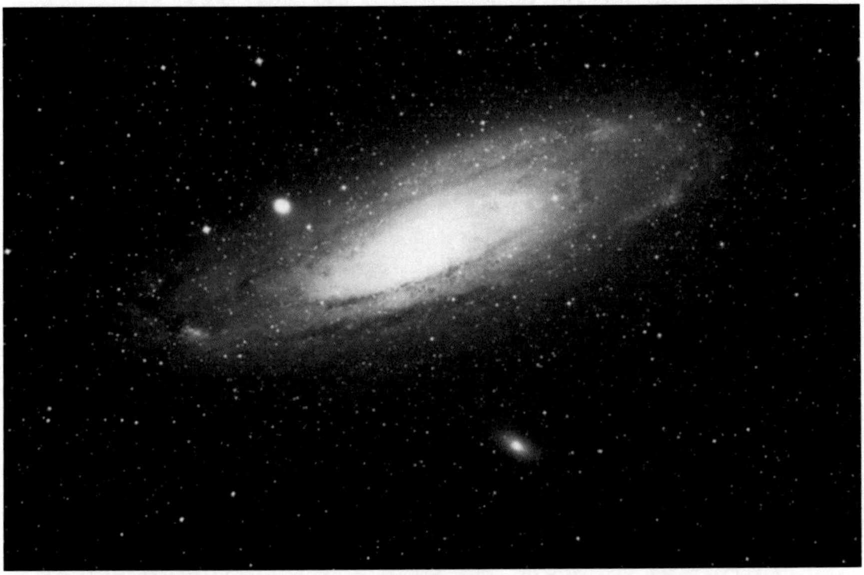

Figure 55. Photo of M31, Andromeda Galaxy, from bedfordnights.com by permission of the author, John Lanoue.

In 1929 Hubble published a study on M31, the great Andromeda Nebula that provided evidence that M31 is a giant stellar system like the Milky Way Galaxy. In 1944 Walter Baade announced the successful resolution into stars of the centre of the Andromeda Galaxy, M31, and its two elliptical companions, M32 and NGC 205. Our Milky Way Galaxy and the larger Andromeda Galaxy are the dominant galaxies in a local cluster of galaxies called the Local Group. The Local Group contains seven reasonably prominent galaxies and perhaps another two dozen less conspicuous members Another spiral in the Local Group--M33, Hubble type Sc and luminosity class III--is notable, but the rest are intermediate to dwarf systems, either irregulars or ellipticals..

The size of the Local Group is larger only by about 50 percent than the 2 million light-years separating the Milky Way system and the Andromeda galaxy, and the centre of mass lies roughly halfway between these two giants.

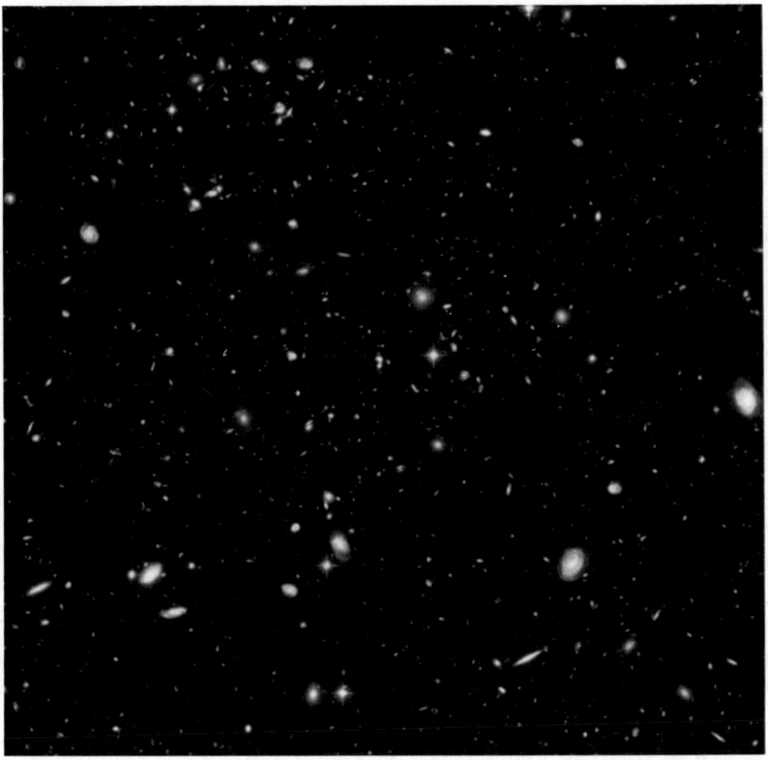

Figure 56. This picture shows the positions of over 2 million galaxies spread across a tenth of the sky. Note that the universe is fairly uniform on large scales. NASA and STScI.

Astronomers have moved from a limited one-galaxy Cosmos to an immense vastness of space populated by billions of galaxies, mostly grander in size and design than the Milky Way system had once been thought to be. The largest scale on which the mass density has been measured with any precision is that of superclusters. A supercluster is an aggregate of several clusters of galaxies, extending over about 10 million parsecs (Mpc). (One parsec equals 3.26 light-years. A light year is the distance which light traveling at 300,000 kilometers/second covers in a year. In the Milky Way Galaxy, wherein the Earth is located, distances to remote stars are measured in terms of kiloparsecs). Our local supercluster is an extended distribution of galaxies centered on the Virgo cluster, some 10-20 Mpc distant. Our Local Group is an outlying member of the Virgo Supercluster.

So our Sun is nowhere near the centre of our Milky Way Galaxy. Our Milky Way Galaxy is not the largest galaxy in our Local Group of Galaxies and Our Local Group of Galaxies is an outlying member of the Virgo Supercluster. There are roughly 100 billion stars in our galaxy and billions of galaxies in the universe. *Did all of this awesome immensity come into being by chance? Atheists insist that it did. Why? Because they don't believe in God so it had to have come about in that manner.*

Chapter 13

THE UNIVERSE IS EXPANDING

Did the universe have a beginning? In studying the galaxies, Hubble made his second remarkable discovery--namely, that these galaxies are apparently receding from the Milky Way and that the further away they are, the faster they are receding (1927).

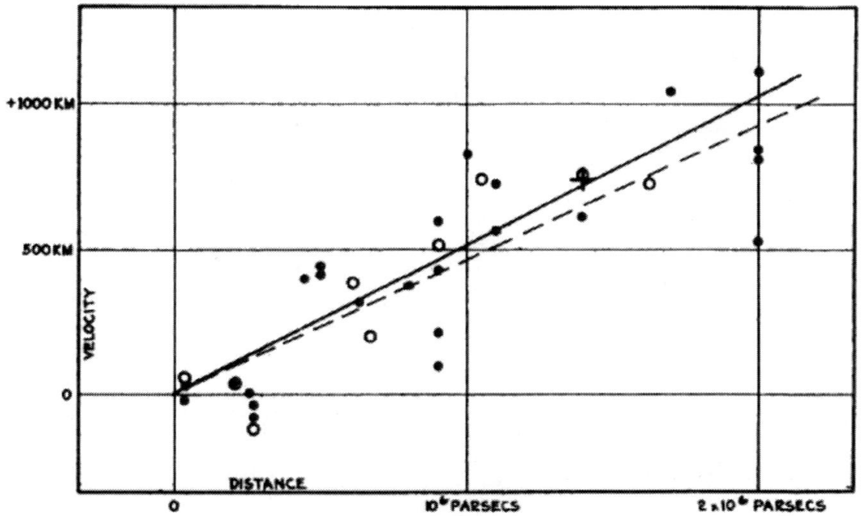

FIGURE 1

Velocity-Distance Relation among Extra-Galactic Nebulae.

Figure 57. From Hubble, E. (1929). "A Relation between Distance and Radial Velocity among Extra-Galactic Nebulae." Proceedings of the National Academy of Science 15: 168-173.

Einstein's Special Theory of Relativity predicts that the wavelength of light emanating from sources traveling at relative speeds that are significant fractions of the speed of light will exhibit a significant increase (shift toward the red end of the spectrum). As early as 1912 V. M. Slipher, working at the Lowell Observatory had noted that many of the spiral nebulae were redshifted. However, until Hubble established that nebulae were at large distances from Earth, there was no obvious interpretation of this information.

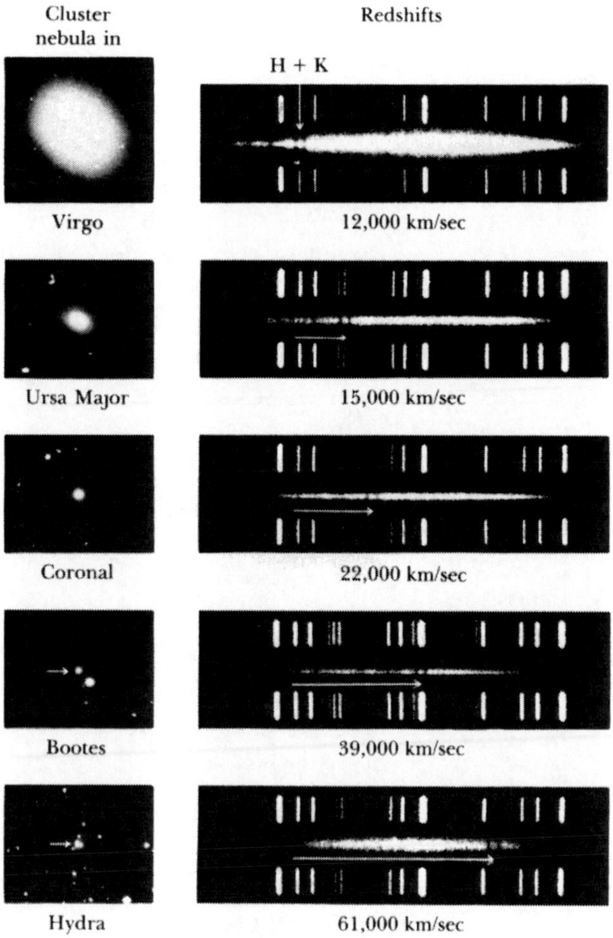

Figure 58. Photographs from the Mount Wilson and Palomar observatories. Reproduced with permission A. P. French and by the Massachusetts Institute of Technology, copyright 1968, 1966.

Because galaxies generally speaking have motions within clusters, a clearer picture emerges if we consider only galaxies at the centre of super clusters. Examples are shown in Figure 58. The H+K is a distinctive marker in stellar spectrum. The faster the relative speed of a galaxy compared to us, the more this gap is shifted towards the red. A substitution of the position of this gap into a simple formula derived within Special Relativity yields the relative speeds of our galaxies. We can then plot the speeds and distances of the observed galaxies:

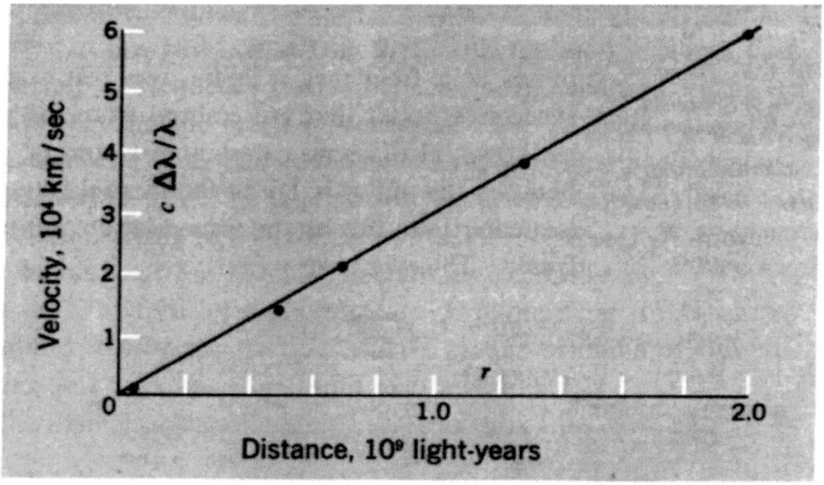

Galaxy in:	*Velocity,* $\times\ 10^4$ *km/sec*	*Distance, light-years*
Virgo	0.12	0.4×10^8
Ursa Major	1.40	5.0×10^8
Corona Borealis	2.14	7.0×10^8
Boötes	3.90	1.3×10^9
Hydra	6.10	2.0×10^9

Figure 59. Reproduced with permission A. P. French and by the Massachusetts Institute of Technology, copyright 1968, 1966.

Hubble's observations made it clear that the universe is expanding. Subsequent to this 1927 publication, there arose two views of this expansion. One of these was that the universe had expanded from an original creation a long time ago. (A straightforward examination of the graph yields the timeframe. Modern estimates, using more precise distance measurements, place the value of H (Hubble's constant), the slope of the straight line in the graph to be between 15 and 30 km (9.3 and 18.6 miles) per second per 1,000,000 light-years. The reciprocal of Hubble's constant lies between 10 billion and 20 billion years, and this cosmic time scale serves as an approximate measure of the age of the universe.)

A second view is that of a steady-state universe. According to this view, the universe is always expanding but maintaining a constant average density, matter being continuously created to form new stars and galaxies at the same rate that old ones become unobservable as a consequence of their increasing distance and velocity of recession. A steady-state universe has no beginning or end in time; and from any point within it the view on the grand scale i.e., the average density and arrangement of galaxies is the same. Galaxies of all possible ages are intermingled. The theory was first put forward by Sir James Jeans in about 1920 and again in revised form in 1948 by Hermann Bondi and Thomas Gold. It's final form was developed by Sir Fred Hoyle.

George Gamow modified the theory of the expanding-universe theory that had been advanced by Friedmann, Edwin Hubble, and Georges LeMaître and named his version the "big bang." In a paper called "The Origin of Chemical Elements" (1948), he and Ralph Alpher attempted to explain the distribution of chemical elements throughout the universe. According to the theory, after the big bang, atomic nuclei were built up by the successive capture of neutrons by the initially formed pairs and triplets. Gamow had a great sense of humour and at one point convinced the future Nobel laureate Hans Bethe to coauthor a paper so that it could be referred to as the Alpher-Bethe-Gamow paper. In explaining his ideas to the general public, Gamow used the crude analogy of a piece of grass covered land that had in "primitive times" been used by a farmer as a cow pasture. How, Gamow asked, could you tell if this had actually happened. Gamow's answer was that you should look for "prehistoric" cowpats. To prove the big bang theory, we also look for "cowpats". After the original explosion, matter existed as a high temperature plasma. No atoms existed. In this ionized state of electrons, protons and neutrons, matter continuously absorbed and emitted radiation. When the plasma cooled sufficiently, it condensed into atoms and ceased to absorb and emit radiation. Effectively, the radiation that was present became disconnected with the matter in the universe.

Chapter 14

EVIDENCE FOR THE BIG BANG

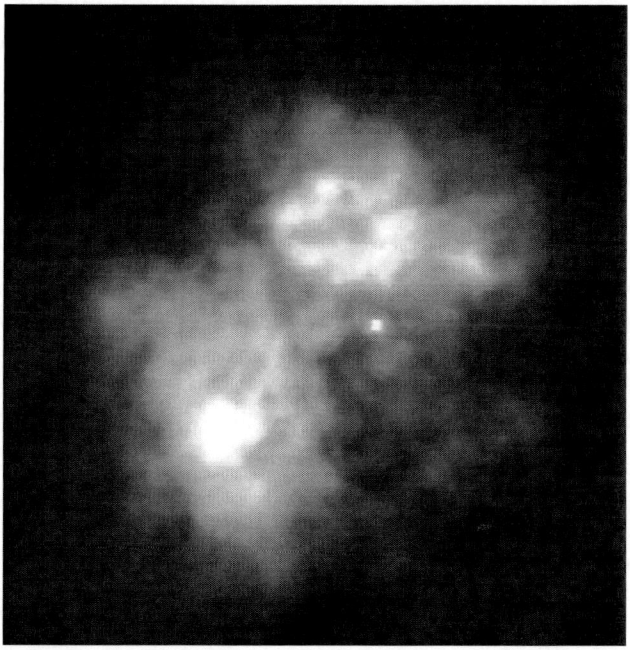

Figure 60. Papillon Nebula N159-5 NASA, ESA, and The Hubble Heritage Team (STScI/AURA) STScI-1999-23.

Every body in the universe emits radiation (See section - Properties of radiation emitted by all bodies.) :

- continuous spectra

- all bodies at the same temperature have the same spectra
- as the temperature changes, the peak in the curve shifts.

In the early universe, there was a soup of charged high energy particles (plasma) that constantly radiated energy and then reabsorbed the energy. At times of around t= 100,000 years nuclei had formed but temperatures were still too high for electrons to attach to them to form atoms. The cloud of 'hot' electrons formed a plasma that filled the universe. Electrons in such a plasma would constantly absorb and reemit all the radiation. The universe cooled, until around three hundred thousand years after its beginning, matter condensed into atoms. The temperature at that time was 3000 K about the same temperature as a red-giant star's surface. Thus the peak of the emitted radiation was in the visible spectrum. Because atoms are electrically neutral, they no longer absorbed the surrounding radiation. This primordial radiation is still with us. The peak of the radiation continued to change as the universe cooled (see figure 10 p.24). It is now centred in the microwave region. For this reason, the radiation is now called the Cosmic Microwave Background Radiation (CMBR).

In the early 1960s physicists at Princeton University, N.J., as well as in the Soviet Union, took up the problem again and began to build a microwave receiver that might detect, in the words of the Belgian cleric and cosmologist Georges Lemaître, "the vanished brilliance of the origin of the worlds."

The actual discovery of the relic radiation from the primeval fireball, however, occurred by accident. In experiments conducted in connection with the first Telstar communication satellite, two scientists, Arno Penzias and Robert Wilson, of the Bell Telephone Laboratories, Holmdel, N.J., measured excess radio noise that seemed to come from the sky in a completely isotropic fashion. When they consulted Bernard Burke of the Massachusetts Institute of Technology, Boston, about the problem, Burke realized that Penzias and Wilson had most likely found the cosmic background radiation that Robert H. Dicke, P.J.E. Peebles, and their colleagues at Princeton were planning to search for. Put in touch with one another, the two groups published simultaneously in 1965 papers detailing the prediction and discovery of a universal thermal radiation field with a temperature of about 3 K.

The Cosmic microwave background radiation is a relic of the early universe background radiation that decoupled from matter when the universe was 350,000 years old. This afterglow of the Big Bang contains 99% of all the radiant energy of the universe, but at the surface of the earth, it is still fainter than the thermal radiation emitted by the earth.

If you attach your TV to an ordinary antenna (not cable or satellite) and look at a channel for which there is no local station, about 1% of the static is due to the CMBR.

It Is Now Known That 1/4 of the Mass of the Universe Is He^4

The early universe contained only light elements perhaps only hydrogen. Stars normally produce light elements by fusion — elements lighter than iron.

The first nuclear reaction to occur in stars is the conversion of hydrogen into helium. Considering the relative amounts of helium and heavier elements, observations indicate that the total mass of helium may be ten times greater than that of the heavier elements; if all elements other than hydrogen have been produced in stars. As stars evolve, however, the conversion of hydrogen into helium is followed by the conversion of helium into heavier elements. The possible chemical composition of a highly evolved star is a series of layers of different chemical composition. A very special type of mass loss would be required to expel 10 times as much helium as heavy elements from these different layers into interstellar space.

It is also difficult to see how the full amount of helium could have been produced. If a quarter of the galactic mass, originally hydrogen, has been converted into helium, it can be shown that essentially all of the mass must have passed through at least one generation of massive stars. The total energy release under such a circumstance would imply that the Galaxy was very much more luminous in the past--one hundred times more luminous for the first 10 percent of its lifetime, for example.

There are complicated big-bang theories but there is only one arbitrary quantity in the simplest theory, and assignment of some arbitrary specified value to any one of the unknowns will determine the others. For a wide range of values of the density of the universe specified at some temperature, the chemical composition after the initial phase is a mixture of hydrogen and helium, with between 20 percent and 30 percent by mass in the form of helium. Most studies in recent years has been concerned with trying to decide whether an initial chemical composition devoid of helium or one with 25 percent helium is most likely to be consistent with present observations.

We are all stardust.

Elements heavier than iron are produced by the absorption of neutrons. This can occur in Red Giant stars and super novae explosions

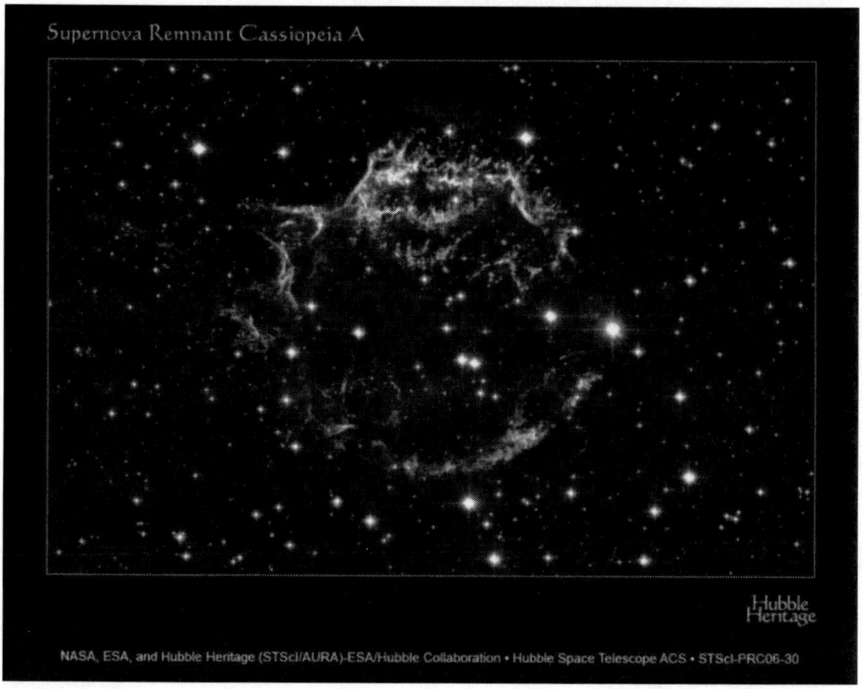

Figure 61.

The star Sanduleak -69 202, out about 169,000 light years in the Large Magellanic Cloud ended its life in a fiery spectacle about 167,000 B.C. (give or take up to a few 1000 years). The light from this explosion arrived at Earth after a journey of 169,000 light years, thus 169,000 years later, on February 23, 1987.

Supernova 1987A [see chapter 8] was the nearest observed supernova since Kepler's Supernova of 1604, which occurred before the invention of the telescope. Supernova 1987A, was one of the most interesting objects for the astrophysicists in the 1980s (some even say of the twentieth century). This supernova first observed Feb 23,1987 probably threw out enough heavy elements to constitute 5 million planets of the size of our Earth.

Ten years after the explosion, the cosmic fireball was large enough —- about one-sixth of a light-year in diameter —- to be resolved from the Earth's orbit with the Hubble Space Telescope. The debris is resolved into two opposing blobs and is dim in the center. The apparent direction of ejection is the same as the short axis of the bright inner ring that surrounds the supernova. This suggests that the explosion is directed out of the plane of the ring. The ring is probably composed of materials lost by the pre-supernova star in the last stages of its evolution. When a new star appeared Oct. 9, 1604 [Kepler's Supernova], observers could use only their eyes to study it. The telescope would not be invented for another four years. A team of modern astronomers has the combined abilities of NASA's Great Observatories, the Spitzer Space Telescope, Hubble Space Telescope and Chandra X-ray Observatory, to analyze the remains in infrared radiation, visible light, and X-rays. The combined image unveils a bubble-shaped shroud of gas and dust, 14 light-years wide and expanding at 6 million kilometers per hour (4 million mph).

Figure 62. This Hubble Space Telescope picture shows Supernova 1987A and its neighborhood. The series of four panels shows the evolution of the SN 1987A debris from February 1994 to February 1996. Material from the stellar interior was ejected into space during the supernova explosion in February 1987. The explosion debris is expanding at nearly 6 million miles per hour.

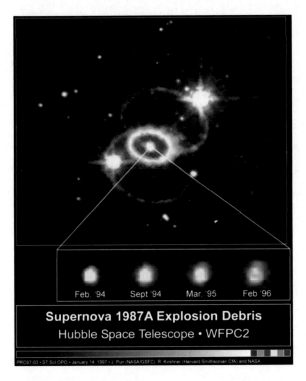

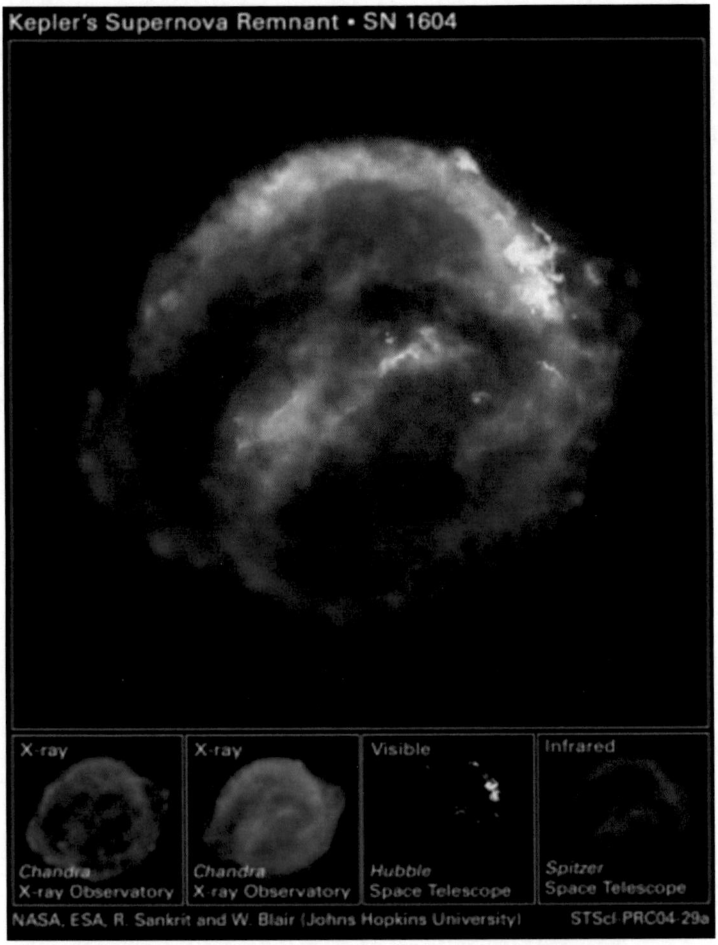

Figure 63.

Observations from each telescope highlight distinct features of the supernova, a fast-moving shell of iron-rich material, surrounded by an expanding shock wave sweeping up interstellar gas and dust.

This is the youngest known supernova remnant in our Milky Way Galaxy, and the strongest extrasolar radio source in the sky. Calculating its expansion back, astronomers have found that the supernova must have blown up around the year 1667.

Measurements of Deuterium at the center of our Milky Way galaxy confirm theoretical models that most deuterium, the heavy isotope of hydrogen containing one proton and one neutron, is primordial (made at the time of the big bang) and not subsequently created in galaxies or stars. A Hofstra-Williams-Colgate-Manchester (UK) team of astronomers have used the National Radio Astronomy Observatory 12-m radio telescope to scan a huge molecular cloud only 30 light years from the galactic center. From their observed ratio of deuterium-to-hydrogen D/H, the researchers (Don Lubowich, Jay Pasachoff, Tom Balonek, and Tom Millar) deduce three things: (1) The D/H ratio is higher than you would expect in the absence of a source of virginal (preexisting- such as at the moment of creation) unprocessed material (high in D, low in heavier elements).

This demonstrates that matter comparatively rich in D is indeed raining down with the cloud onto the plane of our galaxy In other words, the in-falling matter is to the galaxy what comets are to our solar system: specimens of relatively unprocessed, primitive material. (2) For all that, the D/H ratio at the galactic center is lower than in all other places in the galaxy. This is important evidence confirming that D is not made in stars and that what D we see is made by the big bang. (3) From models of D production in quasars, the observed D/H ratio suggests that the Milky Way could not have harbored a quasar for at least a billion years and probably not for four billion years. (Lubowich et al., Nature, 29 June 2000.)

Not just Deuterium (D) but the entire abundance pattern of the light elements D, 3He, 4He, 7Li seen in the most primitive samples of the cosmos conform to the predictions of big bang nucleosynthesis.

Using this data David Schramm and his collaborators determined that the number of neutrino species could be at most 4 and was very likely less than four.

This is a great prediction perhaps of equal importance to the prediction by Gamow of radiation from the early universe.

At the 25th International conference on High Energy Physics (Singapore, 1990), based on the decays of the Z, Carla Jarlskog reported that there would be 2.96±0.06 neutrinos. This confirms Schram's prediction.

(Schramm, David N., American theoretical astrophysicist who was an international leader in the field of cosmology and a distinguished professor (1974-97) at the University of Chicago; by making a cosmic inventory of the material making up the universe, he helped determine that most of the universe consists of unseen and as-yet-unknown forms of matter. He was killed when the plane he was piloting crashed near Denver (b. Oct. 25, 1945--d. Dec. 19, 1997).

SUMMARY OF EVIDENCE FOR THE BIG BANG

The "Big Bang" is supported by three main pieces of evidence – CMBR, the abundance of light elements in the universe and the prediction of the number of generations of quarks and leptons. Because of the strength of the evidence, virtually all scientists abandoned the "Steady State" theory of the universe for the "Big Bang". All of this evidence tells us that the "Big Bang" occurred, but nothing about the absolute beginning. Formation of the lightest nucleus – deuterium (contains one proton and one neutron) occurred roughly 100 seconds after the beginning. But what happened before that?

Chapter 15

BEFORE THE BIG BANG

As we move backwards in time towards the moment of creation, prior to one hundredth of a second, the universe becomes hotter and denser until matter actually changes its phase, that, is it changes its form and properties.

An everyday analogue familiar to all are the phase changes in water.

With increasing temperature we see a succession of phase transitions for water in which its properties change dramatically: the solid phase - ice - melts to the liquid phase - water - and then eventually boils to the gaseous phase - steam. You should notice that steam is 'more symmetric' than water, which is in turn more symmetric than ice. And so it is with matter in our Universe; it begins in a unified or 'symmetric' phase and then passes through a succession of phase transitions until, at lower temperatures, we finally obtain the matter particles with which physicists are familiar today, that is, electrons, protons, neutrons, photons etc.

Electromagnetism is associated with the electric and magnetic forces, that is, phenomena such as electricity and light. It was Maxwell's great achievement at the end of the nineteenth century to unify electric and magnetic effects into one single mathematical theory - electromagnetism.

Weak nuclear force: The weak nuclear force was unified with electromagnetism by Weinberg and Salam in the late seventies, into what is known as electroweak theory.

The mathematical theory of the strong nuclear force is known as quantum chromodynamics (QCD). Models which unify the strong nuclear force with electroweak theory are known as grand unified theories or GUTs.

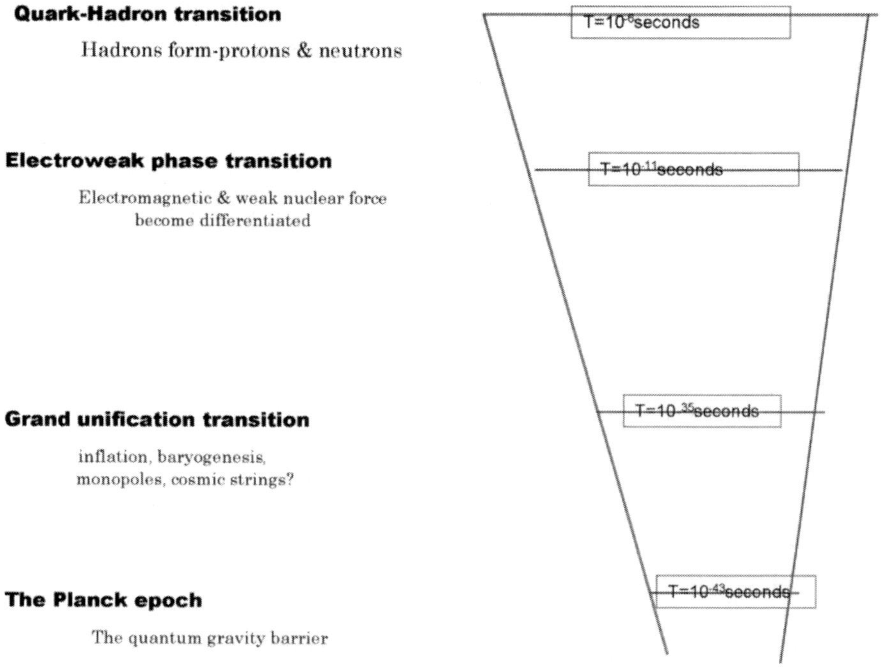

Figure 64. The increase of symmetry in the universe is represented by a unification of the fundamental forces in nature.

Gravity: The weakest force of all - the gravitational force - is not included in the above scheme. The unification of the other fundamental forces with gravity is one of the great intellectual challenges facing theoretical physics. A number of possibilities exist and they are known as TOEs, that is, theories of everything.

Increasing symmetry means that forces that had different strengths become merged with the same strength. and the corresponding particles lose their separate identities. The only difference between the particles are their labels— quantum numbers.

Thus Heisenberg's original idea of the isotropic spin was that if you could neglect the electromagnetic interaction, the neutron and particlc could be regarded as two "states" of the same particle (the nucleon)

In the electroweak merger there are four massless gauge bosons; each corresponding to forces of the same strength and the quarks of each generation become identical. The charge of the u and d quarks are then just labels. Since the only difference between the proton and the neutron are the numbers of u and d quarks, this realizes Heisenbergs idea albeit in a different manner.

At lower temperatures, three of the gauge bosons acquire a mass and the weak interaction decouples from the electromagnetic interaction making the u and d quarks and consequently the proton and the neutron into different particles.

Grand unified theories describe the interactions of quarks and leptons within the same theoretical structure. There is also evidence to suggest that the strengths of the forces do not converge exactly unless new effects come into play at higher energies. One such effect could be a new symmetry called "supersymmetry." A successful GUT will still not include gravity. The problem here is that theorists do not yet know how to formulate a workable quantum field theory of gravity based on the exchange of a hypothesized graviton.

The idea of grand unified theory is to explain the electromagnetic, weak, and strong nuclear forces as a single grand force of nature. The resulting symmetry corresponding to the GUT means that all the particles associated with the basic cluster of the GUT react in the same way.

Since the strong and electroweak forces are unified, it is perhaps not surprising that quarks and neutrons can be found in the same cluster. Because of this "quark" and "lepton" are now just labels and in the Higgs boson cluster we now find strange new entities called leptoquarks, which have both quark and lepton labels. Absorption of such an entity (the X and Y bosons) can change a quark into a lepton and vice versa.

MATTER-ANTIMATTER ASYMMETRY

In the beginning, the universe is dominated by radiation (Gauge Bosons). These bosons can split into particle-antiparticle pairs, but the pairs will recombine into radiation.(Thus the combination has zero lepton and zero baryon number.) As the universe cools, the chance of a gauge boson splitting into a particle-antiparticle pair rapidly diminishes. Nonetheless originally, there is a complete symmetry between matter and antimatter.

If we work out what the universe was like at 10^{-35} seconds (0.00000000000000000000000000000000000 seconds), it turns out that for every billion particle-antiparticle pairs, there was approximately one extra particle. To these few particles, we and the stars owe our existence. Were it not for the infinitesimal initial asymmetry, the universe would consist entirely of radiation.

> We can understand the initial asymmetry and estimate correctly the ratio of matter to radiant energy provided that we have:
>
> A GUT that can change quarks to leptons and leptons to quarks , that is baryon nonconservation
>
> A GUT that has some kind of asymmetry between particle and antiparticle reactions or decay rates.
>
> A universe that cools sufficiently to undergo a phase transition so that the reactions described above no longer take place.

Extraordinary "fine tuning" is needed in so many places. If not for such fine tuning, the world as we know it would not exist. *Why are the laws just right so that this world exists.* Atheists answer that this is one of an infinite number of possible universes and the others do not have the correct properties. This seems like sophistry to me. They do not want to believe in God and will go to any lengths to make fun of believers and to construct tortuous explanations for the existence of the universe..

C and CP

C simply denotes charge conjugation and represents the symmetry between particle and antiparticle. P, or parity like a mirror reverses the direction of particle motion, but preserves its angular momentum. CP thus turns a particle (antiparticle) into antiparticle (particle) with reversed momentum but identical angular momentum. If CP was a symmetry of nature, particle production would always be countered by equal antiparticle production and the universe would consist only of radiation.

In 1956 Lee and Yang realized that C and P separately were violated by the weak interaction. Shortly afterwards, Madam Wu confirmed this experimentally. In 1964 Cronin and Fitch observed CP violation.

Chapter 16

WILL THE UNIVERSE END IN A BIG CRUNCH

The expansion of the universe was faster in the past than it is now. Gravity slows the velocities at which galaxies are flying away from each other. Just as it slows the velocity of a baseball thrown into the air. The motion of the baseball stops at its maximum height. Will the expansion of the universe also come to a halt and start to "fall" back to an eventual "Big Crunch"? To escape this fate the universe has to have more kinetic energy than the total potential energy generated by its own gravitational pull. Hubble's constant tells us the kinetic energy of the universe. The potential energy depends on the density of matter in the universe labeled by the symbol Ω:

$$\Omega = (2/3\Lambda)(c^2/H^2)$$

where …

Λ = Cosmological Constant
c = speed of light
H = Hubble Constant

Ω is a combination of ordinary matter (basically what we see as stars and galaxies) and two other forms that we will discuss "dark matter" and "dark" energy. We will discuss "dark matter" and "dark energy" later.

A 'closed' universe is massive enough that it eventually collapses back onto itself has Ω larger than 1; an 'open' universe, one that expands outwards forever, has Ω less than 1; and a 'flat' universe, perfectly balanced between the two, has Ω = 1.

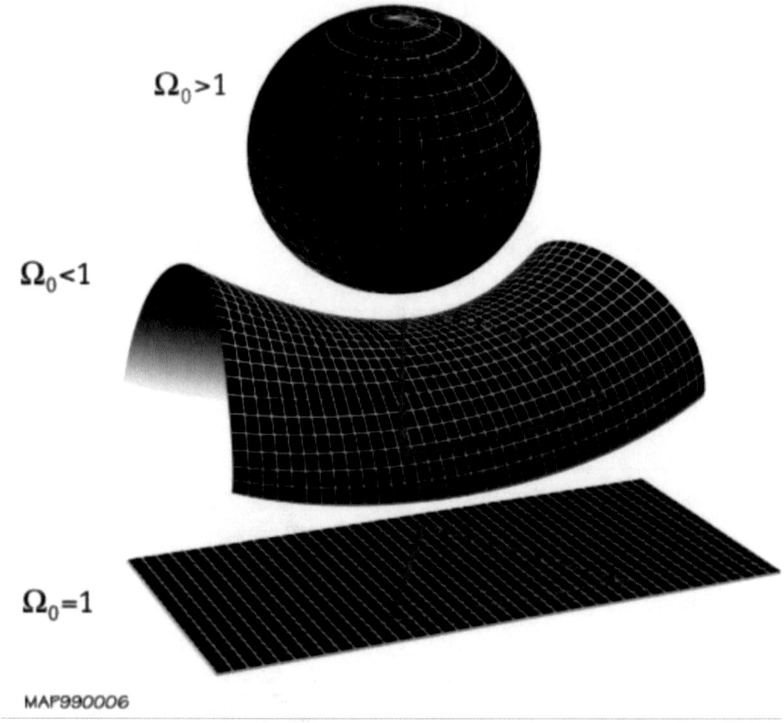

Figure 66. taken from http://map.gsfc.nasa.gov/m_uni/uni_101bb2.html.

To his great chagrin Einstein found in 1917 that with his assumptions, his equations of general relativity--as originally written down--had no meaningful solutions. To obtain a solution, Einstein realized that he had to add to his equations an extra term, which came to be called the cosmological constant (Λ). If one speaks in Newtonian terms, the cosmological constant could be interpreted as a repulsive force of unknown origin that could exactly balance the attraction of gravitation of all the matter in Einstein's closed universe and keep it from moving.

When Einstein later learned of Hubble's discovery of the expansion of the universe and realized that he could have predicted it had he only had more faith in the original form of his equations, he regretted the introduction of the cosmological constant as the "biggest blunder" of his life. Ironically, recent theoretical developments in particle physics suggest that in the early universe there may very well have been a nonzero value to the cosmological constant and that this value may be intimately connected with precisely the nature of the vacuum state.

A first look at the universe would imply that the expansion of the universe will cause the galaxies to move away from each other. As we have seen, cosmologists like to talk about the amount of matter in the universe in terms of Ω. A closed universe is massive enough that it eventually collapses back onto itself has Ω larger than 1; an `open' universe, one that expands outwards forever, has $\Omega$ less than 1; and a `flat' universe, perfectly balanced between the two, has $\Omega = 1$. Many cosmologists like to believe that for the Universe, $\Omega = 1$. However, the amount of visible matter in the universe is about $\Omega = 0.05$.

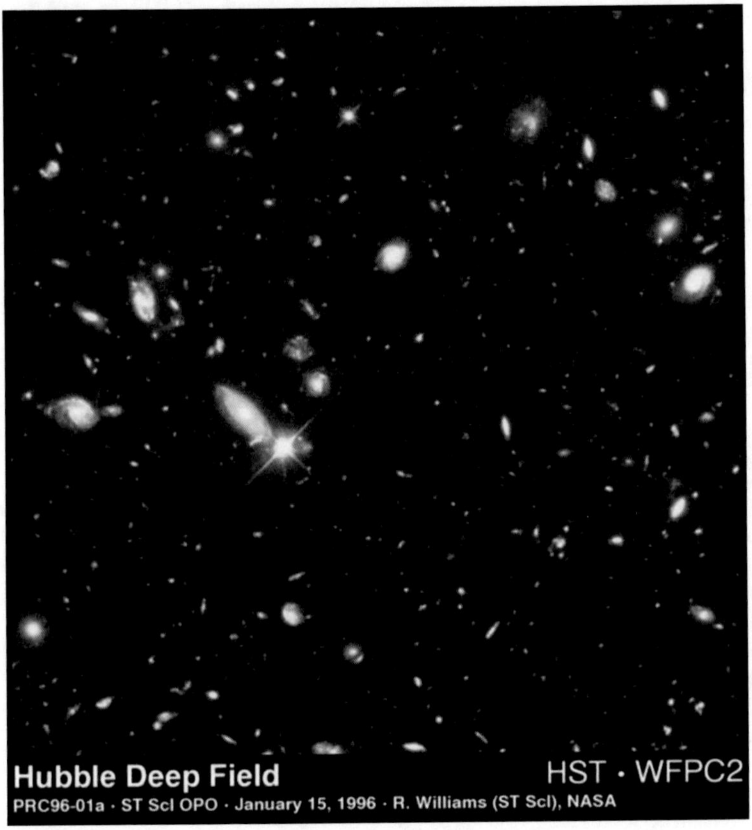

Figure 67.

The density of ordinary matter in the universe is about 3×10^{-31} g/cm3, which is 300 billion billion billion times less dense than water. Now, the size of the observable universe is about 14 billion light years, and using the above value of the density gives you a mass) of about 3×10^{54} g, which is roughly 25 billion galaxies the size of the Milky Way.

Figure 67 is a picture of nearly 10,000 galaxies. "The snapshot includes galaxies of various ages, sizes, shapes, and colors. The smallest, reddest galaxies may be among the most distant known, existing when the universe was just about 800 million years old. The nearest galaxies - the larger, brighter, well-defined spirals and ellipticals - thrived about 1 billion years ago, when the cosmos was 13 billion years old. " [from release by NASA, ESA, and S. Beckwith (STScI) and the HUDF Team]

I am always totally awestruck when I look at this picture. There are 200 billion other stars in our Milky Way galaxy. That means something like 5000000000000000000000 stars in the universe. Beyond my comprehension.

Chapter 17

Dark Matter

Beginning in the 1930's, evidence began to accumulate that there were contributions to Ω in addition to visible matter. Dutch astronomer Jan Oort first discovered the presence of a new non-visible form of matter, called "dark matter" in the 1930's when studying stellar motions in the local galactic neighborhood. By observing the red shifting (See p. 98) of stars moving near the galactic plane, Oort was able to calculate how fast the stars were moving. Since he observed that the galaxy was not flying apart he reasoned that there must be enough matter around that the gravitational pull kept the stars from escaping, much as the sun's gravitational pull keeps the planets in the solar system in orbit. He was able to determine that there must be *three times as much mass* as is readily observed in the form of visible light.

Galaxy Clusters While Oort was carrying out his observations of stellar motions, Fritz Zwicky of Caltech discovered the presence of dark matter on a much larger scale through his studies of galactic clusters. A galactic cluster is an group of galaxies which are gravitationally bound. Using the same method employed by Oort, Zwicky determined the Doppler shifts of individual galaxies in one particular system, the Coma cluster--about 300 million light years away. Zwicky found nearly *10 times as much mass* as observed in the form of visible light was needed to keep the individual galaxies within the cluster gravitationally bound. It was clear to Zwicky, as it had been to Oort, that a large sum of mass was extant which *was simply not visible.*

Invariably, for all galaxies, it is found that the stellar rotational velocity remains constant, or "flat", with increasing distance away from the galactic center. This result is highly counterintuitive since, based on Newton's law of gravity, the rotational velocity would steadily decrease for stars further away from the galactic center.

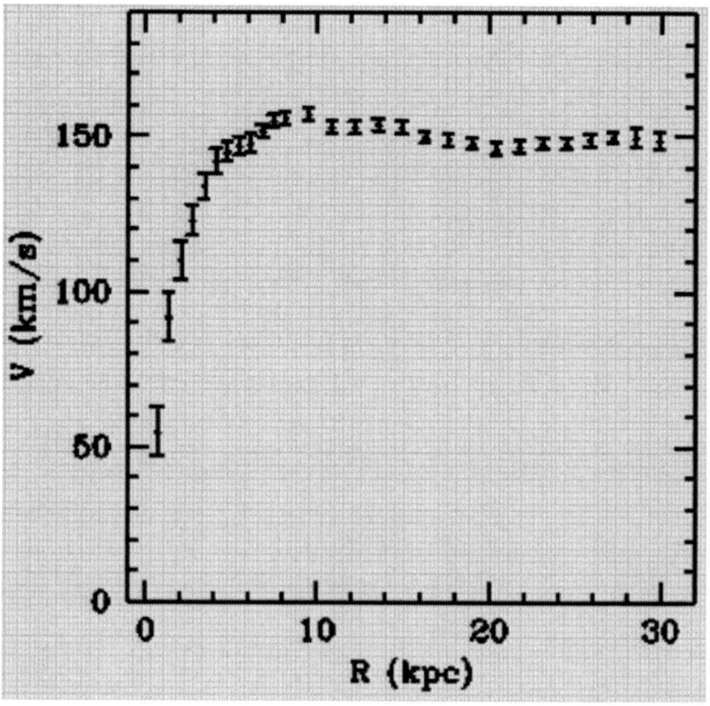

Figure 68. The rotation curve for the galaxy NGC3198 from Begeman, K. G. 1989, AandA, 223, 47.

Analogously, inner planets within the Solar System travel more quickly about the Sun than do the outer planets (e.g. the Earth travels around the sun at about 100,000 km/hr while Saturn, which is further out, travels at only one third this speed). One way to speed up the outer planets would be to add more mass to the solar system, between the planets. By the same argument the flat galactic rotation curves seem to suggest that each galaxy is surrounded by significant amounts of dark matter. It has been postulated and generally accepted, that the dark matter would have to be located in a massive, roughly spherical halo enshrouding each galaxy.

Recall that one of the three pieces of evidence for the big bang is the entire abundance pattern of the light elements D, 3He, 4He, 7Li. The abundance of these light elements seen in the most primitive samples of the cosmos conforms to the predictions of big bang nucleosynthesis. The amount of luminous matter in the universe is significantly less than the mass density implied by Big Bang Nucleosynthesis. This deficit also indicates the existence of dark matter. Could dark matter be ordinary baryonic matter in a form that doesn't shine perhaps brown dwarf stars, black holes, or hot intergalactic gas? Apparently not, according to the calculations of primordial nucleosynthesis, which work only if the density of baryons is less than 0.1 of the critical value ($\Omega_B < 0.1$). Thus the bulk of the dark matter must be composed of an unknown form of matter. Observations show that the dark matter is much less clumped than the visible matter. Therefore, the two kinds must interact only weakly, mainly via the gravitational force. Computer simulations of the formation of large-scale structure show that the non-baryonic dark matter candidates can be divided into two categories depending on the velocity with which the particles were moving when the universe became dominated by matter During this epoch, a rapidly moving particle (e.g., because its mass is small) is considered hot dark matter; a slowly moving particle is considered cold dark matter. Currently, the cold dark matter candidates, or a mixture of hot and cold, give the best agreement between computer simulation results and the observed large-scale structure.

Most cosmologists believe that the unknown matter needed to explain the "missing mass" exists in the form of some yet-undetected elementary particle- a particle that is fundamentally different from ordinary matter. Such a particle would be a relic of some process in the high-energy-physics era, but whether from the grand unification era or some later era is not known. Chief among the theoretical elementary-particle candidates for non-baryonic dark matter are weakly interacting massive particles (WIMPs), axions, and neutrinos with finite mass. The experimental upper limit for the electron neutrino mass is about 7 electron-volts. A sea of primordial neutrinos with this mass would provide sufficient dark mass to make $\Omega = 1$. However, neutrino dark matter would be hot and so does not work well by itself in computer simulations of the observed large-scale structure.

AXIONS

The axion is an unusual particle whose existence has been postulated for reasons related to charge-parity (CP) conservation. If axions actually exist, they do not behave like most particles, which move independently and randomly with different directions and energies. Instead, axions are expected to move coherently, behaving more like a slowly moving sea of particles. Theory allows only a narrow range of possible masses for the axion, near 10^{-5} eV. Nevertheless, if the axion exists with this mass, its total cosmological mass density could still dominate the universe. If axions exist, they could make up the bulk of dark matter. With an estimated 10 trillion of them packed into every cubic centimeter of space in our galaxy, what they lack in mass individually, they would make up for in sheer numbers. Dark matter axions could be detected based on the prediction that axions can change into photons in a strong magnetic field. Two experimental groups are attempting to track down the axion: one in Japan (CARRACK2 at Kyoto University's Institute for Chemical Research), and the other at Lawrence Livermore under the leadership of physicists Leslie Rosenberg and Karl van Bibber. This team consists of researchers from Livermore, UF, UCB, and NRAO.

Chapter 18

SUPERSYMMETRY

There are good theoretical and experimental reasons to suspect that a new symmetry exists in nature, known as supersymmetry, which might enable gravity to be unified with the weak, electromagnetic, and strong forces. If supersymmetry exists, then every fundamental particle of ordinary matter and radiation has a supersymmetric partner particle, as yet undetected. The lightest supersymmetric particle cannot decay (because there are no lighter particles to decay into) and would therefore have survived from the time of the early universe until now. Such a particle's interactions with ordinary matter would be very weak, and current accelerator experiments tell us that the mass of the lightest supersymmetric particle is greater than 20 GeV Thus WIMPs make an ideal candidate for non-baryonic dark matter in the universe. They are imagined to be only weakly associated with luminous matter, for example, forming a loosely bound halo around our galaxy and others.

Supersymmetry solves many problems that exist in nature. One of them involves the mass of the fundamental particles. It is understood that these particles derive their mass through interactions with the Higgs boson. A problem that was proposed by Stephen Hawking was that through the interactions of the Higgs boson with the graviton, the Higgs would acquire an enormous mass – much too large to serve the purposes envisioned in the Standard Model of fundamental particles. The problem arises because the Higgs particle is a boson. Fermion masses can never increase in such an uncontrolled manner. This is because fermion masses are protected from coupling in this manner by *gauge* symmetry. (See chapter 10 "Symmetries and fields")

The symmetry in supersymmetry is that every fermi particle has a partner particle of bosonic type and every bosonic particle has a partner particle of fermionic type. Every particle is an element of a *supermultiplet* in which every boson is partnered to a fermion and vice versa. In exact supersymmetry, the Higgs Boson has the same mass as its partner the Higgsino- the Higgsino as a fermion has a mas protected by its gauge symmetry.

Exact supersymmetry is not possible because it has predictions which contradict experimental evidence. The trick is to break supersymmetry to the extent that the Higgs mass remains small. Interestingly enough the breaking of supersymmetry automatically incorporates gravity into the theory. *This gives us another reason for why supersymmetry is likely to be part of the underlying structure of the universe; it is a means of unifying the gravitational interaction with the rest of the forces.*

In broken local supersymmetry, usually referred to as supergravity, a spin 3/2 partner (gravitino) to the graviton naturally occurs. The contribution to the Higgs mass arising from the coupling of the graviton to the Higgs- boson is nearly cancelled by the contribution of the gravitino.

Once again everything fits together so neatly. It is so remarkable how all the laws in nature so perfectly work together so that our universe can exist. Could this be a giant coincidence?

Beginning with a theory incorporating supersymmetric grand unification of the strong and electromagnetic forces (SUSY GUTS), one can evolve the measured electroweak and strong coupling constants. The coupling constants based upon the charges tell us the strength with which a particular force causes particles to be attracted or pushed apart.

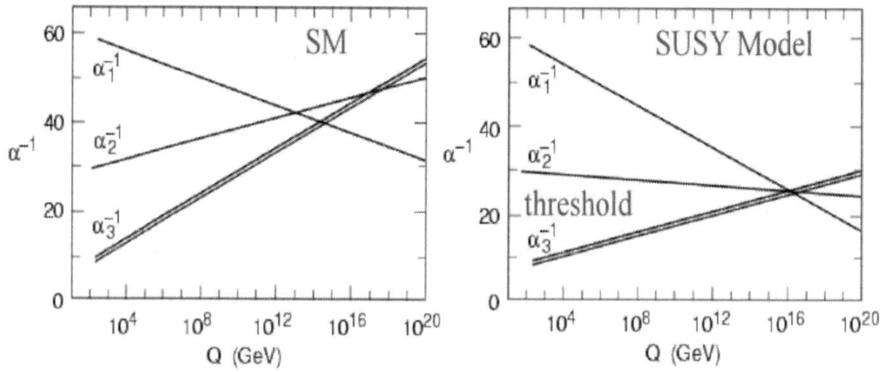

Figure 69.

The fundamental prediction based upon such theories is that the three coupling constants were equal when the universe was very young and diverged a short time after it was formed. Using present data from CERN's LEP electron positron collider, we can work backwards from present values. We find that using the Standard model alone, a single unification point is excluded, but in contrast, the minimal *supersymmetric* standard model leads to a good agreement with a single unification scale.

Chapter 19

PUZZLES

To derive his 1917 cosmological model, Einstein made three assumptions that lay outside the scope of his equations. The first was to suppose that the universe is homogeneous and isotropic in the large (i.e., the same everywhere on average at any instant in time), an assumption that Edward A. Milne later elevated to an entire philosophical outlook by naming it the cosmological principle.

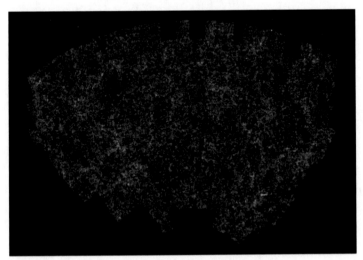

APM Survey picture of a large part of the sky, about 30 degrees across, showing almost a million galaxies out to a distance of about 2 billion light years.
MAP990047

Figure 70.

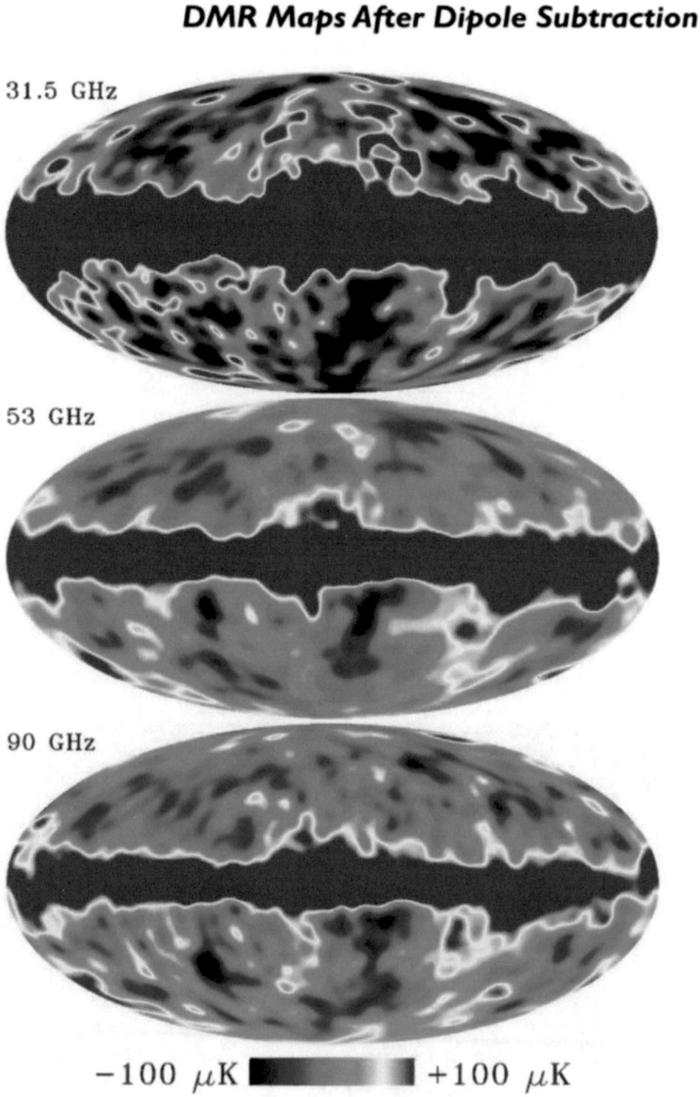

Figure 71. (NASA / WMAP Science Team) shows observations from the COBE satellite. The Milky Way is the horizontal band through the middle of the top picture.

Newton had it implicitly in mind in a letter to Bentley when he took the initial state of the Cosmos to be everywhere the same before it developed "ye Sun and Fixt stars."

The COBE (Cosmic Background Explorer) satellite, developed by NASA's Goddard Space Flight Center, was launched November 18, 1989to measure the diffuse infrared and microwave radiation from the early universe to the limits set by our astrophysical environment.

The cosmic microwave background radiation (CMBR) spectrum was found to be that of a nearly perfect blackbody with a temperature of 2.725 +/- 0.001K. This observation matches the predictions of the hot Big Bang theory extraordinarily well, and indicates that nearly all of the radiant energy of the Universe was released within the first year after the Big Bang.

However, the CMBR was found to have intrinsic "anisotropy" for the first time, at a level of a part in 100,000. These tiny variations in the intensity of the CMB over the sky show how matter and energy was distributed when the Universe was still very young. Later, through a process still poorly understood, the early structures developed into galaxies, galaxy clusters, and the large scale structure that we see in the Universe today.

Dr. John Mather, and Dr. George F. Smoot, of the COBE team received the 2006 Nobel Prize in Physics "for their discovery of the blackbody form and anisotropy of the cosmic microwave background radiation"

In Figure 72, the effects of the Milky Way are removed. The spots reveal the imprints of gigantic primordial structures when the universe was 380,000 years old. The structures revealed here were much larger than 380,000 light years across at that time. Thus even movement of matter and light at the speed of light could not have changed these structures significantly.

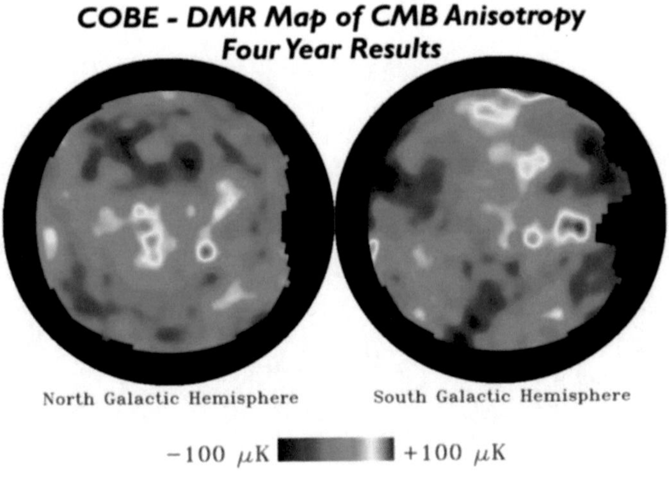

Figure 72. NASA / WMAP Science Team.

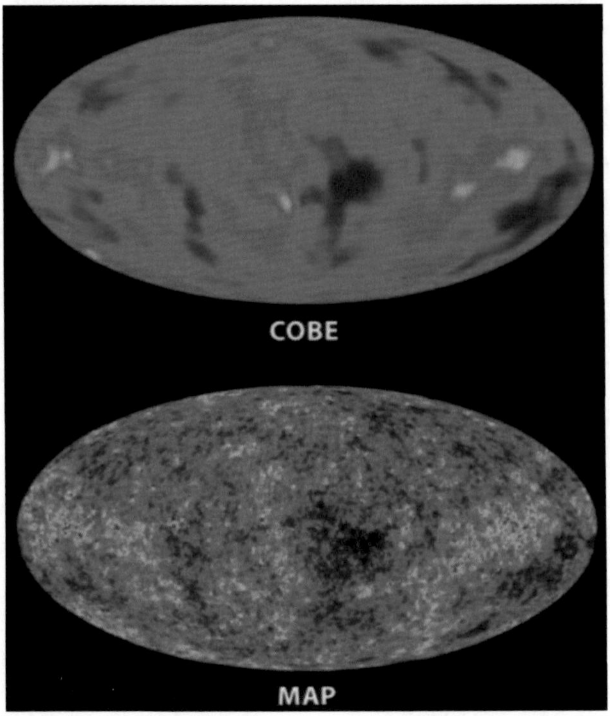

Figure 73. NASA/WMAP Science Team.

Figure 73 shows a comparison between CMBR as observed by COBE and by the more sensitive WMAP..

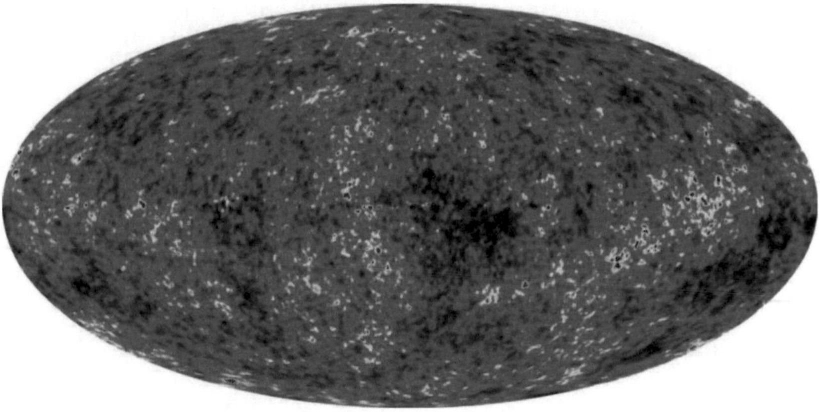

Figure 74. NASA/WMAP Science Team.

The detailed, all-sky picture of the infant universe found in Figure 74 arises from three years of WMAP data. The image reveals 13.7 billion year old temperature fluctuations (shown as color differences) that correspond to the seeds that grew to become the galaxies.

The Wilkinson Microwave Anisotropy Probe (WMAP) is named after Dr. David Wilkinson, a member of the science team and pioneer in the study of cosmic background radiation. The inhomogenious nature of the universe is even clearer in the WMAP results.

Figure 75 shows galaxies on fanlike swaths extending outwards from the Earth. Each dot represents a galaxy. Note that galaxies are not scattered randomly. The universe appears to be clumpy and uneven. The voids and "walls' that form large-scale structures are mapped here by 11,000 galaxies. Our galaxy, the Milky Way is at the center of the figure. Galaxies seem to lie along sheets and strings interspersed with voids that contain very few galaxies.

The 'Great Wall" is the sheet of galaxies that forms the arms of the stick figure at the center.

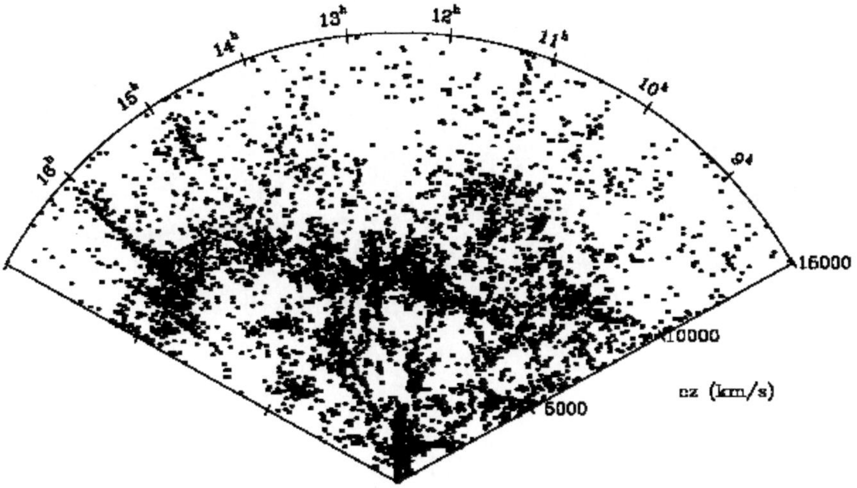

Figure 75. Reproduced with permission John Huchra Harvard-Smithsonian Center for Astrophysics.

If $\Omega = 2$ at 10^{-43} seconds, the universe would rapidly (less than 10^{-40} seconds) close in on itself again to a big crunch.

If $\Omega = 0.5$ at 10^{-43} seconds, the universe would rapidly (less than 10^{-40} seconds) expand to a size many times larger than its present size. Individual particles would all be so far from each other that they could not attract each other and no stars would ever form.

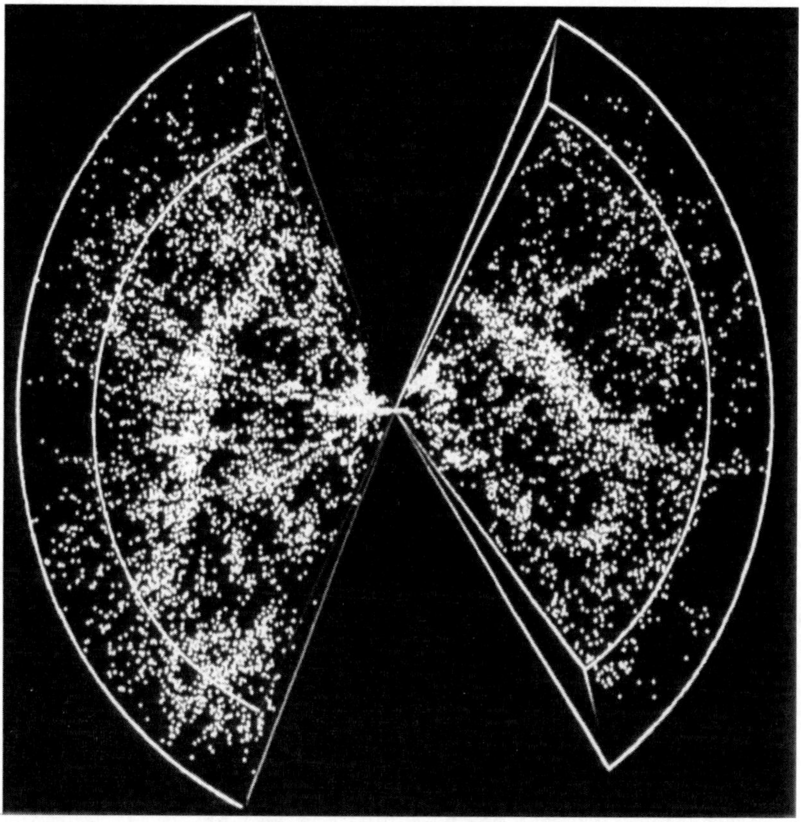

Figure 76.

THE AGE PROBLEM

At 10^{-43} seconds we require Ω almost exactly $=1$ Almost no deviation at all from that value.

Chapter 20

INFLATION

A concept called inflation proposes that the universe went through a huge, rapidly accelerating expansion at extremely early times (somewhere between 10^{-43} and 10^{-32} seconds).

Inflation also adjusts the density to precisely the critical value needed to balance the expansion. Like all worthwhile scientific theories, the idea of inflation is testable. For example, it predicted a particular size distribution for the bumps in the cosmic microwave background radiation. The results from the COBE and WMAP satellites confirm these unique signatures of the early universe.

Before the confirmation of the inflation hypothesis, the combination of luminous matter, nonluminous ordinary matter and dark matter yielded a value of $\Omega = 0.27$. Many physicists such as Stephen Hawking therefore felt that the universe would ultimately collapse into a Big Crunch. Clear evidence for the inflation hypothesis from WMAP means that there is another contribution to Ω; "Dark Energy". (The term "Dark Energy" was coined by Michael Turner in an article for Physical Review Letters.)

Evidence for Dark Energy first emerged in 1998, when a 10-year old study of supernovae took an astonishing turn. The goal had been to measure changes in the expansion rate of the universe, which in turn would yield clues to the origin, structure, and fate of the cosmos, It seemed obvious that the universal law of gravity, operating since shortly after the universe began would be causing the expansion of the universe to slow down. Instead, the study showed that the expansion rate is accelerating.

The precision was arrived at by running the extremely accurate temperature readings obtained by WMAP through hundreds of thousands of computer simulations that model how the universe cooled.

The Early Universe

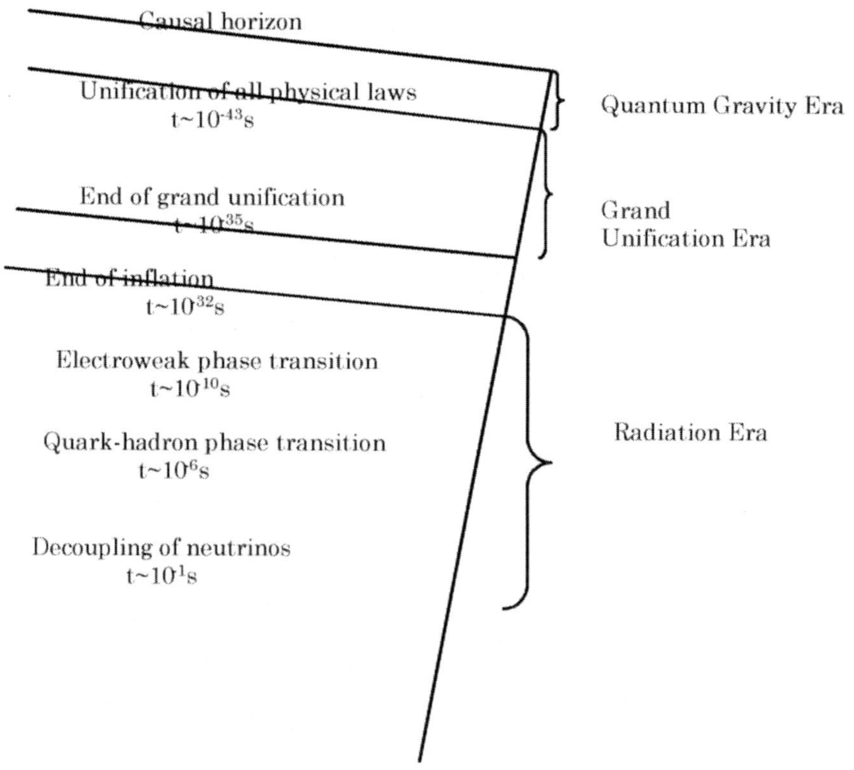

Figure 77.

Working forwards to the present day WMAP scientists show that the first stars appeared 200 million years after the universe began and that the universe is between 13.5 and 13.9 billion years old. Working backwards to the origin, WMAP scientists show that the CMBR first appeared 380,000 years after the universe began.

Combining WMAP results with other astronomical data sets a limit of <less than 0.23 eV on the mass of the neutrino species. Re the reliability of the WMAP results it should be noted that its inferred age of the universe is

consistent with stellar ages, the baryon/photon ratio is consistent with measurements of the [D/H] ratio, and the inferred Hubble constant is consistent with local observations of the expansion rate.

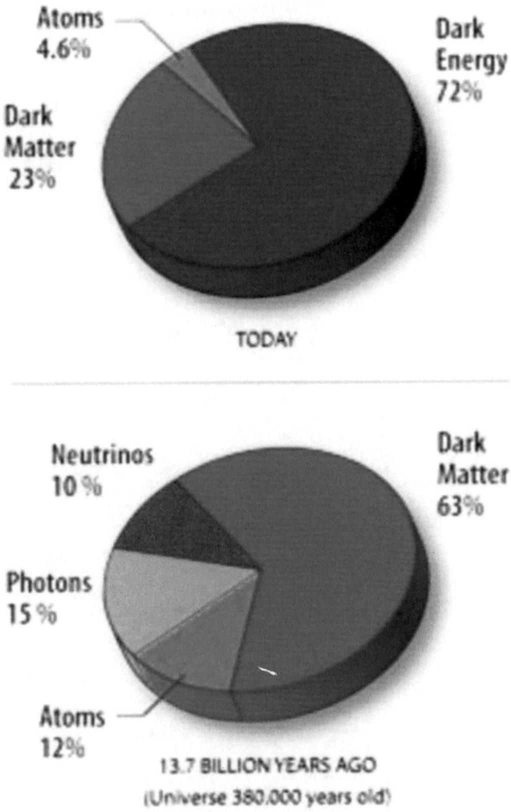

Figure 78. NASA/WMAP Science Team.

Each cosmic theory makes a specific prediction about the patterns in the oldest light in the universe. Like a detective, the WMAP team compared the unique "fingerprint" of patterns imprinted on this ancient light (figure 79) with fingerprints predicted by various cosmic theories and found the match.

At the beginning, the temperature was so high that all the forces except gravity were of equal strength; GUT era. The lowest-energy state (the vacuum) is not symmetric at the low temperatures of the present universe. As time progressed, the temperature decreased, and the vacuum underwent a phase transition from a symmetric state of higher energy. This phase transition is thought to have happened about 10^{-35} seconds after the creation of the Universe. It filled the Universe with a kind of energy called the vacuum energy, which plays the role of an effective cosmological constant. As a consequence gravitation effectively became repulsive for a period of about 10^{-32} seconds. During this period the Universe expanded at an astonishing rate, increasing its size scale by about a factor of 10^{50}.

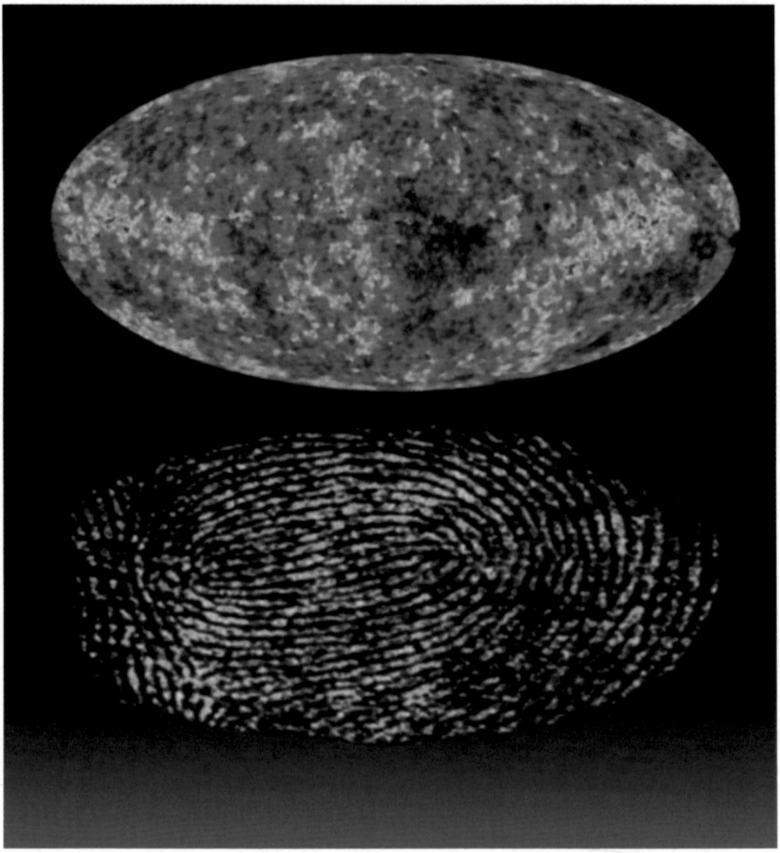

Figure 79. The Universe as Fingerprint NASA/WMAP Science Team.

Inflation beautifully explains three long-standing problems of cosmology. Because inflation can quickly expand an extremely tiny volume into a vastly larger region of space, it would allow a small, uniform patch to expand to cover our entire observable universe, leading to a nearly uniform temperature for the cosmic microwave background radiation. At the same time, there must remain some minimum level of bumpiness even in the uniform patches, because quantum mechanics and the uncertainty principle require it. Inflation magnifies these tiny fluctuations into the cosmic microwave background radiation anisotropy. Inflation takes microscopic quantum noise and blows it up to create the seeds of galaxies and large-scale structures.

A third advantage of inflation is that it forces the spatial curvature of the universe to be negligibly small on a cosmological scale so that space is flat (i.e. Euclidean geometry applies). This flatness is a direct consequence of the tremendous expansion expected during inflation. A small closed surface such as a balloon has an obvious curvature, but if expanded to the size of Earth, its curvature is much less apparent. The absence of curvature in an inflationary universe would imply that today, the density parameter Ω should be close to unity. Thus, an inflationary phase in the early universe naturally solves the fine-tuning problem mentioned above.

Inflation smooths the universe by postulating an early epoch of extremely rapid expansion during which whatever irregularities may have existed prior to inflation are virtually erased. In ordinary inflation, as developed by Guth, Linde, Albrecht, and Steinhardt, this smoothing flattens the universe as well, yielding a universe of critical density. In ordinary inflation, a critical universe could in principle be avoided by shortening the amount of inflation, but in that case the smoothness on large scales remains a mystery, causing inflation to lose most of its appeal.

The 3K cosmic microwave background radiation emanates from an epoch approximately three hundred thousand years after the Big Bang, when the universe was approximately one thousandth its present size. At this time the electrons, because of the cooling of the universe, combined with protons and other nuclei to form neutral hydrogen and other elements. Because of this change in composition from a highly ionized plasma to a neutral gas, the formerly opaque universe becomes virtually transparent. The non-uniformities in the microwave background provide a snapshot of the ripples at that time, which later developed into galaxies and the structure that we observe today.

How the universe began is unknown. There is nothing in the present universe that we can point to as resulting directly or indirectly form the quantum gravity era. We do not understand the physics of quantum gravity and we have no experimental results to explain or to guide us.

The expansion of the universe and the cosmic microwave background point to the existence of a beginning and to the time at which it took place—nothing more. The abundance of D, 3He, 4He, and 7Li come from a relatively late period ($t \approx 100$ seconds). Thus the theory of Alpher and Gamow and the work of Schramm and collaborators are as Guth has stated the theory of the aftermath of the 'big bang'

At its beginning the universe originated in a different state of symmetry than we observe now. As the universe expanded and cooled, it underwent a series of phase transitions associated with breaking different states of symmetry.

The picture of spontaneous symmetry breaking is encoded in a Higgs potential. As the temperature cools below some critical temperature, the minimum of the Higgs potential shifts breaking the symmetry.

Phase transitions occur through the formation of bubbles of the new phase in the middle of the old phase; these bubbles then expand and collide until the old phase disappears completely and the phase transition is complete. A small patch of the early universe begins in the false vacuum. The enormous energy density of the false vacuum corresponds to Einstein's cosmological constant and thus creates a repulsive gravitational field. This field inflates this region exponentially while the rest of the early universe remains microscopic. This huge expansion factor drives the universe towards flatness for the same reason that the Earth appears flat., even though it is really round. A small piece of any curved space, if magnified sufficiently will appear flat.

A short period of inflation can drive the value of Ω very accurately to one, *no matter where it starts out.* Just before inflation occurred, the entire observable universe was less than 10^{-35} light second across. Radiation traveling at light sped easily equalized all the temperatures and densities in the universe. Heisenberg's uncertainty principle requires the existence of fluctuations in the vacuum. These normally occur at the quantum level or on the size smaller than an atomic nucleus (10^{-15} m). But just prior to inflation, the entire universe was 10^{-35} light second across or 10^{-26} m. Thus quantum ripples would be of enormous size on this scale. After inflation, ripples would be magnified by a factor of 10^{50} and so correspond to the lumpiness in the present universe.

The energy of a gravitational field is always negative. The energy of matter is positive. During inflation the total energy; matter plus the energy stored in the gravitational field remains constant. The matter energy density increases by the cube of the linear expansion rate or at least by a factor of 10^{75}; the gravitational energy becomes more and more negative to compensate.

The decay of the false vacuum releases a hot uniform soup of particles; exactly the starting point of traditional big bang theory. *The entire matter content of the universe can develop from just a few grams of primordial matter.*

Guth says that if inflation is right, the universe can properly be called the ultimate free lunch!

The idea of purpose is central to the religious conception of the world. The world must have been created for a purpose, and this purpose must be a part of creation and evident in it. Atheists deny the notion of purpose in the world. It all happened by chance.

For the believer, the universe is beautiful and awesome. How could God have acted otherwise than to establish a coherent set of laws that guide the universe?

INDEX